Foreword

It is with pleasure that I write the Foreword to this publication of Prof. Trisha Dunning. This comprehensive work represents a kaleidoscope of excellence, and all professionals involved in the provision and delivery of diabetes care will find it invaluable in their practice. It is a most useful addition to their knowledge and will positively influence their delivery of care in the context of evidence-based practice and person-centred care.

Each chapter pertinently addresses the key points as outlined at the beginning and is comprehensively referenced. Each of the 19 chapters can be read individually or in sequence to get the comprehensive view.

The burden of diabetes at both an individual and societal level is well documented and therefore this book should prove to be a most useful guide to policy makers at national and international levels.

The author is eminent in the field of diabetes research, care and contemporary policy development and implementation. She is also a regular and respected contributor at international conferences and serves as a member of significant national and international boards. We are indebted to her commitment to the field of diabetes clinical practice and research. She is richly deserving of our congratulations for this work, which I recommend without hesitation.

Anne-Marie Felton
President and co-founder of Foundation of
European Nurses in Diabetes (FEND)
Vice President Diabetes UK
Co-Chair European Coalition on Diabetes (ECD)

Preface

Science and technology has increased our understanding about the pathophysiology of diabetes, its management and the key role of education and self-care in achieving optimal outcomes since it was first described as *diabetes maigre* (bad prognosis) and *diabetes gros* (big diabetes). Qualitative research highlights the importance of considering the individual's beliefs and attitudes, their explanatory models for diabetes and life in general, their social situations and the key central role they play in their care. Translational research is becoming important. Person-centred care is now central to service delivery, care standards and best practice.

Equally importantly, nurses and other health professionals are accountable for the care they provide and must reflect on their own beliefs, attitudes and explanatory models because they affect the care and advice health professionals provide and their ability to establish therapeutic relationships with people with diabetes. The strength of the therapeutic relationship is a significant factor in diabetes outcomes.

However, evidence is not always easy to interpret and may not be readily accessible, despite the advances in education and technology and the increasing number of databases of systematic reviews such as the Cochrane Collaboration, the Joanna Briggs Institute and the bewildering number of management guidelines, many of which make slightly different recommendations that are regularly published.

In other ways, we have made very little progress. The prevalence of obesity, the metabolic syndrome and diabetes are all increasing globally. People are living longer, and there is an increasing prevalence of Type 2 diabetes in developing countries and, worryingly, in children. People with diabetes are still developing devastating complications and premature death.

Care of People with Diabetes was revised to reflect the changes in our understanding of the pathophysiology of diabetes and its complications and diabetes care and education since 2009. It is not possible to include every new piece of information, and I had to leave a great deal of information out; I stress not including work, does not mean it is not interesting, relevant or worthwhile.

A new chapter about diabetes and palliative care has been included. Some information has been removed and some chapters amalgamated. I use the term 'people/person with diabetes' in most places in the text to be consistent with the Position Statement *A New Language for Diabetes* (Diabetes Australia. 2011); however, the term 'patient' still occurs in many places, where it seems appropriate such as referring to people in hospital.

I am indebted to people with diabetes for teaching me so much about the practicalities of life diabetes and how they live with it. I invite readers to reflect on the following words of a young woman with Type 1 diabetes:

> Diabetes is a designer disease. It was designed for people with routine lives – and that's NOT me!

Her words eloquently illustrate the enduring importance of Hippocrates' words, which reflects the essence of person-centred care:

> It is more important to know what sort of person has a disease, than to know what sort of disease the person has.
>
> (Hippocrates circa 460–370 BC)

Both statements highlight the imperative to consider the individual in their life context and involve them in setting relevant goals and planning their care.

I sincerely hope the revised edition of the book will continue to contribute to the vast body of information about diabetes. The book was not intended to take the place of the procedures and policies of health professionals' employing institutions: it will complement them.

The book also complements two of my other books: *Managing Clinical Problems in Diabetes* (2009) and *Diabetes Education: Art, Science and Evidence* (2012), both also published by Wiley-Blackwell. I hope my books will help nurses and other health professionals care for people with diabetes in a holistic, caring and sensitive way and that each person who reads the books will find something of value. Finally,

> *People get off track. Just have the patience to help them get back on track.*
> *That's what's important.*

(Rural health TV programme about type 2 diabetes
and Aboriginal and Torres Strait Islander People.
www.ruralhealth.com.au)

Acknowledgements

I sincerely thank Wiley Blackwell for promoting the book and for supporting it since the first edition was published in 1994.

I work in a supportive team of doctors and nurses and with wonderful academic colleagues. My special thanks go to them for their friendship and critical comment on various sections of the book. In particular, Dr Bodil Rasmussen, Dr Sally Savage, Susan Streat, Nicole Duggan, Michelle Robins, Heather Hart, Patricia Streitberger and Pamela Jones.

I am also grateful to Professor Alan Sinclair for his friendship and advice about managing diabetes in older people, Professor Peter Martin for his advice about palliative care, Lisa-Jane Moody for her comments about hearing impairment and Jessie Joose for her suggestions about nutrition.

I acknowledge the generosity of the Australian Commonwealth Department of Health and Aging for permission to reproduce the figure depicting how the Quality Use of Medicines framework can be applied to diabetes management that appears in Chapter 5.

My thanks also to Dr Sally Savage, Nicole Duggan and Professor Peter Martin for agreeing it would be appropriate to include Table 18.2 and Figure 18.1. The table and figure were first published in *Guidelines for Managing Diabetes at the End of Life* (Dunning, Savage, Duggan, Martin 2010).

I am in awe of the people who undertook the work described in this book and other researchers and clinicians who contribute so much information about diabetes that continues to challenge, inform and inspire me.

I continue to learn a great deal about diabetes from the people who live with diabetes whom I teach and care for, and who participate in my research, and their families. I thank these people for the privilege of working with them and for the information and stories they share.

I appreciate 'drop in' visits from Leigh Olsen, a man with diabetes who scours bookshops and other places for old medical and nursing texts he thinks I will enjoy.

My especial thanks go to Anne-Marie Felton, trailblazer, dear friend and esteemed colleague for 'everything', especially for agreeing to write the foreword for this edition.

I am grateful to, James Rainbird for his careful editing and attention to detail.

Finally, I treasure the support and understanding of my family: the furry four-legged ones and feathered two-legged ones. My special thanks and love go to my husband, John.

List of Abbreviations and Symbols

↑	Increased
↓	Decreased
≤	Equal to, or less than
<	Less than
≥	Equal to, or greater than
>	Greater than
ADA	American Diabetes Association
ADS	Australian Diabetes Society
BG	Blood glucose
BMI	Body mass index
BP	Blood pressure
BUN	Blood urea nitrogen
CAM	Complementary and alternative medicine
CAPD	Continuous ambulatory peritoneal dialysis
CCF	Congestive cardiac failure
CCU	Coronary care unit
CSII	Continuous subcutaneous insulin infusion
DA	Diabetes Australia
DKA	Diabetic ketoacidosis
DUK	Diabetes UK
ECG	Electrocardiogram
EN	Enteral nutrition
FFA	Free fatty acids
GLM	Glucose lowering medicines
HbA_{1c}	Glycosylated haemoglobin
HHS	Hyperosmolar Hyperglycaemic States
HM	Human insulin
IAPO	International Alliance of Patient Organisations
ICU	Intensive care unit
IDF	International Diabetes Federation
IV	Intravenous therapy
LFT	Liver function test
MI	Myocardial infarction
MODY	Maturity onset diabetes of the young

NDSS   National Diabetes Supply Scheme
OGTT   Oral glucose tolerance test
PCOS   Polycystic Ovarian Syndrome
SIGN   Scottish Intercollegiate Guidelines Network
TPN   Total parenteral nutrition
TPR   Temperature, pulse and respiration
TZD   Thiazolidinediones
WHO   World Health Organization

The words are used in full the first time they appear in the text. All abbreviations are widely accepted and recognised.

Chapter 1
Diagnosing and Classifying Diabetes

Cancer, diabetes, and heart disease are no longer diseases of the wealthy. Today they hamper the people and economies of the poorest populations...this represents a health emergency in slow motion.

(Ban Ki Moon, Secretary General of the United Nations)

Key points

- Diabetes is the modern pandemic. It represents a considerable global economic and social burden for the person with diabetes and for health services.
- The prevalence of the metabolic syndrome, Type 1, Type 2 and gestational diabetes is increasing.
- The greatest increase in diabetes prevalence is occurring in Africa, the Middle East and South East Asia.
- The overlapping mechanisms by which obesity leads to the metabolic syndrome and Type 2 diabetes are complex and not yet fully understood.
- Not everybody who is obese has insulin resistance or diabetes
- Central obesity plays a key role in the progression to insulin resistance and Type 2 diabetes.
- Lean people may be at higher risk of morbidity and mortality than obese people.
- Primary prevention and early detection are essential to reduce the personal and community burden associated with the metabolic syndrome and diabetes and their complications.
- Type 2 diabetes is a progressive disease and complications are often present at diagnosis. Thus, insulin will eventually be necessary in most people with Type 2 diabetes.
- The prevalence of obesity, the metabolic syndrome and Type 2 diabetes is increasing in children.

What is diabetes mellitus?

Diabetes mellitus is a metabolic disorder in which the body's capacity to utilise glucose, fat and protein is disturbed due to insulin deficiency or insulin resistance. Both states lead to hyperglycaemia and glycosuria.

The body is unable to utilise glucose in the absence of insulin and draws on fats and proteins in an effort to supply fuel for energy. Insulin is necessary for the complete metabolism of fats, however, and when carbohydrate metabolism is disordered fat metabolism is incomplete and intermediate products (ketone bodies) can accumulate in the blood leading to ketosis, especially in Type 1 diabetes. Protein breakdown also occurs and leads to weight loss and weakness and contributes to the development of hyperglycaemia and lethargy.

The different types of diabetes have different underlying causal mechanisms and clinical presentation: in general, young people are insulin-deficient (Type 1 diabetes), while older people usually secrete sufficient insulin in the early stages but demonstrate resistance to insulin action (Type 2 diabetes). In the early stages of Type 2 hyperinsulinaemia might be present. Type 2 is a progressive disease with slow destruction of the insulin-producing beta cells and, consequently, insulin deficiency.

However, ~10% of older people with presumed Type 2 diabetes have markers of islet autoimmunity and become insulin dependent early in the course of the disease (Turner *et al.* 1997) (see latent autoimmune diabetes (LADA) later in this chapter); Type 2 is becoming increasingly prevalent in children and adolescents as a result of the global obesity epidemic (Barr *et al.* 2005; Zimmet *et al.* 2007). Type 2 diabetes is the most common, accounting for ~85% of diagnosed cases; Type 1 accounts for ~15% of diagnosed cases.

Prevalence of diabetes

Diabetes is a global health problem affecting ~371 million people worldwide (International Diabetes Federation (IDF) 2012) and more than 187 million are unaware they have diabetes. The prevalence is expected to increase to 552 million by 2030 unless the epidemic can be halted. In lower income families, 3 out of 4 people have diabetes. The number of deaths attributed to diabetes in 2012 was ~4.8 million, and global diabetes-related spending was estimated to be >471 billion US dollars (IDF 2012). The three countries with the highest diabetes prevalence are China (92.3 million), India (63 million) and USA (24.1 million).

In Australia, AusDiab data show 100 000 people develop diabetes annually (Cameron *et al.* 2003) and the prevalence continues to increase: 7.5% of people over 25 years and 16.8% of people over 65 have diabetes and a further 16.1% >65 have impaired glucose tolerance (IGT). In addition, >200 000 progress from being overweight to obese, 3% of adults develop hypertension, and 1% develop renal impairment annually, and the average waist circumference increases by 2.1 cm, particularly in women. The prevalence increases annually by 0.8% (Australian Diabetes Society (ADS) 2012). Thus, a significant proportion of the population develops features of the metabolic syndrome with the associated increased risk of Type 2 diabetes and other associated conditions and leads to high health costs (Colagiuri *et al.* 2003; Australian Institute of Health and Welfare (AIHW) 2005).

In the UK, an estimated 2.3 million people have diabetes and up to another 750 000 people have undiagnosed diabetes (SIGN 2010). In Scotland, approximately 228 000 people were registered as having diabetes in 2009; an increase of 3.6% from 2008 (SIGN 2010). The reason for the increased prevalence of Type 2 diabetes is due to many inter-related factors including genetic predisposition, environmental factors and the ageing population. Type 2 is the most common type, accounting for 80–90% of cases.

There is wide variation in the incidence rates of newly diagnosed Type 1 diabetes in children in different populations. However, Type 1 in children and adolescents is increasing, particularly in developed countries (EURODIAB 2000; The DIAMOND Project Group 2006; Soltesz *et al.* 2006). The incidence of Type 1 diabetes in children <15 years on the Western Australian Children's Database has increased gradually over the past 25 years but occurs in peaks and troughs rather than in a linear progression (Haynes *et al.* 2012). For example peak years were 1992, 1997 and 2003 in Australia. The incidence of type 1 appears to fluctuate in five-year cycles and might be influenced by circulating viruses, especially enterovirus infections or other environmental factors (Haynes *et al.* 2012).

The association between ingestion of cow's milk in infancy and pathogenesis of Type 1 diabetes is discussed in Chapter 13. Recently, the role of IRE1∂ in inducing thioredoxin-interacting protein to activate the NLRP3inflammasome and promote programmed pancreatic cell death (Lerner *et al.* 2012). The researchers stated that the findings suggest dietary modification could extend the honeymoon period in Type 1 diabetes or possibly prevent diabetes.

Thus, the economic burden of diabetes and health care costs are high. Over 9% of people admitted to hospital in Australia have diabetes and rates of 11–25% are reported in other countries. The proportion of people with diabetes admitted to hospital is increasing, and they mostly have longer lengths of stay (ADS 2012). Some people, not known to have diabetes, develop hyperglycaemia in hospital. Hyperglycaemia is associated with increased morbidity and mortality, independently of diabetes (Chapter 7). It is not clear whether hyperglycaemia in people without a diabetes diagnosis is due to undiagnosed diabetes/IGT or whether it is an indicator of underlying critical illness. However, because in-hospital hyperglycaemia in non-diabetics may represent undiagnosed diabetes or risk of future diabetes, these people should receive education and be followed up.

Classification of diabetes

Diabetes is broadly classified into Type 1 and Type 2 diabetes and other types.
- Type 1 diabetes has two forms:
  - Immune-mediated diabetes mellitus, which results from autoimmune destruction of the pancreatic beta cells leading to absolute insulin deficiency.
  - Idiopathic diabetes mellitus refers to diabetes forms that have no known aetiologies.

Type 2 diabetes mellitus refers to diseases associated with relative insulin deficiency as a result of progressive beta cell failure and insulin resistance.

- Impaired glucose homeostasis is an intermediate metabolic stage between normal glucose homeostasis and diabetes. It is a significant risk factor for cardiovascular disease and Type 2 diabetes. Thus early detection and management are important. There are two forms:
  (1) Impaired fasting glucose (IFG) where the fasting plasma glucose is higher than normal but lower than the diagnostic criteria.
  (2) Impaired glucose tolerance (IGT) where the plasma glucose is higher than normal and lower than the diagnostic criteria after a 75 g glucose tolerance test. IFG and FPG often occur together and are associated with the metabolic syndrome.
- Gestational diabetes mellitus, which occurs during pregnancy.

- Other specific types, which include diabetes caused by other identifiable disease processes and other factors:
  - Genetic defects of beta cell function such as Maturity Onset Diabetes of the Young (MODY).
  - Genetic defects of insulin action.
  - Diseases of the exocrine pancreas such as cancer and pancreatitis.
  - Endocrine disorders such as Cushing's disease and acromegaly.
  - Medicines, such as glucocorticoids and atypical antipsychotics have been associated with weight gain but the newest second-generation antipsychotic medications such as aripiprazole are weight neutral (Citrome *et al.* 2005). Possible causes of weight gain associated with medicines include food cravings and eating more, changed resting metabolic rate, changes in neurotransmitters and neuropeptides such as leptin, which regulate appetite, and weight loss before medicines are commenced (Zimmermann & Himmerich 2003). Individuals with schizophrenia are generally more overweight than those without.
- Chemical-induced diabetes.

Overview of normal glucose homeostasis

Blood glucose regulation (glucose homeostasis) relies on a delicate balance between the fed and fasting states and is dependent on several simultaneously operating variables including hormones, nutritional status, especially liver and muscle glucose stores, exercise, tissue sensitivity to insulin, and the type of food consumed. Figure 1.1 shows the key features of the fed and fasting states. Insulin release occurs in two phases. The first phase is important to controlling the postprandial blood glucose rise and is lost early in the progression to Type 2 diabetes. Postprandial glucose >7.8 mmol/L is associated with cardiovascular events and plays a role in the development of other co-morbidities (IDF 2011). Insulin action is mediated via two protein pathways: Protein 13-kinase through insulin receptors and influences glucose uptake into the cells; and MAP-kinase, which stimulates growth and mitogenesis.

Anabolism (fed state)	Catabolism (fasting state)
• Driven by Insulin and the incretin hormones	• Driven by a variety of hormones, e.g. catecholamines, cortisol, growth hormone, glucagon
• Insulin release stimulated by the rise in blood glucose	• Increases endogenous glucose output: 80% liver, 20% kidney
• Two phase response	• Induces insulin resistance
• Facilitates glucose uptake	• Reduces glucose utilisation
• Reduces hepatic glucose output	• Insulin output reduced
	• Protective during hypoglycaemia

– Fasting state 12–16 hours after an overnight fast and is an important determinant of day long glycaemia
– Postprandial (fed) state – dynamic regulated by insulin and glucagon especially in the first 30–60 minutes
– insulin is secreted in two phases and regulates the rate of glucose entry into cells and removal from the circulation:

  - Post prandial blood glucose rise is usually transient
  - Peaks 60–90 minutes
  - Usually returns to normal within 3 hours
  - Usually there is very little diurnal variation in the blood glucose level
  - Isolated post prandial hyperglycaemia occurs in IGT

Figure 1.1 Overview of glucose homeostasis showing the key factors operating during the fed and fasting states. Usually the blood glucose is maintained within the normal range by the interplay of the anabolic and catabolic hormones, which are in turn influenced by other hormones and a number of factors such as nutritional status and intake.

Recently researchers identified the interaction of insulin with its primary binding site on the insulin receptor; revealing a conformational switch in insulin once it engages with the receptor (Menting *et al.* 2012). Conformational switching is unusual in the tyrosine receptor kinases. The clinical significance of the finding is not yet clear but it could influence the development of future insulin analogues.

The metabolic syndrome

The metabolic syndrome consists of a cluster of risk factors for cardiovascular disease and Type 2 diabetes. Several researchers have explored the factors that predict diabetes risk including the World Health Organization (WHO), IDF, Diabetes Epidemiology Collaborative Analysis of Diagnostic Criteria in Europe (DECODE 2008), Epidemiology Study on the Insulin Resistance Syndrome (DESIR), US National Cholesterol Education Programme Adult Treatment Panel (NCEP ATP 111), and the European Group for the Study of Insulin Resistance: Relationship Between Insulin Sensitivity and Cardiovascular Disease Risk (EGIR-RISC).

Key features of the metabolic syndrome

- The metabolic syndrome appears to be a result of genetic predisposition and environmental factors, which include high saturated fat diets, inactivity, smoking, hormone imbalances contributing to metabolic stress, maternal obesity, age and some medicines (Bruce & Byrne 2009). These factors represent a cumulative risk and are largely modifiable.
- Central obesity, waist circumference: Europoids >94 cm in men and >80 cm in women; South Asian and Southeast Asian men >90 cm, women >80 cm: (Zimmet, *et al.* 2005); childhood/adolescent Body Mass Index (BMI) 25–29 overweight, >30 obese. Interestingly, Carnethon *et al.* (2012) reported overweight people diagnosed with diabetes live longer than leaner people with diabetes in a prospective study to identify cardiovascular risk factors (n = ~ 2600). The death rate was 1.5 in overweight people compared to 2.8 in lean people after accounting for cardiovascular risk factors such as age, hypertension, hypercholesterolaemia and smoking. The authors acknowledged the limitations of the study. They also noted Asian people are more likely to be normal weight at diagnosis and stressed the need for extra vigilance in leaner people. Significantly, not all obese people develop the metabolic syndrome. See also Chapter 4.
- Raised serum triglycerides >1.7 mmol/L.
- Low serum HDL-c: <1.03 mmol/L males, <1.29 mmol/L women.
- Hypertension: systolic > 130 mmHg or diastolic >85 mmHg in women.
- IFG: >5.6 mmol/L or previously diagnosed diabetes (e.g. gestational diabetes (GDM). IFG is associated with a 20–30% chance of developing Type 2 diabetes within 5–10 years. The chance increases if FPG is also present.

Other key features include:

- Increasing age.
- Insulin resistance. High serum levels of sugar metabolites, amino acids and chlorine-containing phospholipids are associated with reduced insulin sensitivity and insulin secretion and higher risk of Type 2 diabetes (Floegel *et al.* 2012). A small study suggests people who sleep for <4 hours are 30% more insulin resistant than those who sleep longer (Cappuccio & Miller 2012). However, the sample size was a small one and only one participant was female which could be important because men and women respond to sleep deprivation differently. Thus, further research is needed.

- Genetic predisposition and the Developmental Origins of Adult Health and Disease (DOHaD) hypothesis (Barker *et al.* 1990). Maternal obesity at conception alters gestational metabolism and affects placental, embryonic and foetal growth and development (King 2006) and increases the susceptibility of the child to components of the metabolic syndrome (Taylor & Poston 2007; Bruce & Byrne 2009; Armitage *et al.* 2008; Nakamura & Omaya 2012). Epigenetic changes occur during early foetal development when mothers suffer malnutrition during pregnancy. Their children are more likely to develop metabolic syndrome, diabetes, obesity and cardiovascular disease. In addition, the grandchildren of malnourished mothers are more likely to be low weight at birth, regardless of the nutritional status of their mothers, (see www.themedicalbiochemistrypage.org 1996–2012). In addition, under-nutrition increases susceptibility to infection and obesity, or over-nutrition leads to immunoactivation and susceptibility to inflammatory diseases such as diabetes (Dandona *et al.* 2010). Likewise, *Helicobacter pylori* may predispose individuals to diabetes (Haan *et al.* 2012). Haan *et al.* followed 800 Latino non-diabetic adults over age 60 for 10 years; 144 developed diabetes. People who tested positive for *Helicobacter pylori* were 2.7 more likely to develop diabetes compared to other infections.
- Hyperinsulinaemia, which occurs in the presence of insulin resistance and exaggerates the proliferative effects of the MAP-kinase pathway.
- Procoagulent state: elevated plasma fibrinogen and plasminogen activator inhibitor-1 (PAI-1).
- Vascular abnormalities: increased urinary albumin excretion and endothelial dysfunction, which affect vascular permeability and tone.
- Inflammation: both over nutrition and infection induce inflammation. Dietary fats and sugars can induce inflammation by activating an innate immune receptor, Toll-like receptor 4 (TLR4) (Omaye 2012). Recent research suggests 'good' intestinal bacteria have a preventative role and pre- and probiotics help maintain healthy gut and immune systems (www.themedicalbiochemistrypage.org 1996–2012; Nakamura & Omaya 2012). Inflammatory markers such as cytokines, Interleukin, adhesion molecules and TNF-alpha alter endothelial function. C-reactive protein is a significant predictor of cardiovascular disease and possibly depression, and there is an association among diabetes, cardiovascular diseases and depression. In fact some experts suggest depression could be an independent risk factor for Type 2 diabetes (Loyd *et al.* 1997) and accelerates the progression of coronary artery disease (Rubin 2002). Depression is associated with behaviours such as smoking, unhealthy eating, lack of exercise and high alcohol intake, which predisposes the individual to obesity and Type 2 diabetes. Peripheral cytokines induce cytokine production in the brain, which activates the hypothalamic-pituitary-adrenal axis and the stress response, which inhibits serotonin and leads to depression. Inflammation appears to be the common mediator among diabetes, cardiovascular disease and depression (Lesperance & Frasure-Smith 2007; Bruce & Byrne 2009).
- Hyperuricaemia: More recently, liver enzymes such as sustained elevations of alanine aminotransferase (ALT) and gamma-glutamyl transferase (GGT), which are associated with non-alcoholc fatty liver disease and low adiponectin, have been associated with diabetes and cardiovascular disease. Therefore, the relationship is complex. Conversely, normal testosterone levels appear to be protective against diabetes in men, and low testosterone levels in men with diabetes are associated with a significantly increased risk of death (Jones *et al.* 2011). In women high testosterone indicates greater risk of developing diabetes: high oestradiol levels confer increased diabetes risk in both men and women (American Diabetes Association 2007).

Consequences of the metabolic syndrome include:

- A five-fold increased risk of Type 2 diabetes.
- A two- to three-fold increased risk of cardiovascular disease (myocardial events, stroke and peripheral vascular disease).
- Increased mortality, which is greater in men but women with Type 2 diabetes have a greater risk than non-diabetic women.
- Increased susceptibility to conditions such as:
  - Gestational diabetes (GDM)
  - Foetal malnutrition
  - Polycystic ovarian syndrome
  - Fatty liver
  - Gallstones
  - Asthma
  - Sleep problems
  - Some forms of cancer.

The risk of developing cardiovascular disease and Type 2 diabetes increases significantly if three or more risk factors are present (Eckel *et al.* 2005).

The metabolic syndrome in children and adolescents

The prevalence of metabolic syndrome in children and adolescents is usually extrapolated from adult definitions and may not be accurate. However, it is vital that children and adolescents at risk of developing the metabolic syndrome be identified early. Future risk appears to be influenced *in utero* and early childhood by factors such as GDM, low birth weight, feeding habits in childhood, genetic predisposition and socio-economic factors (Burke *et al.* 2005; Nakamura & Omaya 2012).

The IDF proposed that the metabolic syndrome should not be diagnosed before age 10 but children at risk should be closely monitored especially if there is a family history of metabolic syndrome, diabetes, dyslipidaemia, cardiovascular disease, hypertension and obesity, and preventative strategies should be implemented (Weiss & Caprio. 2005; Zimmet *et al.* 2007).

In the 10–16-year-old age range diagnostic features are waist circumference >90th percentile, triglycerides >1.7 mmol/L, HDL-c >1.03 mmol/L, glucose >5.6 mmol/L (OGGT recommended), systolic blood pressure >130 mm Hg and diastolic >85 mm Hg. Adult criteria are recommended for adolescents over 16 years. The long-term impact on morbidity and mortality will emerge as young people with the metabolic syndrome become adults. However, heart disease may be apparent in children as young as 10 (Sinaiko 2006) and early onset of Type 2 diabetes in adolescents is associated with more rapid progression of complications than occurs in Type 1.

Management of the metabolic syndrome in children and adults consists of primary prevention through population-based strategies aimed at early detection, regular follow-up of at-risk individuals and personalised education. Secondary prevention concentrates on preventing the progression to diabetes and cardiovascular disease. Lasting effects demonstrating reduced cardiovascular and Type 2 diabetes risk has been demonstrated in studies such as the Diabetes Prevention Program (DPP), the Finnish Diabetes Prevention Study and the Da Quing IGT and Diabetes Study. These studies showed the importance of multidisciplinary team care, modifying lifestyle factors that contribute to obesity by improving diet and activity levels to reduce weight (10% body weight in the long term), and stopping smoking. Some programmes include health coaching but the cost–benefit has not been demonstrated (Twigg *et al.* 2007). The Transformational Model of Change is frequently used to implement preventative strategies.

Medicines might be required for secondary prevention, for example to control blood glucose and lower lipids, antihypertensives such as statins, and weight management medicines in addition to lifestyle modification. Several medicines have been shown to reduce the incidence of diabetes in people with the metabolic syndrome. These include Metformin 850 mg BD, which showed a 31% risk reduction in the DPP; 100 mg of Acarbose TDS by 25% after three years (STOP-NIDDM); and women with a history of GDM in the TRIPOD trial were less likely to develop diabetes when they were treated with Troglitazone. Troglitazone was withdrawn from the market because of the tendency to cause liver disease. Other thiazolidinediones such as pioglitazone and rosiglitazone do not have the same adverse effects on the liver. Rosiglitazone reduced the risk of prediabetes progressing to diabetes by 60% over three years in the DREAM study but has since been associated with increased risk of MI and Poiglitizone might increase the risk of bladder cancer; the risk appears to be higher with long duration of use (NPS 2012) (see Chapter 5). Orlistat, an intestinal lipase inhibitor taken TDS, reduced the risk of progression to diabetes in obese adults with metabolic syndrome by 37% over four years (XENDOS study). However, compliance with Orlistat is low due to the side effects, see Chapter 5.

The macrovascular risk factors need to be managed proactively and screening programmes are imperative so abnormalities are treated early, see Chapter 8. A 75 g OGGT may be performed initially to diagnose the metabolic syndrome and repeated after 12 months to determine whether glucose tolerance changed, then the test interval can be increased to every two to three years (WHO 1999). However, if an individual demonstrates significant changes in weight gain, OGGT may be performed earlier.

The Consensus Development Conference on Antipsychotic Drugs and Obesity and Diabetes (American Diabetes Association *et al.* 2004) recommended monitoring people on antipsychotic medicines including:

- BMI at baseline and every visit for 6 months then quarterly and treat if weight increases by one BMI unit;
- Blood glucose and lipids at baseline and if weight increases by 7% and then annually;
- HbA$_{1c}$ 4 months after starting antipsychotic medicines and then annually in people with metabolic syndrome or diabetes risk factors.

Type 1 and Type 2 diabetes

Type 1 diabetes

Type 1 diabetes is a disease of absolute insulin deficiency that usually affects children and young adults but can occur in older people where it usually manifests as latent autoimmune diabetes (LADA), see the following section. Recent research has indicated that insulin resistance is also a feature in lean people with uncomplicated Type 1 diabetes (Donga *et al.* 2012). However, Donga *et al.*'s sample was small, eight people using insulin pumps and eight healthy controls matched for age, gender and BMI, thus, the clinical relevance of the finding is not clear.

The symptoms usually occur over a short space of time (two to three weeks) following a subclinical prodromal period of varying duration where the beta cells are destroyed. The precipitating event may have occurred many years prior to the development of the symptoms. Type 1 diabetes can be due to an autoimmune or idiopathic process. Various researchers have demonstrated that exogenous factors play a role in the development of Type 1 diabetes on the basis that <10% of susceptible people develop diabetes and <40% of monozygotic twins both develop diabetes, the >10-fold increase in the incidence of Type 1 diabetes in European Caucasians in the last 50 years, and migration studies that show the incidence of Type 1 has risen in people who migrated from low to high incidence regions (Knip *et al.* 2005). This is known as the trigger-bolster hypothesis. Seasonal variations in incidence of new diagnosis occur.

The EURODIAB sub-study 2 study group researchers (EUROBIAB 1999) suggested low plasma 25-hydroxyvitamin D may be implicated in the development of Type 1 diabetes (1999). Later, Stene & Jones (2003) suggested there was no link between vitamin D supplementation and lower rates of Type 1 diabetes. A systematic review and meta-analysis of observational studies and a meta-analysis of cohort studies undertaken in 2008 suggest vitamin D supplementation in early childhood might reduce the risk of Type 1 diabetes by 30% (Zipitis & Akoberng 2008). A recent prospective study in Spain identified a significant inverse association between vitamin D and risk of Type 2 diabetes (Gonzalez-Molero *et al.* 2012). However, randomised controlled trials are required to clarify whether there is a causal link and the optimal vitamin D dose, duration of treatment, and the best time to begin using vitamin D supplements.

As indicated earlier in this chapter, and in Chapter 13, a range of other environmental triggers has been implicated in the development of Type 1 such as potatoes, cow's milk, and various viruses. Thus, the cause of Type 1 diabetes appears to be multifactorial due to a combination of genetic predisposition and a diabetogenic trigger that induces an immune response, which selectively destroys pancreatic beta cells. Islet cell antibodies (ICA), glutamic acid carboxylase (GAD), or tyrosine phosphatase (IA-2A) antibodies are present in 85% of cases.

Type 1 diabetes in children usually presents with the so-called classic symptoms of diabetes mellitus:

- Polyuria
- Polydipsia
- Lethargy
- Weight loss
- Hyperglycaemia
- Glycosuria
- Blood and urinary ketones.

In severe cases the person presents with diabetic ketoacidosis (DKA) (see Chapter 7). Bed-wetting may be a consequence of hyperglycaemia in children (and older people). Classically, insulin secretion does not improve after treatment but tissue sensitivity to insulin usually does.

Figure 1.2 is a schematic representation of the progression of Type 1 diabetes. It shows the progressive relentless destruction of the beta cells from the time of the initial triggering event. Five to ten per cent of first-degree relatives of people with Type 1 diabetes have beta cell antibodies, usually with normal glucose tolerance, and some progress to diabetes.

Recent studies suggest early infant feeding is associated with the development of Type 1 diabetes-related autoantibodies such as GAD, 1A-2A with a male preponderance and is more common in children of mothers with Type 2 diabetes or coeliac disease and with short term breast feeding (Zeigler *et al.* 2003; Wahlberg *et al.* 2006) (Chapter 13).

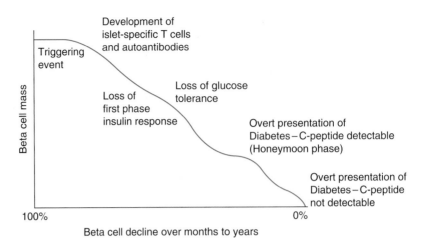

Figure 1.2 Schematic representation of the slow progressive loss of beta cell mass following the initial trigger event in Type 1 diabetes.

Latent autoimmune diabetes (LADA)

LADA is a genetically linked autoimmune disorder that occurs in ~10% of people who are often initially diagnosed with Type 2 diabetes. LADA prevalence varies among ethnic groups (www.actionlada.org). LADA has some features of both Types 1 and 2 diabetes. The UKPDS (1998) identified that one in 10 adults aged between 25 and 65 presumed to have Type 2 diabetes were GADAb positive, and these findings have been evident in other studies (Zinman *et al*. 2004). LADA often presents as Type 2 but has many of the genetic and immune features of Type 1 (see the previous section and Table 1.2).

People with LADA had a different clinical course from Type 2 diabetes: in a 6-year follow up in the UKPDS 84% of people with GADA required insulin compared to 14% of antibody negative people. LADA is primarily an insulin deficiency state, where Type 2 has a long progression to insulin and is characterized by insulin resistance. The clinical features also resemble Type 1 in that people with LADA are not usually obese, are often symptomatic, and do not have a family history of Type 2 diabetes.

However, GADA appears to have a bimodal distribution in LADA identifying two LADA subgroups with different, distinct clinical, autoimmune and genetic features. People with high GADA titers are younger, leaner, insulin deficient, have lower C-peptide and high HbA1c, higher prevalence of other diabetes-specific autoantibodies or other autoimmune diseases such as thyroid disease and lower prevalence of metabolic syndrome than people with LADA and low GADA titers (Buzzetti *et al*. 2007).

There are no current guidelines for managing LADA (Cermea *et al*. 2009) although an expert panel convened by the ADA suggested C-peptide response is an appropriate measure of beta cell function and response to treatment. Management depends on the GADA titers and clinical presentation and should be individualised. Management considerations include:

- Testing lean people presenting with Type 2 diabetes for autoantibodies, especially GADA and C-peptide to correctly diagnose LADA, treat it appropriately with insulin and prevent episodes of ketoacidosis (Niskanen *et al*. 1995; Cermea *et al*. 2009).
- Introducing insulin early to support insulin secretion and protect the remaining beta cells (Cernea *et al*. 2009). Sulphonylureas appear to achieve similar or worse glycaemic control than insulin alone and lead to the early need for insulin, thus Sulphonylureas are not recommended as first line treatment (Cremea *et al*. 2009).

- Thiazolidediones may have a beta cell protective/augmentative effect but their benefit in LADA has not been demonstrated and the contraindications need to be considered.
- Metformin may be contraindicated because insulin resistance is not always a feature of LADA and because of the potential risk of lactic acidosis in susceptible people (Chapter 5).
- Diet and exercise relevant to the individual and the treatment mode.
- Stress management and regular complication screening and mental health assessment (as per Types 1 and 2 diabetes).
- Appropriate education and support.

Type 2 diabetes

Type 2 diabetes is not 'just a touch of sugar' or 'mild diabetes'. It is a *serious*, insidious progressive disease that is often diagnosed late when complications are present. Therefore, population screening and preventative education programs are essential. Type 2 diabetes often presents with an established long-term complication of diabetes such as neuropathy, cardiovascular disease, or retinopathy. Alternatively, diabetes may be diagnosed during another illness or on routine screening. The classic symptoms associated with Type 1 diabetes are often less obvious in Type 2 diabetes, however, once diabetes is diagnosed and treatment instituted, people often state they have more energy and are less thirsty. Other subtle signs of Type 2 diabetes, especially in older people, include recurrent candida and urinary tract infections, incontinence, constipation, symptoms of dehydration and cognitive changes, particularly in information processing speed, and executive function (Spauwen *et al.* 2012). As indicated, insulin resistance often precedes Type 2 diabetes.

Insulin resistance is the term given to an impaired biological response to both endogenous and exogenous insulin that can be improved with weight loss and exercise. Insulin resistance is a stage in the development of impaired glucose tolerance. When insulin resistance is present, insulin production is increased (hyperinsulinaemia) to sustain normal glucose tolerance; however, the hepatic glucose output is not suppressed and fasting hyperglycaemia and decreased postprandial glucose utilisation results in postprandial hyperglycaemia.

Insulin resistance is a result of a primary genetic defect and secondary environmental factors (Turner & Clapham 1998). When intracellular glucose is high, free fatty acids (FFAs) are stored. When it is low FFAs enter the circulation as substrates for glucose production. Insulin normally promotes tryglyceride synthesis and inhibits postprandial lipolysis. Glucose uptake into adipocytes is impaired in the metabolic syndrome and Type 2 diabetes and circulating FFAs as well as hyperglycaemia have a harmful effect on hepatic glucose production and insulin sensitivity. Eventually the beta cells do not respond to glucose (glucose toxicity). Loss of beta cell function is present in over 50% of people with Type 2 diabetes at diagnosis (United Kingdom Prospective Study (UKPDS) 1998) (Figure 1.2). Figure 1.3 depicts the consequences of insulin resistance.

Insulin is secreted in two phases: an effective first phase is essential to limit the postprandial rise in blood glucose. The first phase is diminished or lost in Type 2 diabetes leading to elevated postprandial blood glucose levels (Dornhorst 2001; IDF 2011). Postprandial hyperglycaemia, >7.8 mmol/L two hours after a meal, contributes to the development of atherosclerosis, hypertriglyceridaemia and coagulant activity, endothelial dysfunction, and hypertension, and is a strong predictor of cardiovascular disease and contributes to the development of other diabetes complications (Ceriello 2003; IDF 2011).

Interestingly, the beta cells do respond to other secretagogues, in particular sulphonylurea medicines.

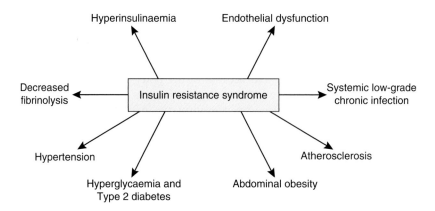

Figure 1.3   Some consequences of the insulin resistance syndrome. These factors lead to increased morbidity and mortality unless diabetes is diagnosed early treatment commenced.

The net effect of these abnormalities is sustained hyperglycaemia as a result of:

• impaired glucose utilisation (IGT);
• reduced glucose storage as glycogen;
• impaired suppression of glucose-mediated hepatic glucose production;
• high fasting glucose (FPG);
• reduced postprandial glucose utilisation leading to postprandial hyperglycemia.

Various tools and risk calculators are used to detect Type 2 diabetes. They encompass some or all of the following risk factors (AUSDRISK Tool; Abassi *et al.* 2012):

• have the metabolic syndrome;
• are overweight: abdominal obesity, increased body mass index (BMI), and high waist-hip ratio (>1.0 in men and >0.7 in women). The limitations of the waist circumference in some ethnic groups are outlined later in the chapter. Elevated FFAs inhibit insulin signalling and glucose transport (see Figure 1.4) and are a source of metabolic fuel for the heart and liver. Binge eating precedes Type 2 diabetes in many people and could be one of the causes of obesity; however, the prevalence of eating disorders is similar in Type 1 and Type 2 diabetes (Herpertz *et al.* 1998);
• are over 40 years of age, but note the increasing prevalence in younger people (see also Chapter 13);
• are closely related to people with diabetes;
• are women who had gestational diabetes or who had large babies in previous pregnancies;
• the children of a woman who had gestational diabetes, maternal obesity or maternal malnutrition;
• are inactive; high levels of sedentary time is associated with 117% increase in the relative risk of Type 2 diabetes and 147% increase in the risk of cardiovascular disease and 49% increased risk of all-cause mortality (Wilmot *et al.* 2012). Occupational sitting time also represents increased risk of Type 2 diabetes (van Ufelen *et al.* 2010).

Other metabolic syndrome-associated risk factors for Type 2 diabetes have already been described. In addition, active and former smoking and acanthosis nigricans are associated with hyperinsulinaemia (Kong *et al.* 2007). Baseline and hypertension progression are independent predictors of Type 2 diabetes (Conen *et al.* 2007). Recent research suggests insulin lack might be partly due to the enzyme PK Cepsilon (PKCe),

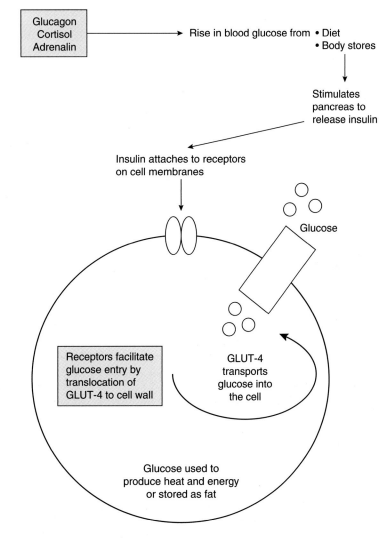

Figure 1.4 Diagrammatic representation of insulin binding, insulin signalling, translocation of GLUT-4 and glucose entry into the cell. GLUT-4 is a glucose transporter contained in vesicles in the cell cytoplasm. Once insulin binds to an insulin receptor GLUT-4 moves to the cell membrane and transports glucose into the cell. During fasting GLUT-4 is low and increases in response to the increase in insulin. Failure of GLUT-4 translocation could explain some of the insulin resistance associated with Type 2 diabetes. The effects of insulin are mediated by two protein pathways: P13-kinase through the insulin receptors (glucose uptake) and MAP-kinase, which stimulates growth and mitogenesis.

which is activated by fat and reduces insulin production. Future medicines may target this deficiency and restore normal insulin function (Biden 2007).

In addition, Swedish researchers Mahdi *et al.* (2012) demonstrated that people with high serum Secreted Frizzled-Related protein 4 (SFRP4) have a 5-fold increased risk of developing diabetes in the following five years. SFR4 plays a role in the inflammatory process and its release from islet cells is stimulated by interleukin-1β. High serum SFRP4 reduces glucose tolerance. SFRP4 is elevated several years before Type 2 diabetes is diagnosed indicating it could be a useful risk marker for Type 2 diabetes independently of other risk factors

Table 1.1   Generally agreed characteristics of Type 1 and Type 2 diabetes mellitus.

	Type 1	Type 2
Age at onset	Usually <30 years[a]	Usually >40 years. But increasing prevalence in children and adolescents
Speed of onset	Usually rapid	Usually gradual and insidious
Body weight	Normal or underweight; often recent weight loss	80% are overweight
Heredity	Associated with specific human leukocyte antigen (HLA-DR3 or 4)[b]	No HLA association Genetic predisposition, which is complex and only beginning to be understood
	Autoimmune disease and environmental triggers	Environmental and lifestyle factors contribute
Insulin	Early insulin secretion Impaired later; may be totally absent	Often preceded by the metabolic syndrome (see section on 'The metabolic syndrome'). Insulin resistance is reversible if appropriate diet and exercise regimens are instituted. Type 2 is associated with slow, progressive loss of beta cell function
Ketosis	Common	Rare
Symptoms	Usually present	Often absent, especially in the early stages. Acanthosis nigricans is common in some ethnic peoples
Frequency	~15% of diagnosed cases	~85% of diagnosed cases
Complications	Common but not usually present at diagnosis	Common, often present at diagnosis
Treatment	Insulin, diet, exercise, stress management, regular health and complication assessment	Diet, GLM, exercise, insulin, stress management, regular health and complication assessment

[a] Increasing incidence of the metabolic syndrome and Type 2 diabetes in children and adolescents.
[b] Occurs in older people; see LADA.

Vitamin D deficiency may also be a risk factor for diabetes independently of other risk factors in longititudinal studies such as the Australian Obesity and Lifestyle (AusDiab) study (Gagnon *et al.* 2011). Given the increasing information about the complexity of Type 2 diabetes pathophysiology, it is unlikely any single intervention will prevent or treat the disease effectively; thus, it is not clear whether vitamin D supplementation is likely to modify diabetes risk. Vitamin D deficiency is very common and is also a marker of general health status and may be indicated to manage other concomitant conditions such as osteoporosis.

The characteristics of Type 1 and Type 2 diabetes are shown in Table 1.1.

Management is discussed in Chapter 2. The majority of people with Type 2 diabetes require multiple therapies to target the multiple underlying metabolic abnormalities and achieve and maintain acceptable blood glucose and lipid targets over the first nine years after diagnosis (UKPDS 1998). Between 50% and 70% eventually require insulin, which is often used in combination with other glucose lowering medicines (GLM), which means diabetes management becomes progressively more complicated for people with Type 2 diabetes, often coinciding with increasing age when their ability to manage may be compromised, which increases the likelihood of non-adherence and the costs of managing the disease for the patient and the health system.

Type 2 diabetes in Indigenous children and adolescents

Type 2 diabetes in children and adolescents is discussed in Chapter 13 but it is a significant problem in Indigenous children and adolescents. Indigenous Australians, like other Indigenous peoples, are at high risk of Type 2 diabetes, especially when they live in remote communities, and it develops at a younger age (Minges *et al.* 2011). Onset is often in early adolescence and frequently asymptomatic. Indigenous children and adolescents with diabetes usually have a family history of Type 2 diabetes, are overweight and have signs of hyperinsulinaemia and acanthosis nigricans. There is a high prevalence of misrovascular and macrovascular complications and the associated morbidity and mortality (Azzopardi *et al.* 2012).

A number of causative factors are implicated including intrauterine exposure to risk during maternal pregnancy, obesity, physical inactivity, genetic predisposition and socioeconomic and environmental factors. Consequently, experts recommend screening Aboriginal and Torres Strait Islander children over age 10 for metabolic syndrome and diabetes. The IDF (2011) criteria for diagnosing Type 2 diabetes in Indigenous children and adolescents are:

- Random laboratory venous blood glucose (BG) >100 mmol/L and polyuria and polydipsia especially when the symptoms occur at night. OR
- Fasting laboratory venous BG > 7 mmol/L performed after fasting for at least 8 hours. OR
- Random laboratory plasma BG .11.1 mmol/L on at least two separate occasions.

Oral glucose tolerance tests (OGTT) are not practical in many remote Indigenous communities. Point-of-care HbA1c might be an alternative but no clear diagnostic recommendations are available for children. Ketones should be checked in newly diagnosed Indigenous children to ensure treatment is appropriate. Management should be individualised taking into account the psychosocial factors that influence adherence.

Gestational diabetes

Diabetes occurring during pregnancy is referred to as gestational diabetes (GDM). GDM occurs in ~5% of all pregnancies (Rice *et al.* 2012). The incidence of GDM is increasing with the global obesity epidemic. GDM refers to carbohydrate intolerance of varying degrees that first occurs or is first recognised during pregnancy. Several factors have been implicated in the development of GDM including diet and lifestyle, smoking, some medicines, older age, genetic background, ethnicity, number of previous pregnancies and recently, short stature (Langer 2006).

People at risk of GDM should be screened for diabetes using standard diagnostic criteria at the first prenatal visit. High risk women have impaired fasting glucose (5.6–6.9 mmol/L) and/or, impaired glucose tolerance (2-hour OGTT 7.8–11.0 mmol/L). Women with HbA1c 5.7%–6.4% are also at increased risk (Rice *et al.* 2102). For more information about GDM refer to Chapter 14.

Maturity onset diabetes of the young (MODY)

Maturity onset diabetes of the young (MODY) is a rare heterogeneous group of disorders that result in beta cell dysfunction. MODY can develop at any age up to 55. It has a genetic basis and at least nine different genes that result in the MODY phenotype, which

Table 1.2 Classification of single gene mutations resulting in MODY (Data from Rice *et al.* [2012]).

Genetic variety	Prevalence: % of overall MODY gene mutations depending on the populations studied	Features
HNFIA	30–50%	Common mutation Progressive beta cell failure > 5 mmol/L BG rise at 2 hours on OGTT (75 gram) Sensitive to sulphonylureas
GCK	30–50%	Common mutation Elevated fasting BG with small, <3 mmol/L, rise at 2 hours on OGTT (75 gram) Mild hyperglycaemia and may not require treatment
HNF-4A	5%	Similar presentation to HNF1A Associated with higher birth weight Transient neonatal hyperglycaemia Progressive beta cell failure Sensitive to sulphonylureas
HNF1B	5%	Associated with renal disease Urogenital tract abnormalities in girls
* INS	< 1%	Varied clinical presentation Usually present with neonatal diabetes but can present in childhood and early adulthood
* IPF1	< 1%	Average age at diagnosis 35 years
* NUEROD1	< 1%	Vary rare Similar to type 2 diabetes Onset mid 20s Development of beta cell failure and reduced insulin production May be overweight
* CEL	< 1%	Very rare Due to exocrine pancreatic dysfunction but pathophysiology is unknown Adult onset ~ age 36
* PAX4	< 1%	Vary rare

*fewer than five families reported with the genes.

suggests MODY is a single entity. MODY accounts for 1%–2% of people diagnosed with diabetes, but the prevalence could be underestimated because population-based screening programmes have not been performed (Gardner & Tai 2012). The different genetic aetiologies vary in age at onset, hyperglycaemia pattern, response to treatment and extra-pancreatic manifestations. The varieties of MODY are shown in Table 1.2.

People with MODY often have a strong family history of diabetes, insulin independence, no insulin autoantibodies and evidence of endogenous insulin production, low insulin requirement and generally do not become ketotic (McDonald *et al.* 2011). However, there are distinct phenotypes which might present differently. Treatment depends on the MODY type but generally includes GLMs, diet and exercise, although insulin may eventually be required. HNFIA individuals are very sensitive to sulphonylureas.

MODY can be difficult to recognise and the diagnosis missed or delayed (Appleton & Hattersley 1996). This can have implications for the individual and their family in commencing appropriate treatment for the specific type of MODY. Genetic counselling is also advisable.

Practice points

(1) MODY is a different disease process from Type 2 diabetes that occurs in young people and has a different genetic and inheritance pattern from Type 2.
(2) The prevalence of Type 2 diabetes in children is increasing and is associated with obesity and insulin resistance (Sinha *et al.* 2002).
(3) MODY has been misdiagnosed as Type 1 diabetes and insulin commenced unnecessarily.
(4) MODY has also been diagnosed instead of Type 1 diabetes in the UK (Health Service Ombudsman 2000).
(5) Type 2 diabetes is a serious, insidious life-threatening disease.

These points demonstrate the importance of taking a careful clinical history and undertaking appropriate diagnostic investigations.

Diagnosing diabetes

Urine glucose tests should not be used to diagnose diabetes; if glycosuria is detected, the blood glucose should be tested. When symptoms of diabetes are present, an elevated blood glucose alone is often sufficient to confirm the diagnosis. See Table 1.3 for diagnostic criteria.

If the person is asymptomatic, abnormal fasting blood glucose values of >7 mmol/L should be demonstrated on at least two occasions before the diagnosis is made (note that some guidelines suggest >6.5 mmol/L). Random plasma glucose >11.1 mmol/L and symptoms are diagnostic of Type 2 diabetes. An oral glucose tolerance test (OGTT) using a 75 g glucose load may be indicated to determine the presence of glucose intolerance if results are borderline. The criteria for diagnosing diabetes according to the World Health Organization are shown in Table 1.3. A protocol for preparing the patient and performing an OGTT are outlined later in the chapter. However, some experts suggest 75 g may be too high a load for some ethnic groups such as Vietnamese.

Abnormal plasma glucose identifies a subgroup of people at risk of diabetes-related complications. The risk data for these complications is based on the 2-hour OGTT

Table 1.3   Diagnostic criteria for non-pregnant adults with diabetes based on the World Health Organization and the American Diabetes Association Guidelines.

Stage	Fasting plasma glucose	Random plasma glucose	Oral glucose tolerance test (OGTT)
Normal	<6.1 mmol/L		2 hour plasma glucose <7.8 mmol/L
Impaired glucose tolerance	Impaired fasting glucose – fasting glucose ≥6.1 and <7.0 mmol/L		Impaired glucose tolerance – 2 hours plasma glucose ≥7.8 and <11.1 mmol/L
Diabetes	≥7.0 mmol/L	≥11.1 mmol/L and symptoms	2 hour plasma glucose >11.1 mmol/L

Note: In this table venous plasma glucose values are shown. Glucose in capillary blood is about 10–15% higher than venous blood. HbA1c can be used to make the diagnosis instead of or as well as venous blood glucose; >6.5% in a laboratory using certified assay method standardised to DCCT criteria.

Practice point

Hyperglycaemia often occurs as a stress response to serious intercurrent illness such as cardiovascular disease and it may be difficult to diagnose diabetes in such circumstances. However, controlling the blood glucose during the illness is important and leads to better outcomes including in non-diabetics (Chapters 7 and 9).

plasma glucose level. However, the fasting glucose of >7.8 mmol/L does not equate with the 2-hour level used to diagnose diabetes. Recently, the ADA and the WHO lowered the fasting level to 7.0 mmol/L to more closely align it to the 2-hour level.

The WHO continues to advocate routine OGTT screening in at-risk individuals to identify people at risk of complications early, in order for early treatment to be instituted. The ADA does not advocate routine OGTT use because it believes that the revised fasting level is sensitive enough to detect most people at risk. Therefore, there could be differences internationally about the routine use of the OGTT. The ADA and the WHO do agree on how the test should be performed. Australia supports the continued use of the OGTT when the diagnosis is equivocal and to detect GDM (Hilton *et al.* 2002; Twigg *et al.* 2007). However, OGTT may not always be practical in remote communities (Azzopardi *et al.* 2012).

A recent study suggested untrained people could perform self-administered OGTT in the community setting using a specific device (n = 18 people without diabetes and 12 with Type 2) OGTT were performed unaided in the home twice, unaided but observed in the clinic and one OGGT/participant was perfumed by a nurse. The results were verified with simultaneous laboratory values of the 0 and 120-minute samples (Bethel *et al.* 2013). A data recorder attached to the test device recorded information about the test. Device failures meant 0 and 120 minutes BG was only available for 141/180 OGTTs independent of the test setting. Self-performed and laboratory values were similar and reproducible. The clinical implications are unclear at this time.

Other prevention measures include providing the public with information about screening and health maintenance programmes, and self-risk assessment lists, for example checklists from the Agency for Healthcare Research and Quality (AHRQ). Checklists can be downloaded from the Internet (http://www.ahrq.gov/ppip/healthywom.htm or http://www.ahrq.gov/ppip/helthymen.htm). The information is based on the US Preventative Services Task Force recommendations.

HbA1c has an accepted place in monitoring metabolic control in people with diabetes. In addition, the WHO, IDF, and the American Diabetes Association (ADA) recommend using HbA1c as screening test for Type 2 diabetes. The Australian Diabetes Society (ADS), Royal College of Pathologists of Australasia and the Australasian Association of Clinical Biochemists released a position statement in 2102 that recommended HbA1c be used to diagnose diabetes if the analysis is performed in a laboratory that meets external quality assurance standards and recommended HbA1c >6.5% (48 mmol/mol) as the diagnostic cut point. Point-of-care HbA1c tests are useful clinical decision-making tools but they are not recommended for diagnosing diabetes. The ADS noted HbA1c <6.5% (48 mmol/mol) does not exclude a diagnosis of diabetes based on existing fasting BG or OGTT criteria. The latter remain the diagnostic tests of choice for GDM, Type 1 diabetes and when people have conditions that affect the HbA1c result (d'smden *et al.* 2012). In November 2012 a Medicare Consultation paper was released in Australia proposing a rebate of

$16.90 when HbA1c was performed as a diagnostic test, but the rebate would be limited to one test per year per person; an additional confirmatory test would be covered if the result was ≥6.5% (48 mmol/mol). The rate of screening in primary care might increase if the rebate is introduced.

Advantages of HbA1c as a diagnostic test are people do not need to fast before blood is collected and the test can be performed at any time of the day. HbA1c measures chronic glycaemia and HbA1c levels are strongly associated with retinopathy, macrovascular outcomes and mortality (d'Emden *et al.* 2012). HbA1c assays are standardised and generally reliable in most countries. However, errors associated with non-glycaemic factors such as haemoglobinopathies and anaemia that affect HbA1c need to be considered when interpreting the findings (Saudek *et al.* 2008).

Other markers of hyperglycaemia and diabetes risk include Fructosamine, glycated albumin and 1,5 anhydroglucitol (1,5-AG), which are associated with the development of diabetes independently of baseline HbA1c and fasting glucose (Juraschek *et al.* 2012). It is not clear what place these markers have in diagnosing or monitoring diabetes as yet, but they could be useful when HbA1c is not reliable such as haemoglobinopathies. In fact, fructosamine is recommended in the latter situation.

Other experts suggests the combination of HbA1c 5.7%–6.4% (39–46 mmol/mol) and fasting plasma glucose 5.6–6.9 mmol/L are likely to reduce the likelihood of missing a diagnosis of diabetes and be more likely to identify people with prediabetes (fasting plasma glucose 6.1–6.9 and HbA1c 6.0%–6.4% (42–46 mmol/mol) who are likely to progress to diabetes (Heianza *et al.* 2012). Abikshyeet *et al.* 2012) suggested salivary glucose could be a useful non-invasive diagnostic and monitoring test for diabetes but acknowledged more research is needed before salivary glucose testing is adopted.

Most prediction models for the risk of developing Type 2 diabetes appear to identify individuals at high and low risk of developing diabetes but extended models that include conventional biomarkers perform better. Some models overestimate risk (Abbassi *et al.* 2012). Thus, it could be important to ensure the screening parameters such as BMI and glycaemic targets are relevant to the target population.

Oral glucose tolerance test (OGTT)

An OGTT is used to diagnose diabetes:

- When fasting and random blood glucose results are equivocal.
- When there is a strong family history of diabetes, especially during pregnancy.
- If the suspicion of diabetes is high but blood glucose tests are normal/equivocal.

An OGTT should not be performed when the person:

- Is febrile;
- Is acutely ill, for example postoperatively, or uraemic;
- Has been immobilised for more than 48 hours;
- Has symptoms of diabetes or an elevated blood glucose before commencing the test.

Rationale for OGTT

Early diagnosis and treatment of diabetes reduces the morbidity and mortality associated with the hyperglycaemia.

Preparing the patient for an OGTT
(1) Give specific oral and written instructions to the patient. A sample is given in Example Instruction Sheet 1 below.
(2) Ensure the diet contains at least 200 g/day carbohydrate for at least 3–5 days before the test.
(3) If possible stop medicines that can influence the blood glucose levels 3 days before the test: some of these will need to be reduced gradually, for example corticosteroids (Chapter 10). People should be informed about the consequences of stopping their medicines and when to resume taking them after the test:
- thiazide diuretics
- antihypertensive medicines
- analgesic and anti-inflammatory medicines
- antineoplastic medicines
- steroids.
(4) Fast from 12 midnight, the night before the test.
(5) Avoid physical/psychological stress for 1 hour prior to, and during, the test.
(6) Avoid smoking for at least 1 hour prior to the test.
(7) Allow the patient to relax for 30 minutes before beginning the test.

Example Information Sheet: Preparation for an oral glucose tolerance test

---

PATIENT INSTRUCTIONS FOR ORAL GLUCOSE TOLERANCE TEST

Date of test: **Name**:
Time: **I.D. label**

Location where test will take place:

(1) Please ensure that you eat high carbohydrate meals each day for 3 days before the test. Carbohydrate foods are: breads, cereals, spaghetti, noodles, rice, dried beans and pulses, vegetables, fruit. These foods should constitute the major part of your diet for the 3 days.
(2) Have nothing to eat or drink after 12 midnight on the night prior to the test day, except water.
(3) Specific information about managing medicines: ....
(4) Bring a list of all the tablets you are taking with you when you come for the test.
(5) Do not smoke for at least one hour before the test.

The test

The test is performed in the morning. You are required to rest during the test, which will take approximately 3 hours to complete. A small needle will be inserted into an arm vein for blood sampling. The needle will stay in place until the test is completed. You will be given 300 mL of glucose to drink. This is very sweet but it is important to drink it all over the 5 minutes, so that the results of the test can be interpreted correctly. Water is permitted.
You will be given a drink and something to eat when the test is finished. The doctor will discuss the results with you.

Test protocol
(1) The person should rest during the test to avoid dislodging the cannula.
(2) Insert a cannula into a suitable vein for blood sampling e.g. the cubical fossa.

(3) The blood glucose should be tested before commencing the test. If elevated, clarify with the doctor ordering the test before proceeding. Collect two milliliters of blood in fluoride oxalate tubes for laboratory analysis at each test time point.

(4) Flush the cannula with normal saline between samples to prevent clots forming in the cannula. One to two milliliters of blood should be withdrawn and discarded before collecting each sample to avoid contaminating the sample with saline left in the tubing.

(5) Collect blood samples at the following times. However, sometimes only a baseline (0) and a two-hour sample are collected:

minutes: −10

0

⇒   75 g glucose, consumed over 5 minutes. Water can be given after the glucose is all consumed. It is very sweet and some people find it difficult to drink.

+30

+60

+120

The glucose used for an OGTT is prepacked in 300 mL bottles containing exactly 75 g of glucose.

(6) Ensure the person has a follow-up appointment with the referring doctor whose responsibility it is to explain the test results and commence or arrange for appropriate management and education.

Screening for diabetes

Because of the insidious nature and increasing incidence and prevalence of Type 2 diabetes, many countries have instituted population-based education and screening and/or case detection programmes in at-risk populations. Fingerprick blood glucose tests are not generally used to diagnose diabetes: see Table 1.3 for the diagnostic criteria. Many programmes also involve checking for obesity and cardiovascular risk factors. At-risk groups include:

- age >55 years;
- high-risk ethnic groups such as indigenous people, Southeast Asians, Indians from the subcontinent;
- women with Polycystic Ovarian Syndrome (PCOS)
- previous GDM;
- family history of diabetes;
- people with symptoms, but symptoms are often absent in Type 2 diabetes;
- older people >65 years;
- People with known diabetes complications such as cardiovascular, erectile dysfunction, and renal disease;
- active smokers (Willi *et al.* 2007).

Screening for Type 1 diabetes is not usually necessary because it presents differently and has a more rapid onset and symptoms are usually present. First-degree relatives of people with Type 1 diabetes can be tested for risk markers (autoantibodies) for diabetes but the preventative strategies applicable to Type 2 diabetes do not apply.

An example of one screening and preventative model of care is shown in Figure 1.5.

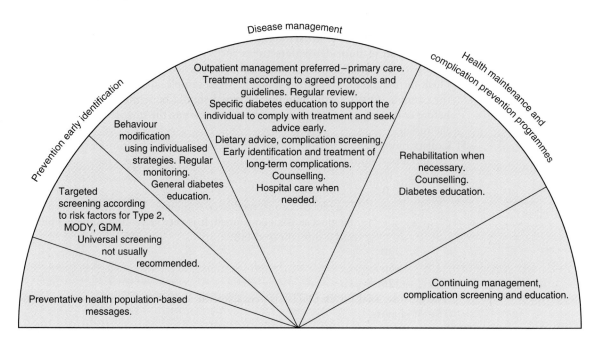

Figure 1.5   Example of a screening and preventative model of health care.

Preventing Type 2 diabetes

A number of clinical trials have demonstrated that it is possible to prevent Type 2 diabetes and may in turn prevent the associated morbidity from long-term complications. Most prevention trials were conducted among people with IGT because it is a strong predictor of Type 2 diabetes. These programmes include the Da Qing Study (Pan 1997), the Oslo Diet and Exercise Program, the Diabetes Prevention Program (DPP) (2002), and the Finnish Diabetes Prevention Study (DPS) (2003), which showed a 58% reduction in the progression to diabetes in people who followed a healthy lifestyle and the effects were still present at the four-year follow up. (Tuomilehto *et al.* 2001). The DPS was stopped early because the intervention was so successful but the researchers continued to follow people who did not develop diabetes for up to 10 years. The intervention group achieved a reduction of ~40% compared to controls.

Elements of these programmes have been adapted and implemented in many countries since the findings were first published, especially the DPP, for example *Go For Your Life* and the Life Programme in Australia. However, a Cochrane review (Nield *et al.* 2008) stated 'There is no high quality data on the efficacy of dietary intervention for the prevention of Type 2 diabetes.' Since causes of the metabolic syndrome and Type 2 diabetes are complex and multifactorial, it is not surprising that dietary interventions in isolation are ineffective.

Key features of the DPS are weight reduction (~5%), reducing fat intake to <30%, with <10% coming from saturated fats, fibre intake of >15 g per 1000 calories and >30 minutes of moderate exercise per day. In the DPS, weight loss and exercise appeared to be more important than dietary goals in preventing diabetes. Achieving weight loss and making dietary changes is difficult and only 2% of participants in the DPS achieved four or five targets but no participant who did so developed diabetes compared to 50% of the control group. Weight management strategies are discussed in Chapter 4.

Studies concentrating on increasing fibre and magnesium to prevent Type 2 diabetes show inconsistent results despite current guidelines to increase the total fibre intake. The type of fibre consumed may be important in that soluble fibre may enhance gastric emptying and reduce the postprandial glucose rise. A meta-analysis revealed lower diabetes risk with increased intake of cereal fibre but no significant association with fruit and vegetable fibre. Thus, including whole grain foods is important in diabetes prevention diets (Krishnan *et al.* 2007) and, as indicated, pre- and probiotics are emerging as important considerations for gut health and preventing immune- and inflammatory-related diseases such as diabetes. An example of a screening and prevention model is shown in Figure 1.5.

Vegetarians appear to have reduced risk of metabolic syndrome and reduced risk of Type 2 diabetes. (Nash 2012). Likewise Mediterranean diets, while not strictly vegetarian, are generally high in fibre, prebiotics and whole grains and are associated with reduced risk of Type 2 diabetes. Avoiding liquid calories such as those in sugar sweetened beverages, fruit juice and alcohol appears to be important. These liquids also lead to dental caries. Rice is the staple food in many countries such as China where white rice is consumed at 3–4 times per day. The Glycaemic Index of white rice is higher than other whole grains and Basmati type rice. Studies suggest the relative risk of developing diabetes is 1.11 for every serving of white rice consumed per day (Hu *et al.* 2012).

Many existing public health screening and prevention models fall into four main categories (Lang & Rayner 2012):

- Sanitary-environmental model.
- Biomedical model that can be individual or population focused.
- Social behavioural model, which rivals the biomedical model. It might not take account of who has the strongest influence on behavior, which may be companies like Coca Cola.
- Techno-economic model, which views health as depending on economic growth and knowledge development.
- Ecological model, which focuses on interactions among factors that impact on health, including climate change, and integrates elements of the other four models. Climate change impacts on factors such as food security/availability, extreme weather events, which displace people and affect their lifestyle and social circumstances (IDF 2012).

The relative merits of these models have not been tested but current policies do not appear to be halting the exponential rise in the prevalence of the metabolic syndrome and diabetes. In fact Simmons *et al.* (2012) suggested screening for diabetes does not reduce deaths. The researchers followed a cohort of nearly 12 000 people at high risk of diabetes for 10 years and found they were no more likely to have died than 4000 people who were not screened, and there were no significant differences between the two groups for deaths specifically attributable to diabetes. Interestingly, benefits for microvascular disease were not analysed. It is unlikely that screening alone *would* reduce risk unless relevant prevention strategies were used and early diagnosis and management incorporated into the model. Likewise, population-wide prevention may not reduce healthcare spending because it does not reduce the risk of serious illness or premature death, because of the number of people who need to receive a particular preventive treatment to prevent a single illness (Reuters Health Information 2013). Targeted prevention programmes that incorporate environmental and social factors and collaborating with local government and religious institutions and other key stakeholders need to be part of prevention programmes.

Two European projects DE-PLAN and IMAGE are addressing implementation processes for diabetes prevention programs and developing a toolkit to help people develop and implement programmes for preventing Type 2 diabetes. The kit includes a practical guideline that targets everybody who could have a role in prevention such as health professionals, teachers, traditional healers, and politicians, it explains key aspects of financial management, how to identify people at risk, as well as educating and training key personnel, and monitoring and quality assurance processes that need to be addressed. It will be interesting to determine whether the toolkit makes a difference in actual practice, since many prevention programmes already encompass all the elements in the tool kit including education.

One important factor that might lead to changes is the Global Monitoring Framework (GMF) for non-communicable disease, which was agreed in November 2012 between the WHO and national governments. The GMF is ambitious and has been dubbed '25 by 25' in recognition of the first target, which is to reduce NCD-related deaths by 25% by 2025. Other targets include reducing the:

- increase in diabetes and obesity;
- prevalence of inactivity by 10%;
- harmful use of alcohol by 10%;
- consumption of salt by 30%;
- prevalence of tobacco use by 30%;
- prevalence of hypertension by 25%.

Signatory countries to the agreement will be required to report their performance against the agreed targets in 2013. The targets reflect metabolic syndrome risk factors such as hypertension, inactivity and smoking. Importantly, one target is to halt the increasing prevalence of diabetes and premature mortality from non-communicable diabetes. Important proposed strategies to help meet the Global Framework is to ensure essential medicines and self-management preventative education are available (IDF 2012).

Meanwhile, research is underway to understand the genetics that predispose people to insulin resistance and Type 2 diabetes and help predict the risk for diabetes to better target prevention and management strategies. Significant progress has been made in identifying the variations in DNA sequence involved in the development of diabetes as part of the Genome-wide study (GWAS). Sixty-five regions of the human genome associated with diabetes have been identified (Morris 2012), however the effects of the variants are too subtle to be used as risk predictors at present.

Research to determine how beta cells and insulin-responsive tissues normally develop and function are also progressing, for example discovering the relationship between the FTP gene and obesity. Animal studies are underway to determine the mechanisms that affect appetite and metabolism and predispose to obesity. Genetic studies are increasing our understanding of the relationship between SHBG levels and diabetes risk. SHBG is a binding protein produced in the liver that transports testosterone, and to oestrogen to some extent, to target tissues. SHBG levels are often low in people with Type 2 diabetes. Previously, researchers assumed that insulin resistance lowered SHBG, however genetic studies suggest low SHBG may have a causal role in Type 2 diabetes (Ding *et al.* 2009).

Preventing Type 1 diabetes

Research for the elusive cure for Type 1 diabetes continues. Approaches include:

- Immune intervention using monoclonal antibodies to prevent the immune system destroying beta cells. People diagnosed early enough to still have some functioning beta cells receive a combination of medicine such as Teplizumab and Otelixizumab. The medicines protect the remaining beta cells and people may need less insulin. The results of clinical trials vary among countries. For example, in Europe and America young, slim people appear to benefit from the medicines; however, people from Asia derive less benefit. Genetic differences, age and BMI might account for the different responses.
- Stem cells: blood stem cells have been used in a similar way to treatment for leukemia in Brazil. Radiation is used to destroy the immune system and fresh blood stem cells are infused to calm the immune system so it no longer destroys beta cells. Early clinical studies show 'promise.' The following is more specifically treatment but it is relevant to stem cell research. In Australia, researchers have isolated stem cells in the adult pancreas and developed a technique to transform the stem cells into insulin-producing beta cells that release insulin in response to glucose. The hope is people with Type 1 diabetes may be able to regenerate their own beta cells if the immune attack that initially caused diabetes can be prevented.
- Reprogrammed liver cells are being researched in animal studies in Israel (Jaekel 2012).

Managing diabetes mellitus

Key points

- The person with diabetes undertakes >90% of their diabetes management, thus they are experts in *their* diabetes and their lives.
- Visits to health professionals occur at regular intervals and mostly concern assessing physical, psychological and metabolic status and making treatment recommendations.
- Diabetes education is the cornerstone of management. The phrase generally refers to people with diabetes BUT it applies equally, if not more so to the health professionals who provide education and care for people with diabetes.
- It is essential to individualise care plans and develop them with the individual concerned.

Management strategies for specific aspects of care are discussed in almost every chapter of the book. This section deals with general management information.

Many 'diabetes care models' have been developed as the framework within which to provide diabetes care. These include the Chronic Disease Model and its derivations such as the Flinders Model used in some Australian states. Research suggests effective diabetes care models need to enable early diagnosis and coordinate diagnosis, treatment and ongoing management, and educate people with diabetes and their health professionals (Renders *et al.* 2012). Effective components of management programs appear to be high frequency of contact with people with diabetes and ability for the people managing the disease (primarily the person with diabetes) to adjust their medicines and are more effective for people with inadequate glycaemic control (HbA1c >8% at baseline) (Pimouguet *et al.* 2010).

Diabetes education is an essential component of diabetes management and the benefit seems to apply equally to groups and individual education and combinations of both (Pimouguet *et al.* 2010) (Chapter 16).

Currently, the Australian Government is evaluating a new care model: the Diabetes Care Project (DCP) in a large randomised control trial involving general practices, nurses and allied health professionals in Queensland, Victoria and South Australia. The DCP consists of two models of coordinated care. General practices that enroll will be randomised to either usual care (control) or intervention 1 or 2. Intervention 1 will test an electronic tool that creates individualised care plans and enables health professionals and the individual to access the care plan and health record and update information, and automated follow-up and review processes. Patient progress will be monitored against their care plan. Health professional compliance with Medicare will also be monitored.

Intervention 2 uses the same electronic tool and a new funding model and encompasses a new team member, the care facilitator. The new funding model is risk adjusted and enables patients to access diabetes educators and allied health professionals. It will be interesting to track progress of this innovative model. The model appears to comply with Pimouguet *et al.* (2010) and Renders *et al.* (2012) criteria for effective models.

The diabetes team

Effective diabetes management depends on having a collaborative multidisciplinary health care team. The person with diabetes is the central player in the team. Good communication among team members is vital and information the patient receives must be consistent between, and within, hospital departments, health services and health professionals to ensure smooth transition among services and avoid confusing the patient with inconsistent information. The team usually consists of some or all of the following:

- Diabetologist;
- Diabetes nurse specialist/diabetes educator and/or diabetes nurse practitioner;
- Dietitian;
- Podiatrist;
- Social worker;
- Psychologist;
- General practitioner.

Other professionals who contribute regularly to the diabetes management:

- Opthalmologist
- Optometrist
- Pharmacist
- Specialists such as vascular and orthopaedic surgeons, neurologists, and urologists, audiologists;
- Cultural/traditional health workers, for example, Aboriginal health workers in Australia and traditional healers in Africa;
- Exercise physiologists;
- Hospital physiotherapists.

The ward staff who care for the patient in hospital and the community also become team members during presentations to hospital and emergency departments and care in home settings including:

- Doctors
- Nurses
- Dietitians
- Community physiotherapists
- Occupational therapists.

It is easy to understand why people with diabetes can be confused about health professional roles and responsibilities and about their own role and responsibilities in diabetes care if they receive conflicting information from health professionals.

Managing diabetes consists of dietary modification, regular exercise/activity and in some cases insulin or GLMs. Diabetes education and regularly assessing metabolic control and complication status is essential. In addition, general health care is very important and includes dental checks, mammograms, prostate checks and preventative vaccinations, for example, fluvax and pneumovax. As indicated many times in this book, it is essential to personalize the care plan and individualise management targets to suit the person's risk status, social situation and capabilities. (Repetition is one important education strategy. Politicians and marketers also use it! Helping people manage their diabetes requires health professionals to be effective marketers, politicians and communicators.)

Aims of management

Diabetes management should be determined within the Quality Use of Medicine framework, see Chapter 4. Management aims for Australia are defined in the National Diabetes Strategy and a number of other specific guidelines such as those described in the Australian Diabetes Society Position Statements, and Clinical Management Guidelines for Diabetes in General Practice. A range of other guidelines produced by various countries and diabetes associations such as the UK, Scotland, the USA and the IDF, some of which are listed in this and other chapters in the book.

The aim of diabetes management is to maintain quality of life and keep the person free from the symptoms of diabetes, and the blood glucose and blood lipids within in an acceptable range. The blood glucose range needs to be determined on an individual basis, usually between 4.0 and 6.0 mmol/L for 90% of tests, especially during acute illness and surgery, young people and during pregnancy and HbA1c <7% (Diabetes Australia (DA 2011/12) and Royal Australian College of General Practitioners (RACGP) 2011/12), Table 1.4. However, higher targets might be more appropriate for people at risk of hypoglycaemia (Chapter 6), older people (Chapter 12) and children (Chapter 13). The aim is to obtain results as near as possible to the target blood glucose range but there must be a balance between the food plan, medication (insulin/GLMs) and exercise/activity. Maintaining emotional well-being is essential (Chapter 1). General management goals (targets) are shown in Table 1.4.

The regimen should affect the person's lifestyle as little as possible, although some modification is usually necessary. People with Type 1 require insulin in order to survive. Obese people with Type 2 can sometimes be treated effectively with a combination of diet and exercise, but research suggests that people managed with diet are not as rigorously monitored and have more hyperglycaemia and hypertension than those on medicines (Hippisley-Cox & Pringle 2004). Many people with Type 2 diabetes require GLMs and usually eventually insulin due to the progressive loss of beta cell function

In the current person-centred empowerment model of diabetes care, the person with diabetes is the pivotal person in the management team. Forming a therapeutic

Table 1.4 Diabetes management targets; but note most current guidelines recommend targets be individualised according to specific microvascular, macrovascular and hypoglycaemia risk (ADS 2012, ADA 2013, DA/RACPG 2011/12, SIGN 2010, NICE 2008).

Glucose: Fasting blood glucose 4–6 mmol/L; HbA$_{1c}$ <7% (53 mmol/mol)

Lipids: LDL-c <2.5 mmol/L; triglycerides <1.5 mmol/L; HDL-c >1.0 mmol/L, total cholesterol <4.0 mmol/L

Blood pressure: 130/80 mmHg; 125/75 mmHg if proteinuiria exceeds 1 g/day: 140/90 if over 65 years.

BMI <25 kg/m^2 (ideal); waist circumference women <80 cm, men <94 cm.

Renal function: Urine albumin excretion 20 mm/min in timed overnight collection; <20 mm/min spot collection; albumin–creatinine ratio <3.5 mg/mmol in women, <2.5 mg/mmol men eGFR.

Alcohol intake: Women, 1 standard drink/day, men, 2 standard drinks/day.

No smoking

Exercise/activity: >150 minutes/week; at least 30 minutes brisk walking or equivalent/day or on at least five days/week

partnership with the individual and accepting their choices is essential to achieving optimal outcomes. Putting the person at the centre of care means respecting their choices, even when the individual elects not to follow advice after receiving adequate information (informed decision-making). Not following advice should not be labeled 'non-compliant or non-adherent.' Accepting the person's decision does not mean the health professional does not continue to provide information and advice. It does mean *they* might need to change the way they do things and try new strategies.

Clinical observation

Diabetes is a balancing act. The individual's physical, psychological, spiritual and social and relationship needs must be balanced to enable people to undertake the necessary self-management to achieve management targets (optimal physical health). In fact, the emphasis should be on balance rather than control. Spirituality, resilience and positive thinking, in particular, are important but neglected aspects of current diabetes management strategies and are key to being able to manage life changes (turning/tipping points), self-empowerment and self-determination (Parsian & Dunning 2008).

Management involves educating the person with diabetes and other family members and carers in order to help them:

- Understand diabetes, be involved in deciding their care plan and adopt relevant self-care strategies necessary to maintain optimal health and meet glycaemic targets.
- Manage the impact of diabetes on their physical, psychological and spiritual functioning to maintain an acceptable quality of life.
- Achieve and maintain an acceptable weight.
- Achieve acceptable blood glucose levels and HbA1c.
- Achieve a normal blood lipid profile.
- Relieve symptoms of diabetes (polyuria, polydipsia and lethargy). This involves helping the person recognise and manage relevant signs and symptoms associated with diabetes and any concomitant condition/s.
- Prevent and/or manage hypolycaemia.
- Manage intercurrent illnesses (sick days).
- Prevent complications of diabetes and of treatment.

Table 1.5 Guidelines for assessing the patient's blood glucose testing pattern. The results should be considered as part of the overall situation not as isolated pieces of data. The target HbA$_{1c}$ is <7% (<6.5% in some countries).

% Haemoglobin A1c	Glucose (mmol/L)		Control
	Fasting	Two hours after food	
4.0–6.0 (~ 31–48 mmol/mol)	4	<7	Excellent or 'too good' high risk of hypoglycaemia[a]
6.0–7.4 (48–58 mmol/mol)	7	9	Upper limit of target range
7.5–9.4 (58–75 mmol/mol)	10	14.5	Increased short- and long-term complication risk.
>9.5 (> 75 mmol/mol)	14	20	Increased short- and long-term complication risk

[a] If fasting glucose is high postprandial glucose is often also high. Postprandial glucose is affected by first phase insulin response, glucagons secretion, muscle and live glucose stores, fat tissue sensitivity to insulin, food intake and digestion and absorption of food from the gut. Both affect the HbA1c level. Fasting and postprandial have the same effect on HbA1c when the HbA1c is 7.3%–8.4%. Fasting glucose has a greater effect when the HbA1c is >8.5%. The higher the HbA1c the greater the effect fasting glucose has on HbA1c.
Note the HbA1c mmol/mol values are the closest approximations to the HbA1c percentage values. The general target is < 53 mmol/mol.

- Maintain a healthy, independent lifestyle where the person is able to manage the necessary self-care tasks to achieve acceptable glycaemic control and have a good quality of life.
- Understand social and legal responsibilities and entitlements such as driving, insurance, National Diabetes Supply Scheme (in Australia).
- Plan for life transitions including stopping driving, moving to supported or aged care facilities and end of life care.

Table 1.4 described the management targets. Table 1.5 provides some glycaemic information to consider when assessing metabolic control. *HbA1c is only part of the overall picture and should NOT be considered in isolation.*

A suggested model for managing diabetes is shown in Figure 1.6. The model is divided into phases and indicates that management, education and counselling are required for life.

Exercise/activity

Exercise plays a key role in the management of Type 1, Type 2 diabetes, and GDM as well as people without diabetes (including health professionals). It increases tissue sensitivity to insulin aiding in the uptake and utilisation of glucose during exercise and for several hours afterwards. The energy sources during exercise are depicted in Figure 1.7.

In addition, regular exercise may have beneficial effects on the risk factors that contribute to the development of diabetes complications especially cardiovascular disease (Boule *et al.* 2001). Exercise:

- Increases cardiovascular efficiency;
- Reduces blood pressure;
- Reduces stress;
- Aids in weight reduction and appetite control;
- Promotes a sense of wellbeing;
- Aids in blood glucose control;
- Improves strength and reduces the risk of falls in older people, which helps them remain independent (anaerobic exercise).

All of these factors also reduce the risk of developing the long-term complications of diabetes. People are advised to have a thorough physical check-up before commencing

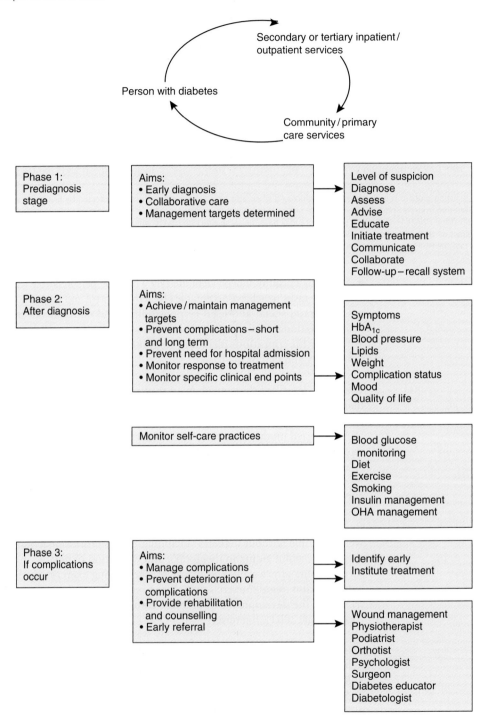

Figure 1.6 Suggested diabetes management model. Most diabetes management occurs in primary care settings in collaboration with secondary and tertiary care services.

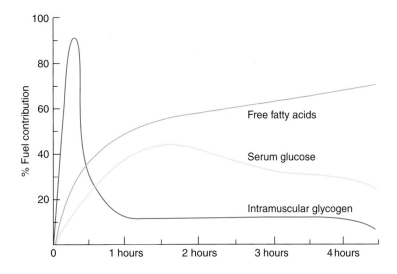

Figure 1.7 Normal energy sources during exercise. *Note*: At rest free fatty acids are the major energy source. As exercise begins muscle glycogen is utilised as the predominant energy source. As exercise continues the blood glucose is utilised, reverting to free fatty acids as the major energy source if exercise is prolonged. Blood glucose is maintained by hormonal regulation of hepatic glucose output and lipolysis.

an exercise programme; in particular, the cardiovascular system, eyes, nerves and feet should be examined. Food, fluid and clothing should be suitable for the type of exercise and the weather.

Insulin/GLM doses might need to be adjusted. Where the duration of the exercise is <30 minutes adjustments are generally not required. Adjustments are often necessary where the duration of the exercise exceeds 30 minutes (Perlstein *et al.* 1997). Exercise should be decided in consultation with the individual and suited to their preferences and physical capabilities. It is advisable that the person tests their blood glucose before and after exercising and to have some carbohydrate available during exercise in case of hypoglycaemia. Infrequent exercise is not advisable; the aim should be to begin with 10–15 minutes exercise and progress to 30–60 minutes of moderate intensity three to five times per week, daily if possible.

Footwear and clothing should be appropriate to the type of exercise and the feet inspected after exercising. Exercise is not recommended in extremes of temperatures, or at periods of hyperglycaemia, especially if ketones are present in the urine or blood. People should discuss their exercise plans with the diabetes team and/or exercise physiologist in order to plan an appropriate routine, adequate carbohydrate intake, and appropriate medication doses. Ensure adequate fluid intake to replace water loss especially in hot weather.

In general, anaerobic exercise (e.g. weight lifting) does not significantly enhance glucose utilisation. It does build muscle mass and improve strength but does not improve

Practice point

Hypoglycaemia can occur several hours after vigorous or prolonged aerobic exercise due to continuing glucose uptake by muscles. People need to be informed about adequate carbohydrate intake and medication dose adjustment as well as recognising and treating hypoglycaemia before and after exercise, see Chapter 5.

cardiovascular fitness and may reduce falls risk in older people. Anaerobic exercise is unlikely to cause an increase in blood glucose. Aerobic exercise (e.g. running, cycling, swimming) uses glucose as the major fuel source and hypoglycaemia can occur. It also confers cardiovascular benefits. Chapter 12 discusses exercise in older people. Falls risks need to be considered in older people.

Specific advice about medications and food intake needs to be tailored to the individual. The relationship between hypoglycaemia and exercise is generally well recognised. Hyperglycaemia can also occur if insulin levels are low when exercising. In this situation the counter-regulatory hormones predominate and increase the blood glucose and extra medicine doses might be needed. Insulin is easier to titrate in such circumstances.

Exercise for the person in hospital

(1) Encourage as much mobility/activity as the person's condition allows.
(2) Increase movement and activity gradually after a period of being confined to bed.
(3) Consider postural hypotension and differentiate it from hypoglycaemia to ensure correct management is instituted.
(4) Consult the physiotherapy department for assistance with mobility, chair or hydro-therapy exercises.
(5) Consider having the occupational therapist undertake a home assessment to ensure safety at home, for example, following a stroke.

Practice point

Be aware that resuming normal activity after a period of prolonged inactivity, for example in rehabilitation settings, constitutes unaccustomed exercise and can result in hypoglycaemia, especially if the person is on insulin/GLM and is not eating well or is malnourished. Exercise/activity increases the basal energy requirement by ~20%.

Diabetes education

Diabetes education is an integral part of diabetes management. Regular support and contact with the diabetes care team assists people to self-manage their diabetes by providing advice and support when necessary. For more details see Chapter 16.

Practice points

(1) People with Type 2 diabetes do not become Type 1 when insulin is needed to control blood glucose. The current accepted term is insulin-treated or insulin-requiring diabetes. The basic underlying pathophysiology does not change and usually enough endogenous insulin is produced to prevent ketosis occurring except during severe intercurrent illness.
(2) Type 2 diabetes is characterised by progressive beta cell destruction and insulin is eventually required by >50% of people (UKPDS 1998).
(3) People with LADA often require insulin soon after diagnosis, because they are insulin deficient not insulin resistant.

Complications of diabetes

Many people with diabetes are admitted to hospital because they have an active diabetes complication. The presence of a diabetic complication can affect the duration of the admission and the patient's ability to care for him or herself. Hence diabetic complications contribute to the overall cost of health care for these patients. In addition, they represent significant physical and mental lifestyle costs to the person with diabetes and their family.

Complications can be classified as acute or long term. Acute complications can occur during temporary excursions in blood glucose levels. Long-term complications occur with long duration of diabetes and persistent hyperglycaemia, especially in the presence of other risk factors. In Type 2 diabetes long-term complications are frequently present at diagnosis. Often there are few symptoms and both the diagnosis of diabetes and the coexisting complication/s can be overlooked (Chapter 8).

Acute complications

(1) Hypoglycaemia (refer to Chapter 6).
(2) Hyperglycaemia:
   • diabetic ketoacidosis (refer to Chapter 7)
   • hyperosmolar states (refer to Chapter 7).
(3) Infections can occur if blood glucose control is not optimal. Common infections include dental disease, candidiasis and urinary tract infections.
(4) Fat atrophy/hypertrophy and insulin allergy occur very rarely with modern highly purified insulins and correct injection site rotation.

Long-term complications

Two important studies, the DCCT in 1993 and the UKPDS in 1998 (DCCT 1993; UKPDS 1998) demonstrated the relationship between the development and progression of the long-term complications of Type 1 and Type 2 diabetes, respectively. In addition, the UKPDS demonstrated the importance of controlling blood pressure to reduce the risk of cardiovascular disease. Diabetes management guidelines and metabolic targets are regularly revised as new evidence emerges.

Current management targets are shown in Table 1.4.
(1) Macrovascular disease or disease of the major blood vessels, for example:
   • myocardial infarction
   • cerebrovascular accident
   • intermittent claudication.
(2) Microvascular disease or disease of the small blood vessels associated with thickening of the basement membranes of the small blood vessels, for example:
   • retinopathy
   • nephropathy.
(3) Neuropathy: diabetes can also cause damage to the central and peripheral nerves:
   • *peripheral*: decreased sensation in hands and particularly the feet, which can lead to ulcers, Charcot's arthropathy and amputation.
   • *autonomic*: erectile dysfunction, atonic bladder, gastroparesis, mononeuropathies.
(4) Complications of pregnancy: diabetes during pregnancy carries risks for both mother and baby:
   • *mother*: toxaemia, polyhydramnous intrauterine death, and Caesarian section
   • *baby*: congenital malformations, prematurity, respiratory distress, hypoglycaemia at birth.

A number of other factors might play a role in the development of diabetic complications. For example, studies are under way to determine the role of free radicals or reactive oxygen species (ROS), advanced glycated end products (AGE), changes in cellular signalling and endothelial humoral components that determine coagulation status and the tendency to form microthrombi. Long term complications are discussed in Chapter 8.

It is the responsibility of all health professionals involved in providing care to comprehensively assess the patient including the presence of complications to determine their self-care potential and devise an appropriate achievable management plan in consultation with the individual, and to be involved in preventative teaching about reducing risk factors for the development of diabetic complications. Health professionals need to be proactive about identifying opportunities for health screening and education.

Practice points

(1) Hyperglycaemia and insulin resistance commonly occur in critically ill patients, even those who do not have diabetes (van den Berghe *et al.* 2001; ADS 2012).

(2) It is important to control these states in people with diabetes during illness because of the extra stress of the illness and/or surgery, and their compromised insulin response. Elevated blood glucose in these situations in people without diabetes will require decisions to be made about the diagnosis of diabetes after the acute episode resolves.

Aim and objectives of nursing care of people with diabetes

In hospital

Being hospitalised is more common for people with diabetes than those without, and they are more likely to stay longer (ADS 2012). Current diabetes management guidelines are heavily weighted towards screening and primary care management but recently the ADS (2012) and other diabetes professional associations released guidelines for managing people with diabetes in hospital and these guidelines should be used to guide care. Specific nursing care is described in most other chapters of the book.

Factors that complicate diabetes management during illness

- Age.
- Gender.
- Type and duration of diabetes.
- Presence of diabetes complications.
- Nutritional status.
- Potentially erratic insulin absorption, especially in Type 1.
- Haemodynamic changes in blood flow.
- Counter-regulatory stress response to illness, hospitalisation, treatment, pain, psychological stress and fear.
- Timing of meals and snacks as well as during TPN, fasting and renal dialysis and especially in relation to medicine administration.

- Duration of time between insulin administration and meals.
- Effect of medications on the gut, especially narcotics for pain relief. Glucose requirements may need to be increased to compensate for slow transit times, to supply sufficient energy and prevent hypoglycaemia.
- Increased white cell count and impaired leukocyte function as a result of hyperglycaemia might not indicate the presence of infection.
- Presence of 'silent' disease such as MI, UTI and few classic symptoms of Type 2 diabetes, hypoglycaemia or hyperglycaemia.
- Delayed wound healing and strength of healing tissue.
- Increased risk of thrombosis.
- Development of ketoacidosis and/or hyperosmolar states if hyperglycaemia is not reversed.
- Impaired cognitive function and lowered mood can make problem-solving, self-care, and learning difficult.
- Depression.

People's stories

(1) People with diabetes worry that hospital staff will make mistakes, especially with their medication doses and administration times and managing hypoglycaemia.
(2) They dislike being made to feel incompetent and not trusted by staff who 'take over' the self-care tasks they usually perform for themselves, and who do not believe what they say.
(3) Conversely, some people prefer the nurses to take on diabetes slef-care tasks because it is an opportunity to 'let go of' the responsibility for a short time.
(4) They find judgmental attitudes about eating sweet things demeaning, especially when they are accused of dietary indiscretions when their blood glucose is high.
(5) They dislike being labelled non-compliant, or uncooperative, if they have difficulty learning and remembering information.

Aims and objectives of nursing care

Aims

To formulate an individual nursing management plan so that the person recovers by primary intention, maintains their independence and quality of life as far as possible and does not develop any complications of treatment and, in some cases, helping them prepare for a peaceful death.

Recognise the importance of support from the family and other key individuals to the individual's well-being, self-care capacity and ability to take responsibility for their disease.

Rationale

Early diagnosis of diabetes and monitoring for short- and long-term complications enables early treatment and improved outcomes. The nurse's understanding of the pathophysiology and classification of diabetes and its complications will improve the care they provide.

Objectives

(1) Establish a therapeutic relationship based on respect, equality and trust. The therapeutic relationship is essential to healing.
(2) To assess the person's:
  - usual care plan;
  - physical, mental and social status;
  - usual glycaemic control;
  - ability to care for themselves;
  - knowledge about diabetes and its management;
  - the presence of any diabetes-related complications including lowered mood and depression;
  - acceptance of the diagnosis of diabetes;
  - presence of concomitant disease processes;
  - medicine regimen including complementary medicines.
(3) To encourage independence as far as the physical condition allows in hospital (test own blood glucose, administer own insulin, select own meals).
(4) To obtain and maintain an acceptable blood glucose range that minimises hypoglycaemia or hyperglycaemia and keeps the person free from distressing symptoms and fluctuating blood glucose levels.
(5) To prevent complications occurring as a result of hospitalisation (e.g. falls associated with hypo- and hyperglycaemia and a range of other factors).
(6) To observe an appropriate management plan in order to achieve these objectives.
(7) To inform appropriate health professionals promptly of the patient's admission, for example, diabetes nurse specialist/diabetes educator, dietitian, or podiatrist.
(8) To ensure the patient has the opportunity to learn about diabetes and its management, particularly self-management and particularly when their usual care changes and new medicines are commenced.
(9) To plan appropriately for discharge including managing medicines and undertaking or referring the person for a home medicine review if they meet the criteria and ensuring they have the equipment necessary to manage their diabetes (medicines, blood glucose meter, insulin devices).
(10) To prevent further hospitalisations as a result of diabetes.

Technology and diabetes management

Technology increasingly supports diabetes management and self-care and health professional learning. Electronic media such as the Internet enables users to retrieve and store information, exchange information by participating in virtual communities and networks of practice and communicate with the people they care for (Harno 2013). For example, health information services, peer communities, practice guidelines, risk assessment tools, self-management tools, research publications and counselling are available online. Telephone general health care advice services often manned by specially trained nurses and diabetes-specific call centres.

In addition electronic media enable people with diabetes to be monitored remotely via teleconferences/telemedicine and by exchanging information such as blood glucose data between the individual and the health professional via email or mobile phone. Electronic patient registers and medical records are a reality in some countries. Research suggests a nurse-led multidisciplinary team can manage a group of people with diabetes in online disease management programmes (Tang *et al.* 2012) and patients are generally satisfied with electronic monitoring (Mehrotra *et al.* 2013), but it is possible to misdiagnose the condition and some doctors are not prepared to make a diagnosis without examining the patient.

Some doctors use smart phones to photograph health issues such as wounds to track wound healing, and eye health and for teaching purposes.

Some specific diabetes management technology includes:

- A range of increasingly sophisticated blood glucose meters, some with connectivity to other electronic systems such as mobile phones and insulin pumps and some with inbuilt management algorithms.
- Insulin delivery systems such as pumps.
- Automated support algorithms for adjusting medicine doses and carbohydrate intake.
- Non-invasive devices to detect nocturnal hypoglycaemia.
- Automated, portable system to control blood glucose overnight in people with Type 1 diabetes.
- Online HbA1c converter tool that converts HbA1c percentages to mmol/mol/.
- Health behaviour tracking systems such as stairs climbed, kilojoules burned, some of which link to smart phones, which become like a personal trainer.
- Many mobile phone apps such as symptom checkers and risk calculators that help people in a range of ways.
- Electronic decision-support tools for people with diabetes and health professionals including computer-generated reminders. Interestingly, the latter appear to be more effective if they are delivered on paper and if there is space on the reminder for the clinician to document the reminder content or advice (Ariditi Rege-Walther *et al.* 2012).

There is no doubt there will be more the exciting technological advances that will enhance the care of, for, and by people with diabetes. However, like most health care options there are risks and benefits that need to be considered. Some risks to consider include:

- Not all information on the Internet is accurate or appropriate. People with diabetes need help to identify reliable sites such as the websites of diabetes organisations like Diabetes UK, Diabetes Australia, the American Diabetes Association and service providers such as Government websites, Mayo Clinic and sites that display the Hon Code symbol.
- Internet information may improve knowledge but it may not change behaviours (Chapter 16) or health professional practice because social, cultural and behavioural context are not part of the learning process (Kinson 2012) although socialisation might be a feature of online group activities and support groups.
- A combination of education about how to use management guidelines, decision support tools and patient registers can lead to improved outcomes for people with Type 2 diabetes in general practice settings (Barlow 2013).
- Adequate back up and data management systems need to be in place so important data are not lost or accessible to people not involved in the individual's care. That is, stringent, monitored security systems must be in place wherever confidential information is stored, including on mobile phones.
- Medicolegal issues such as breeches of privacy and confidentiality for example storing personal patient information, including research data, on smart phones. There are very significant implications for individuals whose data are not protected and the health professional concerned if the smart phone is lost or stolen.
- Using/communicating patient information without consent including in tele/video health professional management conferences, case discussions, publications and presentations.

A sobering final comment

OPTIMISE, the Optimal Type 2 Diabetes Management Including Benchmarking and Standard Treatment Trial (Hermann *et al.* 2012) compared physician's individual performance with a peer group to determine whether benchmarking and assessing change in three quality indicators of vascular risk: HbA1c, LDL-C and systolic blood pressure improved the quality of Type 2 diabetes care in primary care settings (n = 3980). The findings show HbA1c targets were only met in 52.2%; 34.9% for LDL-C and 27.3% for systolic blood pressure. Other studies show older physicians are less likely to follow guidelines or use new medicines (Tung 2011) and nurses have inadequate diabetes knowledge (Livingstone & Dunning 2010) including about medicines and in aged care settings (Dunning *et al.* 2012).

These findings are very concerning, even allowing for the many confounding variables that affect the ability of people with diabetes to meet targets. As suggested in Chapter 16, patient-related targets may not be the best measure of health professional performance and more appropriate measures should be considered. If they are the best measure of health professional performance, health professionals must examine their care practices, behaviours and attitudes and the care systems in which they operate, to determine whether/how these factors affect their performance. For example, general practitioners identified treatment costs to the patient and reluctance to commence insulin as barriers to their ability to achieve optimal management targets in a cluster randomised trial in Asia-Pacific that involved educating doctors about how to use diabetes guidelines (Reutens *et al.* 2011).

A great deal of time and money is spent on health professional education; if health professionals are ineffective more than 50% of the time, we need to determine whether education programmes adequately train health professionals to deliver diabetes education and care, and/or are delivered in a manner suitable to health professionals' learning needs. Another consideration is inherent weaknesses in the literature and varying interpretations of the same literature base. For example, most guidelines are developed using the same literature but recommendations often differ. In addition, the exclusive nature of randomised trials means the findings might not be relevant in all clinical practice settings.

References

Abassi A., Peelen L., Corpeleinj E. *et al.* (2012) Risk models for risk of developing Type 2 diabetes: A systematic literature search and independent external validation study. *British Medical Journal*, **345** e5900.

Abikshyeet P., Ramesh V., Oza N., (2012) *Glucose estimation in the salivary secretion of diabetes mellitus patients Diabetes Metabolic and Obesity Targets and Therapies* **25**, 149–154.

American Diabetes Association, American Psychiatric Association, American Association of Clinical Endocrinologists, North American Association for the Study of Obesity (2004) Consensus Development Conference on Antipsychotic Drugs and Obesity and Diabetes. *Diabetes Care*, **27**, 596–601.

American Diabetes Association (ADA) (2003) Evidence based nutrition principles and recommendations for the treatment and prevention of diabetes and related complications. *Diabetes Care*, **26** (Suppl. 1), S51–S61.

American Diabetes Association (2007) *Preventing Diabetes* (www.diabetes.org/diabetes-basics/prevention/ (accessed January 2013).

Appleton, M. & Hattersley, A. (1996) Maturity onset diabetes of the young: A missed diagnosis. *Diabetic Medicine*, (Suppl. 2), AP3.

Ariditi C., Rege-Walther A., Wyatt M., Durieux P. & Burnard B. (2012) Computer-generated reminders delivered on paper to healthcare professionals: Effects on professional practice and health care outcomes. Cochrane Database of Systematic Reviews, 12, doi/10.1002/14651858.CD001175.pub3/full.

Armitage J., Poston L. & Taylor P. (2008) Developmental origins of obesity and the metabolic syndrome. *Frontiers of Hormone Research*, **36**, 73–84.

Audit Commission (2000) *Testing Times: a Review of Diabetes Mellitus Services in England and Wales*. Audit Commission, London.

Australian Diabetes Society (1990–1996) *Position Statements*. Australian Diabetes Society, Canberra.

Australian Diabets Society (2012) Guidelines for Routine Glucose Control in Hospital. Australian Diabetes Society, Canberra.

Australian Institute of Health and Welfare (2005) *Costs of Diabetes in Australia, 2000–01*. (AIHW) Cat. No. CVD 26). Canberra.

Australian Type 2 Diabetes Risk Assessment Tool (AUSDRISK) www.diabetesaustralia.com.au/.../ AUSDRISK%20Web%2014%20July%2010.pdf (accessed December 2012).

Azzopardi P., Brown A., Fahy R. *et al.* (2012) Type 2 diabetes in young Indigenous Australians in rural and remote areas: Diagnosis, screening, management and prevention. *Medical Journal of Australia*, **187** (2), 32–36.

Barlow J. (2013) Improving management of type 2 diabetes: Findings of the Type2Care clinical audit. *Medical Journal of Australia*, **42** (12), 57–60.

Barr, E.L., Magliano, D.J., Zimmet, P.Z. *et al.* (2005) *The Australian Diabetes, Obesity and Lifestyle Study (AusDiab). Tracking the Accelerating Epidemic: Its Causes and Outcomes*. International Diabetes Institute, Melbourne.

Bethel M., Price H., Sourij H. *et al.* (2013) Evaluation of self-administered oral glucose tolerance test. *Diabetes Care* (Epub ahead of print January 15th 2013).

Biden, T. (2007) Major breakthrough in understanding type 2 diabetes. Interview in *Nursing Review*, November 2007, 10.

Boule, N., Haddard, E., Kenny, G., Wells, G. & Sigal, R. (2001) Effects of exercise on glycaemic control and body mass index in Type 2 diabetes mellitus: A meta-analysis of controlled clinical trials. *Journal of the American Medical Association*, **286**, 1218–1227.

Burke, V., Beilin, U. & Simmer, K. (2005) Predictors of body mass index and associations with cardio-vascular risk factors in Australian children: A prospective cohort study. *International Journal of Obesity*, **29**, 15–23.

Bruce K. & Byrne C. (2009) The metabolic syndrome: Common origins of a multifactorial disorder. *Postgraduate Medical Journal*, **85**, 614–621.

van den Berghe, G., Wouters, P., Weekers, F. *et al.* (2007) Intensive insulin therapy in critically ill patients. *New England Journal of Medicine*, **345** (19), 1359–1367.

Buzzetti R., Di Pietro S., Giaccari A. *et al.* (2007) Non-insulin requiring autoimmune diabetes study group. High titer autoantibodies to GAD identifies a specific phenotype of adult-onset autoimmune diabetes. *Diabetes Care*, **30**, 932–936.

Cermea S, Buzzetti R & Pozilli P. (2003) ß-cell protection and therapy for latent autoimmune diabetes in adults. *Diabetes Care*, **32**, Suppl 2, S546–5262.

Ceriello, A. (2003) The postprandial state and cardiovascular disease: Relevance to diabetes mellitus. *Diabetes Metabolism Research Reviews*, **16**, 125–132.

Cappuccio F. & Miller M. (2012) A new challenge to widely held views on the role of sleep. *Annals of Internal Medicine*, **157** (8), 593–594.

Carnethon M., De Chavez P., Biggs M. *et al.* (2012) Association of weight status with mortality in adults with incident diabetes. *Journal American Medical Association*, **308** (6), 581.

Chiasson, J., Josse, R., Gomis, R. *et al.* (2002) Acarbose for prevention of type 2 diabetes mellitus: The STOP-NIDDM randomized trial. *Lancet*, **359**, 2072–2077.

Citrome, L., Blonde, L. & Damatarca, C. (2005) Metabolic issues in patients with severe mental illness. *South Medical Journal*, **98** (7), 714–720.

Conen, D., Ridker, P., Mora, S., Buring, J. & Glynn, R. (2007) Blood pressure and risk of developing type 2 diabetes mellitus: The Women's Health Study. *European Heart Journal*, **28** (23), 2937–2943.

Dandona P., Ghanim A., Chaudhuri A., Dhindsa S. & Kim S. (2010) Macronutrient intake induces oxidative and inflammatory stress: Potential relevance to atherosclerosis and insulin resistance. *Experiential Molecular Medicine*, **42**, 245–253.

DECODE Study Group (2001) Glucose tolerance and cardiovascular mortality: Comparison of fasting and two hour diagnostic criteria. *Archives of Internal Medicine*, **161**, 397–405.

d'Emden M., Shaw J., Colagiuri S. *et al.* (2012) The role of HbA1c in the diagnosis of diabetes mellitus in Australia. *Medical Journal of Australia*, **197** (4), 220–221.

DCCT (Diabetes and Control and Complications Trial Research Group) (1993) The effect of intensive insulin treatment on the development and progression of long term complications of insulin depend-ent diabetes. *New England Journal of Medicine*, **329**, 977–986.

Diabetes Australia, (DA) Royal Australian College of General Practitioners (RACGP) (2011/12) *Diabetes management in general practice: Guideline for Type 2 diabetes*. DA and RACGP, Canberra.

Ding E, Song Y, Manson J.. (2009) Sex hormone-binding globulin and risk of type 2 diabetes in women and men. *New England Journal of Medicine* 361, 1152–1163.

Dornhorst, A. (2001) Insulinotrophic meglitinide analogues. *Lancet*, 358 (9294), 1709–1716.

Dunning T., Savage S., Rasmussen B., Wellard S. (2012) Managing diabetes medicines in residential aged care facilities: Balancing competing challenges. *Proceedings OEC 42*. IDF Western Pacific Region Congress, Kyoto, Japan.

EURODIAB Substudy 2 Study Group (1999) Vitamin D supplement in early childhood and risk for Type 1 (insulin-dependent) diabetes mellitus. *Diabetologia*, 42 (1), 51–54.

EURODIAB ACE Study Group (2000) Variation and trends in incidence of childhood diabetes in Europe. *Lancet*, 355, 873–876.

Gagnon C., Lu Z.X. & Magliano D. (2011) Serum 25-hydroxyvitamin D, calcium intake and risk of type 2 diabetes after 5 years results from a national population-based prospective study (the Australian Diabetes, Obesity and Lifestyle Study) *Diabetes Care* 34, 1133–1138.

Gardner D. & Tai E. (2012) Clinical features and treatment of maturity onset diabetes of the young (MODY) *Diabetes, Metabolic Syndrome and Obesity* 25,101–108.

Jones H. (2011) Increase in deaths in men with type 2 diabetes and testosterone deficinecy may be prevented by testosterone replacement. *Science Daily* http://www.sciencedaily.com/releases/2011/04/1104130090030.htm (accessed January 2013).

Gonzalez-Molero I., Rojo-Martinez G., Gauterrez-Repiso C. *et al.* (2012) Vitamin D incidence of diabetes: A prospective cohort study. *Clinical Nutrition* 31 (4), 571–573.

Harno K. (2013) The advance of health information technology: Traveling the Internet superhighway. Chapter 12 in Dunning T. (ed.) *Diabetes Education: Art, Science and Evidence*. Wiley Blackwell, Chichester, pp. 200–214.

Haynes A., Bulsars M., Bower C., Jones T. & Davis E. (2012) Cyclical variation in the incidence of childhood type 1 diabetes in Western Australia (1985–2010). *Diabetes Care*, DOI: 10.2337/dc12-0205.

Health Service Ombudsman (2000) *Errors in the Care and Treatment of a Young Woman with Diabetes*. The Stationery Office, London.

Heianza Y., Arase Y., Fujihara K. *et al.* (2012) Screening for pre-diabetes to predict future diabetes using various cut-off points for HbA1c and impaired fasting glucose: The Toranomon Hospital Health Management Centre study 4. *Diabetic Medicine* DOI: 10.111/j.1464-5491.2012.03686.x.

Herpertz, S., Albus, C. & Wagener, R. (1998) Cormorbidity of eating disorders. Does diabetes control reflect disturbed eating behaviour? *Diabetes Care*, 21 (7), 1110–1116.

Hilton, D., O'sourke, P., Welbourn, T. & Reid, C. (2002) Diabetes detection in Australian general practice: A comparison of diagnostic criteria. *Medical Journal of Australia*, 176, 104–107.

Hippisley-Cox, J. & Pringle, M. (2004) Diabetics treated with diet only have more complications. *Lancet*, (http://www.medscape.com/viewarticle/484479 5.8.2004).

Hu E., Pan A., Malik V., Sun O. (2012) White rice consumption and risk of type 2 diabetes: Meta-analysis and systematic review. *British Medical Journal*, 344, e1454. doi: http://dx.doi.org/10.1136/bmj.e1454 (acessed April 2012)

(IDF) International Diabetes Federation (2006) *The IDF Consensus Worldwide Definition of the Metabolic Syndrome*. IDF, Brussels www.idf.org (accessed December 2007).

(IDF) International Diabetes Federation (2011) *Guideline for management of post-meal glucose in diabetes*. IDF, Brussels www.idf.org (accessed December 2007).

(IDF) International Diabetes Federation (2012) *Diabetes and Climate Change Report*. IDF Brussels.

IMAGE Project (2012) New standards in the prevention of type 2 diabetes: The IMAGE project. *European Diabetes Nursing* 9 (2), 62–65.

Kinson, Janet (2012) Lecture presented at the Diabetes UK annual professional conference, Glasgow. *Practical Diabetes* 29 (6), 247–251.

Juraschek S., Steefes M., Miller E., & Selvin E. (2012) Alternative markers for hyperglycaemia and risk of diabetes. *Diabetes Care* 35, 2265–2270.

Knip, M., Veijola, R., Virtanen, S. *et al.* (2005) Environmental triggers and determinants in type 1 diabetes. *Diabetes*, 54 (Suppl. 2), s125–s126.

Krishnan, S., Rosenberg, L., Singer, M. *et al.* (2007) Glycaemic index, glycaemic load and cereal fiber intake and risk of Type 2 diabetes in US Black Women. *Archives of Internal Medicine*, 167 (21), 2304–2309.

Kong, A., Williams, R., Smith, M. *et al.* RIOS Net Clinicians (2007) Acanthosis nigricans and diabetes risk factors: Prevalence in young persons seen in southwestern US primary care practices. *Annals of Family Medicine*, 5 (3), 202–208.

Lang T. & Rayner G. (2012) Ecological public health: The 21st century's big idea. *British Medical Journal* **345**, 17–20.

Langer, O. (2006) Management of gestational diabetes: Pharmacological treatment options and glycaemic control. *Endocrinology Metabolic Clinics of North America*, **35**, 53–78.

Lerner L., Upton J.P., Praveen P. *et al*. (2012). IRE11∂ induces Thioredoxin-Interacting Protein to activate the NLRP3 inflammasome and promote programmed cell death under irremediable stress. *Cell Metabolism* **16** (2), 250–264.

Lesperance, F. & Frasure-Smith, N. (2007) Depression and heart disease. *Cleveland Clinic Journal of Medicine*, **74** (Suppl. 1), S63–S66.

Livingston R. & Dunning T. (2010) Practice nurses' role and knowledge about diabetes management within rural and remote Australian general practice. *European Diabetes Nursing*, **7**, 55–61.

Loyd, C., Wilson, R. & Forrest, K. (1997) Prior depressive symptoms and onset of coronary heart disease. *Diabetes*, **46**, 3A.

McDonald T., Coldclough K. & Brown R. (2011) Islet autoantibodies and discriminate maturity-onset diabetes of the young (MODY) from type 1 diabetes. *Diabetic Medicine* **28** (9), 1028–1035.

Mahdi T., Hanzelmann S., Salehi A. *et al*. (2012) Secreted Frizzled-Related Protein 4 reduces insulin secretion in type 2 diabetes. *Metabolism* **18**, 625–633.

Mehrotra A., Paone S., Maritch D., Albert S. & Shechik G. (2013) A Comparison of e-visits and physician office visits for sinusitis and urinary tract infections. *Journal of Internal Medicine* **173** (1), 72–74.

Menting J., Whittaker J., Margetts M., *et al*. (2013) How insulin engaged its primary binding site. *Nature*, **493**, 241–245.

Mingea K., Zimmet P. & Magliano D. (2011) Diabetes prevalence and determinants in Indigenous Australian populations: A systematic review. *Diabetes Research and Clinical Practice*, **93**, 139–149.

Morris A. (2012) Large scale association analysis provides insight into the genetic architecture and pathophysiology of type 2 diabetes. *National Genetics* **44**, 981–990.

Nakamura Y., Omaye S. (2012) Metabolic diseases and pro-and prebiotics: Mechanistic insights. *Nutrition & Metabolism* **DOI**: 10.1186 9 (60), 1743–7075.

Nield L., Summerbell C., Hooper L., Whittaker V., Moore H. (2008) *Dietary advice for the prevention of type 2 diabetes mellitus in adults (review)* http://www.thecochranelibrary.com (accessed August 2012).

Niskanen, L., Tuomi, T., Groop, L. & Uusitupa, M. (1995) GAD antibodies in NIDDM. Ten-year follow-up from diagnosis. *Diabetes Care*, **18** (12), 1557–1565.

Pan, X., Li, G., Hu, Y. *et al*. (1997) Effects of diet and exercise in preventing NIDDM in people with impaired glucose tolerance. The Da Qing IGT and Diabetes Study. *Diabetes Care*, **20**, 537–544.

Perlstein, R., McConnell, K. & Hagger, V. (1997) *Off to a Flying Start*. International Diabetes Institute, Melbourne.

Pimouguet C., Le Goff M., Thiebaut R., Dartigues J. & Helmer C. (2010) Effectiveness of disease self-management programs for improving diabetes care: A meta-analysis. *Canadian Medical Association Journal* DOI: 10.1503/cmaj.091786.

Renders C., Valk G., Griffin S., Wagner E., Eijk T. & Assendelft, W. (2012) Interventions to improve the management of diabetes mellitus in primary care outpatient and community settings. Cochrane Database of Systematic Reviews (1), CD001481.

Reuters Health Information (2013) Think preventative medicine will save money? Think again. http://www.medscape.com/viewarticle/778384 (accessed January 2013).

Reutens A., Hutchinson R.& van Binh T. *et al*. (2011) The GIANT study: A cluster-randomised controlled trial of efficacy of education of doctors about type 2 diabetes mellitus management guidelines in primary care practice. *Diabetes Research and Clinical Practice*, **98** (1), 38–45.

Rice G., Illanes S. & Mitchell M. (2012) Gestational diabetes mellitus: A positive predictor of type 2 diabetes? *International Journal of Endocrinology* DOI: 10.1155/2012/72163.

Rubin, R. (2002) Was Willis right? Thoughts on the interaction of depression and diabetes. *Diabetes Metabolism Research Reviews*, **18**, 173–175.

Saudek C., Herman W., Sacks D. *et al*. (2008) A new look at screening and diagnosing diabetes mellitus. *Journal of Clinical Endocrinology and Metabolism*, **93** (7) 2447–2453.

Simmons R., Echouffo-Tcheugui J., Sharp J. *et al*. (2012) Screening for type 2 diabetes and population mortality over 10 years (ADDITION-Cambridge): a cluster-randomised controlled trial. *The Lancet*, **380** (9855),1741–1748.

Sinha, R., Fisch, G., Teague, B. *et al*. (2002) Prevalence of inpaired glucose tolerance among children and adolescents with marked obesity. *New England Journal of Medicine*, **346** (11), 802–810.

Soltesz, G., Patterson, C. & Dahlquist, G. (2006) Global trends in childhood obesity. International Diabetes Federation (IDF) *Diabetes Atlas*, 3rd edn IDF, Brussels, pp. 154–190.

Stene, L. & Joner, G. (2003) Use of cod liver oil during the first year of life is associated with lower risk of childhood-onset type 1 diabetes: A large, population-based, case-control study. *The American Journal of Clinical Nutrition*, 78 (6), 1128–1134.

Tang P., Overhage M., Chan S. *et al.* (2012) Online disease management of diabetes: Engaging and motivating patients online with enhanced resources-diabetes (EMPOWERE_D): A randomized controlled trial. *Journal of the American Medical Association*, DOI: 10.1136/amiajnl-2012-001263.

The Agency for Healthcare Research and Quality, www.ahrq.gov/ppip (accessed 12/1/2008).

Torgerson, J., Hauptman, J., Boldrin, M. & Sjostrom, L. (2004) XENical in the prevention of diabetes in obese subjects (XENDOS) study: A randomized study of orlistat as an adjunct to lifestyle changes for the prevention of type 2 diabetes in obese patients. *Diabetes Care*, 27,155–161 (erratum in (2004) 27, 856).

The DIAMOND Project Group (2006) Incidence and trends of childhood type 1 diabetes worldwide 1990–1999. *Diabetic Medicine*, 23, 857–866.

Tuomilehto, J., Eriksson, J. & Valle, T. (2001) Prevention of type 2 diabetes mellitus by changes in lifestyle among subjects with impaired glucose tolerance. *New England Journal of Medicine*, 344, 1343–1350.

Tung A. (2011a) The mystery of guideline non-compliance: Why don't doctors do the right thing? *Anaesthesiology* 503:3–10.

Turner, N. & Clapham, C. (1998) Insulin resistance, impaired glucose tolerance and non-insulin-dependent diabetes pathologic mechanisms and treatment: Current status and therapeutic possibilities. *Progress in Drug Research*, 51, 33–94.

Turner R., Stratton I, Horton V. *et al.* (1997) UKPDS 25 autoantibodies to islet cell cytoplasm and glutamic acid carboxylase for prediction of insulin requirement in type 2 diabetes. UKPDS Study group. *Lancet*, 350, 1288–1293.

Twigg, S., Kamp, M., Davis, T., Neylon, E. & Flack, J. (2007) Prediabetes: A position statement from the Australian Diabetes Society and Australian Diabetes Educators Association. *Medical Journal of Australia*, 186 (9), 461–465.

UKPDS (United Kingdom Prospective Diabetes Study) (1998) Intensive blood glucose control with sulphonylureas or insulin compared with conventional treatment and risk of complications in patients with Type 2 diabetes (UKPDS 33). *Lancet*, 352, 837–853.

van Ufelen J., Wong J. & Chau J. (2010) Occupational sitting and health risks: a systematic review. *American Journal of Preventative Medicine* 39, 379–388.

www.themedicalbiochemist.org (1996–2012) *Obesity: Metabolic and Clinical Consequences* (accessed October 2012).

Wahlberg J., Vaarala O. & Ludvigsson J. ABIS-study group (2006) Dietary risk factors for the emergence of type 1 diabetes-related autoantibodies in 2 1/2 year-old Swedish children *British Journal of Nutrition* 95 (3), 603–608.

Weiss, R. & Caprio, S. (2005) The metabolic consequences of childhood obesity. *Best Practice & Research Clinical Endocrinology & Metabolism*, 19 (3), 405–419.

Willi, C., Bodenmann, P., Ghali, W., Faris, P. & Cornuz, J. (2007) Active smoking and the risk of Type 2 diabetes: A systematic review and meta-analysis. *Journal of the American Medical Association*, 298, 2654–2664.

Wilmot E., Edwardson C., Achana A. *et al.* (2012) Sedentary time in adults and the association with diabetes, cardiovascular disease and death: Systematic review and meta-analysis. *Diabetologia* DOI: 10.1007/00125-012-2677-z.

World Health Organization (WHO) (1999) *Definition, Diagnosis and Classification of Diabetes Mellitus and its Complications: Report of a WHO Consultation. Part 1: Diagnosis and Classification of Diabetes Mellitus.* WHO, Geneva.

Zimmermann, U. & Himmerich, H. (2003) Epidemiology, implications and mechanisms underlying drug-induced weight gain in psychiatric patients. *Journal of Psychiatric Research*, 37, 193–220.

Zinman, B., Kahn, S., Haffner, S. *et al.* (2004) Phenotypic characteristics of GAD antibody-positive recently diagnosed patients with type 2 diabetes in North America and Europe. *Diabetes*, 53 (12), 3193–3200.

Zimmet, P., Alberti, G. & Shaw, J. (2005) Mainstreaming the metabolic syndrome: a definitive definition. *Medical Journal of Australia*, 183 (4), 175–176.

Zimmet, P., Alberti, G., Kaufman, F. *et al.* & IDF Consensus Group (2007) The metabolic syndrome in children and adolescents – An IDF consensus report. *Paediatric Diabetes*, 8, 299–306.

Further reading

Conen, D. (2007) Blood pressure may predict incident type 2 diabetes in healthy women. *European Heart Journal* (published online 9–10-2007).

Dean, L. & McEntyre, J. (2004a) The genetic landscape of diabetes. http>//www.ncbi.nlm.nih.gov/books/bv.fegi?call=bv.View.ShowTOC&rid=diabetes. (TOC accessed January 2008).

Dean, L, McEntyre, J. (2004b) The genetic landscape of diabetes (http>//www.ncbi.nlm.nih.gov/books/bv.fegi?call=bv.View.ShowTOC&rid=diabetes. TOC accessed January 2008).

Donga E., van Dijk M., Hoogma R., Corssmit E. & Romijn J. (2012) Insulin resistance in multiple tissues in patients with type 1 diabetes mellitus on long term continuous subcutaneous insulin infusion. *Diabetes Metabolism Research Reviews*. DOI: 10.1002/dmrr.2343.

Dunstan, D., Zimmet, P., Welborn, T. *et al.* (2002) The rising prevalence of diabetes and impaired glucose tolerance: The Australian obesity and lifestyle study. *Diabetes Care*, **25**, 829–834.

Engelau M & Gregg E.(2012) Diabetes screening does not reduce deaths. *The Lancet* **380** (9855) www.thelancet.com/journals/lancet/.../PIIS0140-6736(12)X6048-3 (accessed December 2012).

Eltisham, S., Hattersley, A., Dunger, A. & Barrett, T. (2004) First UK survey of paediatric type 2 diabetes and MODY. *Archives of Diseases in Childhood*, **89**, 526–529.

Floegal A., Stefan N., Yu Z., *et al.* (2012) Identification of serum metabolites associated with risk of type 2 diabetes using a targeted metabolomic approach *Diabetes* DOI; 10.2337/db12-0495.

Hermans M., Brotons C., Elisaf M. *et al.* (2012) Optimal type 2 diabetes mellitus management: The randomized controlled OPTIMISE benchmarking study: Baseline results from six European countries. *European Journal of Preventative Cardiology* DOI: 10.1177/2047487312449414.

Lindstrom, J., Ilanne-Parikka, P. & Peltonen, M. (2006) Sustained reduction in incidence of type 2 diabetes by lifestyle intervention: Follow-up of the Finnish Diabetes Prevention Study. *Lancet*, **368**, 1673.

Maynard, J., Rohrscheib, M., Way, J., Nguyen, C. & Ediger, M. (2007) Non-invasive Type 2 diabetes screening: Supervision substudy to fasting plasma glucose and A_{1c}. *Diabetes Care*, **30** (5), 1120–1126.

Nichols, G. (2007) Preventing and predicting diabetes. *Medscape Diabetes and Endocrinology* (posted 8.10.2000).

Nilsson, C., Ursing, D., Torn, C., Aberg, A. & Landin-Olsson, M. (2007) Presence of GAD-antibodies during gestational diabetes predicts type 1 diabetes. *Diabetes Care*, DOI: 10. 2337/dc07–0157.

Oomichi, T., Emoto, M., Tabata, E. *et al.* (2007) Impact of glycemic control on survival of diabetic patients on chronic regular hemodialysis: A 7-year observational study. *Diabetes Care*, **29**, 1496–1500.

Pradhan, A., Rifai, N., Buring, J. & Ridker, P. (2007) Hemoglobin A1c predicts diabetes but not cardiovascular disease in nondiabetic women. *The American Journal of Medicine*, **120** (8), 720–727.

Schultz, M. (2007) Fiber and magnesium intake protects against developing type 2 diabetes. *Archives of Internal Medicine*, **167**, 956–965.

Snitker, S., Watanabe, R. & Avi, L. *et al.* (2004) Changes in insulin sensitivity in response to troglitazone do not differ between subjects with and without the common functional pro12Ala perixisome proliferator-activated receptor gamma2 gene variant: results from the Troglitazone in Prevention of Diabetes (TRIPOD) study. *Diabetes Care*, **27**, 1365–1368.

Spanwen, P., Kohler, S., Verhey, F., Stenhonwer, C. & van Boxtel, M. (2012) Effects of type 2 diabetes on 12-year cognitive change. Results from the Maastricht Aging study. *Diabetes Care*, DOI; 10.2337/dc12-0746.

Chapter 2
Holistic Assessment, Nursing Diagnosis, and Documentation

Every person who requires health care has a unique set of needs.

Key points

- An holistic diabetes assessment, education and management plan must:
  - Encompass the physical, emotional, spiritual, family, social, and environmental factors relevant to the individual and be developed in collaboration with them and significant family members and carers.
  - Include general nursing and health care needs as well as diabetes management.
- Incorporate diabetes-specific factors likely to affect self-care, health professional care and outcomes.
- Develop and document individual care plans based on the best available evidence and communicate them to other relevant health professionals, family and carers, keeping in mind the individual's right to privacy.
- Evaluate outcomes relevant to the overall management goals, agreed metabolic targets as well as short-term goals formulated within the overall plan for a specific episode of care such as an admission to hospital.
- Discharge planning and transitional care among health services should be part of the care plan.

Rationale

Best practice diabetes education and care relies on a combination of the best available evidence, intuition, and clinical judgement, effective communication skills and the informed participation of the person with diabetes. Careful assessment enables physical, psychological, spiritual and social issues that impact on care to be identified and

Care of People with Diabetes: A Manual of Nursing Practice, Fourth Edition. Trisha Dunning.
© 2014 John Wiley & Sons, Ltd. Published 2014 by John Wiley & Sons, Ltd.

incorporated into nursing management and discharge/transition plans. Life balance and emotional well-being are essential to achieving metabolic targets.

Significantly, many care standards now include person-centred and family-centred care. However, fee-for-service payment models do not encourage health professionals, especially doctors, to spend time with patients, yet person-centred care depends on health professionals having sufficient time to address the whole patient and his or her concerns. At present, most systems expect the individual to engage with the healthcare system, but often systems and processes are not integrated or accessible.

Holistic nursing

Holistic care aims to heal the whole person using art and science to support the individual to mobilise their innate healing potential: that is, to become empowered. Healing occurs when the individual embraces and transforms traumatic life events and is open to and/or recognises his or her potential (Dossey *et al.* 1995, p. 40). Transcending traumatic life events such as the diagnosis of diabetes or a diabetes complication is part of the spiritual journey to self-awareness, self-empowerment, and wholeness. Significantly, spirituality is not the same as religion, although it may encompass religion (Dossey *et al.* 1995, p. 6; Parsian & Dunning 2008; Dunning 2013).

Thus, in order to achieve holistic care, nurses must consider the individual's beliefs and attitudes because the meaning people attach to their health, diabetes, and treatment, including medicines, affects their self-care behaviour and health outcomes. At least eight broad interpretations of illness have been identified: challenge, enemy, punishment, weakness, relief, irreparable loss/damage, value adding, and denial (Lipowski 1970; Dunning 1994; Dunning & Martin 1998). In addition, the author has identified other explanatory models during routine clinical care: diabetes is an opportunity for positive change; and diabetes is a visitation from God.

Care models

Wagner *et al.* (1996a) suggested that many care models have limited effectiveness and reach because they rely on traditional education methods and do not support self-management and transition among services. The essential elements needed to improve outcomes encompass:

- Evidence-based planned care including management guidelines and policies.
- Appropriate service and practice design that encompasses prevention and expedites referral and communication among services.
- Systems to support self-management.
- Process to ensure practitioners are knowledgeable and competent, collaborate and communicate effectively, have sufficient time to provide individual care and are supported to do so and where health professional roles are clearly defined and complementary.
- Clinical information systems that enable disease registries to be maintained, outcomes to be monitored, relevant reminders to be sent to patients and performance to be evaluated (Wagner *et al.* 1996a).

Many current diabetes management models such as the Lorig and Flinders models, the Group Health Cooperative Diabetes Roadmap, Kaiser-Permanente in Colorado, nurse-led case management, and various shared care models including computer programs

(Interactive Health Communication Applications (IHCA)) encompass these elements and improve patient adherence to management strategies and satisfaction. However, their application is still limited by time and resource constraints, including timely patient access to health professionals.

Research suggests Internet-based support can improve patient-practitioner communication and collaboration, and enhance a patient's sense of being valued and secure (Ralston *et al.* 2004). However, more research is needed to determine the best way to use these programmes and their effects in specific patient groups (Murray *et al.* 2005). Generally, patients have a better understanding of what is expected of them if they receive both written and verbal information (Johnson *et al.* 2003). The font size, colour and language level of any written material provided including instructions for procedures and appointments and health professional contact details needs to be appropriate to the age, education level, and culture of the individual concerned (see Chapter 16).

In addition, health professionals must clearly promote a patient-centred approach to care (National Managed Care Congress 1996) that is evident within the service. For example, patients are involved in decisions about their care and see the same doctor each time they attend an appointment. They should also be involved in service planning and deciding what constitutes quality care and what metrics to use to measure quality (Jones 2013). Most patients want to be cared for by knowledgeable, competent and caring health professionals who are approachable and expert communicators; yet these issues that are so important to patients are not included in quality metrics.

Patient satisfaction surveys fall short of demonstrating person-centred care; although such surveys often seek information to help them make services more 'patient friendly' they often reflect selection bias and contain multiple confounders, and many are not validated in any appropriate way. In addition, patient satisfaction does not reflect person-centred care or quality care.

Although patient-centred care is difficult to define and achieve, often because it is a subjective concept and, as indicated, because of time constraints, it generally refers to:

- personalised care rather than 'one target fits all:' diabetes management guidelines are beginning to encompass individualised management targets;
- ensuring care considers the individual's social, mental, physical, social situation as well as their goals, explanatory models, capability (physical, mental, spiritual and linguistic) and health and general beliefs, experiences, religion and culture;
- delivering care that is culturally sensitive and relevant to the individual, but which is also family-centred (Joint Commission 2010);
- using effective communication strategies that account for any disabilities the individual might have and using translators sensitively. Effective communication is a two way process in which messages are negotiated until the information is correctly understood by everybody involved in the communication;
- developing strategies to help the patient trust their health professionals (Wagner *et al.* 1996a) and vice versa!
- helping patients acquire the information they need to make informed decisions (McCulloch *et al.* 1998);
- improving patient adherence to management recommendations (Wagner *et al.* 1996b): also see Chapters 15 and 16;
- making collaborative decisions with the patient and communicating them to relevant people.

Kleinman *et al.* (1978) suggested some simple questions that can help create shared understanding between people with diabetes and health professionals. The questions are still relevant today and are in fact recommended by the Joint Commission roadmap for hospitals concerning advocacy and person- and family-centred care (2010). Such questions encompass:

- What do you think caused your illness/problem/s?
- Why do your think the problem started when it did?
- How is the problem affecting you?
- How serious do you think the problem is?
- What sort of treatment do you think will help?
- What do you want the treatment to do (outcomes)?
- What are your main concerns about the problem?
- How can I/we help?

These questions can be supplemented with clarifying questions and by checking assumptions.

Specific programs that train health professionals how to deliver patient-centred care improve patient trust in doctors (Lewin *et al.* 2001; McKinstry *et al.* 2006), and the delivery of patient information (Kinnersley *et al.* 2007). In addition, patients may need specific education about how to ask relevant questions during consultations, and how to participate in making management decisions. Both parties may need education about how to negotiate the complex nature of shared decision-making to balance the imperative for evidence-based care with the need to incorporate the individual's values and preferences (Kilmartin 1997). In order to assist the process, the Foundation for Informed Decision-Making in the USA (2007) developed a series of interactive videos and written materials for patients about a range of common medical conditions.

In order to deliver person-centred care it is necessary to undertake a thorough assessment, use appropriate questions and clinical reasoning to identify the patient's needs and management guidelines to determine whether the recommended treatment is likely to benefit the individual, whether the benefits outweigh the risks, and whether the individual can/will adhere to the recommendations including their self-care capacity, and then recommend appropriate treatment options to the individual.

Characteristics of an holistic nursing history

The nursing history is actually the individual's story and health professionals are privileged to learn part of that story. The art of 'story listening' is essential to compiling a useful patient history. The history/story:

- includes demographic data (age, gender, social situation);
- collects units of information about past and current individual and family health, and family and social relationships (see Figure 2.1) to enable individual care plans to be formulated considering the person's goals and expectations:
  - ○ obtains baseline information about the person's physical and mental status before and after and the presenting complaint;
  - ○ collects information about the person's general health and diabetes-related beliefs and attitudes and the meaning they attach to, and the importance they place on symptoms;
- Should be concise to enable information to be collected in a short time;
- Should focus on maintaining the person's independence while they are in hospital (e.g. allowing them to perform their own blood glucose tests).

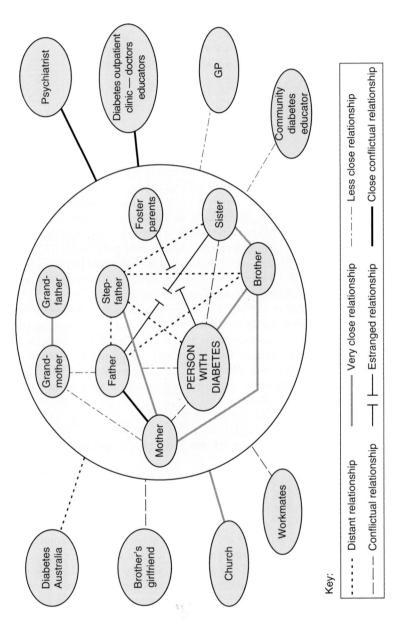

Key:

⋯⋯⋯ Distant relationship	—— Very close relationship	– · – · – Less close relationship
— — Conflictual relationship	⊣ ⊢ Estranged relationship	━━ Close conflictual relationship

Figure 2.1 Example of a combination of a genomap (information inside the circle) and an ecomap (information outside the circle) of a 50-year-old woman with Type 2 diabetes and a history of childhood molestation and sexual abuse. It shows a great deal of conflict within and outside the family and identifies where her support base is.

The findings should be documented in the medical record (one should think about that term – does it reflect person-centred care?) and communicated to the appropriate caregivers. There is an increasing trend towards electronic data collection and management process that enable information to be easily and rapidly transferred among health professionals. Some systems enable patients to access their health information. Most modern electronic blood glucose meters have a facility for marinating a record of blood glucose test results that can be downloaded into computer programs. These systems have the capacity to significantly improve health care; however, consideration must be given to the privacy and confidentiality of all personal information and appropriate access and storage security mechanisms should be maintained according to the laws of the relevant country.

Note: A guideline for obtaining a comprehensive nursing history follows. However, it is important to listen to the patient and not be locked into 'ticking boxes' so that assumptions can be checked and non-verbal messages and body language noted and clarified, and vital and valuable information is not overlooked.

Most of the information is general in nature, but some is specifically relevant to diabetes (e.g. blood glucose testing and eating patterns). The clinical assessment in the example guideline is particularly aimed at obtaining information about metabolic status.

Assessing the person with diabetes does not differ from assessing people with any other disease process. Assessment should take into account social, physical and psychological factors in order to prepare an appropriate nursing care plan, including a plan for diabetes education and discharge/transition. Any physical disability the patient has could affect their ability to self-manage their diabetes (inject insulin, inspect feet, test blood glucose). Impaired hearing and psychological distress and mental illness may preclude people attending group education programmes. Management and educational expectations may need to be modified to accommodate disabilities.

If the person has diabetes, however, metabolic derangements may be present on admission, or could develop as a consequence of hospitalisation. Therefore, careful assessment enables potential problems to be proactively identified, alerts to be flagged if necessary, a coordinated collaborative care plan to be developed and appropriate referral to other health professionals (medical specialist, podiatrist, diabetes nurse specialist/diabetes educator, dietitian, and psychologist) to take place. A health 'problem list' that ranks problems in order of priority can also assist health professionals to plan individualised care that addresses immediate and future management goals. The first step in patient assessment is to document a comprehensive health history.

Nursing history

A nursing history is a written record of specific information about a patient. The data collected enable the nurse to plan appropriate nursing actions considering the individual patient's worldviews and needs. A good patient care plan will enable consistent care to be delivered within, and among, nurses and service departments. An example patient assessment chart follows. It was formulated to collect relevant diabetes-specific data, which could be used in conjunction with other relevant tools such as those shown in Table 2.1. Some electronic data management systems enable some information to be collected electronically from existing records when the patient has attended the service before.

Example Health Assessment Chart

Formulated for people with diabetes in hospital but most issues are relevant in any health care setting. Other systems-based assessment may also be necessary, for example respiratory, renal, nervous, and gastrointestinal systems.

A. Demographic data

Name ....
Age ....   Gender   ☐ Male   ☐ Female
Type of diabetes   ☐ Type 1   ☐ Type 2   ☐ Other ....
Duration of diabetes .... years
Known allergies ....

Social

Language spoken: ....
Command of English/language of relevant country: ☐ Written   ☐ Spoken
Important cultural practices, e.g. fasting, dietary requirements, practices related to dying and death
Marital status ....
Living arrangements   ☐ With partner   ☐ Alone   ☐ Other
Support systems ....
Age and health status of significant other/carer) ....
Work type ....
Responsibility in the home ....
Hobbies ....
Education level ....
Religion and religious practices e.g. prayer ....
Spiritual practices e.g. meditation

Meals

Regular meals   ☐ Yes   ☐ No
Food allergies ....

Usual diet ....
Appetite generally .... currently ....
Who does the cooking ....
Who does the shopping ....
Eating out ....
Current nasogastric tube .... TPN .... IV ....
Alcohol consumption   ☐ Yes   ☐   No How much ....
                                                                  How often ....

Smoking

☐ Yes   ☐ No   Cigarettes/pipe ....
How many per day .... Marijuana: ....

Current medications

Record dose and dose frequency for each medicine, when they administer it in relation to food and exercise, whether they miss doses, if so how often and why, whether they alter doses, if so how often and why.

Check insulin injection sites

Insulin delivery system used ....
Insulin administration technique/accuracy ....
Preparing injection using usual system ....
Patient can name type/s of insulin   ☐ Yes   ☐ No. Do they adjust their insulin dose?

Why? ....…............. What criteria do they use to adjust doses? ....…..............
Complementary therapies: name of the product/therapy, why they are using it and what they are using it for.
If on insulin or oral hypoglycaemic agents: ask whether they have hypoglycaemia.
How often?
Do they ever lose consciousness during a hypoglycaemic episode?
Do they recognise the signs and symptoms of hypoglycaemia?
What signs/symptoms do they experience?
When does it usually occur?
What is the blood glucose level before they treat the hypo?
How do they treat the hypo?
Do they always have some form of glucose with them? ....….........................…........

Usual activity level

Sports ....
Gardening ....
Walking ....
Other ....

Sleep pattern

Approximately how long do they sleep for?
Do they have trouble getting to sleep?
Do they have trouble staying asleep?
Do they need to get up at night to go to the toilet? ....….................................... How often?
Can they go back to sleep after going to the toilet?
What prevents them from sleeping?
Do they use anything to help them sleep? ....…............. What? ....…..........

Disabilities

What activities are limited ....
To what degree ....
(1)   General ....
(2)   Hearing ....…..................
(3)   Related to diabetic complications ....
Reduced vision   ☐ glasses   ☐ contact lenses   ☐ registered blind
Neuropathy (a)   Peripheral ....
                   (b)   Autonomic ....
Vascular   (a)   Cardiac ....
                   (b)   Legs and feet ....
Kidney function ....
Sexuality   (a)   Erectile dysfunction ....
                   (b)   Sexual difficulties ....
(4)   Mobility and flexibility
(5)   Dexterity (fine motor skills)

Self-monitoring of diabetes status (testing methods)

....
Tests own blood glucose   ☐ Yes   ☐ No
Tests blood ketones during illness   Yes ☐   No ☐
Testing frequency ....
System used
Blood glucose meter type ....
Testing accuracy ....

Psychological status

Anxiety
Depression

Adjustment to diabetes

☐ Anxious ☐ Denial ☐ Depression ☐ Well adjusted
Usual mental state .... Current mental state ....
Current stressors ....
Coping mechanisms ....

Diabetes knowledge

Previous diabetes education   ☐ Yes   ☐ No How long ago ....
Attendance at education support groups   ☐ Yes   ☐ No
Name of group ....

Patient's stated reason for being in hospital

....
....

B. Clinical and laboratory examination

A detailed physical examination is essential. Particular attention should be paid to the following areas.

(1) General inspection

- Conscious state
- Temperature, pulse and respiration
- Blood pressure lying and standing; note any postural drop
- Height
- Weight and history of weight gain/loss; BMI, ...Waist circumference
- Hydration status, skin turgor
- Presence of diabetic symptoms, thirst, polyuria, polydipsia, lethargy
- Full urinalysis
- Blood glucose
- Presence of ketones in blood ☐   urine ☐

(2) Skin

- Pigmentation (Acanthosis nigricans)
- Skin tone/turgor, colour
- Presence of lesions, rashes, wounds, ulcers
- Inspect injection sites, including abdomen; note any thickening, lumps, bruises

(3) Mouth

- Mucous membranes (dry/moist)
- Lips
- Infection, halitosis
- Teeth: evidence of dental caries, loose teeth, red gums, incorrectly fitting dentures

(4) Feet and legs

- Temperature of feet and legs, noting any differences between two legs and parts of the feet and legs
- The skin of the feet and legs may be hairless and shiny due to poor circulation
- Muscle wasting
- Ulcers or pressure areas on soles of feet and toes, including old scars
- Loss of pain sensation that may be due to nerve damage; estimate the size and depth of any ulcers using a template filed in the medical record, note their location and how long they have been present
- Presence of oedema

- Infection including fungal infection; inspect between the toes
- Condition of nails and general cleanliness of feet
- Type of footwear
- Record podiatry contact or referral, if any

Laboratory tests

Full blood count
Glucose
HbA$_{1c}$
Lipid profile
Kidney function
Liver function
Urea and electrolyte
Other relevant tests

Table 2.1   Some commonly used assessment instruments. The content of the instruments, the purpose of the assessment, and the particular patient population should be considered when selecting instruments, even when they are valid and reliable. Some are available in languages other than English. Details of most of the diabetes-specific instruments can be found on http://www.musc.edu/dfm/RCMAR/Diabetes Tool.html (2006) and Garrett *et al.* (2001).

Generic instruments	*Diabetes-specific instruments*
Sickness Impact Profile (Bergner *et al.* 1976)	Audit of Diabetes-dependent Quality of Life (ADDQoL) (Bradley *et al.* 1999)
Nottingham Health Profile (Hunt & McKenna 1985)	Appraisal of Diabetes Scale (ADS) (Carey *et al.* 1991)
Short Form Health Survey (SF-36) (Ware *et al.* 1992)	Diabetes Health Profile (DHP-1, DHP-18) (Meadows *et al.* 1996)
Quality of Life After Acute Myocardial Infarction (Oldridge *et al.* 1991)	The Diabetes Impact Measurement Scale (DIMS) (Hammond & Aoki 1992)
K10+ depression scale, which is sometimes used as part of the psychosocial profile developed by the Department of Human Services, Victoria, Australia	Diabetes Quality of Life (DQOL) (Jacobson *et al.* 1988) Diabetes Specific Quality of Life Scale (DSQOLS) for Type 1 diabetes (Mulhauser *et al.* 1998)
Perceived Therapeutic Efficacy Scale (PTES)	Questionnaire on Stress in Diabetic Patients (QSD-R) (Duran *et al.* 1995)
Spiritual Assessment Tool (Dossey *et al.* 1995)	Well-being Enquiry for Diabetics (WED) (Mannucci *et al.* 1996)
Hospital Anxiety and Depression Scale (HADS)	
Self Assessment Health Status (EQ-5D)	Problem Areas in Diabetes (PAID) (Polonsky *et al.* 1995)
Center for Epidemiological Studies Depression Scale (CESD) (Radloff 1997)	Diabetes Treatment Satisfaction Questionnaire (DTSQ) (Bradley 1994)
Patient Health Questionnaire (PHQ-9) (Pfizer Inc 2003)	Diabetes Care Profile (DCP) (Fitzgerald *et al.* 1996) Diabetes-39 Questionnaire (D-39) (Boyer & Earp 1997)
	Spirituality Questionnaire for young adults with diabetes (SQ) (Parsian & Dunning 1997, which is not listed on the RCMAR website)

Note: permission to use some of these tools may be needed before the tools can be used and specific training in analysing and interpreting the data is needed with some instruments. Other useful instruments include pain scales, falls risk tools, activities of daily living and mental assessment such as Folstein's Minni Mental. The Victorian Department of Human Services (now Department of Health and Aging, DOHA) (2006) produced a range of profiles such as the Psychosocial Profile, which encompasses mental health and well-being, and the Health Behaviours Profile that are used in many Australian DOHA funded projects.

Other important information to obtain might include functional status, whether the person has an advanced care plan and other proxy decision-making tools and what special provision might be required to fulfill religious observances e.g. fasting for Ramadan or Buddhist lent, and how to care for the body after death. These issues are often difficult to discuss but they are an essential part of person-centred care.

Instruments to measure health status

Some specific instruments can be very helpful to determine health status, quality of life (QOL), beliefs and attitudes, and satisfaction. QOL is a complex, multifactorial, and individual construct encompassing the individual's physical, social and mental functioning, satisfaction with life and whether/how these factors are affected by illness and its management (Salek 1998). Significantly, social well being is strongly correlated with emotional well being. A range of instruments generally designated as generic and disease-specific is available. Generic instruments were designed for use in a wide range of patients and populations. Disease-specific instruments have a narrower focus on particular illnesses, in this case, diabetes; see Chapters 4, 12 and 15.

Table 2.1 presents an overview of generic and diabetes specific instruments commonly used to collect important subjective information from individuals about their health status and beliefs. The instruments have all been extensively validated.

Documenting and charting patient care

Documenting in the health record

Documentation is an essential part of health management. Alternative methods of documenting care are emerging, for example charting by exception, where only events outside the normal expected progress are recorded. This form of charting requires supportive documentation in the form of guidelines, flow charts, care plans and care maps. They can avoid duplication and streamline documentation. The use of care pathways is becoming increasingly common in Australia and in the UK (O'Brien & Hardy 2000).

Other ways of documenting holistic care incorporate genomaps and ecomaps (see Figure 2.1), which can effectively convey a great deal of information about the social relationship and support base aspects of an individual's life (Cluning 1997). They are particularly useful for long-term chronic diseases such as diabetes where these factors affect management outcomes; see Chapters 15 and 16. They also record information that is often passed on anecdotally during handover or in the 'corridor', which means vital information that could assist in planning care is not available or is misinterpreted.

Genograms illustrate how an individual relates to other people in the family and ecomaps place the family in the context of the wider social situation in which they live. Ecograms and ecomaps can be simple or convey complex and detailed information. Together they give a great deal of information about:

- the individual's environment
- their relationships with people in their environment
- family structure
- family and extended support
- family health history
- family functioning
- health service utilisation
- social orientation.

This information helps determine how social support and other networks influence the person's self-management and the assistance they can rely on, for example to manage serious hypoglycaemia and intercurrent illness.

Care plans

The employing institution's policy regarding the method of documentation should be followed. Good documentation enables the required care to be communicated to all staff. In the future, changes will occur to the methods of documenting care, for example focus charting and flow charts may replace narrative notes. Flow charts are designed to enable all healthcare providers to document care on a single care plan, which reduces duplication and may enhance communication. Many health services now use electronic documentation and communication processes.

Standardised care plans of common medical and nursing diagnosis are being developed to serve as blueprints and may reduce the time spent on documentation. Despite the fact such care plans encompass 'charting by exception,' they are not consistent with personalised care. For example, a patient consulted the author about her electronic 'personalised' care plan that was generated in primary care by her general practitioner, who printed a copy of the care plan for her to keep. She did not understand what the information meant. The care plan contained the standard blood glucose, lipid, blood pressure and weight targets and indicated she should have no more than one glass of alcohol per day. When the information was explained to her she became very upset and agitated, crumpled the care plan into a ball and threw it in the bin. She said: 'well it is not personalised for me. I am a former alcoholic. I have not had any alcohol for 5 years, now my target is one glass a day. If I had one glass I could not stop.'

The move towards computerised or 'paperless' documentation is daunting and exciting but due consideration must be given to data security. Confidential information should be labelled as such in the medical record. Extra care is required with mobile technology such as smart phones, laptops and palm pilots to ensure patient confidentiality is protected if any patient data are stored and/or communicated via these media.

Nursing notes

Due consideration needs to be given to standard policies for good documentation and the laws governing privacy and confidentiality and people's right to access their medical records. Medical notes are a record of the patient's encounter with a service provider in any setting and hospital admission, the care they received and the outcomes of the care provided, and acts as a guide for discharge planning. Handwritten documentation should be written legibly and objectively. Medical records are not legal documents but can subpoenaed for a court hearing. In such cases, good documentation can help the health professional recall the situation.

Documentation should contain the following:

- The condition of the patient recorded objectively; for example, describe wounds in terms of size and depth.
- Quantification of the patient's condition, recording swelling, oedema, temperature, pulse, and respiration (TPR) and blood pressure (BP) using objective measures.
- All teaching the patient receives and that still required.
- The patient's response to treatment.

- All medications received and any associated adverse events.
- Removal of all invasive medical devices (e.g. packs, drains, IV lines).
- Psychological, spiritual, and social factors.

Clinical observation

In some cases it is possible to refer to standard protocols in medical records if there is a set procedure documented and regularly revised, for example there is a standard procedure for performing an oral glucose tolerance test. The documentation could note relevant details such as the time, date and person's name and then state 'OGGT performed according to the standard protocol'. Where any deviation from the protocol occurred it should be recorded. If required, the standard protocol could be produced.

Documenting metabolic status ('diabetic charts')

The purposes of 'diabetic charts' are:

- To provide a record of blood glucose measurements so the blood glucose pattern can be identified and used to adjust insulin/glucose lowering medicine (GLM) doses, dose forms, and the dose regimen.
- To record blood ketone measurements to detect risk of ketoacidosis especially in Type 1 diabetes.
- To provide a record of the dose and time insulin and other GLMs were administered.
- To record episodes of hyper or hypoglycaemia and how they were managed.

Frequency of blood testing depends on the patient's status and the management plan (see Chapter 3).

Practice point

A common error is that medication doses are not recorded on the 'diabetic chart,' which makes it difficult to interpret the blood glucose pattern without the medication information.

Nursing responsibilities

(1) Write legibly. Avoid using unauthorised abbreviations. Insulin doses should be documented as 'units' not u/s.
(2) Accurately record all medication doses and dose intervals.
(3) Record hypoglycaemic episodes (symptoms, treatment, time, activity and food omission) in the appropriate column. Hypoglycaemia should also be documented in the patient's unit record.
(4) Do not add unnecessary details.
(5) Sign and include the date and time of all entries.

Figure 2.2 depicts example charts for (a) frequent testing and (b) testing 4-hourly or less often.

(a)

DIABETIC FREQUENT MONITORING													IDENTIFICATION

DATE	TIME	INSULIN		BLOOD SUGAR	URINE								NURSING COMMENTS E.g. Adverse reactions or food omission
		TYPE	DOSE		GLUCOSE						ACETONE	PROTEIN	
					0 %	1/10 %	1/4 %	1/2 %	1 %	2 %			

(b)

INSTRUCTIONS
TYPE OF INSULIN, BLOOD GLUCOSE AND
URINE TESTS MUST BE RECORDED IN FULL.

IDENTIFICATION

Date		0700	1100	1600	2100	COMMENTS
	Insulin type					
	Dose					
	Blood glucose mmol/L					
	Urine glucose					
	Ketones					
	Insulin type					
	Dose					
	Blood glucose mmol/L					
	Urine glucose					
	Ketones					

Figure 2.2 Sample diabetes record charts for (a) 2-hourly testing (e.g. when using an insulin infusion); (b) 4-hourly or less frequent testing.

Documentation by people with diabetes

People with diabetes also document a great deal of information about their disease. They use a variety of written and electronic record-keeping methods including blood glucose monitoring diaries, complication screening records and other management information such as medication lists and the results of investigative procedures. These records are a vital part of the documentation process. They not only supply written information, they also contain a great deal of information about an individual's self-care ability, for example a blood glucose diary covered with blood smears could mean the person is having difficulty placing the blood on the strip. Discussing the issue with the patient might reveal that they often get the shakes and their vision is blurred due to hypoglycaemia. It is important, however, that all such assumptions are checked.

Importantly, the information in the individual documents must be valued and used in the clinical encounter. It is a tangible record of the hard work of self-care.

References

Cluning, T. (1997) Social assessment documentation: genomaps and ecomaps. In *Nursing Documentation: Writing What We Do* (ed. J. Richmond), Chapter 7. Ausmed Publications, Melbourne.

Dossey, B., Keegen, L., Guzzetta, C. & Kolkmeier, L. (1995) *Holistic Nursing: A Handbook for Practice.* Aspen Publishers, Maryland, pp. 20–21.

Dunning, P. (1994) Having diabetes: young adult perspectives. *The Diabetes Educator*, **21** (1), 58–65.

Dunning, P. & Martin, M. (1998) Beliefs about diabetes and diabetes complications. *Professional Nurse*, **13** (7), 429–434.

Dunning, T. (2013) Turning points and transitions: Crises and opportunities. Chapter 8 in *Diabetes Education: Art, Science and Evidence* (ed. T. Dunning) Wiley Blackwell, Chichester pp 117–131.

Foundation for Informed Medical Decision Making (2007) http:// www.fmdm.org/decision_sdms.php (accessed December 2007).

Hunt, S. & McKenna, J. (1985) Nottingham Health Profile. http://.www.eygnus-group.com/cidm/risk/html (accessed January 2008).

Johnson, A., Sandford, J. & Tyndall, J. (2003) Written and verbal information versus verbal information only for patients being discharged from acute hospital settings to home. *Cochrane Database of Scientific Reviews*. Issue 4 Art No Cd003716. DOI; 10. 1002/14651858. CD 003716.

Kilmartin, M. (1997) Evidence is lacking on shared decisions. *Journal of Health Services Research and Policy*, **2** (2), 112–121.

Kinnersley, P., Edwards, A., Hood, K. *et al.* (2007) Interventions before consultations for helping patients address their information needs. *Cochrane Database of Scientific Reviews*, Issue 3, Art. No. CD 004565. DOI 10. 1002/14651858. CDOO4565.pub2.

Kleinman, A., Eisenberg, L. & Goode, B. (1978) Culture, illness and care: Clinical lessons from anthropological and cross cultural research. *Annals of Internal Medicine* **88** (2), 251–258.

Lewin, S., Skea, Z., Entwistle, V., Zwarenstein, M. & Dick, J. (2001) Interventions for providers to promote a patient-centred approach in clinical consultations. *Cochrane Database of Systematic Reviews*, Issue 4, Art. No. CDOO 3267. DOI 10. 1002/14651858.CDOO3267.

McCulloch, D., Price, M., Hindmarsh, M. *et al.* (1998) A population based approach to diabetes management in a primary care setting: Early results and lessons learned. *Effective Clinical Practice*, **1**, 1222.

McKinstry, B., Ashcroft, R., Car, J., Freeman, G. & Sheik, A. (2006) Interventions for improving patients' trust in doctors and groups of doctors. *Cochrane Database for Systematic Reviews*, Issue 3, Art. No. CDOO4134. DOI: 10. 1002/14651858.CDOO4134.pub2.

Murray, E., Burns, J., See Tai, S., Lai, R. & Nazareth, I. (2005) Interactive health communication applications for people with chronic illness. *Cochrane Database of Systematic Reviews*, Issue 4, Art. No. CDOO4274. DOI: 10. 1002/4651858.CDOO4274.pub4.

National Managed Health Care Congress (NHCG) (1996) *The Disease Management Strategic Research Study and Resource Guide*. NHCG, Washington.

O'Brien, S. & Hardy, K. (2000) Impact of a care pathway driven diabetes education programme. *Journal of Diabetes Nursing*, **4** (5), 147–150.

Parsian, N. & Dunning, T. (2008) Spirituality and coping in young adults with diabetes. *Diabetes Research and Clinical Practice*, **79** (182), S82–S121.

Ralston, J., Revere, D. & Robins, L. (2004) Patients' experience with a diabetes support program based on an interactive electronic medical record: Qualitative survey. *British Medical Journal*, **328**, 115–162.

Salek, S. (1998) *Compendium of Quality of Life Instruments*. John Wiley & Sons, Chichester, UK.

The Joint Commission (2010) *Advancing Effective Communication, Cultural Competence, and Patient- and Family-Centered Care: A Roadmap for Hospitals*. Oakbrook Terrace, IL, USA: The Joint Commission.

Wagner, E., Austin T., Davis, C. *et al.* (1996a) Improving outcomes in chronic illness. *Managed Care Quarterly*, **4** (2), 1225.

Wagner, E., Austin, T., *et al.* (1996b) Organising care for patients with chronic illness. *The Milbank Quarterly*, **74** (4), 51–54.

Further reading

Bradford, K. (2013) Patients need to be involved in quality metrics. *Primary Care Progress blog* primarycareprogress.smallworldlabs.com/blogs/16?year=2013 (accessed February 2013).

Garratt, A., Schmidt, L. & Fitzpatrick, R. (2002) Patient-assessed health outcome measures for diabetes: A structured review. *Diabetic Medicine*, **19**, 111.

Chapter 3
Monitoring Diabetes Mellitus

Key points

- Regular assessment of the individual's physical, emotional, social, spiritual, relationship status, and their capability to perform their usual activities of daily living and self-care is essential to enable proactive management strategies to be implemented.
- Structured regular complication screening programmes that encompass mental health, self-care, driving safety, and a structured medication review should be undertaken at least annually. In some cases the health and well-being of spouses need to be considered, especially older spouses who provide care and support.
- Diabetes education and management programmes should be evaluated and revised regularly to ensure they remain current. People with diabetes should be involved in the evaluation processes.
- The people with diabetes has a responsibility to undertake appropriate self-care to manage their disease.

Rationale

Proactive monitoring programmes enable blood glucose and lipid patterns, complication status, and self-care capability to be identified and the management regimen appropriately tailored to the individual. The accuracy of blood glucose self-monitoring technique and appropriate maintenance of equipment is an important aspect of the individual's ability to manage their diabetes and helps ensure management decisions are based on the best available data when used in conjunction with laboratory investigations and physical and mental assessment. Self-monitoring enables people with diabetes to identify the effects of diet, exercise and other factors on their blood glucose levels, and gives them greater insight into and control over their disease.

Care of People with Diabetes: A Manual of Nursing Practice, Fourth Edition. Trisha Dunning.
© 2014 John Wiley & Sons, Ltd. Published 2014 by John Wiley & Sons, Ltd.

Monitoring and meeting management targets is also a key quality management activity, and funding and the service accreditation processes are often based on health professionals and governments meeting targets and complying with guidelines and care standards. The new Non-Communicable Disease Global Monitoring Framework ((IDF 2012) was discussed in Chapter 1. In addition, health services in Australia will have to demonstrate person-centred care in all of the 12 new accreditation standards. These regulatory expectations put pressure on service managers, clinicians, clerical staff and ultimately people with diabetes.

Introduction

Monitoring blood glucose is an important part of diabetes management. The results obtained form the basis for adjusting medication, food intake, and activity levels. Urine glucose is not a reliable method of assessing metabolic control, but *might* still be useful for some people and in some countries where no other method is available, provided the renal threshold for glucose has been established. Most glucose circulating in the blood is reabsorbed in the renal tubules, however the capacity to reabsorb glucose is exceeded during hyperglycaemia and glucose appears in the urine. The renal threshold for glucose is fairly constant, about 10 mmol/L, but may be higher in older people and during pregnancy (Sonksen *et al.* 1998). Glucose in the urine represents the amount of glucose that collects in the urine since the bladder was last emptied and is therefore, a retrospective value.

> ### *Practice point*
>
> Urine glucose testing cannot detect hypoglycaemia.

People with diabetes are expected to, and do, manage their diabetes at home; that is they are responsible for over 90% of diabetes management decisions. Thus, each individual is an expert in his/her diabetes. People should be encouraged to continue to self-monitor blood glucose in hospital if they are well enough to do so. If health professionals perform the test they should always inform the patient about the result unless they are too ill to understand the information. In addition blood glucose testing time can be used as a teaching opportunity and an opportunity to assess the individual's testing technique. The results of blood and urine tests are only useful if the tests are accurately performed.

Monitoring 1: Blood glucose

> ## Key points
>
> - Follow correct procedure when performing tests.
> - Perform meter control and calibration tests regularly.
> - Clean and maintain equipment regularly.
> - Record and interpret results according to the clinical situation.

The role of blood glucose monitoring in the care of diabetes

Blood glucose monitoring provides insight into the effectiveness of the diabetes management plan. It enables direct feedback to the patient about their blood glucose. Some experts suggest the cost and time associated with blood glucose self-monitoring is not cost effective, even when patients are taught to adjust their management regimen. For example, the DiGEM investigators undertook a randomised control trial involving people with treated Type 2 diabetes over age 25 treated with diet or GLMs, which showed no statistically significant difference in HbA_{1c} at 12 months but there was a significant change in total cholesterol (Farmer 2007). Subjective parameters such as quality of life and sense of control were not measured. Other researchers also show that people who monitor their blood glucose are younger at diagnosis and present with a higher HbA_{1c} than people who do not test (Franciosi *et al.* 2005; Davis *et al.* 2006).

In contrast, the ROSSO study (Schneider *et al.* 2006) showed metabolic control improved in people with Type 2 diabetes who performed frequent blood glucose tests, and demonstrated a 51% lower risk of death and a 32% lower risk of microvascular and macrovascular complications. In addition, people who monitored were more aware of their blood glucose levels and sought advice from health professionals sooner. Likewise, Karter *et al.* (2006) demonstrated improved HbA_{1c} after home blood glucose testing was instituted in the Kaiser Permanente study.

Other researchers show lower rates of self-blood glucose monitoring in men and people with low education level, those who do not have health insurance, in countries where equipment is not subsidised, as well as those not on insulin, those taking GLMs, having less than two consultations with the doctor annually, and not attending diabetes education programmes (Centers for Disease Control and Prevention (CDC) 2007).

These studies suggest there may be gender and age differences in the rates of blood glucose self-monitoring, but the rates are similar in different countries. Nevertheless, most management guidelines continue to recommend blood glucose self-monitoring as an integral part of the management plan. Testing frequency should be individualised depending on glycaemic control and health status in Type 2 diabetes but at least daily when insulin and/or GLMs are used. People with Type 1 should monitor at least TDS (Canadian Diabetes Association 2008).

Blood glucose testing is performed to:

- Monitor the effectiveness of diabetes therapy and guide adjustments to the food plan, OHAs/insulin dose, exercise/activity, mental well being and quality of life; see Chapter 2.
- Detect hyperglycaemia, which can be confirmed by laboratory blood glucose tests and elevated HbA_{1c} levels, a marker of the average blood glucose over the preceding three months, and more recently, A_{1c}-derived average glucose.
- Achieve blood glucose targets, which has a role in preventing or delaying the onset of diabetes-related complications and maintaining independence and quality of life.
- Diagnose hypoglycaemia, including nocturnal hypoglycaemia, which can present as sleep disturbances, snoring, restlessness or bad dreams.
- Establish the renal threshold for glucose to determine the reliability of urine testing in those rare cases where people still test their urine glucose.
- Achieve 'tight' control in pregnancy and thereby reduce the risks to both mother and baby.
- Provide continuity of care following hospitalisation.

Blood glucose monitoring is of particular use in:

- Frequent hypoglycaemic episodes and hypoglycaemic unawareness.
- Unstable or 'brittle' diabetes.
- Managing illnesses at home and when recovering from an illness.
- GDM, pregnancy and in neonates born to women with GDM and diabetes.
- Establishing a new treatment regimen.
- Stabilising OHA and/or insulin doses:
  - patients with renal failure, autonomic neuropathy, cardiovascular or cerebrovascular insufficiency where hypoglycaemia signs can be masked or not recognized;
  - during investigations such as angiograms and surgical procedures;
  - detecting actual or potential medicine/medicine or medicine/herb interactions;
  - during travel.

Clinical observation

In the home situation, blood glucose testing enables the person with diabetes to take more responsibility for and control over their disease and is a tool they can use to maintain their quality of life. It is not a means by which health professionals control people with diabetes. It is only one aspect of an holistic, individualised assessment; see Chapter 2.

The target blood glucose range and frequency of testing should be assessed individually when people with diabetes are in hospital. The aim is to achieve a blood glucose pattern as close to normal as possible. Generally accepted blood glucose targets are: pre-meal < 5 mmol/L and two-hour post prandial <7.8 mmol/L (IDF 2007). However, the management regimen must target both fasting and post prandial blood glucose to achieve optimal control and reduce the risks associated with hyperglycaemia see Chapters 1, 7 and 8. Hyperglycaemia in hospitalised people with and without diabetes is associated with more morbidity and mortality in general, surgical, IVU and cardiology settings (Australian Diabetes Society (ADS) 2012). ADS guidelines generally recommend blood glucose range between 5 and < 10 mmol/L in most situations, but the individual's needs must be considered.

Increasing emphasis is being placed on reducing post prandial hyperglycaemia because it is associated with increased risk of retinopathy, cardiovascular disease, increased risk of cancer and impaired cognitive function in older people (IDF 2007). Significantly, elevated postprandial hyperglycaemia is present before Type 2 diabetes is diagnosed and partly accounts for why cardiovascular complications are frequently present at diagnosis. Management of postprandial hyperglycaemia is discussed in Chapters 5 and 8. Likewise, glucose variability is also associated with diabetes complications and mortality, therefore, the aim is to try to reduce swings in blood glucose between hyperglycaemia and hypoglycaemia (Chapter 7). The medicine regimen is often intensified when the individual is in hospital to reduce optimise metabolic control. Such intensification is associated with lower 30-day readmission/emergency presentation risk and lower HbA_{1c} on outpatient follow-up (Wei *et al.* 2013).

Although the focus is on achieving optimal blood glucose control to prevent or delay the onset of diabetes complications, optimal control is often not achieved. The person is usually blamed for not 'complying' with recommendations. However, the progressive nature of Type 2 diabetes and clinical inertia also play a part (Grant *et al.* 2004). Clinical inertia refers to health professionals recognising a problem but failing to act. Like 'non-compliance', clinical inertia is a derogatory term for a complex phenomenon where behaviours are influenced by factors such as competing demands in the clinical setting including time constraints and patients presenting with multiple problems that cannot all be addressed at the same time (Parchman *et al.* 2007). However, clinician inertia combined with patient non-adherence might increase the risk of poor control and may be mutually causative.

Factors that influence blood glucose levels

(1) Food: times of last food intake, quantity and type of carbohydrate/fibre consumed in relation to meals and activity.
(2) Exercise: timing with respect to food, medication and insulin doses, injection site, type of exercise and blood glucose level when commencing exercise.
(3) Intercurrent illness, for example, influenza, urinary tract infection.
(4) Medications used for diabetes control blood glucose: oral agents, insulin.
(5) Other medicines, for example, corticosteroids, oral contraceptives, beta blockers, and non-prescription medications that contain glucose, ephedrine, pseudoephedrine or alcohol, for example, cold remedies and glucose lowering complementary medicines see Chapters 5 and 19.
(6) Alcohol: type, relationship to food intake, amount consumed.
(7) Insulin type, injection site, injection technique.
(8) Complementary medicines/therapies, for example, glucose lowering herbs, stress management techniques, see Chapter 19.
(9) Emotional (emotional dwelling) and physical stress – not only stress itself but medications used to treat stress.
(10) Accuracy of monitoring technique.
(11) Pregnancy in people with diabetes and gestational diabetes.
(12) Childhood: erratic swings in blood glucose levels are common.
(13) Adolescence: hormonal factors during adolescence can make control difficult.
(14) Renal, liver, and pancreatic disease.
(15) Other endocrine disorders, for example, thyroid disease, Cushing's disease, and acromegaly.
(16) Parenteral nutrition.
(17) Obtaining the blood sample from unwashed fingers, for example, after the patient or health professional treated a hypoglycaemic event with oral glucose.

Clinical observation

Insulin absorption can be delayed if insulin is injected into an oedematous or ascitic abdomen. The delayed absorption can affect the blood glucose level. The thigh or upper arm may be preferable sites in this instance.

Guidelines for the frequency of blood glucose monitoring
(1) In care settings, capillary blood glucose tests should be performed only by adequately qualified health professionals or the person with diabetes.
(2) Medical staff and sometimes diabetes educators are usually responsible for interpreting the results and adjusting the diabetes management plan. Over time, many people with diabetes become expert at adjusting their insulin doses to

account for carbohydrate intake (Dose Adjustment for Normal Eating (DAFNE)) and during illness and exercise.

The following recommendations are guidelines only; the policies and procedures of the employing institution should be followed and the regimen should be tailored to the individual's needs and hospital setting, for example frequent monitoring is required when IV insulin infusions are used and in surgical and ICU settings.

Suggested protocol in hospital settings.   Blood glucose tests performed before meals and before bed (e.g. 7 a.m., 11 a.m., 4 p.m. and 9 p.m.) in order to obtain a profile of the effectiveness of diabetes therapy. Occasionally, urine glucose will be measured at these times for 24 hours to establish the renal threshold. As indicated, testing two hours after food, especially in Type 2 diabetes, may be preferable in order to provide information about glucose clearance from the blood stream after a meal as an indicator of cardiovascular risk. Blood glucose tests may be performed at 2 a.m. or 3 a.m. for two to three days if the blood glucose is high before breakfast and there is a possibility of nocturnal hypoglycaemia; see Chapter 6.

Blood ketones should be monitored in all patients with Type 1 diabetes and in Type 2 people during severe stress, for example surgery, infection, and myocardial infarction if blood glucose tests are elevated. Urine ketone tests might still be used in some places but are a less reliable indicator of ketosis than blood ketones. Each person's needs should be assessed individually and the testing schedule tailored to individual requirements where work routines and staffing levels allow. One way to achieve an individualised monitoring regimen is to allow the patient to perform their own blood glucose tests where their condition permits them to do so.

Regimen for patients on insulin.   Initially, for 48 hours, monitor at 7 a.m., 11 a.m., 4 p.m. and 9 p.m. to assess the effectiveness of the prescribed insulin therapy. Review after 48 hours and alter the testing frequency if indicated. If the insulin regimen is altered, review again after 48 hours.

Note: The timing of blood glucose monitoring depends on the insulin regimen and the action profile of the prescribed insulin; see Chapter 5.

Patients using insulin pumps and those on IV insulin infusions require more frequent monitoring.

Patients on oral GLM.   Initial monitoring as for insulin-treated patients. Review after 48 hours and reduce monitoring frequency to twice daily, daily or once every second or third day, alternating the times of testing, as indicated by the level of control and the general medical condition of the patient.

Patients managed on diet and exercise.   Initially, twice daily monitoring, decreasing to daily or once every second or third day, unless the patient is having total parenteral nutrition (TPN), diagnostic procedures, is undergoing surgery or is actually ill.

In the acute care setting, patients are usually ill and require at least 4-hourly monitoring. The frequency can often be reduced in rehabilitation, mental health and care facilities for older people, and in the end stages of life.

Special circumstances.   These might require a prescription from the medical staff. They include:

(1) Insulin infusion: tests are usually performed every 1–2 hours during the infusion and reviewed every 2 hours. Reduce to 3–4 hourly when blood glucose levels are stable (see Chapter 5).

(2) People on corticosteroid therapy because these medicines induce insulin resistance and increase hepatic glucose output, which might be greater in people who already have insulin resistance and hyperglycaemia and may be a risk factor for hyperosmolar states; see Chapters 7, 10 and 18. Ketones should also be monitored in Type 1 diabetes because some corticosteroids also induce lipolysis and increase the risk of ketoacidosis.

   (a) Non-diabetic patients: regularly screen for hyperglycaemia. The effects on blood glucose depend on the formulation, dose, dose frequency and duration of action, and the response of the individual to the particular preparation used. Often the blood glucose increases during the day and is higher in the afternoon (Dunning 1996; Diabetes UK 2012). Oral preparations have a greater impact on blood glucose than IV preparations, which usually do not cause a great rise in the blood glucose.

   (b) People with diabetes: see protocols in the preceding sections 'Regimen for patients on insulin', 'Patients on GLMs' or 'Patients managed on diet and exercise'.

(3) TPN guidelines suggest:

   (a) Routine blood glucose testing for the first 48 hours: 7 a.m., 11 a.m., 4 p.m. and 9 p.m., until the patient is stable on TPN, then revert to protocol in section Regime for patients on insulin or Patients on oral hypoglycaemic agents.

   (b) Monitor blood for ketones: 7 a.m., 11 a.m., 4 p.m. and 9 p.m.

Practice point

Never prick the feet of an adult because it causes trauma and increases the risk of infection. Heel pricks can be performed on babies.

Blood glucose meters

Blood glucose meters are devices used to monitor blood glucose in the home or at the bedside in hospital. The first capillary blood glucose meter was introduced in 1974. Over the following decades the technology of both meters and test strips has changed rapidly. Staff should become familiar with the system used in their place of employment. Consult the diabetes educator/specialist team or manufacturer for specific advice.

Where meters are used, a blood glucose meter quality management programme with a centralised coordinator is desirable (Figure 3.1). As part of such a programme it is recommended that:

- Individual nurses and other users demonstrate competence to use the system in operation.
- Meters are subject to regular control testing and calibration according to the manufacturer's recommendations and are calibrated as required, usually when a new pack of strips is opened, and are appropriately cleaned and maintained, and that these processes are documented.
- A procedure for dealing with inaccurate results and meter malfunction is in place.

Most meters can be programmed to read in mmol/L or mg/dL, which is used in the United States. Most meters also store a record of blood glucose tests and other information that can be downloaded into computer software programs that enable the data to be displayed in a range of ways. Increasingly they include other functions that enable personalised information to be entered and decision aids to help people with diabetes manage their diabetes.

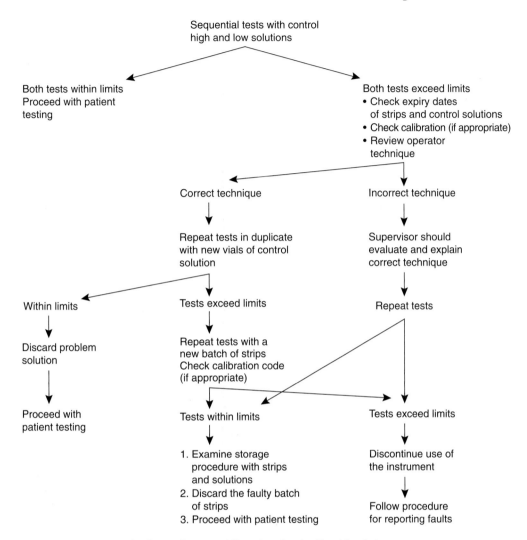

Figure 3.1 An example of a quality control flow chart for checking blood glucose meters.

Modern meters are small and light, easy to operate, and only require a very small amount of blood. Particular meters are designed specifically for particular target audiences such as children and older people, who have different requirements. For example, large result display screens and 'talking' meters for vision-impaired people. Test strips require a minimal amount of blood. Therefore, many of the systems errors associated with early meters have been eliminated. However, inaccuracies still occur and are mostly due to technique errors.

Meter technology changes rapidly and health professionals need to be aware that the system in use in the hospital may be different from the system the person uses at home, and should be aware that:

• Although blood glucose readings obtained from the fingertip most closely correlate with arterial glucose, there are usually small differences in test results between capillary and venous blood.

- There are often small differences between blood glucose tests performed on different meters at the same time. Several factors account for the difference such as squeezing the finger to obtain a second drop of blood. Usually a difference of ~3% is acceptable. People may need to be reassured that their meter is not at fault. The individual's needs and understanding and likely reaction need to be considered before comparing results on different meters in the presence of the person with diabetes.
- Alternative site testing (from sites other than the fingertip such as the forearm, abdomen and thigh) are available and cause less discomfort but only yield a small quantity of blood ~3 mL. However, blood glucose levels vary among different sites. For example, there is a lag in increases and reductions in blood glucose by up to 30 minutes at the forearm compared with the fingertip, which can lead to delay in detecting and treating hypoglycaemia (Jungheim & Koschinsky 2002). Less variation occurs between the palm and ball of the thumb.
- Heat and light affect strip accuracy.

Practice point

'Glucometer' is not a generic term for blood glucose meters. It was the name of a specific meter that has not been available on the market for at least 10 years. A more appropriate term is 'blood glucose meter' or use the name of the particular meter.

Continuous glucose monitoring systems

The technology to enable continuous glucose monitoring is developing rapidly towards the ultimate 'closed loop system'. Fingerprick blood glucose tests may miss many hypoglycaemic and hyperglycaemic levels: continuous blood glucose monitoring systems enable 'real-time' continuous blood glucose levels to be identified. Sampling generally occurs from interstitial and tissue sites. Interstitial glucose concentrations are often lower than capillary concentrations during the night compared with capillary glucose (Monsod *et al.* 2002. However, continuous monitoring enables the trend toward hyperglycaemia or hypoglycaemia (trend analysis) to be monitored and preventative action to be taken.

Continuous glucose monitoring system (CGMS)

The original CGMS system consists of a pager-sized glucose monitor, disposable subcutaneous glucose sensor and a cable connecting these two components to a communication system that stores data, which is downloaded into a computer software program that enables the results to be displayed in graph form. Glucose concentrations are measured every 10 seconds: an average of those values is saved in the meter every five minutes for 72 hours. CGMs is usually performed over three days.

Glucose targets can be assigned, the duration and frequency of hypo- and hyperglycaemic episodes and modal time determined using modern software. This provides important information that can help health professionals and patients understand the differences between their home blood glucose testing results and HbA$_{1c}$ and detect unrecognised hypoglycaemia. Previously, CGMS was primarily used to determine blood glucose profiles before using insulin pumps, during GDM, in paediatrics, and to detect unrecognised hypoglycaemia rather than for routine home monitoring because of the cost.

CGM meters are still more expensive than other blood glucose meters but the technology has advanced significantly. Four CGM systems were recently introduced and show real time glucose levels on the monitor every five minutes and have hypo- and hyperglycaemia alarms. A significant advantage of CGM is the ability to monitor glucose variability and adjust diabetes management regimen to reduce it because glucose variability is associated with increased risk of complications and mortality; Chapter 8. HbA_{1c} does not measure glucose variability. The four CGMS meters are not all available in every country at the time of writing. The four CGMs meters are:

- Freestyle Navigator (Abbott Diabetes Care).
- Gardian Real-Time (Medtronic MiniMed).
- Dexcom SEVEN (Dexcom).
- GlucoDay (Menarini).

A competent trained team is essential to correctly attaching CGMS, explaining the system to the individual and ensuring they are competent to operate it. Currently CGM is not recommended for routine use in people with diabetes (SIGN 2010).

A system that links CGMS and an insulin pump has been developed, which makes personalised, intensive management possible for those who can afford it. The CGMS system is attached to the body or inserted into the body. Blood glucose information is transferred to the insulin pump, which controls the insulin dose (Kim *et al.* 2012).

Interpreting different results

Patients often comment that their blood glucose results are different from the results obtained using the meter in the outpatient clinic and doctor's rooms or at when they retest their blood glucose after a few minutes. Blood glucose meter tests only reflect individual points in time and may not detect fluctuations in blood glucose especially post prandially and overnight. CGMS is useful to detect such fluctuations.

Different meters give different results even when the tests are performed correctly and close together in time but generally should not differ by more than $< 5\%$. Squeezing the finger to obtain a drop of blood can dilute the sample with tissue fluids and affect the accuracy of the test result.

Likewise, capillary glucose values are likely to differ from laboratory values reported on venous blood. Capillary glucose is ~5% higher than venous glucose. Laboratory values can be affected by glycolysis. Glucose in whole blood decreases by ~5–7% per hour because of the glycolytic enzyme activity in red blood cells. Thus, venous samples should be sent to the laboratory promptly or kept at 4 °C for short periods if it is not possible to transport the sample immediately. Preservatives such as fluoride in blood tubes slow but do not stop glycolysis in blood samples.

People are often confused by the different ways of reporting blood glucose (mmol/L or mg/dL) and HbA_{1c} (% and mmol/mol). Meter blood glucose results may not give an accurate indication of the average blood glucose level or of the minute fluctuations that occur minute-by-minute. Discrepancies between blood glucose meter readings and HbA_{1c} could be used as an opportunity to explore testing technique, other factors that affect the results of both testing methods and the individual's feelings about diabetes and its management. The differences may be a sign of underlying stress, especially in adolescents (Rose *et al.* 2002); see Chapter 13.

Practice point

Incorrect operator technique, inadequate quality control testing, incorrect meter calibration, and using out-of-date test strips are the major causes of inaccurate results using blood glucose meters.

Reasons for inaccurate blood glucose results

Inaccurate blood glucose readings can occur for the following reasons:

(1) Meters and test strips
- using the incorrect strip for the meter;
- using the incorrect calibration or code, although several meters no longer need to be coded;
- using an unclean meter;
- low or flat battery;
- inserting the strip incorrectly or facing the wrong way;
- insufficient blood on the strip will give a false low reading with some older meters;
- quality control tests/calibration are not performed;
- strips used after the expiry date;
- failure to wash hands before testing, especially if sweet substances have been handled;
- humidity and high temperatures affect some meters and/or strips.

If in doubt, repeat the test or confirm biochemically.

Practice points

- It is not necessary to swab the finger with alcohol prior to testing because it can dry the skin. Alcohol swabbing does not alter the blood glucose results (Dunning *et al.* 1994).
- The hands should be washed in soap and water and dried carefully before testing, especially if the person has been handling glucose, for example, in an accident and emergency department/casualty when the person presents with hypoglycaemia.

Monitoring blood ketones

A 10-second capillary blood ketone testing meter is a useful adjunct to blood glucose testing for people with Type 1 diabetes during illness and enables them to detect ketosis and institute treatment or seek a health professional early to prevent ketoacidosis, see Chapter 7. Blood ketone testing is increasingly being used in the clinical setting for the same reasons, as well as giving an indication of the adequacy of the treatment during illness (Wallace *et al.* 2001; ADS 2012).

Blood ketone monitoring is required during sustained hyperglycaemia and can reduce attendances at emergency departments, for example, SIGN (2010) quoted a 50% reduction in the need for a hospital admission for DKA in people testing blood ketones compared with people using urine ketone testing, but the event rates in most trials are small (SIGN 2010). Thus, many guidelines still indicate there is not enough evidence to recommend routine ketone testing in Type 1 Type 1 or Type 2 diabetes. However, there is enough clinical experience to suggest it is warranted in acute illness including in hospital.

Blood ketones are raised after fasting, in the morning, during starvation, may indicate a UTI in non-diabetic patients, after hypoglycaemia not due to excess insulin, some inborn errors of metabolism and ketoacidosis, which is most commonly due to diabetes. Ketosis characteristic of untreated Type 1 diabetes and can occur in LADA and Type 2 diabetes. The main ketone bodies are:

- Acetoacetate, which is an end product of fatty acid metabolism.
- Acetone, which is formed from spontaneous decarboxylation of acetoacetate. Acetone is volatile and is expelled in expired air. It is the ketone responsible for the acetone smell of ketoacidosis.
- Beta-hydroxybutyrate (B-OHB), which is a reduced form of acetoacetate and the major ketone formed in acidosis.

Acetoacetate and beta-hydroxybutyrate are important energy substrates for many tissues especially the brain, particularly during fasting and inadequate food intake. Blood ketone testing for B-OHB is more reliable than urine ketone testing (Fineberg *et al.* 2000). Currently available urine ketone test strips do not measure B-OHB and laboratory ketone testing often does not do so either, unless it is specifically requested.

The ketone meter measures capillary B-OHB, which is the most abundant ketone body and the best guide to the patient's metabolic status: Levels >1 mmol/L require further action, for example, extra insulin, levels >3 mmol/L require medical assessment.

Blood glucose testing checklist

Nursing actions

(1) Assemble materials and prepare environment according to hospital policy and testing system used:
- test strip removed from vial and cap replaced immediately or open foil package;
- dry cotton or rayon ball or tissue to blot the test site if required;
- disposable fingerpricking device or a device with disposable end cap to avoid the possibility of cross-infection from blood left on the device.
(2) Explain procedure to patient.

Obtaining a drop of blood

(3) Wash patient's hands with soap and warm water, dry carefully.
(4) Choose a site on any finger, near the side or tip. Avoid using the pad of the finger where nerves and arteries are concentrated: it is more painful.
(5) Prick finger firmly, using a fingerprick device.
(6) 'Milk' along the length of the finger to well up blood at the puncture site. Avoid squeezing too hard.
(7) Allow the drop of blood to fall onto the strip or be drawn up by capillary action, depending on the type of meter and strips in use.
(8) Dispose of sharps into an appropriate sharps container.

Documenting the results

(1) Record test results on diabetes chart and in any other pertinent record.
(2) Communicate results to appropriate person, for example, the doctor and the patient.

Tips

(a) Warm hands bleed more readily.
(b) If peripheral circulation is deficient, obtaining blood can be difficult. Trap blood in fingertip with one hand, by milking the length of the finger and applying pressure with finger before pricking.
(c) Excess squeezing can dilute the red cells with plasma and lead to inaccurate results.
(d) Check with biochemistry result if the result does not match the clinical picture.

Table 3.1 Blood ketone levels and potential management. It should be noted that these levels are an indication and are not evidence-based (Data from Laffel, L. & Kettyle, W. [2000]).

Blood ketone level (B-OHB)	Potential management
Normal <0.5 mmol/L	
Elevated 0.5–1.5 mmol/L and blood glucose ≥16 mmol/L	Ketosis risk/impending ketosis; insulin dose may need to be increased
	Food intake might be low due to fasting, poor intake or anorexia
Acidosis >1.5 mmol/L and blood glucose >16 mmol	Ketones established and ketoacidosis risk; medical review required
	Insulin required, possibly as an IV infusion
	Infection could be present

People with Type 1 diabetes are advised to test for ketones during illness, hyperglycaemia, pregnancy, if polyuria, polydipsia, and lethargy are present and if they have abdominal pain. Abdominal pain is common in ketoacidosis and usually resolves as the ketosis clears. If it persists it could indicate an abdominal emergency; see Chapter 7. Type 1 patients with hyperglycaemia and HbA_{1c} >8.5%, in association with B-OHB, are insulin deficient and at risk of ketosis. Normal blood B-OHB is 0–0.5 mmol/L. Table 3.1 depicts normal and abnormal ketone levels and suggests the management required.

Testing for ketones is important during illness in:

- all people with Type 1 diabetes;
- people with Type 2 who are severely ill;
- during fasting
- after severe hypoglycaemia:
  ○ severe stress;
  ○ TPN feeds high in glucose or lipids;
  ○ in the operative period.

The rate of fall of B-OHB using blood ketone strips can potentially avoid these situations and improve self-care and enable preventative action to be taken early to avoid ketoacidosis. Blood ketone strips can be used as an indicator of the adequacy of the treatment in acute care settings.

Clinical observation

Lower than actual capillary blood glucose levels can be recorded using some blood glucose meters in the presence of moderate-to-heavy ketosis. The reason for this finding is not clear. As a consequence, health professionals and patients can underestimate the severity of the hyperglycaemia, miss developing ketoacidosis, and delay appropriate treatment.

Practice points

(1) Ketones are present in non-diabetic individuals during fasting and can be detected in 30% of first voided morning urine specimens of pregnant women.

(2) Ketone test strips using nitroprusside reagents (used on urine test strips) give false-positive ketone results in the presence of sulphydryl drugs such as captopril.

(3) Insulin replacement corrects the acidosis by facilitating the conversion of B-OHB into acetoacetate and indicates the ketosis is resolving. However, urine ketone tests can indicate the ketones are still high. That is, urine ketone clearance lags behind actual blood ketone levels.

(4) Urine ketone test strips give false-negative results when they have been exposed to the air for some time, have passed their expiry date and if the urine is highly acidic, such as in a person taking large doses of vitamin C.

Monitoring 2: Urine glucose

Key points

Urine glucose testing is not recommended except in countries that do not have ready access to blood glucose meters or for people who cannot afford to buy a blood glucose meter. (Meters are sometimes supplied without charge in some countries but strips have to be purchased).

If it is used:

• Establish renal threshold to determine the reliability of urine tests.
• Fluid intake, hydration status, urine concentration and time since last voiding affect results.
• Double voiding is unnecessary.
• However, a full urinalysis can provide important clinical information such as the presence of infection, which is often silent in people with diabetes, haematuria and indicates jaundice.

In the presence of normal kidney function, glycosuria is correlated to the blood glucose concentration. Glycosuria occurs when the tubular maximum reabsorption is exceeded, usually around 8–10 mmol/L blood glucose. The test reflects the average glucose during the interval since the person last voided, rather than the level at the time the test is performed. This is called the renal threshold for glucose and varies within and between individuals. The renal threshold may be changed by:

- increasing age
- renal disease
- long-standing diabetes.

Therefore:

- The blood glucose can be elevated without glycosuria being present.
- Traces of glucose in the urine can indicate loss of control.
- The renal threshold can be low in children and glycosuria present when blood glucose is normal.

It is important to establish the renal threshold during a period of good control (normoglycaemia) by simultaneously testing blood and urine glucose.

Practice points

- Urine glucose monitoring is not an accurate reflection of the blood glucose level. In addition, it does not give warning of impending hypoglycaemia.
- A negative urine glucose finding does not indicate hypoglycaemia.
- Double voiding prior to testing is not necessary.

Indications for urine glucose tests

(1) If a person refuses to monitor their blood glucose or cannot afford the equipment.
(2) When the aim is to avoid glycosuria.

Monitoring kidney function

Diabetic nephropathy is the leading cause of end-stage renal disease thus early identification of declining renal function is imperative; see Chapter 8. Twelve- and 24-hour urine collections are used to monitor kidney function and detect early kidney damage by monitoring creatinine clearance rates and microalbumin excretion rates. Microalbuminuria reflects abnormally elevated albumin level not detectable on urine dipsticks. It is the earliest marker of the onset of kidney and cardiovascular damage and predicts deteriorating renal function (Krolewski *et al.* 1995). Up to 30% of newly diagnosed people with Type 1 diabetes already have high urine albumin levels; of these ~75% have microalbuminuria and 25% have overt nephropathy. People with Type 2 in the MICRO-Hope study (HOPE 2000) had a 20% risk of progression from normal to microalbuminuria to nephropathy over 5 years, which is similar to Type 1.

Early diagnosis and treatment can delay the onset by 24 years and decrease the need for dialysis and increase life expectancy (Borch-Johnsen *et al.* 1993). Seventeen per cent of people with essential hypertension develop proteinuria despite satisfactory treatment (Ruilope *et al.* 1990).

Methods of screening for microalbuminuria

Several methods are available and include:

- Timed 12- or 24-hour urine collections.
- Spot urine tests. The first voided morning specimen is often used for initial screening (Jerums *et al.* 1994).
- Random urine tests using dipsticks or automated urine analysers to measure microalbumin and calculate the microalbumin–creatinine ratio (normal level in males is <2 mg/mmol and <2.8 mg/mmol in women). These tests should be negative for protein (Sheldon *et al.* 2002).
- Micral-Test dipstick tests (Boehringer Mannheim, GmbH Mannheim, Germany) is an immunochemical- based urinary dipstick used to test for microalbuminuria and can be used in the ward situation. Compared to radioimmunoassays, Micral-Test has a sensitivity of 92.2% , specificity of 92.3% and a positive predictive value of 37.8% in predicting an albumin excretion rate >20 m/minute (Jerums *et al.* 1994). However, it is not often used clinically in Australia.
- Glomerular filtration rate (GFR). The degree of reduction in the GFR is linked to the development of renal disease. GFR is used as the index to classify the severity of renal disease; see Chapter 8.
- Serum creatinine, which is used as a surrogate marker of GFR is relatively inaccurate (Chadban *et al.* 2003). Significantly, serum creatinine is not reliable in older people; especially those with lean muscle mass who can have creatinine in the normal range despite severely compromised renal disease (Mathew 2003).
- Estimated GFR (e-GFR) is calculated using a predictive equation that uses serum creatinine, age, and gender. It is less accurate in Chinese people and possibly other Asian peoples and Indigenous Australians (Zuo *et al.* 2005). In the US, the Modification of Diet in Renal Disease (MDRD) is a valid method of determining e-GFR and classifying renal disease (National Kidney Foundation 2002). e-GFR may be unreliable in the following situations:
  - acute changes in kidney function;
  - people on dialysis;
  - high protein and high vegetable diets and those who take creatinine supplements;
  - skeletal muscle diseases such as paraplegia and amputees.
  - those with high muscle mass;
  - in the presence of severe liver disease;
  - when the e-GFR is >60 mL/min/1.73 m^2;
  - children <18 years;
  - Asian peoples;
  - Maori and Pacific Islander peoples;
  - Aboriginal and Torres Strait Islander peoples.

Microalbuminuria is diagnosed when the urine albumin level is >30 mg/dL and is expressed as the quantity of albumin excreted in a given time (>20 m/minute) or as a concentration (>20 m/L urine). Most experts prefer the albumin–creatinine ratio because the other tests can be affected by the concentration of the urine.

Nurses have a role in screening and detecting declining renal function and educating the person about appropriate preventative measures. If timed urine collections are needed, the procedure for collecting the urine should be explained to the patient carefully. Written instructions should be supplied if the collection is to be performed at home. Collections are best obtained at a period of good control and normal activity, not during illness or menstruation; therefore, the urine is often collected on an outpatient basis. The opportunity can be taken during a hospital admission to collect 12- or 24-hour timed urine collections when people repeatedly fail to collect them as outpatients. In some cases the first early morning voided specimen will be collected ~50 mL.

Ensure the correct containers are used for the collection and the specimen is correctly labelled.

Monitoring 3: Additional assessment

In addition to blood and urine testing, diabetic status is assessed by:

(1) Psychological and emotional health and wellbeing (Chapter 15).
(2) Self-care capacity.
(3) Regular weight checks. Height is also required to calculate BMI. Waist circumference is preferred and sometimes arm circumference in older people.
(4) Regular physical examination, especially:
  - blood pressure (lying and standing to detect any postural drop that could indicate the presence of autonomic neuropathy);
  - eyes (retina) and visual acuity;
  - cardiac status;
  - feet;
  - kidney function;
  - driving safety, especially in older people.
(5) Regular education about:
  - diet;
  - self-monitoring techniques;
  - injection sites;
  - general diabetes information, especially new technology and research findings that need to be discussed in the context of the individual; see Chapter 16;
  - changes to diabetes care as a result of research.

Specific age groups such as children (Chapter 13) and older people (Chapter 12) require additional assessment such as physical and mental functioning and psychological status (Chapter 15).

Practice point

Normal ranges for the tests described differ among laboratories depending on the assay methods used. It is helpful if people attend the same pathology service to have blood and urine tests performed.

Nursing responsibilities

(1) To have a basic knowledge of the tests in order to be able to explain them to the patient.
(2) Ensure patients who are required to fast are given appropriate *written* instructions before the test about their medications and any other preparation required.
(3) To ensure the correct collection technique, appropriate amount of blood and correct tubes are used.

(4) Mix the sample by inverting the tube two or three times if an anticoagulant tube is required. Vigorous shaking causes haemolysis of red blood cells, which affects the results.
(5) To ensure the specimen reaches the laboratory within 30 minutes of collection or be refrigerated to prevent glycolysis occurring and consequent inaccurate results.
(6) To ensure results are available for medical evaluation.
(7) To know the effects of illness and stress on the results of the test.
(8) To ensure the appropriate sterile blood collection technique is used.
(9) To ensure appropriate disposal of used equipment, and to protect themselves from needlestick injury.
(10) To ensure patients are given their medication and something to eat after completing tests when fasting is required and that they are informed about when to recommence any medications that were temporarily stopped, and the doses to take.

Blood glucose

Venous glucose is measured to:

• Screen for and diagnose diabetes.
• Monitor effectiveness of and determine the need for glucose lowering medicines and the dose and dose frequency.
• Evaluate glycaemic control.
• Confirm high/low capillary glucose result.

Glycosylated or glycated haemoglobin (HbA$_{1c}$)

It is most useful to have the HbA$_{1c}$ result at the time the person is assessed by the doctor/diabetes educator. Blood can be drawn from a vein and measured in the laboratory before the clinic/doctor visit so the result is available at the time of the consultation. Alternatively, blood can be drawn from a fingerprick sample at the time of the visit using devices such as the DCA 2000 (Bayer) analyser.

Circulating blood glucose attaches to the haemoglobin in the red blood cells and undergoes an irreversible non-enzymatic interaction with amino groups of lysine and valine residues in haemoglobin (Amadori reaction) whereby the glucose becomes permanently fixed to the haemoglobin (glycosylation). The glycosylated haemoglobin, HbA$_{1c}$ (A$_{1c}$ in the US) can be measured and quantified to give an indication of the average blood glucose concentration over the preceding 3 months (normal 4–5.9%) and to predict risk of long-term diabetes complications (Bloomgarden 2007; Kilpatrick *et al.* 2007). Currently, four main assays and ~20 different measurement methods are used that measure different glycated products and report different units (% HbA$_{1c}$, % HbA$_1$, and total GHb) (Colman *et al.* 2008). The four assay methods are: ion-exchange chromatography, electrophoresis, affinity chromatography, and immunoassay.

Fasting prior to obtaining the blood sample for HbA$_{1c}$ is not necessary. Tests are usually performed at least three months apart but can be done sooner to gauge the effect of a treatment modification and in research.

Kirkpatrick *et al.* (2007) pointed out that HbA$_{1c}$ is a proxy measure of average blood glucose and can be misleading because individuals are higher or lower glycosylators at specific mean blood glucose levels, which emphasises the importance of considering the individual and the overall clinical picture.

Current assay methods use a mixture of glycated haemoglobins to determine the HbA$_{1c}$. Representatives from the American Diabetes Association, The European Association for the Study of Diabetes, the International Diabetes Federation and the International Federation of Clinical Chemistry and Laboratory Medicine (IFCC) have been discussing methods of standardising HbA$_{1c}$ measurement for a number of years and released a consensus statement in Milan in 2007 (Consensus Committee 2007).

Key recommendations were:

- Standardising the method of measuring HbA_{1c} and the reference system used to report results.
- The IFCC reference system is the only currently valid method of measuring HbA_{1c} and should be used as the basis to standardise HbA_{1c} measurements.
- The results should be reported in IFCC units (mmol/mol) and derived national Glycohaemoglobin. Standardisation Program Units (NGSP) (%) should be calculated using the IFCC-NGSP master equation.
- Laboratories should be able to maintain a CV <3% at HbA_{1c} between 6 and 9% and manufacturer's assays should have a CV <5% (Colman *et al.* 2008).
- If the ongoing 'average plasma glucose study' using frequent capillary glucose measurements and continuous glucose monitoring due to be published in early 2008 fulfills its priori-specified criteria, an A_{1c}-derived average glucose value (ADAG) should also be reported (Nathan 2007). The ADAG value is calculated from the individual's A_{1c} result to deduce an estimate of their average blood glucose (O'siordan 2007).
- That clinical guidelines be revised and glycaemic targets be expressed as IFCC units, derived NGSP units, and ADAG.

Consequently education programmes for health professionals and people with diabetes are being developed and a smart phone app is available to convert % HbA_{1c} to mmol/mol, the new measurement units.

Glycaemic targets should not be considered independently of other risk factors for complications such as hyperlipidaemia, hypertension and smoking, age and comorbidities. HbA_{1c} targets differ slightly among various guidelines. It is generally accepted that targets should be:

- As low as possible to reduce the likelihood of microvascular complications. Most recommend <6.5% or <7% for most people with Type 2 diabetes.
- Individualised for specific patients after discussing the risks and benefits with them. For example, children, older and frail people, and those with limited life expectancy might require higher targets (<8%) and those at very high risk of microvascular complications may need lower targets (range 7–7.5%).
- Avoid adverse events such as frequent hypoglycaemia.

Practice points

- People who experience frequent hypoglycaemic episodes may have a low HbA_{1c} that might not reflect their complication risk.
- HbA_{1c} results should be evaluated as part of the total clinical picture and not viewed in isolation.
- HbA_{1c} does not represent the blood glucose profile, but gives an average level. It is considered to be the 'gold standard' for monitoring metabolic control.

Table 3.2 lists some factors that might affect HbA_{1c} results.

Fructosamines
The fructosamines are a group of glycosylated blood and tissue proteins that reflect the average blood glucose levels within the preceding three weeks. Fructosamine results can be lower in patients with low serum albumin, cirrhosis of the liver or haemoglobinopathies.

Table 3.2 Non-glycaemic factors that can affect results of glycosylated haemoglobin assays.

False high	False low
Chronic alcohol abuse	Anaemia
Foetal haemoglobin	Abnormal haemoglobins such as
Hyperlipidaemia	HbS, HbC, HbD found in some
Hyperbilirubinaemia	ethnic groups
Renal failure	Chronic blood loss
Splenectomy	Haemolysis
	Haemorrhage
	Recent blood transfusion

Fructosamine estimations are not performed very often but they are useful for monitoring:

- diabetes during pregnancy;
- initial response to diabetes medication;
- patients with chronic anaemia;
- patients with haemoglobinopathies.

Serum lipids

Serum lipids are usually elevated if the blood glucose is elevated. Three classes of lipids are measured as shown with the target range in brackets:

(1) Cholesterol (<4.0)
(2) Triglycerides (<1.5)
(3) Lipoproteins:
- very low-density lipoprotein (VLDL)
- low-density lipoprotein (LDL) (<2.5)
- high-density lipoprotein (HDL) (>1.0).

Although it is generally accepted that fasting blood lipid levels are most useful, recent research suggests non-fasting levels correlate more closely with cardiovascular risk (Bansal *et al.* 2007; Vardo *et al.* 2007). However, there are many forms of hypertriglyceridaemia and more research is needed to determine the exact relationship with atherosclerosis. High lipids, especially elevated triglycerides and LDL, and low HDL is a common lipid profile in people with poorly controlled Type 2 diabetes, which may be secondary to hyperglycaemia, and is a clinical useful measure of the need for lipid-lowering medications such as fibrates, fish oil concentrates or nicotinic acid depending on the type of lipid abnormality present; see Chapter 5.

Alcohol should not be consumed for 24 hours before the blood sample for serum lipid measurements is taken.

C-peptide

C-peptide is the connecting peptide, which determines the folding of the two insulin chains during insulin production and storage in the pancreas. It splits off in the final stages and can be measured in the blood. It is used to measure endogenous insulin production, to determine the type of diabetes (along with various antibodies; see Chapter 1) if it is not clear in the clinical presentation. C-peptide is present in normal or elevated amounts in Type 2 diabetes, indicating that insulin is being produced and that diet and/ or OHAs with exercise could achieve acceptable control. However, progressive beta cell loss occurs in Type 2 diabetes and C-peptide levels fall proportionally.

C-peptide is absent or low in people with Type 1 diabetes and can be a useful indicator in slow onset Type 1 diabetes (LADA) occurring in adults (Cohen 1996); see Chapter 1. C-peptide is not changed by injecting exogenous insulin. Fasting results are most useful.

Islet cell antibodies

Islet cell antibodies (ICA) are found in most newly diagnosed people with Type 1 diabetes, indicating that diabetes is an autoimmune disease. The beta cells of the pancreas are the specific target in diabetes and other pancreatic functions are not affected. In the laboratory, impaired insulin release can be demonstrated when ICA are present but the clinical implication is still unclear.

ICA are present in the prediabetic state before the disease is clinically obvious. They can also be present in close relatives who are at high risk of developing diabetes if they have ICA.

GAD antibodies are also present in 80% of people with Type 1 diabetes and enable it to be distinguished from Type 2 diabetes (Cohen 1996); see Chapter 1.

Creatinine clearance and urea

As indicated, creatinine clearance is used to estimate renal function. It is also used to determine nutritional status in relation to protein especially during TPN and continuous ambulatory peritoneal dialysis (CAPD). An increase in the blood urea nitrogen (BUN) may indicate impaired renal function; however, the BUN can also be increased if the patient is dehydrated, has internal bleeding or is on steroids. Anorexia, a low protein diet and fasting can lead to a decrease in urea.

Self-care

The key aspects of self-care are discussed in Chapter 16. Generally assuming responsibility for self-care is an iterative process that falls into three main categories:

(1) Focusing on diabetes after diagnosis to acquire the knowledge and skills, master the self-management tasks and make life adjustments needed to perform diabetes self-care, which involves individuals and their family/carers. It takes time to accept diabetes and master these significant life changes. Some people take a long time, others adapt quickly depending on social, environmental and a range of other factors.
(2) Activating resources, which encompasses being able to identify relevant resources and using them effectively to support their self-care activities. Resources might be family, friends, health professionals, Internet and other media as well as local resources such as libraries, churches, meals on wheels and transport.
(3) Living with diabetes: people cope with diabetes and successfully integrate it into their lifestyle and grow as individuals (Schulman-Green *et al.* 2012). This essential stable phase can easily be disrupted by life events and when a complication develops, and the person needs to readapt.

Nurses can ask four simple questions to help make a decision about an individual's diabetes self-care capacity:

(1) Does the individual have the knowledge and skills to manage their diabetes to the best of their ability?
(2) Has the individual access to appropriate resources, equipment, support and health professional advice?
(3) Is the individual satisfied with their life at present?
(4) Are their cultural issues that need to be considered?

Nurses are in an ideal situation to help determine the barriers to optimal self-care and potential medicine non-adherence (Chapter 5). Barriers might be physical, financial/economic, psychological, cognitive, health literacy/numeracy, social and environmental (Baumann & Dang 2012). Motivational interviewing, active listening, reflecting, clarifying, being present in the moment (fully focused on the individual and their story) and involving the individual in making management decisions and setting goals and targets is essential.

The annual review

The annual review is a structured nursing and medical review undertaken in general practice to:

- review management goals;
- assess diabetes complication status;
- determine whether referral to one of more specialists is warranted.
- revise the immunisation schedule;
- undertake other important monitoring process as indicated (Diabetes Australia/Royal Australian college of General Practitioners 2011/12).

Many of the assessments discussed in this chapter are encompassed in the annual review.

References

Australian Diabetes Society (ADS) (2012) *Position statement individualization of HbA1c targets for adults with diabetes mellitus*. ADS, Canberra.

Bansal, S, Buning S, Rifai N. *et al* (2007) Fasting compared with nonfasting triglycerides and risk of cardiovascular events in women. *Journal of the American Medical Association*, **18** (298), 309–316.

Baumann, L. & Dang, T. (2012) Helping patients with chronic conditions overcome barriers to care. *Nurse Practitioner* **37** (3), 32–38.

Bloomgarden, Z. (2007) Glucose variability. Comment on sessions presented during the 67th American Diabetes Association, Scientific Sessions June 22–26, Chicago, Illinois. http://www.medscape.com/viewarticle/560754 (accessed January 2008).

Borch-Johnsen, K., Wenzel, H., Vibert, G. & Mogensen, C. (1993) Is screening and intervention for microalbuminuria worthwhile in patients with IDDM? *British Medical Journal*, **306**, 1722–1725.

Canadian Diabetes Association (2008) *Reduce your risk of serious complications associated with diabetes*. www.canadiandiabetes association.ca (accessed on 9 January 2008).

Chadban, S., Briganti, E. & Kerr, P. (2003) Prevalence of kidney disease in Australian adults: the AusDiabe kidney study. *Journal of the American Society of Nephrologists*, **14** (7) (Suppl. 2), S121–S138.

Cohen, M. (1996) *Diabetes: A Handbook of Management*. International Diabetes Institute, Melbourne.

Colman, P., Goodall, I., Garcia-Webb, P., Williams, P. & Dunlop, M. (2008) Glycohaemoglobin: a crucial measurement in modern diabetes management. Progress towards standardization and improved precision of measurement. *EMJA* http://www.mja.com.au/public/issues/jul21/colan/colman. html (acessed February 2008).

Consensus Committee (2007) Consensus Statement on the Worldwide Standardisation of the Haemoglobin A_{1c} Measurement. The American Diabetes Association, European Association for the Study of Diabetes, International Federation of Clinical Chemistry and Laboratory Medicine, International Diabetes Federation. *Diabetes Care*, **30**, 2399–2400.

Davis, T., & Bruce, D. (2006) Is self-monitoring of blood glucose appropriate for all Type 2 diabetic patients? The Freemantle Diabetes Study. *Diabetes Care*, **29**, 1764–1770.

RACGP/DA (Royal Australian College of General Practitioners & Diabetes Australia) 2011/12) *Diabetes Management in General Practice: Guidelines for Type 2 Diabetes* DA & RACGP, Canberra.

Diabetes UK (2012) *End of life diabetes care*. Diabetes UK, London.

Dunning, T., Rantzau, C. & Ward, G. (1994) Effect of alcohol swabbing on capillary blood glucose. *Practical Diabetes*, **11** (4), 251–254.

Dunning, T. (1996) Corticosteroid medications and diabetes mellitus. *Practical Diabetes International*, **13** (6), 186–188.

Farmer, A. (2007) Self-monitoring of blood glucose does not improve HbA_{1c} levels in patients with non-insulin treated diabetes: The DIGEM study. Presented during the 67th American Diabetes Association, Scientific Sessions June 22–26, Chicago, Illinois. Also published in the *British Medical Journal Online* June 6, 2007.

Fineberg, S. (2000) Comparison of blood beta-hydroxybutyrate and urine ketones in 4 weeks of home monitoring by insulin-requiring children and adults. American Diabetes Association Scientific Meeting, USA, June.

HOPE (Outcomes Prevention Evaluation Study Investigators) (2000) Effects of ramipril on cardiovascular and microvascular outcomes in people with diabetes. *Results of HOPE and MICRO-HOPE substudy. Lancet*, **355**, 253–259.

International Diabetes Federation (IDF) (2007) *Guideline for Management of Postmeal Glucose*. IDF, Brussels.

International Diabetes Federation (IDF) (2012) The Global NCD Framework. IDF, Brussels.

Jerums, G., Cooper, M., O'srien, R. & Taft, J. (1994) ADS Position Statement 1993: Microalbuminuria and diabetes. *Medical Journal of Australia*, **161**, 265–268.

Jungheim, K. & Koschinsky, T. (2002) Glucose monitoring at the arm: Evaluation of upper dermal blood glucose kinetics during rapid systemic blood glucose changes. *Hormone Metabolism Research*, **34**, 325–329.

Kilpatrick, E., Rigby, A. & Atkin, S. (2007) Variability in the relationship between mean plasma glucose and HbA_{1c}: Implications for the assessment of glycaemic control. *Clinical Chemistry*, **53**, 897–901.

Kim H.S., Shin J.A., Chang J.S. *et al.* (2012) Continuous glucose monitoring: current clinical use. *Diabetes Metabolism Research Reviews* **28** (Suppl 2), 73–78.

Laffel, L. & Kettyle, W. (2000) Frequency of elevations in blood b-hydroxybutyrate (B-OHB) during home monitoring and association with glycaemia in insulin-treated children and adults. *Proceedings, ADA Scientific Meeting*, USA.

Monsod, T., Flanagan, D. & Rife, F. (2002) Do sensor glucose levels accurately predict plasma glucose concentrations during hypoglycaemia and hyperinsulinaemia? *Diabetes Care*, **15**, 899–893.

Nathan, D. (2007) The problem with ADAGE (A1c-derived average glucose equivalent). 67th American Diabetes Association, Scientific Sessions June 22–26, Chicago, Illinois.

O'siordan, M. (2007) Average blood glucose instead of HbA_{1c}? Change appears to be coming for diabetes care. *Heartwire*, July 3. http://www.medscape.com.viewarticle/559262 (accessed December 2007).

Parchman, M., Pugh, J., Romero, R. & Bowers, K. (2007) Competing demands or clinical inertia: The case of elevated glycosylated hemoglobin. *Annals of Family Medicine*, **5** (3), 196–201.

Rose, M., Fliege, H., Hildebrandt, M., Schirop, T. & Klapp, B. (2002) The network of psychological variables in patients with diabetes and their importance for quality of life and metabolic control. *Diabetes Care*, **25**, 35–42.

Ruilope, L., Alcazar, J., Hernandez, E. & Rodico, J. (1990) Does an adequate control of blood pressure protect the kidney in essential hypertension? *Journal of Hypertension*, **8**, 525–531.

Schneider, M., Heinemann, B., Lodwig, L. *et al.* (2006) The ROSSO Study group: self-monitoring of blood glucose in Type 2 diabetes and long term outcome: An epidemiological study. *Diabetologia*, **49**, 271–278.

Schulman-Green D., Jases S. & Martin F. (2012) Self-management in chronic illness. *Journal of Nursing Scholarship* **44**, 136–144.

SIGN (Scottish Intercollegiate Guidelines Network) (2010) SIGN, *Management of Diabetes: a national Guideline*, Edinburgh.

Sonksen, P., Fox, C. & Judd, C. (1998) *Diabetes at Your Fingertips*. Class Publishing, London, p. 105.

Varbo A, Benn M, Tybjaerg-Hansen A. *et al.* (2007) Nonfasting triglycerides and risk of myocardial infarction, ischemic heart disease, and death in men and women. *Journal of the American Medical Association*, **18** (298), 299–308.

Wallace, T., Meston, N., Gardnert, S. & Matthews, D. (2001) The hospital and home use of a 30-second hand-held blood ketone meter: Guidelines for clinical practice. *Diabetes Medicine*, **18** (8), 640–645.

Wei N., Wexler D., Nathan D. & Grant R. (2013) Intensification of diabetes medication and risk for 30-day readmission. *Diabetes Medicine* **30** (2), e56–62.

Zuo, L., Ma, Y. & Zhou, Y. (2005) Application of GFR – estimating equations in Chinese patients with chronic kidney disease. *American Journal of Kidney Diseases*, **45**, 463–472.

Further reading

Garg, S., Potts, R., Ackerman, *et al.* (1999) Correlation of fingerstick blood glucose measurements with Glucowatch biographer glucose results in young subjects with Type 1 diabetes. *Diabetes Care*, **22**, 1708–1714.

Kolb, H., Schneider, B., Heinemann, L., Lodwig, V. & Martin, S. (2007) Is self-monitoring of blood glucose appropriate for all Type 2 diabetic patients? Comment on the the Freemantle Diabetes Study. *Diabetes Care*, **30**, 183–184.

McGowan, K., Thomas, W. & Moran, A. (2002) Spurious reporting of nocturnal hypoglycaemia by CGMS in patients with tightly controlled Type 1 diabetes. *Diabetes Care*, **25**, 1499–1503.

Weinstein, R., Schwartz, S., Brazg, R. *et al.* (2007) Accuracy of the 5-day Freestyle navigator Continuous Glucose Monitoring system: Comparison with frequent laboratory reference measurements. *Diabetes Care*, **30**, 1125–1130.

Chapter 4
Nutrition, Obesity and Exercise

Key points

- Obesity is an increasing global health issue.
- Obesity is associated with more than 30 medical conditions and affects many other conditions. Weight loss can improve some obesity-related conditions including the metabolic syndrome, Type 2 diabetes, hypertension, and reduce cardiovascular risk.
- The relationship between weight, health outcomes and life expectancy is complex and is affected by genetic make-up and, significantly, environmental factors, which may play a more dominant role.
- Population-based and targeted screening and prevention programmes are required to address the problem.
- Dietary advice for people with diabetes is applicable to the whole population. However, specific dietary advice should be individualised
- Diet and exercise continue to be the cornerstone of diabetes management even when medicines are required.
- Regular dietary assessment is advisable.

Rationale

Good nutrition is vital to health and well being and is an essential basis of diabetes management. Obesity is a significant health problem and a major risk factor for serious disease including Type 2 diabetes. Managing obesity is difficult. Regular nutritional assessment is important to maintain the optimal health of people with diabetes as their general health, age and diabetes-related circumstances change.

Care of People with Diabetes: A Manual of Nursing Practice, Fourth Edition. Trisha Dunning.
© 2014 John Wiley & Sons, Ltd. Published 2014 by John Wiley & Sons, Ltd.

The importance of good nutrition

Good nutrition is essential to health. Inadequate nutrition leads to many diseases and affects the primary condition and response to treatment (Sydney-Smith 2000). Sixty per cent of deaths are related to nutritional factors, for example, diabetes-associated cardio-vascular disease (Middleton *et al.* 2001). In particular, micronutrients and protein intake are often inadequate and mineral deficiencies are common in Australia, especially in people living in poverty.

Diets low in vitamins and minerals are also deficient in antioxidants that modulate oxidative tissue damage. Oxidative tissue damage is implicated in the development of long-term diabetes-related complications and is compounded by smoking, excess alcohol intake and chronic inflammatory diseases; see Chapter 8. Vitamins C, E, and A and some plant chemicals (phytochemicals) are naturally occurring antioxidants derived from a well-balanced diet.

Obesity

Obesity is defined as excess body fat and is now recognised as a disease in its own right (Marks 2000; James & Coster 2011). Obesity is emerging as a complex phenomena caused by a number of inter-related factors including high fat energy-dense diets, inadequate amounts of exercise, and genetic, hormonal and environmental factors (Brunner & McCarthy 2001; Bouchard *et al.* 2004; Freyling 2007; Unger & Scherer 2010). The estimated risk of becoming obese using data from the Framlingham Study suggests a normal weight person has a 50% long-term risk of becoming overweight and 25% risk of becoming obese (Reynolds *et al.* 2005). However, a number of studies suggest underweight might confer greater health risks, especially in older people (Diehr *et al.* 1998, 2008).

A recent study suggests normal weight people with Type 2 diabetes are more likely to die from any cause than heavier people with Type 2 diabetes over 10–30 years after adjusting for demographic factors, smoking and cardiovascular risk (Carnethon *et al.*2012). Cardiovascular mortality risk in normal weight individuals was higher by 50% and non-cardiovascular risk more than double of than those in overweight individuals, which is consistent with the so called 'obesity paradox.' Unlike most researchers, Carnethon (2012) measured BMI when diabetes was diagnosed, which helped control for the effect of diabetes duration on complication status. However, lower body weight might be associated with underlying illness or nutritional deficiencies that predisposes individuals to morbidity and mortality risk.

Some medicines such as corticosteroids, antipsychotics, birth control medicines, insulin, sulphonylureas, and thiazolidinediones (TZDs) contribute to weight gain; see Chapter 5. There is increasing evidence that ethnicity, environmental factors, social isolation, being teased about weight, low self-esteem and low global self-worth contribute to obesity in children (Goodman & Whitaker 2002; Eisenberg *et al.* 2003). Contributing environmental factors include sedentary behaviour including excess television viewing (Wilmot *et al.* 2012), insufficient physical activity, which might be influenced by living in unsafe areas, and high consumption of fast foods (Burdett & Whitaker 2005).

The prevalence of overweight and obesity are increasing globally but there are differences among populations and among ethnic groups within populations. Rates of overweight and obesity are also increasing in children and adolescents. A child with one overweight parent has a 40% chance of becoming overweight and the risk increases to 80% when both parents are overweight. A recent Dutch study showed that more than 75% of severely obese children younger than 18 already has one or more cardiovascular risk factors. Significantly, 62% of severely obese children younger than 12 years have one or more cardiovascular risk factors. Many also have hypertension, low HDL cholesterol and impaired fasting glucose (Chapter 13).

Obesity prevents people from undertaking many self-care tasks and activities of daily living and increases the burden on joints leading to pain and discomfort that limits exercise capability. In addition, obesity makes it difficult for health professionals to perform some preventative health care interventions such as cervical smears and mammograms, and overweight women are more likely to have false-positive results in these tests than non-obese women (Elmore *et al.* 2004).

Overview of the pathogenesis of obesity

As indicated, environmental factors play an important role in the development of obesity and its related diseases. A simplistic explanation is: increased food intake leads to weight gain and obesity, which lead to insulin resistance and impaired insulin action in muscle, liver and fat tissue. The pancreas compensates by secreting extra insulin (hyperinsulinaemia). In the long term the beta cells become exhausted and hyperglycaemia and hypertriglyceridaemia develop (James & Coster 2011). In addition, a novel hypothesis suggests diet-induced obese people homeostatically guard their weight (Spreadbury 2012).

Abdominal fat is not inert. It produces signalling molecules, adipokines, which exacerbate endothelial dysfunction. A number of adipokines are produced; see Table 4.1. In addition, the endocannabinoid (CRB) neuroregulatory system influences the activity of other neurotransmitter systems including hormone secretion and modulates immune and inflammatory responses. Likewise, understanding of the role of

Table 4.1 Effects of adipokines and changes that occur in the presence of abdominal obesity, which demonstrates their role in the development of insulin resistance, Type 2 diabetes and cardiovascular disease.

Name of adipokine	Effects in the body	Effect of increasing abdominal obesity on adipokine levels
Tumour necrosis factor-alpha	Disrupts insulin signalling processes in the cell membranes Reduces endothelial vasodilatation by reducing nitric oxide	Higher
Interleukin-6	Stimulates rate of C-reactive protein release from the liver Induces insulin resistance Damages endothelial function	Higher
Plasminogen Activator Inhibitor-1	Enhances prothrombotic state	Higher
Leptin	Regulates: • appetite • energy expenditure • insulin sensitivity Stimulates the sympathetic nervous system Acts as a signalling factor in hypertension	Higher
Adiponectin	Improves tissue sensitivity Anti-inflammatory Reduces atherogenesis	Lower
Angiotensinogen	Contributes to hypertension	Higher

leptin-resistance on satiety mediators and white adipose tissue in regulating body metabolism, insulin sensitivity, and food intake has increased rapidly over the past few years (Spreadbury 2012).

The CRB system consists of many endocannabinoids including CB_1 and CB_2. CB_1 occurs through the body including in the brain, adipose tissue, vascular endothelium and sympathetic nerve terminals. CB_2 mostly occurs in lymph tissue and macrophages. In addition, a number of endocannabinoid subtypes exist whose function is yet to be determined. Endocannabinoids regulate metabolism in a number of ways. Blocking CB_1 reduces food intake, abdominal fat, triglycerides, LDL, C-reactive protein (CRP), and insulin resistance, and it increases HDL.

Activating CB_1 has the opposite effect. Data from the RIO-Europe Trial showed significant weight reductions and reduction in cardiometabolic risk factors such as waist circumference, triglyceride levels and elevated HDL using the CB_1 blocker, Rimonabant, compared to controls (van Gaal 2005). The latter effects occurred independently of weight loss. People taking Rimonabant averaged 4.7 kg weight loss after a year and were more likely to achieve a 10% weight loss than controls.

White adipose tissue has many functions including acting as a storage depot for triglycerides. It is regarded as an endocrine organ that secretes a range of adipokines, which influence weight, inflammation, coagulation, fibrinolysis, tissue response to insulin, and contributes to the development of metabolic syndrome and Type 2 diabetes. Energy balance is impaired and obesity results if white adipose tissue function is disrupted (Iqbal 2007); see Table 4.1. Ghrelin is produced in the stomach and mediates hunger. Restricting calories and exercising increases Ghrelin levels (Leidy *et al.* 2007).

Adipose tissue has a major role in hormone metabolism such as synthesising oestrogen in postmenopausal women, which is protective against osteoporosis (Moyad 2004). Likewise, replacing testosterone preserves skeletal muscle and reduces abdominal obesity in non-obese men over 50 years whose testosterone level is <15 nM (Allan 2009). Thus, it contributes to overall well-being.

The significance of abdominal obesity

People with central or abdominal obesity are at increased risk of obesity-related diseases such as metabolic syndrome, Type 2 diabetes, dyslipidaemia, fatty liver, and therefore, are at significant risk of cardiovascular disease. Obesity is a risk factor for shortened life expectancy in younger but not older people (Heiat *et al.* 2001) and the importance of overweight and obesity as predictors of health status decline in people >65 years. In fact, some research indicates being overweight is associated with better quality of life and health status in older people (Stevens 2000).

Waist circumference is significantly correlated with triglyceride levels, CRP, cholesterol and glucose, but not HbA_{1c} in healthy women (Behan & Mbizo 2007). Likewise, the INTERHEART Study Group (2005) demonstrated that waist circumference is strongly related to myocardial infarction but the level of risk is unclear. Physical fitness may reduce the inflammation associated with abdominal obesity and reduce cardiovascular risk (Zoeller 2007).

Various cardiovascular risk scores have been developed based on parameters such as age, gender, total cholesterol, LDL, systolic blood pressure, being treated for hypertension and smoking, for example, The Framlingham Risk Score (Expert Panel on Detection, Evaluation, and Treatment of High Blood Cholesterol in Adults (2002) and the Systemic Coronary Risk Evaluation (SCORE) (Third Joint Taskforce of European and Other Societies on Cardiovascular Disease Prevention in Clinical Practice (2003).

However, a 12-year US study of people in their sixties suggests obese people live as long as people of normal weight and are less likely to develop diabetes or lipid abnormalities if they are fit. However, at BMI >30 people experience difficulty performing usual activities of daily living and develop other obesity-related disorders such as musculoskeletal disease that cause pain, lower muscle strength and reduce cardiovascular fitness (ABC Health and Well Being 2007). Thus, the focus on weight management must also include reducing/managing obesity-related disability.

Other obesity-related diseases include osteoarthritis, rheumatoid arthritis and other musculoskeletal diseases, some forms of cancer, for example, breast, oesophagus, colorectal, endometrial and renal cell cancers, sleep apnoea and daytime sleepiness (Chapter 10), gout, urinary stress incontinence, and surgical complications. Significantly, maternal obesity is associated with a higher incidence of birth defects (Chapters 1 and 14).

Nutrition, obesity and stress

There is a complex association among nutrition, stress and overweight/obesity. Stress affects eating behaviour: most people eat more and gain weight; 30% reduce weight (Stone & Brownell 1994) but the reasons for the increased intake are unclear. Likewise, Fiegal *et al.* 2002) found people are concerned about life stress and 50% eat more calorie dense food when they are stressed, and undertake less activity. A suggested mechanism for the effect of stress on weight is that cortisol levels increase during stress, which stimulates appetite: managing stress reduces stress-related intake. In addition, chronic low level stress reduces insulin sensitivity and contributes to abdominal obesity and the metabolic syndrome.

Significantly, 45% of women and 23% of men think they are overweight and 20% of underweight women think they are overweight and are dieting to lose weight (Better Health Channel, January 2008). People use a range of self-initiated strategies to lose weight, which are often successful initially, but regain half to two thirds of the weight lost in the first 12 months and nearly all within 5 years. In contrast, the NHANES 1999–2002 showed 58% of people who lost >5% of their bodyweight maintained the weight loss for up to 5 years.

Factors associated with weight gain in NAHANES included:

- Mexican-American peoples;
- significant weight loss;
- fewer years since reaching their maximum weight;
- long time spent watching TV: children and adults;
- attempting to control weight;
- sedentary lifestyle;
- frequent attempts to diet were associated with increased risk of developing an eating disorder.

Ethnic differences could partly explain the different findings. In addition, people who are supported to lose weight are more likely to stay motivated than those who 'go it alone.' Self-perception and body image influence quality of life and mood and there is a pervasive association among perception of being overweight, depression and disordered body image.

Methods of measuring weight

Measuring obesity is difficult. A number of methods are used. Each has advantages and disadvantages.

Crude weight

Weighing people is the simplest way to estimate obesity using height/weight standards. It does not take into account muscular builds at different heights or that lean body mass weighs more than fat tissue. Mild obesity = 20–40% overweight; moderate obesity = 41–100%, and severe obesity = twice the actual weight for height. Crude weight and BMI are useful to track weight changes over time but weighing is best undertaken using the same scales at the same rime of day wearing the same clothing.

Body mass index

The Body Mass Index (BMI), sometimes referred to as Quetelet's Index, is a simple method of assessing obesity but, like crude weight, it does not take into account muscular builds at different heights. However, despite the limitations BMI >30 generally indicates excess adipose tissue. BMI should be interpreted according to growth charts in children. BMI is calculated using the following formula: weight in kilograms divided by height in metres squared.

Waist-hip ratio

The waist-hip ratio (WHR) is measured with the person standing and specifically measures abdominal obesity. The waist is defined as the largest abdominal circumference midway between the costal margin and the iliac crest. A WHR >90 in men and >80 in women is generally regarded as an accurate predictor of obesity-related disorders, independently of the BMI. WHR can be affected by postprandial status, time of day, and depth of inspiration to an unknown degree. It includes both intra-abdominal fat (the area of interest) and subcutaneous fat, but it is not clear how to adjust the WHR for subcutaneous fat. There are also differences among ethnic groups that need to be considered. It is useful to record the WHR on a regular basis.

Other ways of measuring body fat include:

- Dual energy X-ray absorptiometry (DEXA), which is often used in research and to determine risk of osteoporosis. Lean body mass, skin fold thickness, densitometry hydrostatic weighing and bioelectrical impedance analysis are other ways to measure obesity.
  Strategies used to measure food consumption:
  A number of tools are used to estimate food intake over various time periods. These include:

- Food records: the individual keeps a detailed record of their intake for varying periods from three to seven days. Maintaining a food record can be burdensome and requires the person to be literate. In addition, actually recording intake often influences the person to consider what they eat and change their usual eating pattern.
- Food frequency questionnaires (FFQ) to retrospectively estimate usual dietary intake over time, usually 6–12 months. Information is collected about specific types of food and the quantities and frequency with which they are consumed. Short (60 foods) and long (100 foods) FFQs are used. FFQs must be culturally relevant and a number of culturally relevant forms exist. Modified FFQs identify dietary fat, fibre, fruit, and vegetable intake.
- Dietary recall, often over 24-hours to estimate current intake. Accuracy is influenced by the individual's ability to recall the type and quantity of food consumed. Most people underestimate their intake.
- Visual estimation, where trained observers monitor an individual's food choices, classifies foods using a rating scale and estimates serving sizes. This is intimidating

and may influence the individual's food selection. Nurses can undertake this type of monitoring process.
- Plate waste methodology, which has been used extensively in studies of food intake in school children but is not practical in clinical practice.

Managing obesity and diabetes

Obesity and Type 2 diabetes are chronic conditions and long-term management strategies are needed. Usually a combination of strategies is most effective especially when they are developed in consultation with the individual. In the first instance, energy-dense food intake such as simple carbohydrates and saturated and trans fats should be reduced, exercise increased, and possibly more sleep (Lamberg 2006). Exercise needs to be enough to increase total energy expenditure to 160–180% of the resting metabolic rate (Erlichman *et al.* 2002). Increasing exercise with or without a weight loss diet induces a modest weight loss. People with diabetes should have a thorough physical assessment before undertaking exercise and weight loss programmes that need to be individualised for best effect. Along with diet, exercise prescriptions (Elfhag *et al.* 2005) and wearing a pedometer (Richardson *et al.* 2008) can help the individual achieve weight loss.

Counselling and behavioural strategies that encompass support, exercise and dietary counselling are effective and in Australia are supported through some health benefit funds. For example, commercial diet-oriented weight loss programmes such as *Step into Life, Lifestyle Integrated Functional Exercise* (LIFE), *Mass Attack Weight Loss Program, Lite n' Easy, ClubOptiSlim*. Some of these programmes deliver nutritionally balanced portion controlled low fat meals to the individual's home.

Prepared low-energy meals or meal replacements that replace some or all of the individual's diet can be useful as an initial weight loss strategy or to avoid refeeding syndrome after severe calorie restriction or bariatric surgery. However, they can be expensive in the long term. Avoiding fructose and corn syrup, which are common forms of sugar added to foods and non-alcoholic beverages in the USA.

Self-help programmes often combine lifestyle change, computer-assisted interventions, packaged programmes such as Internet correspondence courses, and take-home weight loss kits. Self-help programmes are difficult to measure but Latner (2001) claimed 45% of people using such programmes lose weight and keep it off. Knowledgeable clinicians can support individuals likely to benefit from a self-help approach (Tan *et al.* 2006).

Significantly, public health programmes that involve health providers, legislators, the food industry, and health insurers are needed and must include children and adolescents. Weigh loss strategies may need to include strategies to keep people physically active in the longer term and recent research suggests it could be important to minimise exercise variation because maintaining exercise at a consistent level moderates age-related weight gain in proportion to the amount of exercise performed (Williams 2008). Even fit people tend to gain weight with increasing age, thus the amount of exercise may need to be increased to reduce age-related weight gain (Williams 2008).

Significantly, stopping exercise leads to weight gain.

Malnutrition and under-nutrition

The focus in diabetes prevention and management is usually on obesity (overnutrition) but malnutrition is a significant problem, especially in older people. Malnutrition prevalence ranges from 10–30% in the community, 20–50% in acute care settings, 30–50% in rehabilitation settings and 40–70% in aged care facilities in Australia (Dietitians Association of Australia 2009). Malnutrition is associated with increased costs and adverse outcomes and is often under-recognised. Importantly, overweight people can be malnourished.

Dietary management: diabetes

Diet and exercise is the mainstay and first line of treatment of Type 2 diabetes to control blood glucose and manage cardiovascular and other health risks. The aim is to achieve a healthy weight range for the individual. The aim is to achieve an appropriate weight within the healthy weight range for the individual, but focusing on weight might mean that *under-nutrition* is not considered, which, as indicated, might confer more health risks than overweight, especially in older people.

Expert dietary advice is essential but the changing role of the nurse and the focus on the preventative aspects of healthcare mean that nurses have a responsibility to develop knowledge about nutrition and its role in preventing disability and disease. A number of basic screening tools can be used to identify dietary intake and nutritional characteristics and can be incorporated into usual nursing assessment and patient care plans and enables useful information to be communicated to the dietitian.

The general dietary principles apply to the whole population as well as all people with diabetes. Precise advice depends on the individual's age, gender, lifestyle, eating habits, cultural preferences and nutritional requirements. It is important that realistic targets are negotiated with the patient, particularly if weight control is necessary. The goal is to achieve gradual progressive weight loss to reduce weight by 5–10%, which is usually achievable and improves the health profile (Pi-Sunyer 2006).

The effect of medications, fasting for procedures, and gastrointestinal disturbances such as diarrhoea and vomiting, on food absorption and consequently blood glucose levels is an important consideration especially during illness.

Optimal nutritional care is best achieved by collaboration among the individual and their family, nurses, other health professionals and the dietitian to decide the most appropriate management regimen. Nurses have the greatest continuous contact with the patient in hospital; consequently they have an invaluable role in nutritional management by:

(1) Identifying patients at high risk of nutritional deficiencies for example poor nutritional intake and/or unintentional weight loss. Approximately 30% of all patients in hospital are undernourished (Kondrup *et al*. 2003a). People with Type 1 diabetes who have repeated admissions to hospital for ketoacidosis (Chapter 7) might have an eating disorder that could be triggered by underlying psychological stress or unrealistic perceptions of obesity. Sensitive discussion with the individual and his or her family and relevant investigations are needed.

(2) Screening patients' nutritional characteristics to identify actual and/or potential problems, for example:
   • Inappropriate, erratic, and over-eating, and those with eating disorders. Screening processes should be connected to relevant actions. For example, if the person is eating appropriately, arrange for regular screening at specified intervals. If the person is at risk of an eating disorder, an appropriate nutrition plan needs to be determined. If functional, metabolic, or diabetes-related complications are present, standard nutrition plans may not be appropriate and dietitian advice will be needed (Kondrup *et al*. 2003b). The following factors need to be considered when deciding the level of risk: the current condition, whether the condition is stable (weight loss/gain can be assessed from the health history), the significance of the condition and whether it is likely to deteriorate or improve, and any disease processes that affect nutritional status such as appetite, diabetes complications, and hyperglycaemia. Managing eating disorders is challenging because people often do not consider their eating behaviour as a problem, or deny they have an eating problem. Repeated episodes of ketoacidosis (DKA) could indicate an eating disorder and needs to be investigated. Young people with diabetes often run their blood glucose levels high to lose weight, which puts them at risk of DKA

(see Chapters 7 and 13). Cognitive behaviour therapy may be a useful strategy when the eating disorder is mild to moderate. The complex underlying issues need to be ascertained and managed.

- Those with domestic, financial, and/or employment problems.

(3) Providing ongoing patient monitoring on a meal-to-meal basis.

Example questions to ask when taking a diet history are shown below. The questions should be asked sensitively as part of a nutritional assessment.

Do you have regular meals?

- It is important to clarify what the individual means by 'regular' and whether they skip meals and if they do when and why. For example, a nurse with diabetes working in the operating theatre might find it difficult to always predict when the operation will finish.

Do you have a good breakfast?

- Poor morning appetite can indicate nocturnal hypoglycaemia and catecholamine production to maintain the falling blood glucose.
- People who do not eat breakfast often snack later in the day on energy-dense foods and can be protein-deficient.
- Missing breakfast interferes with work performance.

How often do you eat takeaway foods?

- Takeaway foods tend to be high in fat, salt and sugar and low in fibre, protein and essential vitamins and minerals.

Do you eat cream biscuits, chocolates or lollies?

- This question is a way of checking the individual's intake of sugar and fat.

Can you tell me some of the foods you eat that contain carbohydrate?

- Regular carbohydrate intake is important when the individual is using insulin or insulin oral glucose lowering medicines. A minimum of 130g carbohydrate per day is required to meet the brain demand for glucose (ADA Guidelines).

The information collected from screening, investigations and questions provides the basis from which nursing staff can quickly and effectively refer patients to the dietitian who can support nursing staff by:

- Setting dietary management goals for the individual consistent with their health status, lifestyle and healthcare goals.
- Identifying possible nutritional problems. Estimating caloric intake is difficult because people generally underestimate their caloric intake by as much as 50% despite trying to keep accurate food records (Fabricatore 2004) but three-day food records can be helpful to health professionals and the person with diabetes.
- Identifying causes of possible nutritional problems and suggesting strategies to overcome them.
- Counselling and educating the patient about how to reduce the risks associated with these problems.
- Supporting nursing and medical staff on an ongoing basis to ensure most effective nutritional management is achieved and maintained (Dunning & Hoy 1994).

The person with diabetes is in control of what they eat and their activity level and must be actively engaged in planning meals and exercise regimens.

Dietary requirements change with increasing age, activity level, health status, pregnancy, and lactation, and during specific disease processes, for example, renal and cardiac disease.

Method of screening for dietary characteristics and problems

Nutritional status

(1) Identify whether the person is overweight or underweight and whether the person's health is affected by their weight status. For example, calculate BMI and/or waist-hip ratio.

(2) Review any current haematological and biochemical measurements, which reflect the person's nutritional status such as haemoglobin and serum albumin levels, creatinine, folate and cholesterol. Clinical signs such as tiredness, fatigue and obesity can indicate inadequate protein intake and can be confirmed by blood urea nitrogen (BUN) and serum creatinine levels. Low creatinine suggests protein intake is low. Low BUN and creatinine suggests a catabolic state such as hyperglycaemia. Consider coeliac disease in people with Type 1 diabetes; see Chapter 10.

Recent research indicates malnourished patients have a longer length-of-stay, are older and have increased mortality rates compared with well-nourished patients. Most malnourished patients are not identified as being at risk (Middleton *et al.* 2001). Clues to nutritional deficiency are:

- Weight loss.
- Low lymphocyte count.
- An illness lasting longer than three weeks.
- Serum albumin <3.5 g/dL. Note serum albumin usually falls during acute illness and is not a stand-alone measure of nutritional deficiency.
- A comprehensive nutrition history and assessment including medicines and possible food-medicine interactions, malabsorption, oral health, anorexia, dysphagia, mental health and functional ability to identify factors that could contribute to under-nutrition, which are likely to be multifactorial.

If a patient is identified as being malnourished, their nutritional status should be monitored by weighing them regularly, using the same scales and with the person wearing similar clothing, by monitoring nitrogen balance and using appropriate screening tools such as those listed below. Nutritional supplements may be needed.

Dietary characteristics

The tools and questions described earlier in this chapter can be used to determine:

- the regularity/irregularity of meals and/or snacks;
- whether the person consumes foods and fluids containing refined sugar;
- whether the person omits any of the major food groups.

If one or more problems are identified the person should be referred to the dietitian for further dietary analysis and advice.

Screening tools

Screening tools are used to measure overall risk of malnutrition rather than food consumption and include:

- Malnutrition Screening Tool (MST), which is widely used in Australia.
- Malnutrition Universal Screening Tool (MUST) for adults (Malnutrition Advisory Group (MAG 2000).
- Simplified Nutritional Assessment Questionnaire (SNAQ).
- Nutritional Risk Screening (NRS-2002) for hospital settings.
- Mini Nutritional Assessment (MNA©) for the elderly (Vellas *et al.* 1999).

- The Healthy Eating Index (HEI) and Modified HEI for children and adolescents (Feskanich *et al.* 2004).
- Biomarkers to identify specific food components in body fluids or tissue, which independently reflect intake of the particular food.

Principles of dietary management for people with diabetes

A number of dietary guidelines have been developed such as the American Diabetes Association, the Diabetes and Nutrition Group of the European Association for the Study of Diabetes, The Canadian Diabetes Association, Diabetes UK, the Indian Council of Medical Research, National Heath and Medical Research Council (NHMRC) and Diabetes Australia. The macronutrient content of these guidelines varies despite the fact they are all evidence-based and largely draw on the same evidence. Not surprisingly, socio-economic factors and food availability appear to influence the dietary advice health professionals provide and what people consume, perhaps more than nutrition guidelines (Kapur & Dunning 2007).

Diets such as the traditional Mediterranean, Okinawan, Dietary Approaches to Stop Hypertension (DASH) antihypertensive, anti-inflammatory diet, South Beach diet, Atkins type diet, Omniheart, Onish, and Onish Zone (A to Z) diets all appear to improve metabolic risk factors by reducing lipids and weight to various degrees (Carey *et al.* 2005; Gardner *et al.* 2007; Fung 2007; Tay *et al.* 2008) although they include different combinations of macronutrients. Interestingly, ancestral diets high in acellular carbohydrates could promote an inflammatory microbiota and could be the primary cause of leptin resistance and obesity (Spreadbury 2012). Likewise, consuming high fat dairy products may reduce obesity risk in Europeans compared to Americans.

The difference could partly be attributed to the different feeding practices adopted in the two countries. Dairy farms are more likely to be highly industrialised in the US where the cows are kept indoors and fed on high protein energy-dense fodder and have little or no exercise. Thus, the milk from US cows has a higher fat content that cows raised on traditional European dairy farms. Ruminant fat consists of more than 400 different fatty acids and is the most complex form of fat in the human diet. These findings are interesting considering NHMRC and other guideline recommendations to consume low fat dairy products where possible.

Likewise, vegetarian and vegan diets, which are high in fibre, low in saturated fat and have a low glycaemic index and lower haem iron, are associated with reduced risk of Type 2 diabetes, less weight gain and better cardiovascular outcomes. However, vegetarian diets may lack essential B group vitamins and iron, thus supplements might be required. Vegetarian people treated with Metformin are at increased risk of vitamin B12 deficiencies because Metformin affects absorption of vitamin B 12; see Chapter 5. Although iron is found in vegetables such as spinach and pumpkin, from eggs it is not absorbed as well as haem iron from red meat. Thus, iron supplements might be required (Marsh 2008).

There are various methods of counting carbohydrate, for example, exchanges, portions and carbohydrate counting that help ensure an even distribution of carbohydrate and appropriate ratio of carbohydrate to exercise and glucose lowering medicines doses and administration times when planning meals for individuals. An exchange is equal to 15 g and a portion 10 g of carbohydrate. Exchanges are sometimes used in the UK while Australia often uses glycaemic index (GI) and glycaemic load.

More recently, portions are making a comeback in programmes such as The German Diabetes Training and Treatment Program (DTTP) and its counterpart the Dose Adjustment for Normal Eating Program (DAFNE). These programmes are being widely adopted and adapted, for example, OzDAFNE in Australia and in group education programmes such as the Royal Derby Hospital in the UK (Shorrock & Hannah 2011).

Using the information they learn in such programmes, people with diabetes estimate their carbohydrate intake based on 10 g portions and calculate their short-acting insulin doses as a ratio to carbohydrate consumption. Basal insulin doses are adjusted to address preprandial and bedtime blood glucose targets, see Chapter 1. HBA_{1c} reductions of ~1% and improved quality of life have been demonstrated without increasing hypoglycaemia or weight (Muhlhauser *et al.* 2002; DAFNE Study Group 2002).

In general, people with diabetes should:

- Eat foods high in complex carbohydrate with low GI (50–60% of total intake), high fibre unprocessed foods. Rapidly digested carbohydrates cause a rapid rise in blood glucose and a greater demand on the pancreas to release insulin to maintain the normal blood glucose range. Low GI foods are associated with a lower risk of diabetes and the related complications (Brand-Miller *et al.* 2003). GI is a method of ranking foods based on their immediate effect on the blood glucose level. Foods that enter the blood stream quickly have a high GI, for example, sugars. Foods that enter more slowly are known as low GI, for example, cereals. The GI is the area under the glucose response curve measured after ingestion of a test food and multiplied by 100. Foods with a GI <55 are classified as low GI, 56–69 as moderate GI, and >70 are high GI foods. In general, the lower the GI, the smaller the impact on the blood glucose level.

However, many factors affect the rate at which carbohydrate is absorbed including the types of sugar and starch in food, the degree of processing, cooking methods and the presence of other nutrients such as fat and fibre and the particular combination of foods. Foods high in fat have a low GI because the fat delays their digestion and they are absorbed slowly, but high fat foods are not recommended.

Low GI foods are the preferred basis of a well-balanced diet. They slow food absorption from the gut so the postprandial glucose load is reduced, cause satiety and help control weight, reduce HBA_{1c}, improve insulin sensitivity and help control lipids (Brand-Miller *et al* 2003).

People with diabetes are advised to include low GI foods in at least one meal each day. Simple sugars do not have to be excluded using the GI food plan. The move to GI-based diets is not universal and GI can be difficult for some people to understand. Generally, if people are accustomed to working in portions or exchanges and have reasonable metabolic control they should not be expected to change, particularly if they are elderly. Scientists are currently undertaking research to reduce the GI of some foods such as rice by altering their amylopectin structure to improve consumer acceptability (Rahman *et al.* 2007).

GI is not related to the quantity (portion size) of carbohydrate, which is measured by glycaemic load (GL). GI is taken into account when determining GL. That is GI indicates how rapidly the food enters the blood as glucose and the GL indicates how much carbohydrate is in a portion/serving; both are important to understanding the effect of a particular carbohydrate on blood glucose. The type of dietary fibre influences GI, water-soluble fibres such as hemicellulose, mucilages, gums and pectins have low GI because they slow digestion and absorption of carbohydrate.

Recent advances in blood glucose meter and insulin pump technology and other technological advances include algorithms that calculate insulin doses based on the insulin to carbohydrate ratio, correction factors, and illness and activity levels. Carbohydrate counting is very important when people use insulin pumps.

- Be low in fat (<10% of total energy value), especially saturated fat and trans fatty acids; see Tables 4.2 and 4.3 which depict the main types of dietary fats and their effects on blood lipids, respectively. Some fat is necessary to supply essential fatty acids and fat-soluble vitamins A, D, E, and K. Despite an overall reduction in dietary fat, the mean Australian serum cholesterol has not fallen since 1980 (National Heart Foundation 2008). Omega 3 and 6 fatty acids are crucial to healthy brain function, normal growth and development and skin and hair growth, bone health, regulating metabolism, and

Table 4.2 Dietary fat comes from animal and plant sources and has various effects on blood lipids. Triglycerides are the most abundant dietary fat.[a] Cholesterol and phospholipid dietary fats have a small but significant impact on serum cholesterol.

Saturated fatty acids (SFA)	Monounsaturated fatty acids (MUFA)	Polyunsaturated fatty acids (PUFA)	Trans fatty acids (TFA)
Not essential fatty acids[b]	Not essential fatty acids[b]	Omega-3 (Eicosapentaenoic acid (EPA and Docosahexaenoic acid (DHA) and omega-6 (Gamma-Linolenic acid GLA) are essential fatty acids (EFA)[c]	Can be MUFAs or PUFAs. TFA are formed when hydrogen is added to vegetable oils but small amounts are found in animal fats. Some dietary supplements contain TFA. Amounts >0.5 must be listed on the label in the US.
With cholesterol contributes to hypercholesterolaemia	Small beneficial effect on lipoproteins	Has a beneficial effect on cholesterol. Increasing omega-3 intake lowers LDL and triglycerides but not as much as reducing dietary SFA. Different omega-3 may have different effects on serum cholesterol. Reduce platelet aggregation and risk of myocardial infarction. Retard deposition of atherosclerotic plaque and have anti-inflammatory effects. May help reduce abdominal fat in insulin-resistant people. Improves morning stiffness in rheumatoid arthritis and has additive effects with anti-inflammatory medicines. High doses may increase the risk of bleeding. Omega-9 might reduce cancer risk and reduces abdominal fat but it also increases LDL, cholesterol and triglycerides so it may not be cardioprotective (Jepersen 2001)	Increase LDL reduce HDL and lipoprotein (a)

[a] Provides SFAs, MUFAs and PUFAs.

[b] Can be obtained from protein and carbohydrate if necessary.

Serum cholesterol is more responsive to changes in dietary SFAs than PUFAs or cholesterol.

TFAs are found in foods containing hydrogenated vegetable oils and fat from ruminant animals.

[c] Omega-6 is derived from linoleic acid; omega-3 is derived from alpha-linolenic acid. All other longer chain PUFAs can be synthesised in the body from these precursors. Omega-3, -6, and -9 compete for the same desaturase enzymes. The desaturase enzymes show preference for the omega-3, -6, and -9 in that order so that synthesis of some EFAs might only occur when the intake of omega-3 and -6 EFAs is low.

Table 4.3 Effect of high carbohydrate, alcohol and fibre on blood fats.

Carbohydrate	Fibre[a]	Alcohol	Non-nutrient components[b]
Increases VLDL and triglycerides	Reduces cholesterol	Increases triglycerides and VLDL and possibly cholesterol	HMG-CoA-like activity
Lowers HDL		Small increase in HDL	Reduces cholesterol and LDL

[a]Effects depend on the type of fibre. Insoluble fibres only have a small effect on lipoproteins; soluble fibre has a favourable effect.
[b]For example allicin, saponins, isoflavonoids, phyto-oestrogens, and anthocyanins. Individually they only have a small LDL lowering effect but combining several components may produce a cumulative effect.

maintaining reproductive function. Omega 6 fatty acids have an important role in modulating the inflammatory response by generating eicosanoids (prostaglandins and leukotrienes) and cytokines (interleukins). For example, gamma-linolenic acid (omega 6) synthesised from linolenic acid reduces inflammation. There is strong evidence that replacing saturated fatty acids with omega 3 and 6 reduces cardiovascular disease in people with diabetes and non-diabetics (Eddy 2008). Dietary sources are not high in gamma-linolenic acid. Some are found in green leafy vegetables and nuts. The richest sources are borage oil, blackcurrant and evening primrose oil and breast milk. The conversion of linolenic acid into gamma-linolenic acid is inefficient in older age, diabetes, high alcohol consumption, eczema, viral infections, excess fat intake, hypercholestrolaemia and deficiency of vitamin B6, zinc, magnesium, calcium and biotin. Deutsch (2007) suggested *Euphasia superba* (krill) is a better source of omega-3 than plant sources and rapidly reduces C-reactive protein, a marker of inflammatory disease. However, compared to fish oils, krill oil has less omega 3, so larger doses are needed and krill is more expensive. Sources of omega 3, 6, and 9 are shown in Table 4.4.

- Contain adequate protein (15% of total intake).
- Be low in simple sugar, less than 25 g/day.
- Ensure a variety of food is eaten daily from each of the five food groups.
- Ensure that complex carbohydrate is consumed at each meal to reduce the postprandial blood glucose rise and the likelihood of hypoglycaemia in patients on insulin or diabetes medication.
- Limit salt. A typical western diet contains about ~10 g of salt per day and 75% of salt consumed is added salt. The National Health and Medical Research Council (NHMRC) (2003) and The Heart Foundation recommend an upper level of 6 g of salt per day. (The 2003 NHMRC Guidelines have been reviewed and should be available in 2013 but the content is expected to be similar). High salt diets are leading causes of cardiovascular disease and hypertension (WHO 2002) and reducing salt intake reduces blood pressure.
- Reduce alcohol. Small amounts of alcohol (0.5–1 drink/day) can reduce cardiovascular risk and post prandial blood glucose levels if consumed with the evening meal containing carbohydrate. Greater quantities impairs glucose metabolism and contributes to hyperlipidaemia, In Australia, the current recommendation is two standard drinks per day for men and one standard drink per day for women.

Goals of Dietary Management

The goals of dietary management are to:
- improve the person's overall health;
- attain optimal body weight;

Table 4.4   Sources of omega-3, -6 and -9 essential fatty acids. And daily intake recommended (RDI) by the National Health and Medical Research Council (2006). A variety of foods high in essential fatty acids should be consumed each day.

Omega-3 (EPA) RDI 50–200 mg/day	Omega-6 RDI 150–1500 mg/day	Omega-9 RDI <50 g/day
Fresh tuna	Safflower	Olive oil
Halibut	Evening primrose	Avocado
Sardines	Sunflower	Almond
Mackerel	Corn and maize	Apricot
Herring	Hempseed	Canola
Trout	Walnut	Peanut
Krill	Pumpkin seed	Butter
Cod liver oil[a]	Borage	Lard
	Blackcurrant	Eggs
	Soya bean	Milk
	Flax and linseed	Coconut

RDI = recommended daily intake. The RDI varies among publications. Consider the quantity of EPA and DHA in omega-3 supplements rather than the total quantity of fish oil in the product. Different types of fish contain different quantities of omega-3.
Consider the risk of bleeding before recommending supplements if the person is on anticoagulant medicines or has bleeding conditions.
[a]Cod liver oil may be contraindicated in pregnancy without medical advice.

- attain lipid and blood glucose levels as close to normal as practical considering hypoglycaemia risk and its consequences: see Chapter 6;
- ensure normal growth and development in children;
- decrease the risk of diabetes- and obesity-related complications and comorbidities;
- identify nutrition-related disorders that can affect diabetes management and interpreting investigative procedures, for example, anaemia.

Dietary management: obesity

Public health strategies are required to have a significant impact on the health, wellbeing and obesity levels of the population; see Chapter 1. Individual dietary advice should be age-, gender- and culture-specific and achievable, which means addressing environmental issues such as access to healthy food, safe, accessible areas to exercise and accurate, understandable food labels.

As well as diet and exercise, a combination of behaviour change strategies tailored to the individual, and support are required. Diets high in fruit, vegetables, whole grains, legumes, and low in fat are generally safe and effective and promote fullness and satiety (National Institute of Health 2000). However <20% of people trying to lose weight consume these foods.

As indicated, commercial weight loss programmes such as Weight Watchers, The slim-fast plan, Dr Atkin's New Diet and the Rosemary Conley Program result in significant weight loss and lower WHR after six months compared to controls who gained an average of 0.6 kg. However, the improvements were not sustained after the trial was completed. More sustained benefit was noted in programmes that included a support group (Truby & Baic 2006).

Other popular diets include the following, which all have advantages and disadvantages. People with diabetes should be advised to discuss these diets with a dietitian and/or their doctor before they try them:

- High protein-low carbohydrate (ketogenic) diets.
- Meal replacement plans where 1–2 meals per day are replaced with meal supplements.
- Dairy diet. Preliminary data suggest 3 servings/day of calcium-rich food enhances weight loss through a variety of mechanisms but more research is needed to confirm these preliminary results (Zemel 2003).

Fish oil supplements (3 g fish oil containing 1.8 g polyunsaturated fatty acids) have been shown to reduce adiposity and atherogenic risk factors in a randomised controlled trial of women with Type 2 diabetes (Rizkalla 2007). However, fish oil may affect the INR in patients taking anticoagulants.

If the BMI is >30 or BMI >27 and diabetes or cardiovascular risk factors are present and diet and exercise is ineffective, medicines such as lipase inhibitors (Xenical) or serotonin reuptake inhibitors such as Sibutramine can be used but they only reduce weight by ~10%. Sibutramine can increase blood pressure (Donohoe 2008). Research into future weight loss medicines is likely to focus on the hormones involved in regulating satiety (leptin, ghrelin and CRBs). Fucoxanthin, an antioxidant obtained from brown seaweed, which is commonly used in Asian cuisine, has been shown to induce weight loss and increase omega-3 fatty acid levels in rats (Miyashita 2006) but its application in humans is unknown.

Bariatric surgery

Gastric bypass surgery (bariatric surgery) is increasingly being recommended for people with Type 2 diabetes who have a body mass index >35 where lifestyle and medical treatments for obesity and uncontrolled diabetes have not been effective, provided they are fit and over 18 years (Proietto *et al.* 2012). Bariatric surgery refers to a variety of surgical procedures that induce weight loss by:

- reducing the size of the stomach to restrict the amount of food that can be consumed;
- delaying digestion and absorption of food in the intestines;
- causing a feeling of fullness and satiety due to stimulation of nerves in the stomach or through the hormones that control hunger, or both.

Types of procedures include:

- adjustable gastric banding (the most commonly used procedure);
- partial or sleeve gastrectomy;
- gastric bypass (Roux-en-Y) and bilopancreatic diversion (see Table 4.5).

Who is suitable for bariatric surgery?
People most suited to bariatric surgery:

- have Type 2 diabetes;
- are obese with a BMI .35;
- have tried lifestyle and medical treatments with no success (significant weight loss);
- are over 18 years;

Table 4.5 Bariatric surgical procedures and the postulated weight loss mechanisms. Complication rates are reported to be low: 1% for gastric banding to between 2 – 10% for the other more complex procedures. Risks increase with increasing age, degree of obesity and concomitant medical conditions.

Bariatric procedure	Outline of the procedure	Postulated weight loss mechanism
Adjustable gastric band	An adjustable gastric band is paced around the upper section of the stomach that creates a small pouch that can only hold a small amount of food.	Restricts the quantity of food consumed
Sleeve gastrectomy	Removal of two thirds of the stomach	Restricts the quantity of food consumed. Affects hunger by stimulating nerves or altering hormones that induce satiety.
Gastric bypass: Roux-en-Y procedure		Restricts the quantity of food consumed Affects hunger by stimulating nerves or altering hormones that induce satiety. Delays digestion and reduces absorption of nutrients.

- are fit enough to undergo surgery;
- understand the procedure and the commitment needed for ongoing care and followup and to maintain lifestyle changes after surgery;
- obese adults with a high risk of Type 2 diabetes and BMI > 35 and another obesity-related-condition or BMI > 40 who meet the other preceding criteria.

The benefits and risks associated with bariatric surgery for people with diabetes has not been established and should be considered on an individual basis.

Bariatric surgery appears to improve blood glucose control through weight loss, reduced insulin resistance and improved insulin sensitivity (Proietto *et al.* 2012). Blood glucose normalises in up to 75% of people, especially if they had Type 2 diabetes for a short period before undergoing surgery. Procedures such as gastric bypass that involve the small intestine appear to induce hormonal effects apart from weight loss that improves blood glucose control within a few days.

Bariatric surgery effectively reduces weight and improves quality of life and lowers the risk of comorbidities after two years compared to controls (Adams 2006) and, with 12 months of medical therapy prior to bariatric surgery, achieved glycaemic control in obese people with uncontrolled Type 2 diabetes (n = 150) (Schauer *et al.* 2012).

Schauer *et al.* did not find significant differences in total and LDL cholesterol levels 12 months post-bariatric surgery or a significant reduction in the number of medicines needed to manage hyperlipidaemia. Adverse events included blood clots requiring surgery, nausea and vomiting, and gastric leak after sleeve gastrectomy. However, they did not report any deaths, serious hypoglycaemia, malnutrition or excessive weight loss.

However, some serious adverse events can occur over time and include:

- The gastric band slipping or, less commonly, the band eroding into the stomach wall.
- Vitamin and mineral deficiencies, due to inadequate nutrition or reduced absorption (Encinosa *et al* 2006).

Improved mood has been demonstrated using the Beck Depression Inventory (Mitka 2003). Several procedures are used such as Roux-en-Y gastric bypass, stapled gastroplasty, and adjustable gastric banding all of which reduce the stomach size and control caloric intake. Although the risks are high, people lose weight and blood glucose levels normalise (Encinose *et al.* 2006). Despite these promising findings, long-term outcomes are not yet available and it is not clear whether glucose control will be maintained in the long term. Significantly, access to an experienced interdisciplinary team is essential for ongoing follow up and to minimise complications.

Complementary weight loss programmes

Many complementary weight (CAM) loss strategies are similar to conventional programmes and these are beneficial and effective. However, many CAM medicines have limited evidence of any benefits (Egger 2005) and some are dangerous, for example, weight loss products that contain ephedra should be avoided and have been banned in some countries. Likewise, creams, soaps, and body wraps are unlikely to lead to weight loss. They may improve body image and self-concept and help the individual mentally. Hypnosis and acupuncture may be useful adjuncts to some other strategies.

People also use topical creams and 'anticellulite' (fat) preparations to improve their body image and research is continuing into the effectiveness such medicines. Caruso *et al.* (2007) reported 11% reduction in waist circumference compared to 5% after 12 weeks in controls with equal reductions in women and men using a 1200-calorie balanced diet, a walking programme and 0.5% topical aminophylline cream applied to the waist BD. The diet and exercise could confound the results. Likewise, the study was not blinded. Thus, there is no compelling evidence to recommend using currently available anticellulite preparations and some that contain aminophylline could affect heart rate and rhythm, which might be undesirable in people with diabetes.

In Australia, weight control products (complementary and conventional) must conform to the Weight Management Industry Code of Practice (http://www.weightcontrol. org/browse.asp?page=349). People should be advised to check whether products conform to this Code before they purchase the product. In addition websites the show the HonCode logo are likely to contain accurate, unbiased information.

Factors associated with making dietary changes

Kapur *et al.* (2008) described a number of factors associated with positive dietary changes in India. These included:

- being older;
- a shorter time since being fit and of acceptable weight;
- having strong family support;
- having a less busy work life;
- being conscious of their health;
- having received dietitian advice and frequent visits to a dietitian;
- being interested in overall health not just diabetes.

Motivational interviewing in addition to diet and exercise leads to weight loss in African-American in a randomised prospective trial in women. HbA$_{1c}$ was correlated

Table 4.6   Medicines whose absorption can be modified by food.

Reduced absorption	Delayed absorption	Increased absorption
Aspirin	Aspirin	Diazepam
Cephalexin	Cefaclor	Dicoumarol
Erythromycin	Cephalexin	Hydrochlorothiazide
Penicillin V and G	Cimetidine	Hydrochlorothiazide
Phenacetin	Digoxin	Metoprolol
Tetracycline	Indoprofen	Nitrofurantoin
Theophylline	Metronidazole	Propranolol

with weight loss at six months but was not sustained at 18 months (Smith-West 2007). Galuska *et al.* (1999) demonstrated cost savings in people being counselled and suggested frequent reminders and support were essential.

These findings suggest important issues for health professionals to consider when developing weight management strategies and delivering dietary advice. They might also indicate that health professionals also need to make some behaviour changes and become better educated about nutrition and how to deliver dietary and weight loss advice.

Nursing responsibilities

(1) To assess dietary and nutritional characteristics and problems such as poor intake, under- or overweight, and unexplained weight loss/gain and refer to a dietitian as required, for example at a change from tablets to insulin, if there are frequent high or low blood glucose levels, the diagnosis of a complication such as renal disease, if the patient displays inadequate knowledge, or when the person requests a referral.

(2) To observe and, if necessary, record food intake, with particular reference to carbohydrate intake of patients on glucose lowering medication.

(3) To promote general dietary principles to patients in accordance with accepted policies and procedures.

(4) To ensure the meals and carbohydrate content are evenly spaced throughout the day.

(5) To ensure adequate carbohydrate intake for fasting patients and those with diminished intake to avoid hypoglycaemia.

(6) Administer medicines at an appropriate time in relation to food.

(7) To know that the absorption of some medicines can be modified by food especially antibiotics and their effectiveness may be diminished or increased (see Table 4.6). The pharmacological response to medicines is influenced by the individual's nutritional status. In turn, medicines can affect the nutritional status. The sense of smell and taste play a significant role in adequate dietary intake. Both these senses diminish with age and can be changed by disease processes and some medicines. Gastrointestinal (GIT) disorders can lead to malabsorption, pH changes alter the bioavailability of nutrients and medicines, inhibit medicine binding and chelation and impair the metabolism and excretion of medicines (NHMRC 1999). Interactions can also occur with commonly used dietary supplements; see Chapter 19 and the International Bibliographic Information on Dietary Supplements (National Institute of Health).

(8) To observe for signs and symptoms of hyper- and hypoglycaemia, and correct the blood glucose level by appropriate nutritional management as part of the management plan.

Table 4.7   Some food-medicine interactions[11]

Food	Medicine	Possible effects
Black liquorice in large doses	Digoxin Diuretics Calcium channel blockers	Irregular heart rhythm Hypertension High serum sodium Muscle pain Weakness
Aged cheese such as brie, parmesan, Roquefort Sauerkraut Over ripe avocadoes Pepperoni	MAO antidepressants	Hypertension
Grapefruit juice	Calcium channel blockers Lipid-lowering medicines Some oral contraceptives Some psychiatric medicines	Modifies medicine metabolism
Orange juice	Aluminium-containing antacids Antibiotics	Increases aluminium
Milk and other dairy products	Tetracycline Digitalis Laxatives containing bisacodyl	Enhanced effects
Oatmeal and high fibre cereals	Many oral medicines including antihypertensive agents	Can affect absorption
Leafy and green vegetables high in vitamin K	Warfarin and other anticlotting medicines	Interferes with blood clotting
Caffeinated foods such as tea, coffee, chocolate	Asthma medications Quinolone antibiotics Some oral contraceptives	Excessive excitability
Alcohol	Medicines containing pseudoephedrine Antidepressant medicines Antipsychotics Muscle relaxants Sedatives Glucose-lowering medicines	Excitability Sedation Hypoglycaemia
High salt foods	Steroids	Fluid retention
Iodine-rich food	Thyroid medicines	Reduced efficacy Might affect blood glucose through its effect on the thyroid

see also Chapter 5.

Note: Alcohol interacts with almost all medicines. Some medicines increase the risk of nutritional deficiencies. For example, metformin leads to vitamin B-12 deficiency; cholestyramine increases excretion of folate and vitamins A, D, E, and K; and antacids interfere with the absorption of many essential minerals. Thus, the person being prescribed medicines should be advised about when to take them in relation to food. People at high risk of a food–medicine interaction are older, taking medicines for chronic diseases such as diabetes, have hypertension, depression hypercholesterolaemia, renal disease, or congestive heart failure.

Inadequate nutrition and low protein stores can delay the healing process. Some food-medicine interactions are shown in Table 4.7.

'Sugar-free' foods

'Sugar-free' usually refers to the sucrose content of foods. Other sugars are often used to sweeten foods labelled sugar-free (e.g. dextrose, fructose, maltose, lactose, galactose).

Recent evidence suggests fructose, which is used to sweeten most soft drinks, causes a greater increase in triglycerides and LDL than glucose (American Dietetic Association 2004; Havel 2007). The study was undertaken in overweight and obese individuals but the findings are likely to apply to non-obese people because fructose is more likely to pass into the lipogenic pathway than glucose after being metabolised in the liver. More research is needed to confirm these findings to determine the percentage of total energy consumption at which fructose has an atherogenic effect. These foods may not be appropriate for people with diabetes. Low calorie and artificially sweetened foods are generally recommended.

Alternative sweeteners

Alternative sweeteners elicit a pleasurable sensation without affecting the blood glucose and are generally safe if used at the recommended doses. They may also play a role in reducing dental caries (American Dietetic Association 2004). They are an acceptable alternative to sugar for people with diabetes. However, a small amount of sugar included in a balanced diet does not adversely affect the blood glucose. There are two types of alternative sweeteners: non-nutritive (or artificial) and nutritive. Non-nutritive sweeteners are kilojoule free, for example:

- Saccharin
- Acesulphame-K
- Aspartame (Equal)
- Cyclamate
- Isomalt
- Neotame
- Sucralose (Splenda)
- Alitame
- Neotame

These products are safe to use. If used in cooking they are best added after cooking because heat can change the taste. The best choices for pregnant women are Acesulphame-K, Alitame, Aspartame, and Sucralose.

Nutritive sweeteners are usually derived from different types of carbohydrate and products containing these sweeteners are often labelled 'carbohydrate modified'.

Nutritive sweeteners include:

- Sorbitol
- Fructose (Sweetaddin)
- Mannitol
- Xylitol
- Maltilol
- Isomalt
- Polydextrose (Litesse)
- Maltodextrin (hydrolysed corn syrup)
- Thaumatin

Many nutritive sweeteners are sugar alcohols, for example, sorbitol. These sweeteners can cause diarrhoea in high doses. Likewise, 'diet' products containing alternative sweeteners can be high in fat.

Stevia (*Stevia rebaudiana*), a herb much sweeter than sugar, is being promoted as a suitable sugar alternative for people with diabetes and may have glucose lowering effects but it has not been extensively evaluated in clinical practice. Only very small quantities are required. Larger doses may cause diarrhoea.

Food additives

Many people are allergic to food additives, which can result in sensitivities or in severe cases, analphylaxis. Different additives are used for different classes of foods. A list of food additives and their code numbers can be obtained from www.foodstandards. gov. au. Types of additives include acidity regulators, antioxidants, bulking agents, colourings, flavourings, emulsifiers, gelling agents, humectants, preservatives, and thickeners. Some of these additives are also used in some medicines.

It is important to learn to read labels and to get to know the alternative names for foods and additives that commonly cause allergies such as cow's milk, soy, nuts, and gluten as well as alternative names for fat and sugar. Key information on a food label people need to look for includes:

- The nutrition claims, for example, fat free, high fibre, low fat, reduced fat, cholesterol free, low in salt, low in sugar and sugar free.
- How to interpret the list of ingredients.
- How to interpret the allergy information.
- The country of origin.
- Use by dates and storage recommendations.
- Understand the nutrition information.
- How to interpret information about recommended daily intake.
- Understanding the figures and symbols such as the GI symbol, genetically modified foods, and the Heart Foundation tick.

These key aspects should be part of routine dietary advice or the person can be referred to Reid (2007) www.healthyfoodguide.com.au for further information.

Alcohol

Alcohol reduces hepatic glucose output but does not have a direct affect on insulin secretion or glucose disposal (Shai 2007). It is recommended that alcohol consumption be limited because of its potential to affect blood glucose and contribute to or mask hypoglycaemia (see Chapter 6). Sweet alcoholic drinks can lead to *hyper*glycaemia, while the alcohol itself leads to *hypo*glycaemia. The hypoglycaemic effect may depend on the nutritional state and glucose stores. Alcohol should *never* be consumed on an empty stomach.

Alcohol supplies considerable calories and provides little or no nutritional value. In addition, alcohol clouds judgment and can lead to inappropriate decision-making. Drunkenness can resemble hypoglycaemia and treatment of hypoglycaemia may be delayed. Appropriate education about hypoglycaemia risk with alcohol consumption is essential. Alcohol has a range of other physical effects including liver cirrhosis, malnutrition and peripheral neuropathy.

Although moderate amounts of alcohol may reduce cardiovascular risk, the current recommended intake still applies: in Australia two standard drinks per day for men and one standard drink per day for women. See also Chapter 10.

Exercise/activity

Exercise has an important role in controlling the blood glucose and increasing overall fitness. It should be combined with a suitable diet. Higher levels of sedentary behaviour are associated with 112% increased risk of developing diabetes, 147% increased risk of developing cardiovascular disease and 49% risk of all cause mortality (Wilmot *et al.* 2012). There is an association between occupational sitting and health outcomes including diabetes, cardiovascular disease and mortality (van Uffelen *et al.* 2010). However, although TV viewing is often cited as a risk factor for diabetes and other diseases, it is a poor measure of overall sedentary behaviour and may underestimate the true effect of over all sitting-related sedentary behaviour (Wilmot *et al.* 2012). However, people who watch a lot of TV often eat large quantities of energy-dense snacks that increase their risk of obesity and consequently obesity-related diseases. Thus exercise programmes should include information about how to reduce occupational and TV-related sitting.

People commencing an exercise programme should first have a medical assessment. Structured aerobic and resistance training programmes improve blood glucose levels and lower HbA$_{1c}$ by ~0.6% and reduce cardiovascular risk in Type 2 diabetes (Krause & Levine 2007). A 1% reduction was associated with 15–20% reduction in major macrovascular events and 37% reduction in microvascular events. In addition, exercise has mental health benefits such as improved body image and feelings of self-worth (Goldfield *et al.* 2007).

Exercise capacity is an independent predictor of non-fatal cardiac events and mortality of patients referred for treadmill testing (ETT) (Peterson *et al.* 2008). For example, low exercise capacity is associated with increased risk of MI on ETT but it is not clear whether limited exercise capacity indicates underlying cardiovascular disease or whether it is a marker of cardiovascular events.

Exercise can result in hypo- or hyperglycaemia. Under normal circumstances exercise stimulates hepatic glucose output and glucose utilisation to maintain glucose in the normal range. However, if exercise occurs in times of metabolic stress the sympathetic drive can be stimulated, which leads to reduced glucose utilisation (van de Veire *et al.* 2006).

Before exercising, people should check their blood glucose levels. It is important to make a gradual start to the exercise. Strenuous activity can cause hypoglycaemia; extra carbohydrate may be needed.

Various strategies are suggested to help people begin and maintain an exercise/activity regimen. The beneficial effects of exercise are less evident if exercise is the sole focus of the intervention (Conn *et al.* 2007). Effective strategies include:

- Providing exercise education.
- Setting achievable goals and focusing on achieving one goal at a time.
- Providing individual supervision is as effective as group programmes and is more acceptable to some people.
- Suggesting written 'exercise prescriptions' that take account of the individual's interests, gender, age and capabilities.
- Wearing a pedometer, especially when combined with a step goal diary. Reduction in BMI of 0.38 kg/m^2 and reductions in blood pressure by 3.8 mm Hg have been described (Bravata *et al.* 2007). A recent meta-analysis suggests people lose an average of 0.05 kg representing 2–3% of body weight over 12 months and continues if the individual continues to wear the pedometer (Richardson *et al.* 2008). People often hope to lose much more weight than this so it is important that they realise even small weight loss is beneficial and to set reasonable goals. Steps walked increased from ~2000 to ~4000 per day on average in Richardson *et al.*'s meta-analysis. Pedometers provide feedback on the number of steps a person takes per day but exercise duration, intensity and frequency and the long-term benefits are unknown.

- Combining exercise with rehabilitation programmes.
- Tai Chi, particularly in older people and those in wheelchairs has a range of benefits such as: improved muscle strength, flexibility, balance and range of movement; lower risk of falls; improved cardiovascular fitness, and reduced cholesterol and abdominal fat. In addition people have a younger vital age (ICCMR 2008); see Chapter 19. More recently, combination programmes such as Lifestyle Integrated Functional Exercise (LIFE) that teach the principles of balance and lower limb strength training, have been shown to be beneficial, especially for older people (Clemson *et al.* 2012). Such programmes help reduce falls and improved functional capacity.

References

Adams, T., Walker, J., Litwin, S. & Pendelton, R. (2006) Two-year improvement in morbidity following gastric bypass surgery. NAASO: *The Obesity Society Annual Scientific Meeting*, Dallas, Texas. Abstract 16-0R October.

Allan, C. (2009) Testosterone reduces visceral fat gain in non-obese older men. *Journal of Clinical Endocrinology and Metabolism*. 30: 139–146.

American Dietetic Association (ADA) (2004) Guidelines for the use of nutritive and non-nutritive sweeteners. *ADA*, **104** (2), 255–275.

Behan, K. & Mbizo, J. (2007) The relationship between waist circumference and biomarkers for disease in healthy non-obese women. *American Society for Clinical Pathology*, **38** (7), 422–427.

Better Health Channel (2008) *Better Health Channel Fact Sheet: Weight Loss – Common Myths*. Available at: htpp://www.betterhealth.vic.gov.au/bhcv2/bhcarticles.nsf/pages/Weight_loss_common (accessed January 2008).

Brand-Miller, J, Hayne S, petocz P, Coalgiuri S. (2003) Low glycaemic index diet in the management of diabetes: a meta-analysis of randomized controlled trial. *Diabetes Care*, **26** (8), 2261–2267.

Bravata, D., Smith-Sprangler, C. & Sundaram, V. (2007) Using pedometers to increase physical activity and health. *A systematic review. Journal of the American Medical Association*, **298**, 2296–2304.

Bouchard, L., Drapeau, V., Provencher, V. & Lemieux, S. (2004) Neuromedin beta: A strong candidate gene linking eating behaviours and susceptibility to obesity. *American Journal of Clinical Nutrition*, **80** (6), 1478–1486.

Burdette, H. & Whitaker, R. (2005) A national study of neighbourhood safety, outdoor play, television viewing, and obesity in preschool children. *Pediatrics*, **116** (3), 657–662.

Dietitians Association of Australia (2009) Evidence based practice guidelines for the nutritional management of malnutrition in adult patients across the care continuum. *Nutrition and Dietetics*, **66** Supp, S4–S10.

Donohoe, M. (2008 Weighty matters: Public health aspects of the obesity epidemic. *Medscape Obstetrics and Gynaecology and Women's Health*. Available at http://www.medscape.com.viewarticle/566056 (acccessed January 2008).

Carnethon, M., de Chaves, P. & Biggs, M. *et al.* (2012) *Association of weight status with mortality in adults with incident diabetesJournal of the American Medical Association*, **308**(6), 581–590

Carey, V., Bishop, L. & Charleston, J. (2005) Rationale and design of the optimal macronutrient intake heart (Omni-Heart) trial. *Clinical Trials* **2** (6), 529–537.

Caruso, M., Pekarovic, S., Raum, W. & Greenway, F. (2007) Topical treatments for fat reduction do they work? A best evidence review. *Diabetes Obesity and Metabolism*, **9**, 300–303.

Clemson, L., Fiatarone Singh M. *et al.* (2012) Integration of balance and strength training into daily life activity to reduce falls in older people (the LIFE study): Randomized parallel trial. *British Medical Journal* 345e4547 DOI:10.1136bmj.e4547.

Deutsch, L. (2007) Evaluation of the effect of Neptune krill oil on chronic inflammation and arthritis symptoms. *Journal of American College of Nutrition*, **26** (1), 39–48.

Conn, V. & Hafdahl, A. (2007) Metabolic effects of interventions to increase exercise in adults with Type 2 diabetes. *Diabetologia*, **50**, 913–921.

DAFNE Study Group (2002) Training in flexible, intensive insulin management to enable dietary freedom in people with Type 1 diabetes: Dose adjustment for normal eating (DAFNE) randomized controlled trial. *British Medical Journal*, **325**, 746.

Diehr, P., Bild, D. & Harris, T. (1998) Body mass index and mortality in non-smoking older adults. The cardiovascular effects. *Journal of Public Health*, **88**, 623–629.

Diehr, P., O'seara, E., Fitzpatrick, A. & Newman, A. (2008) Weight, mortality, years of healthy life and active life expectancy. *Journal American Geriatric Society*, **56** (1), 76–83.

Dunning, T. & Hoy, S. (1994) What To Do Till the Dietitian Gets There. Servier Australia, Melbourne.

Eddy, S. (2008) Omega-6 and 9 fatty acids. *Journal of Complementary Medicine*, **7** (2), 34–39.

Egger, G. & Thorburn, A. (2005) Environmental policy approaches: Methods of dealing with obesity, in Clinical Obesity in Adults and Children, 2nd edn (eds Kopleson, P., Caterson, I. & Deitz, W.), Blackwell Publishing, Oxford.

Erlichman, J., Kerbey, A. & James, W. (2002) Physical activity and its impact on health outcomes. Paper 2: prevention of unhealthy weight gain and obesity by physical activity: An analysis of the evidence. *Obesity Review*, **3**, 273–287.

Elmore, J., Carney, P. & Abraham, L. (2004) The association between obesity and screening mammography accuracy. *Archives of Internal Medicine*, **164**, 1140–1147.

Feskanich, D., Rockett, H. & Colditz, G. (2004) Modifying the healthy eating index to assess diet quality in children and adolescents. *Journal of the American Dietetic Association*, **104** (9), 1375–1383.

Fung, T. (2007) DASH-style diet may reduce risk of CHD and stroke. *American Heart Association Scientific Sessions*, Abstract 2369. November 5th.

van Gaal, L., Rissanen, A. & Scheen, A. (2005) RIO-Europe Study group. Effects of the cannabinoid-1 receptor blocker rimonabant on weight reduction and cardiovascular risk factors in overweight patients: 1-year experience from the RIO-Europe Study. *Lancet*, **365**, 1389–1397.

Galuska, D., Will, J., Serdula, M. & Ford, E. (1999) Are health care professionals advising obese patients to lose weight? *Journal of the American Medical Association*, **282**, 1576–1578.

Gardner, C., Kiazand, A. & Alhassan, S. (2007) Comparison of the Atkins, Zone, Ornish and LEARN diets for change in weight and related risk factors among overweight premenopausal women: The A to Z Weight Loss Study: A randomized trial. *Journal of the American Medical Association*, **297**, 969–977.

Goldfield, G., Mallory, R., Parker, T., Cunningham, T. & Legg, C. (2007) Effects of modifying physical activity and sedentary behaviour on psychosocial adjustment in overweight/obese children. *Journal of Pediatric Psychology*, **32** (7), 783–793.

Havel, P. (2007) Fructose but not glucose consumption linked to atherogenic lipid profile. *American Diabetes Association 67th Scientific Sessions*, Abstract 0062-0R June.

ICCMR (2008) International Council Complementary Medicine Research, march. 29–31, Sydney.

Iqbal, O. (2007) Endocannabinoid system and pathophysiology of adipogenesis: Current management of obesity. *Personalised Medicine*, **4** (3), 307–319.

James, D. & Coster, A. (2011) Identifying the enemy in the battle against diabetes and obesity. *Diabetes Management Journal*, **37**, 68.

Kapur, K., Kupur, A., Ramachandran, S. *et al.* (2008) Barriers to changing dietary behaviour. *Journal of the Association of Physicians in India*, **56**, 27–32.

Kapur, K. & Dunning, T. (2007) Global nutritional recommendations: A combination of evidence and food availability. *Practical Diabetes International*, **24** (9), 1–8.

Kraus, E. & Levine, B. (2007) Aerobic and resistance training improves glycaemic control in Type 2 diabetes. *Annals of Internal Medicine*, **147**, 357–369; 423–425.

Kondrup, S., Allison, S., Elia, M., Vallas, B. & Plauth, M. (2003a) EPSEN guidelines for nutrition screening 2002. *Clinical Nutrition*, **22** (4), 415–421.

Kondrup, J., Rasmussen, H. & Hamberg, O. (2003b) Nutritional risk screening (NRS 2002): A new method based on an analysis of controlled clinical trials. *Clinical Nutrition*, **22**, 321–336.

Lamberg, L. (2006) R$_x$ for obesity: eat less, exercise more, and – maybe get more sleep. *Journal of the American Medical Association* http://www.medscape.com/viewarticle/566056 (accessed February 2008).

Latner, J. (2001) Staff help in the treatment of obesity. *Obesity Review*, **2**, 87–97.

Malnutrition Advisory Group (MAG) (2000) MAG – Guidelines for Detection and Management of Malnutrition. British Association for Parenteral and Enteral Nutrition, Redditch, UK.

Marks, S. (2000) Obesity management. *Current Therapeutics*, **41**, 6.

Marsh K. (2008) Vegetarian diets and diabetes. *Diabetes Management Journal*, **26**, 14–15.

Middleton, M., Nazarenko, G., Nivison-Smith, I. & Smerdely, P. (2001) Prevalence of malnutrition and 12-month incidence of mortality in two Sydney teaching hospitals. *Medical Journal of Australia*, **31**, 455–461.

Mitka, M. (2003) Surgery for obesity: Demand soars amid scientific, ethical questions. *Journal of the American Medical Association*, **289**, 1761–1762.

Miyashita, K. (2006) Brown seaweed may burn away brown fat. American Chemical Society 232*nd* National Meeting and Exposition, San Francisco, 10–14th Sept.

Moyad, M. (2004) Fad diets and obesity-Part 1: Measuring weight in a clinical setting. *Urology Nurse*, **24** (2), 114–119.

Muhlhauser, I. & Berger, M. (2002) Patient education –evaluation of a complex intervention. *Diabetologia*, **45**, 1723–1733.

National Health and Medical Research Council (NHMRC) (1999) Diet for Older Australians. Commonwealth of Australia, Canberra.

National Health and Medical Research Council (NHMRC) (2003) *Dietary Guidelines for Australian Adults*. NHMRC Ref. No. N29-N34.

National Health and Medical Research Council (NHMRC) (2006) Healthy eating Club Fact Sheets: fat & cholesterol. www.healthyeatingclub.org/info/articles/fats-chol/index.htm (accessed January 2008).

Peterson, P.N., Magid, D.J. & Ross, C. (2008) Association of exercise capacity on treadmill with future cardiac events in patients referred for exercise testing. *Archives of Internal Medicine*, **168**, 174–179.

Pi-Sunyer, F. (2006) Use of lifestyle changes, treatment plans and drug therapy in controlling cardiovascular disease and obesity. *Obesity*, **14** (Suppl 3), 135S–142S.

Proietto J., Aly A., Barton M., Spalding A., Hagger V. (2012) Diabetes Australia position statement on bariatric surgery. *Diabetes Management Journal*, **39**, 26–30.

Rahman, S., Morell, M., Topping, D. *et al.* (2007) Low glycaemic response cereals for enhanced human health. *International Diabetes Monitor*, **19** (3), 21–25.

Reynolds, S., Yasuhukio, S. & Crimmins, E. (2005) The impact of obesity on active life expectancy in older Americans. *Gerontologist*, **45**, 438–444.

Richardson, C., Newton, T., Abraham, J., Sen, A. & Swartz, M. (2008) A meta-analysis of pedometer-based walking interventions and weight. *Annals of Family Medicine*, **6** (1), 69–77.

Reid, C. (2007) www.healthyfoodguide.com.au

Rizkalla, S. (2007) Fish oil supplements cut adiposity in Type 2 diabetes. *American Journal of Clinical Nutrition*, **86**, 1670–1679.

Schauer, P., Kashyap, S. & Wolski, K., *et al.* (2012) Bariatric surgery versus intensive medical treatment in obese patients with Type 2 diabetes. *New England Journal of Medicine*, DOI 10.1056/NEJM oa1200225.

Shorrock, I. & Hannah, J. (2011) Carbohydrate counting and insulin dose adjustment –group education for people with Type 2 diabetes. *Journal of Diabetes Nursing*, **15** (6), 239.

Stevens, J. (2000) Impact of age on associations between weight and mortality. *Nutrition Review*, **58**, 129–137.

Smith-West, D. (2007) Motivational interviewing improves weight loss in women with Type 1 diabetes. *Diabetes Care*, **30**, 1018–1087.

Spreadbury, I. (2002) Comparison with ancestral diets suggest dense acellular carbohydrates promote an inflammatory microbiota, and may be the primary dietary cause of leptin resistance and obesity. *Diabetes, Metabolic Syndrome and Obesity*, **2012** (5), 175189.

Stone, A. & Brownell, K. (1994) The stress eating paradox: Multiple daily measurements in adult males and females. *Psychological Health*, **9**, 425–436.

Sydney-Smith, M. (2000) Nutritional assessment in general practice. *Current Therapeutics*, **41** (9), 13–24.

Tay, J., Brinkworth, G. & Noakes, M. (2008) Metabolic effects of weight loss on a very-low-carbohydrate diet compared with an isocaloric high-carbohydrate diet in abdominally obese subjects. *American Journal of Cardiology*, **51**, 59–67.

Truby, H. & Baic, S. (2006) Randomised controlled trial of four weight loss programmes in the UK: Initial findings from the BBC "diet trials". *British Medical Journal*, **332**, 1309–1314.

Third Joint Taskforce of European and Other Societies on Cardiovascular Disease Prevention in Clinical Practice (2003) European guidelines on cardiovascular disease prevention in clinical practice. *European Journal of Cardiovascular Prevention Rehabilitation*, **10** (Suppl. 1), S1–S78.

van Uffelen J., Wong J. & Chau J. (2010) Occupational sitting and health risks: A systematic review. *American Journal of Preventative Medicine*, **39**, 379 – 388.

Unger, R. & Scherer P. (2010) Gluttony, sloth and the metabolic syndrome: A roadmap to lipotoxicity. *Trends in Endocrinology and Metabolism*, **216**, 345–352.

van de Veure, N., de Winter, O., Gir, M. *et al.* (2006) Fasting blood glucose levels are related to exercise capacity in patients with coronary artery disease. *American Heart Journal*, **152** (3), 486–492.

Vellas, B., Guigoz, Y. & Garry, P. (1999) The Mini Nutritional Assessment (MNA) and its use in grading nutritional state of elderly patients. *Nutrition*, **15**, 116–122.

Williams, P. (2008) Asymmetric weight gain and loss from increasing and decreasing exercise. *Medicine Society for Sports Exercise*, **40** (2), 296–302.

Wilmot E., Edwardson C., Achana F. *et al.* (2012) Sedentary time in adults and the association with diabetes, cardiovascular disease and death: A systematic review and meta-analysis. *Diabetologia* DOI:10.1007/s00125-012-2677-z

World Health Organisation (WHO) (2000) The World Health Report – Reducing Risk, Promoting Healthy Life. WHO, Geneva, Switzerland.

Zemel, M. (2003) Role of dietary calcium and diary products in modulating adiposity. *Lipids*, **38**, 139–146.

Zhong X.L. & Sikaris K. (2011) Vitamin D deficiency and diabetes: A review of recent data from the AusDiab study. *Diabetes Management Journal*, **37**, 18–19.

Further reading

Australian Government (1991) Australian Dietary Guidelines Australian Government Publications, Canberra.

Barclay, A. (2012) Fructose. *Diabetes Management Journal*, **39**, 1213.

Block, G. (1982) A review of validations of dietary assessment methods. *American Journal of Epidemiology*, **115**, 492–505.

British Diabetic Association (1992) Dietary recommendations for people with diabetes. *Diabetic Medicine*, **9**, 189–202.

Encinosa, W., Bernard, D., Steiner, C. & Chen, C. (2006) Healthcare utilization and outcomes after bariatric surgery. *Medical Care*, **44**, 706–712.

Grontved A. & Hu F.B. (2011) Television viewing and risk of Type 2 diabetes, cardiovascular disease and all-cause mortality: A meta-analysis. *Journal of the American Medical Association*, **305**, 2448 – 2455.

Jespersen, I. (2001) The effect of dietary oils on blood lipids and the risk of ischemic heart disease with special emphasis on olive oil. A literature review. *Ugeskr Laeger*, **163** (35), 4736–4740.

Katan, W. (1990) Biochemical indicators of dietary intake. *European Journal of Clinical Nutrition*, **52**, S5.

Keleman, L., Jacobs, D. & Cerham, J. (2005) Association of dietary protein with disease and mortality in a prospective study of postmenopausal women *American Journal of Epidemiology*, **161** (3), 239–249.

National Cholesterol Education Program (NCEP) Expert Panel on Detection, Evaluation and Treatment of High Blood Cholesterol in Adults (2002) (Adult Treatment Panel 111) Final Report. *Circulation*, **106** (25), 3143–3421.

National Institutes of Health (NIH) Office of Dietary Supplements IBIDS database. Available at: http://grande.nal.usda.gov/index.php (accessed January 2008).

Tsai, A. & Wadden, T. (2005) Sytematic review: An evaluation of major commercial weight loss programmes in the United States. *Annals of Internal Medicine*, **142**, 56–66.

Weiss, E. (2007) Certain factors associated with weight regain after weight loss. *American Journal of Preventative Medicine Online June 5th 2007*. Available at: http://healthaffairs.org/blog/author/anneweiss/ (accessed December 2012).

Chapter 5
Medicines Management

All things are poison and nothing is without poison. Only the dose distinguishes the killer from the cure.

(Paracelsus circa 1493–1541)

Key points

- Medicines should be managed within the principles of the Quality Use of Medicines and pharmacovigilance.
- Understanding the pharmacology of the different glucose-lowering medicines and other medicines enables meals, activity, and medicine administration times to be planned appropriately to suit the individual.
- Medicines are the cause of many preventable adverse events including death of people in hospital.
- Medicine-related outcomes need to be proactively monitored according to management targets, the indications for their use, and individual benefits and risks.
- Type 2 diabetes is a progressive disease of beta cell decline and insulin will eventually be needed by >50% of people with Type 2 diabetes.
- Polypharmacy is common in diabetes, especially Type 2 and older people, and could be considered best practice, but it increases the risk of adverse events including medicine interactions.
- Medicine-related non-adherence is common, complex and multifactorial. It has its basis in patient and health professional-related issues as well as environmental and system-related issues.
- People with diabetes frequently use complementary medicines/therapies (CAM), which needs to be considered when selecting diabetes management options.

Care of People with Diabetes: A Manual of Nursing Practice, Fourth Edition. Trisha Dunning.
© 2014 John Wiley & Sons, Ltd. Published 2014 by John Wiley & Sons, Ltd.

Introduction

The main 'diabetes medicines' listed below are discussed in this chapter. Other medicines are described in the relevant chapters: likewise, the management targets for blood glucose, HbA_{1c}, lipids, blood pressure and weight are described in Chapter1.

(1) Oral glucose-lowering medicines (GLM)
(2) Insulin
(3) Lipid lowering agents
(4) Cardiovascular agents
(5) Antiplatelet agents.

The author prefers to use the term 'medicines' rather than 'drugs', which is reserved for describing illegal drugs. Medicines should be managed within a quality use of medicine framework (QUM), which is an holistic risk management approach that encompasses all types of medicines and recommends using non-medicine options first. The other key principle is pharmacovigilance to reduce the risk of adverse events and monitor medicine use appropriately to achieve optimal outcomes. People with diabetes also frequently use complementary medicines (CAM) and these are discussed throughout the book but principally in Chapter 19. Medicines are also mentioned in other chapters throughout the book where relevant.

Quality Use of Medicines (QUM)

The information in this section was adapted from *The Quality Use of Medicines in Diabetes* (QUM) (2005) a paper developed by the Pharmaceutical Health and Rational use of Medicines (PHARM) Committee, a Committee of the Australian Commonwealth Department of Health and Ageing (DOHA). The figure is reproduced with DOHA's permission. The Australian medicines system has been reviewed and revised since 2005 and PHARM no longer exists, but QUM is still central to medicines use and policies in Australia and has been adopted in many other countries. QUM also encompasses complementary medicines (Dunning 2005).

QUM aims to help health professionals and consumers make the best possible use of medicines to improve their health outcomes. QUM recognises the central role of the consumer in medicines use and that many people maintain their health without using medicines, while for others medicines are important to their health and well-being. It also recognises that medicines may be needed for prevention as well as treatment. QUM means:

- 'Selecting management options wisely;
- Choosing suitable medicines if a medicine is considered necessary;
- Using medicines safely and effectively,' which includes monitoring the outcomes, dose adjustments, undertaking structured medicine reviews and de-prescribing when indicated (DOHA, 2002).

Thus, QUM highlights health professional's responsibility for safe, effective medicines use in addition to the need to consider patient adherence, which is influenced by health professionals' knowledge, attitudes, behaviours and communication and teaching skills.

Quality Use of Medicines and Diabetes

Medicines are central to effective diabetes management to control metabolic abnormalities and managing the complications of diabetes and other concomitant conditions. However, even when medicines are required, lifestyle factors, diet, exercise and smoking cessation, are necessary to achieve optimal outcomes. Prevention programmes have a central, primary and ongoing role (DOHA 2001).

Medicines are used in four main areas in diabetes:

(1) *Primary prevention* focuses on lifestyle factors to prevent or delay the need for medicines in those at risk of diabetes and its complications. However, medicines may be needed for prevention, for example, lipid-lowering and antihypertensive medicines, and flu vaccine to prevent intercurrent illness in at-risk individuals.
(2) *Secondary prevention* where medicines are usually necessary to reduce the risk of diabetes complications such as renal disease, atherosclerosis, and retinopathy.
(3) *Clinical care* which involves using medicines to achieve optimal metabolic, psychological and quality of life targets by appropriately selecting management options including choosing suitable medicines if they are required, obtaining informed consent, enhancing informed decision-making by ensuring people have the information and skills needed to actively participate in medicine self-management, and monitoring the outcomes to ensure medicines are used safely and effectively. Educating the individual with diabetes and their carers and supporting them to manage their diabetes generally, and medicines in particular, are key aspects of QUM. Medicines prescribed for other conditions, self-initiated non-prescription medicines and CAM use need to be considered as part of a holistic assessment and care plan. Significantly, polypharmacy is usually necessary to achieve optimal outcomes for/with people with diabetes and may be considered best practice. However, polypharmacy increases the complexity, risks and costs of the management regimen. Therefore, as few medicines as possible should be used. Insulin, and sometimes other medicines, are needed at diagnosis in Type 1 diabetes and for many people with Type 2 and LADA. Type 2 diabetes is a progressive disease and, consequently the medication regimen becomes progressively complex with increasing duration of the diabetes.
(4) *Clinical trials* commonly investigate new medicines and other interventions before they are licensed for use to ensure they are safe and efficacious, and to determine cost-benefit. Information from trials is also used to develop clinical practice guidelines and consumer and health professional information. Health professionals are often asked to help recruit participants for clinical trials. The fact that an individual is participating in a clinical trial should be clearly documented in the person's medical record.

QUM is a useful framework for reducing polypharmacy and duplicate prescribing and for de-prescribing because it encompasses prevention using non-medicine options, regular medication reviews, and effective communication among health professionals and with people with diabetes (National Prescribing Service 2000).

Medicines are selected taking into account:

- The individual's social, physical and mental health status.
- Whether there is a suitable non-medicine option.
- The risks and benefits of using medicines for the individual including health literacy and functional and cognitive ability.
- Dosage, dose interval, and duration of treatment.

- Other medicines, CAM and therapies that the individual might be using or considering.
- The process required to monitor the outcomes of medicine use, including adverse events, medication self-management and other relevant self-care such as blood glucose monitoring, processes for communicating the medication plan among the relevant health professionals when the individual makes transitions among health providers and services, and strategies for regularly reviewing the continued benefits and risks of the medication regimen and the individual's self-care capacity.
- The costs to the individual, the community, and the health system. A process for integrating QUM into existing care is shown in Figure 5.1.

Oral Glucose-Lowering Medicines (GLM)

Different OHAs target the various underlying abnormalities of glucose homeostasis in Type 2 diabetes (Chapter 1). They are not appropriate for Type 1 diabetes. Type 2 diabetes is a progressive disease of beta cell decline, thus the medication regimen needs to be constantly monitored and adjusted and medicines included and de-prescribed as necessary. The UKPDS study (Turner *et al.*1999) showed monotherapy was ineffective in 75% of people with Type 2 diabetes. Importantly, an appropriate diet and exercise regimen are essential regardless of whether medicines are required.

Sulphonylureas were the first GLMs to become available in the 1940s. The Biguanides followed in the 1950s. The value of these medicines has been established and they have been consistently improved over time with new generations of the original sulphonylureas. In addition, new classes of GLMs have been introduced, some of which might extend the life of the remaining beta cells and delay the need for insulin (Dornhorst 2001).

GLMs target the different underlying abnormalities of glucose homeostasis associated with Type 2 diabetes. These GLM are:

- Biguanides, which reduce hepatic glucose production and might improve peripheral glucose disposal and promote weight loss. It activates the energy regulating enzyme AMP-kinase in liver and muscle. Metformin is the medicine of first choice in overweight people with Type 2 diabetes (UKPDS 1998). Biguanides are insulin sensitisers.
- Sulphonylureas and Glitinides, which are secretagogues that stimulate insulin release from the beta cells. Therefore, the beta cells must be capable of responding by producing insulin. First generation sulphonylureas such as Chlorpropraminde and Tolbutamide are now rarely used in many countries and have been removed from the market in others. Secretagogues might be first-line treatment in people who are not overweight or who have contraindications to Metformin.
- Alpha-glucosidase inhibitors, which slow carbohydrate digestion and glucose absorption from the gut by inhibiting alpha-glucosidases in the brush border of the small intestine. Alpha-glocosidaises are essential to the release of glucose from complex carbohydrates. Alpha-glocosidaises reduce postprandial glucose levels.
- Meglitinides, which act on the same beta cell receptor as the sulphonylureas but are chemically different.
- Thiazolidinediones (TZD), which increase whole-body sensitivity to insulins by activation of nuclear receptors and prompting esterifiation and storage of free fatty acids in subcutaneous fat tissue. They reduce daytime preprandial hyperglycaemia, and have some effect on the fasting blood glucose. The two main TZDs are Rosiglitazone and Pioglitazone. The latter can be added to Metformin and sulphonylureas or substituted for these medicines if the individual is intolerant of them.

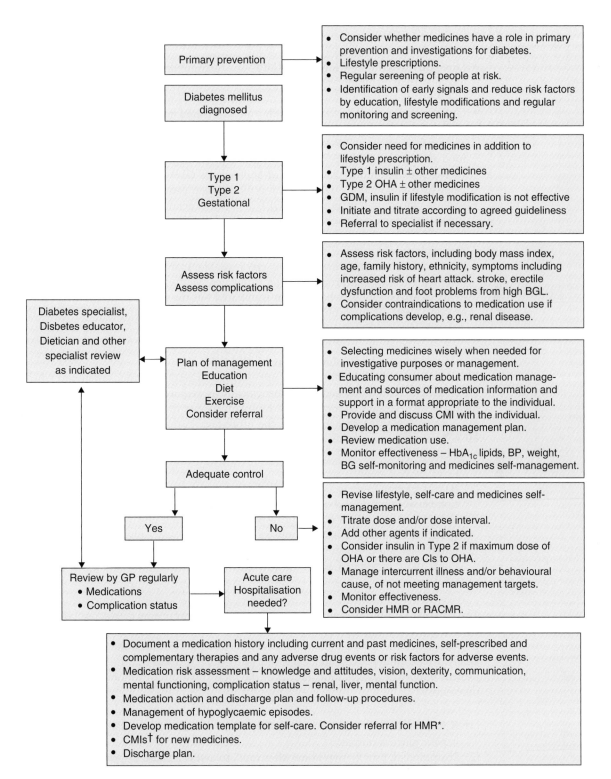

Figure 5.1 The Quality Use of Medicines process applied to diabetes care reproduced from the Quality Use of Medicines in Diabetes Pharmaceutical Health And Rational use of Medicines (PHARM) Committee, Commonwealth Department of Health and Ageing (2005). The medication regimen should be reviewed each time a new medicine is required, if an adverse event occurs, and at least annually as part of routine diabetes complication procedures (included with permission). *HMR = home medicines reviews, †CMI = consumer medicines information.

- Dipeptidyl peptidase-4 inhibitors (DPP-4), which inhibit the activity of DPP-4, an enzyme that prolongs the activity of endogenous glucagon like peptide 1 (GLP-1).
- GLP-1 agonists, GLP-1 is an incretin hormone secreted in the gut in response to food. GLP-1 amplifies insulin secretion from the beta cells and inhibits inappropriate glucagon secretion. GLP-1 also slow gastric emptying, which slows post prandial food absorption and helps control postprandial blood glucose, and reduces appetite. GLP-1 agonists mimic the activity of endogenous GLP-1 but are more resistant to being broken down by DDP-4, which prolongs their action.
- Sodium-glucose cotransporter-2 (SGLT-2) acts independently of insulin secretion or action and target glucose reabsorption and induce glycosuria (Whaley *et al.* 2012). Some SGLT-2 agents have been approved for use in Europe and the US but they are not yet approved in other countries.
- Insulin. Various insulin preparations are available. Insulin can be used alone or in combination with metformin. In Type 2 diabetes, Metformin and sometimes sulphonylureas are continued when insulin is initiated but the risk of hypoglycaemia must be considered when insulin and suphonylureas are combined (NHS 2008; SIGN 2010; ADA&ESAD 2012; NPS 2012).

The commonly available GLM are listed in Table 5.1.

Blood glucose and HbA_{1c} monitoring are essential to assess whether, when and which GLM should be commenced and when insulin is required. When GLMs are commenced it is necessary to monitor the blood glucose in order to appropriately adjust the dose and dose interval. However, the other factors that affect blood glucose and HbA_{1c} must be considered. Normal endogenous insulin secretion consists of two components:

(1) Basal secretion, a constant low secretion rate to suppress hepatic glucose production between meals and overnight (fasting).
(2) Bolus secretion, which occurs in response to increasing glucose levels after meals (postprandial). These insulin boluses also consist of two phases: first phase, an initial high spike, which is lost early in the development of Type 2 diabetes, and a lower more prolonged second phase. Insulin release is influenced by DPP-4 and GLP-1.

The different GLMs and insulins target the different components of glucose homeostasis. Testing the blood glucose is a key to determining medicine effectiveness. HbA_{1c} only provides an overall average blood glucose level and does not account for glucose variability, which influences complication risk (see Chapters 3 and 8). Thus, both measures provide important information as part of the total situation. Key blood glucose testing times are:

(1) Before breakfast to assess the fasting blood glucose, an indicator of overnight hepatic glucose output.
(2) Postprandial, usually two hours after food, to assess glucose disposal. Postprandial hyperglycaemia is common in Type 2 diabetes because of the loss of first phase insulin response early in the course of the disease.

Sometimes testing at both of these times will be required and sometimes overnight (2–3 a.m.) to detect nocturnal hypoglycaemia; see Chapter 6.

Table 5.1 Oral hypoglycaemic agents, dose range and dose frequency, possible side effects, the duration of action and main site of metabolism based on pharmaceutical company prescribing information for each medicine, NIH 2008, ADA/EASD 2012, NPS 2012 guidelines. There are many brand names for the main classes of GLMs and their availability and the brand names differ among countries; not all the GLM brands or generic GLMs are shown in the table.

Medicine	Usual daily dose	Frequency	Possible side effects	Duration of action (DA)	Site of metabolism
(1) Sulphonylureas: these are sulphonamides, urea derivatives that close K ATP channels on beta cell plasma membranes and increase insulin secretion Reduce HbA$_{1c}$ by 1–2% when used as monotherapy			Some blunt myocardial ischaemic preconditioning		
Glibenclamide					
Daonil 5 mg	2.5–20 mg	Up to 10 mg as a single dose	Side effects rarely encountered include:Nausea, anorexia, skin rashes Severe hypoglycaemia especially in elderly and those with renal dysfunction	DA: 6–12 h Peak: 6–8 h	Liver
Euglucon 5 mg Glimel 5 mg		>10 mg in divided doses Taken with, or immediately before food			
Glipizide					
Minidiab 5 mg	2.6–40 mg	Up to 15 mg as a single dose >15 mg in a twice daily dosage Taken immediately before meals	GIT disturbances Skin reactions Hypoglycaemia (rare)	DA: Up to 24 h Peak: 1–3 h	Liver
Gliclazide					
Diamicron MR (a sustained release preparation)	30–120 mg Dose increments should be two weeks apart Should not be crushed	Daily	Hypoglycaemia	Released over 24 hours	Liver
Glimepiride (Amaryl)	1–4 mg	2–3 per day	Hypoglycaemia	DA: 5–8 h	Liver
(2) Biguanides activate Amp-kinase and reduce hepatic glucose production Reduce HbA1c by 1–2% when used as monotherapy					

(Continued)

Table 5.1 Continued.

Medicine	Usual daily dose	Frequency	Possible side effects	Duration of action (DA)	Site of metabolism
Metformin Diaformin 500 mg Diabex 500 mg Glucophage 500 mg	0.5–1.5 g May be increased to 3–0g	1–3 times/day Taken with or immediately after food	GIT disturbances Lactic acidosis Hypoglycaemia with other OHAs Decreased B_{12} absorption	DA: 5–6h	Unchanged in urine
Combination sulphonylurea and biguanide Glucovance: Metformin (M) and Glibenclamide (G): M 250 mg G 1.25 mg M 500 mg, G 2.5 mg M 500 mg G 5 mg Combination Metformin and Rosiglitazone (TZD) e.g. Avandamet in various dose combinations Combination Metformin and Sitagliptin (DPP-4) e.g. Janumet in various dose combinations			Hypoglycaemia especially in older people Side effects associated with each medicine		Liver
(3) *Meglitinides close K-ATP channels on beta cell plasma membranes and increase insulin secretion* Repaglinide Nataglinide	0.5–16 mg	2–3 per day	Hypoglycaemia with other OHAs Weight gain GIT disturbance		Liver
(4) *Thiazolidinediones activate the nuclear transcription factor PPAR-γ and increase insulin sensitivity* Reduce HbA_{1c} by 0.5–1.4% Rosiglitazone: 4, 8 mg Pioglitazone: 15, 30, 45 mg	4–8 mg	Daily	Oedema, weight gain, CCF, heart failure Raised liver enzymes, Fractures Rosiglitazone: pregnancy risk in women with polycystic ovarian disease, increased LDL-C and MI risk Pioglitazone: might increase bladder cancer risk	DA: 24 h	Liver
(5) *Alpha-glucosidase inhibitors* Acarbose: 50, 100 mg Reduce HbA_{1c} by 0.5–0.8%	50–100 mg	TDS with food	GIT problems, for example, flatulence, diarrhoea Hypoglycaemia		Faeces and urine

Class and medicines	Dose	Timing	Notes	Excretion
(6) DPP-4 inhibitors *increase postprandial GLP concentration, which increases insulin secretion and reduces glucagon secretion* Reduce HbA1c 0.5–0.8% Sitagliptin (Januvia) Vildagliptin Saxagliptin Linaglyptin Alogliptin	100 mg per day in BD regimen in combination with Metformin, or a sulphonylurea (experience is with glimepride) or a TZD (experience is with pioglitazone) Moderate renal failure 50 mg Severe renal disease 25 mg	With or without food	Do not cause hypoglycaemia – reduce dose of sulphonylurea if used as dual therapy to reduce hypoglycaemia risk associated with sulphonylureas Safety with insulin has not been established More research is needed in older people	Unchanged in urine
(7) GLP-1 receptor agonists Reduces HbA_{1c} by 0.5–1% Exenatide, Bydureon Lixisenaride	Once to three times per day depending on the medicine: Lixisenatide is administered daily Bydureon can be administered one/week		Flatulence and abdominal bloating	
Sodium-glucose cotransporter-2 (SGLT-2) Dapagliflozin Canagliflozin			Increased incidence of urinary tract and genital infections Possibility of polyuria in volume sensitive people	

Note: Only some of the many trade named formulations are listed. Formulations in each class have similar actions although there are minor differences among them. The table is a guide only. Specific prescribing information for each medicine should be consulted as well as relevant regulatory authority licensing and approvals. Combination medicines such as Glucovance (Metformin and Glibenclamide) may be useful in reducing the overall number of medicines an individual needs to take.

Biguanides

Biguanides are the medicine of first choice for overweight people with Type 2 diabetics when the HbA_{1c} is >7%. Metformin effectively lowers all-cause mortality and diabetes complications among overweight people with diabetes (UKPDS 1998). It is also used to manage insulin resistance associated with PCOS, where it may delay the progression to Type 2. Metformin is the most commonly used Biguanide. It acts by:

- impairing the absorption of glucose from the gut;
- inhibiting hepatic glucose output;
- increasing glucose uptake in peripheral tissues (muscle and fat);
- increasing the effects of insulin at receptor sites;
- suppressing the appetite (mild effect).

Practice points

(1) Biguanides do not stimulate the production or release of insulin, and therefore are unlikely to cause hypoglycaemia.
(2) They have favourable effects on the lipid profile and slow glucose absorption from the intestine.
(3) They do not stimulate the appetite and are unlikely to cause weight gain.
(4) They have similar effects on HbA_{1c} as sulphonylureas (Table 5.1).

Possible side effects

(1) Nausea and/or diarrhoea occur in 10–15% of patients. Most patients tolerate Biguanides if they are started at a low dose, the tablets are taken with or immediately after food, and the dosage is increased gradually.
   - Lactic acidosis is the most significant side effect but it is rare and could be prevented by appropriate assessment, monitoring and prescribing; see Chapter 7. It occurs in at-risk people during acute infections, acute kidney injury and decompensated heart failure, which are independently associated with lactic acidosis (Iedema & Russell 2011). Although lactic acidosis is rare, 48 cases were reported to the Australian Adverse Drug Reactions Advisory Committee (ADRAC) between 1985 and 2001. Of these, known risk factors were present in 35 of the 48 cases (Jerrall 2002). Salpeter *et al.* (2006) found no cases of lactic acidosis in a systematic review of comparative trials and cohort studies (n = 59,320 patient years of metformin use). Salpeter *et al.* estimated the upper limit of true incidence of lactic acidosis per 100,000 patient years was 5.1 in people using Metformin and there was no difference in lactate levels for Metformin compared with non-Metformin therapies. However, the true clinical incidence is unknown and could be higher because not all adverse events are reported. Nisbet *et al.* (2004) identified 13 cases of lactic acidosis possibly related to Metformin since 2000. Of these, two died, three required dialysis for renal failure, and one had severe neurological deficits and required nursing home care. The average age was 67 and average serum creatinine was 0.31 mmol/L (normal 0.05–0.11 women; 0.06–0.12 men mmol/L). Nisbet *et al.*'s study highlights the importance of appropriate clinical assessment before prescribing or represcribing medicines, especially in older people. The risk of lactic acidosis is increased in people with diseases likely to cause hypoxia such as alcohol abuse and liver, renal, and cardiac disease. However, Ekstrom *et al.* (2012) found a reduced risk of all-cause mortality in an

observational study of people on Metformin monotherapy with eGFR 45–60 ml/min/1.73 squared and no increased risk of all-cause mortality, acidosis, serious infection or cardiovascular disease in people with eGFR 30–45 ml/min/1.73 squared (n = 51675). The authors concluded the benefits of Metformin outweigh the risks. Early signs of lactic acidosis include:

anorexia

nausea and vomiting

abdominal pain

cramps

- weight loss
- lethargy
- respiratory distress.

(2) Biguanides should not be prescribed:
- during pregnancy;
- for people with chronic renal failure;
- Type 1 diabetes;
- any disease likely to cause hypoxia such as severe respiratory diseases and hepatic or cardiovascular disease.

There is some evidence that at higher doses and longer duration of use, Metformin inhibits absorption of vitamin B_{12}. The metformin dose is the strongest predictor of vitamin B_{12} deficiency (Ting *et al.* 2006). However, Ting *et al.* did not assess calcium intake or measure vitamin B_{12} metabolites (homocysteine and methylmalonic acid), which could have affected the results. Nevertheless, Vitamin B_{12} deficiency should be considered in people at high risk of malnourishment, for example, older people and those with eating disorders, people who have been on Metformin for long periods of time especially at high doses, and those with malabsorption syndromes such as coeliac disease.

Biguanides should be ceased for two days before IVP, CAT scans and investigations that require IV-iodinated contrast media to be used (Calabrese *et al.* 2002).

Sulphonylureas

Sulphonylureas can be used alone or combined with Metformin. They can be used as first line therapy in non-obese people who are intolerant of, or have contraindications to, Metformin (SIGN 2010). They are usually well tolerated but there is a tendency for people to gain weight, especially with older sulphonylureas, although these are rarely used nowadays. Weight gain occurs to a less extent with newer sulphonylureas (Inzucchi 2002). They generally have a rapid onset of action except for long-acting formulations. Hypoglycaemia is a risk especially in older people on long-acting agents, although these are rarely used and are no longer available in some countries. However, Glibenclamide is available in combination with Metformin (Glucovance). People with renal impairment and those who are malnourished are also at risk of hypoglycaemia.

Sulphonylureas act by:

- stimulating insulin secretion from the pancreatic beta cells;
- increasing the effects of insulin at its receptor sites;
- sensitising hepatic glucose production to inhibition by insulin.

Possible side effects

(1) Hypoglycaemia may result due to over-secretion of insulin if the dose of the medicine is increased, food is delayed, meals are missed, or activity is increased; see Chapter 6.

(2) Liver dysfunction.
(3) Nausea, vomiting.
(4) Various skin rashes.
(5) Increased appetite.
(6) Rarely, agranulocytosis and red cell aplasia can occur.

Note: points 2–6 are very uncommon. Sulphonylureas are contraindicated in pregnancy although they are used during pregnancy in some countries. They are mostly metabolised in the liver and severe liver disease is a contraindication to their use. Caution should be taken in people who are allergic to 'sulphur medicines' because the sulphonylureas have a similar chemical makeup.

Meglitinides

These medicines increase insulin secretion at meal times and they should only be taken with meals, usually 2–3 times per day. They have the same effect on the beta cell receptor but a different chemical structure. They are short acting and have a low hypoglycaemic risk but hypoglycaemia is possible. They have not been assessed for beneficial effects on reducing micro-and macrovascular disease and are generally more expensive then other GLMs (SIGN 2010).

Meglitinides target early phase insulin secretion, which is essential for postprandial glucose and control the postprandial glucose load (Dornhorst 2001). In this way they initiate an insulin response pattern close to normal. They can be used in combination with Biguanides and possibly Thiazolidinediones (TZD). The two main formulations are Repaglinide and Nataglinide. These medicines are rarely used in Australia because they are not listed on the PBS. However, because of their short duration of action and the requirement to take them with meals they could be very useful in older people at high risk of hypoglycaemia.

Thiazolidinediones

The thiazolidinediones (TZD) are also known as peroxisome-proliferator-activated receptor (PPAR-γ. TZDs lower fasting and postprandial blood glucose by increasing insulin sensitivity in muscle, fat, and liver cells. Some improve lipid profiles, enhance insulin sensitivity and may restore the beta cell mass. They are given as a daily dose. It takes several days before they show an effect. There are two forms Pioglitazone and Rosiglitazone. Pioglitazone can be used as dual therapy in combination with Metformin OR a sulphonylurea in Type 2 diabetes when the HbA_{1c} is >7% when combining Metformin and a sulphonylurea is contraindicated. Pioglitazone can be combined with insulin in Type 2 diabetes if the HbA_{1c} is >7% despite treatment with OHAs and insulin, OR insulin alone OR if Metformin is contraindicated. Rosiglitazone can be combined with Metformin AND a sulphonylurea in Type 2 diabetes when the HbA_{1c} is >7% despite maximum tolerated doses of these medicines.

TZDs reduce HbA_{1c} by ~1–2% (Ko *et al.* 2006) with similar improvements to adding insulin. If adding a TZD does not adequately reduce HbA_{1c} to <8 5% in three months, insulin should be commenced (Nathan & Buse 2006). It is usual to start at low dose and monitor the person closely for signs of heart failure especially those with pre-existing cardiovascular disease. Significant cardiovascular disease is a contraindication to TZDs.

Rosiglitazone might prevent or delay the transition to Type 2 diabetes in at-risk individuals (DREAM 2006). However, subsequent modelling of the DREAM data suggests people taking Rosiglitazone to prevent diabetes would end up taking more medicines than those who start medicines after diabetes is diagnosed and are at risk of

TZD side effects (Montori & Isley 2007). SIGN (2010) stated there is no convincing evidence that Rosiglitazone as monotherapy has benefits over Metformin and sulphonylureas.

Pioglitazone is associated with the risk of bladder cancer in people who use the medicine for over 12 months (Lewis *et al.* 2011). The risk is greater in people with bladder cancer or a history of bladder cancer. People should be advised of the risk when discussing their medicine options. Pharmaceutical companies have revised their product information to reflect the risk.

Side effects
- Localised oedema, which can be significant and may occur to a greater extent in people treated with TZD and insulin (SIGN 2010).
- Congestive cardiac failure and heart failure. People with diabetes are 2.5 times more likely to develop heart failure than non-diabetics (Nichols *et al.* 2001) and TZDs increase the risk of heart failure. Rosiglitazone doubles the risk among those with pre-existing cardiovascular disease (Home *et al.* 2009). Both TZDs are contraindicated in people with New York Heart Association Class III or IV heart failure. The person should be closely monitored for signs of heart failure such as oedema and rapid weight gain, and importantly, informed about these risks.
- Myocardial infarction and death associated with Rosiglitazone (Nissen & Wolski 2007). This report caused significant debate among diabetes experts and stress for patients prescribed Rosiglitazone. The risk appears to be small (DREAM 2006). The information should be used in the context of individual risk. For example, Rosiglitazone might increase the risk of MI in people with ischaemic heart disease, those on insulin or nitrates, those with an atherogenic lipid profile, and those at high risk of MI (ADRAC 2007). Pioglitazone does not appear to carry the same risk because it has fewer adverse effects on lipids (Dormandy *et al.* 2005). The RECORD study (2009) suggested there is a possible increase in cardiovascular events with Rosiglitazone in people with existing heart disease, but the association was not statistically significant. The European Medicines Agency (EMA) (2010) reviewed all medicines containing Rosiglitazone that concluded the risks of Rosiglitazone outweigh the benefits and recommended marketing authorisation for all products containing Rosiglitazone be suspended across the European Union (http://bit.ly/Rosi2011). Likewise the US Federal Drug Administration (FDA) added information about the cardiovascular risks of Rosiglitizone to the physician labelling and medication guide (US FDA 2011).
- Reduced red and white cell count.
- Weight gain, especially deposition of subcutaneous fat, while visceral obesity is reduced. Weight gain appears to continue as long as TZDs are continued. Gains between 2 and 5 kg are reported (Dormandy *et al.* 2005). However, insulin also causes weight gain (~3 kg), as do sulphonylureas (~4 kg). Weight gain is lower when patients are taking Metformin before a TZD is added (Strowig *et al.* 2004).
- Hypercholesterolaemia, especially LDL-C (Rosiglitazone).
- Liver damage although it is uncommon. TZDs are contraindicated if liver disease is present or serum transiminase is >2.5 times the upper limit of the normal. Liver function tests should be performed before starting a TZD and then monitored regularly while the patient remains on TZDs. Signs of liver toxicity include nausea, vomiting, jaundice, dark urine, and right upper abdominal discomfort.
- Macular oedema (European Medicine Agency Press 2005). Macular oedema is a known complication of diabetes and there some reports the condition worsens with TZD.
- Fractures occurring in the arms and lower leg usually in women (Meier *et al.* 2008), however the risk is small. Fracture risk may be significant in older women at risk of

osteoporosis and increase the risk of falls if the fractures occur in the feet or legs. People prescribed TZD, especially women, should be informed about the risk.

- Women with polycystic ovarian disease should be counselled about contraception because TZDs may improve fertility in these women.
- They are contraindicated in pregnancy and during breast feeding.
- Care should be taken in lactose intolerant people because TZDs contain a small amount of lactose.
- Hypoglycaemia is possible because TZDs reduce insulin resistance and enhance the effectiveness of endogenous insulin.

These data suggest a thorough assessment, including a medication review, is warranted before commencing TZDs. Health professionals and people with diabetes should be alert to the possibility of silent MI.

Alpha-glucosidase inhibitors

These medicines are usually taken in a TDS regimen.

They act by slowing glucose uptake of many carbohydrates by inhibiting alpha-glucosidase, which slows the metabolism of complex and simple carbohydrates in the brush border of the proximal small intestine so glucose absorption is spread over a longer time frame. Alpha-glucosidase inhibitors reduce fasting and postprandial glucose (Rosak & Mertes 2012).

Their major side effects are due to the arrival of undigested carbohydrate in the lower bowel – bloating, flatulence, and diarrhoea. These symptoms can be distressing and embarrassing and people often stop their medications because of these side effects. Taking the medicines with meals, starting with a low dose and increasing slowly to tolerance levels, and careful explanation to the patient can reduce these problems.

Hypoglycaemia is possible if alpha-glucosidase inhibitors are combined with other GLMs. They may be contraindicated or need to be used with caution in people with gastrointestinal disease such as gastroparesis, coeliac disease, and irritable bowel syndrome.

> ### *Practice point*
>
> Oral glucose may not be an effective treatment for hypoglycaemia occurring in people on alpha-glucosidase inhibitors because absorption from the gut will be delayed. IM Glucagon is an alternative.

The incretin hormones

The incretins enhance glucose-mediated insulin secretion by the beta cells. Approximately 60% of insulin secreted in response to food is due to the activity of incretins. The incretin effect is due to peptide hormones released by K and L cells in the intestine directly into the blood stream. The incretins include:

(1) Glucose-dependent insulinotropic peptide (GIP) secreted by the K-intestinal cells. Postprandially, GIP levels are ~10 times higher than GLP-1 and have similar

insulinotrophic actions when the glucose level is >6 mmol/L, but its effects are limited at blood glucose levels >7.8 mmol/L. GIP does not inhibit glucagon secretion.

(2) Glucagon-like peptide (GLP-1) is secreted by the L-cells in the intestine. It primarily regulates postprandial glucose by slowing gastric emptying and reducing glucagon. It reduces appetite and may induce weight loss (SIGN 2010) and it may stimulate beta cell proliferation (Abraham *et al*. 2002). GLP-1 binds to its specific receptor but has a very short half-life (60–90 seconds) because it is rapidly broken down by dipeptidyl peptidase-4 (DPP-4). Exanetide, liragulitide and Lixisenatide are GLP-1 receptor agonist analogues and may improve metabolic control in people with BMI >30 kg/m squared with Type 2 diabetes. Lixisenatide is administered daily. GLP-1 agonists may not be beneficial in people with inadequate glycaemic control for >10 years: insulin may be the medicine of choice in these people (SIGN 2010).

(3) DPP-4 inhibitor analogues are oral GLMs such as Sitagliptin, Vildagliptin and Saxagliptin that inhibit the action of DDP-4 and consequently increase postprandial GLP concentration, which increases insulin secretion, reduces glucose-dependent glucagon secretion and reduces HbA1c 0.5–0.8% (Nathan & Buse 2006: Inzucchi *et al*. 2012). DPP-4 are listed in most countries as add-on therapy with Metformin or a sulphonylurea where a combination of the latter two medicines is contraindicated and particular prescribing recommendations may apply in particular countries (NICE 2008; SIGN 2019; NPS 2011). Recently, The European Commission approved the combination of Metformin and Linagliptin, a DPP-4 inhibitor.

Side effects

- The effects on long term outcomes are not yet known. Side effects include nasopharyngitis and upper respiratory tract infections, which are common, and hypersensitivity reactions.
- Pancreatitis has been reported with Sitagliptin and Vildagliptin although a causal association has not yet been confirmed (NPS 2011 and 2012).
- Vildagliptin and Saxagliptin should be avoided in people with renal impairment, creatinine clearance <50 ml/mim.
- Vildagliptin is not recommended in people with liver disease. Sitagliptin should be used cautiously in people with liver disease.
- Sitagliptin has been associated with anaphalyxis, angioedema, rashes, urticaria and exfoliative skin conditions but these side effects are rare (NPS 2011).
- Weight gain can occur when the gliptins are used with a sulphonylurea.
- Hypoglycaemia can occur when the gliptins are used with a sulphonylurea.
- Gastrointestinal side effects.

New medicines for type 2 diabetes

Sodium-glucose cotransporter-2 (SGLT2) inhibitors

SGLT2 inhibitors are a new class of GLM that target renal glucose reabsorption and induce glucose excretion in the urine independently of insulin secretion or action and are used in type 2 diabetes (Whaley *et al*. 2012). Trials show SGLT2 medicines reduce hyperglycaemia, fasting and postprandial blood glucose and HbA_{1c}, hypertension and weight. They have a low hypoglycaemia risk and may be able to be combined with insulin and other GLMs (Whaley *et al*. 2012). SLGT2 include Dapagliflozin and Canagliflozin and are administered one per day.

Side effects

Clinical experience with SLGTs is limited at present. Reported side effects include:

- Increased incidence of urinary tract infections, which could put individuals with automomic neuropathy affecting the bladder at particular risk.
- Increased incidence of genital fungal infections.
- Polyuria in volume-sensitive people, which could predispose them to dehydration e.g. older people.
- Canaglifozin may appears to be less effective in people with renal impairment.
- Concerns have been raised about the risk of cardio-and cerebrovascular disease because of the effects on cholesterol.
- Canaglifozin increases LDL cholesterol but it also increases HDL though it is not clear whether the benefits outweigh the risks at this stage.

Canaglifozin was approved by the FDA in March 2013. The US FDA did not approve Dapagliflozin in 2012 because of safety concerns such as increased risk of breast and bladder caner but it was approved in Europe in 2012 under the brand name Forxiga.

Antibody 2H10

Antibody 2H10 appears to slow or reverse the progression to Type 2 diabetes in mice. 2H10 may block a protein called vascular endothelial growth factor (BVEGF-B), which influences fat transport and storage in body tissue such as the heart. Thus, 2H10 appears to target insulin resistance. However, the antibody is in the very early stage of medicine development and has not yet been tested in humans.

Medicine interactions

Some possible interactions between GLMs and other commonly prescribed medicines are shown in Table 5.2. Some medicines interact with GLM and can cause hypo- or hyper-glycaemia. A number of mechanisms for the interactions are known and they include:

- displacing the medicine from binding sites;
- inhibiting or decreasing hepatic metabolism;
- delaying excretion;
- reducing insulin release;
- antagonising insulin action.

Potential medicine and herb or herb/herb interactions and food/medicine interactions should also be considered when introducing a new medicine or reviewing the medicine regimen; see Chapter 19. For example, over 95 medicines administered by mouth can interact with grapefruit including antihypertensive agents, some antibiotics, cancer and cardiovascular medicines (Bailey 2012) and interactions can occur even if grapefruit is taken several hours before taking the medicine. In addition other citrus fruits may also interact but have not been widely studied to date. Interactions can also lead to micro-nutrient deficiency (Braun & Rosenfeldt 2012).

Potential interactions have not yet fully emerged for TZIs and the incretins (gliptins). Medicines that alter hepatic enzymes have the potential to cause interactions with these GLMs because they are metabolised in the liver. Medicines that interfere with access to the gut by alpha-glucosidase inhibitors can inhibit their action, for example, charcoal, digestive enzymes, Cholestyramine, Neomycin, and some CAM medicines such as slippery elm.

Table 5.2 Potential medicine interactions between glucose-lowering medicines and other medicines (Data from Shenfield [2001]).

Medicine	Possible mechanism
Medicines that increase blood glucose	
Clonidine	Adrenergic response
Clozapine	Impaired insulin secretion
Corticosteroids	Oppose insulin action
Diuretics, especially Thiazides	Oppose insulin action
Nicotinic acid	Unknown
Nifedipine	Delays insulin action
Oral contraceptives	Unknown
Phenytoin	Impairs insulin secretion
Glucocorticoids	Cause insulin resistance and weight gain
Antipsychotics, especially atypical antipsychotics	
Sugar-containing medicines, for example, cough syrup	Increase blood glucose
Medicines that lower blood glucose	
ACE inhibitors	Enhance insulin action
Alcohol	Reduce hepatic glucose production
Fibrates such as gemfibrosil	Unknown
MOA inhibitors	Unknown
Salicylates in high doses (some herbal medicines contain salicylic compounds)	Unknown

Practice points

(1) The clinical relevance of some postulated medicine interactions is uncertain.
(2) Other miscellaneous interactions that should also be considered are:
  - beta blockers can mask tachycardia and other signs of hypoglycaemia resulting in delayed recognition and treatment increasing the risk of hypoglycaemic coma.
  - chronic alcohol consumption can stimulate the metabolism of sulphonylureas and delay their effectiveness, cause hypoglycaemia, mask signs of hypoglycaemia, and with Metformin, predispose the individual to lactic acidosis. It may also increase the bioavailability of ACE-1.

Combining GLMs and insulin

Any combination of currently available GLM only lowers HbA_{1c} by ~3% (American Association of Endocrinologists 2011, thus people with HbA_{1c} >10% are unlikely to achieve management targets using GLM alone. Therefore, insulin is assuming an increasingly important role in Type 2 diabetes. As indicated, most people with Type 2 diabetes have progressive beta cell dysfunction and a decline in beta cell mass. Proposed mechanisms for these defects include the interplay among a range of factors that reduce beta cell mass and secretory function such as hyperglycaemia, elevated free fatty acids, and inflammatory processes associated with adipocyte-derived cytokines. Apoptosis appears to be a key underlying mechanism (Leiter 2006). In addition, lifestyle factors, concomitant diseases, and often medicines, compound the metabolic abnormalities. In some cases medication non-adherence may be a factor and should be assessed in a non-judgmental manner.

Goudswaard *et al.* (2004) showed continuing Metformin when insulin is commenced is associated with lower HbA_{1c} (by up to 0.6%) and less weight gain without increasing hypoglycaemia risk. Continuing sulphonylurea when initiating a daily insulin dose was associated with a greater HbA_{1c} reduction than monotherapy. Likewise, continuing Metformin, sulphonylurea or both when insulin is commenced, results in lower insulin requirements compared with monotherapy.

Various algorithms are available for initiating insulin and continuing one or more GLM (NICE 2008; SIGN 2010; DA-RACGP 2011/12; NPS 2012). The medicines selected and the dose and dose regimen must be tailored to the individual's needs. Generally bedtime NPH or a basal insulin analogue should be used when adding insulin to Metformin and/or a sulphonylurea depending on the hypoglycaemia risk (SIGN 2010).

Practice points

- GLMs, including insulin, are not substitutes for healthy eating, weight management and regular exercise.
- Medication administration times should be planned so that GLMs are administered with or before, meals to reduce the risk of hypoglycaemia.

When should insulin be initiated in Type 2 diabetes?

Commencing insulin should be a planned, proactive decision and should not be delayed. Some experts refer to 'tablet failure' as a reason for initiating insulin. The choice of words should be considered carefully when conveying the need for insulin to a person with diabetes: they may interpret 'tablet failure' to mean *they* have failed (Diabetes Australia 2011/12).

Clinical observations

- The challenge for health professionals is to balance the optimal time to initiate insulin with the time the individual is ready to accept insulin.
- Culture, literacy, beliefs, experience, and social situation are some of the factors that affect people's readiness to accept insulin.
- Interestingly, doctors, and probably other health professionals, frequently do not follow recommended guidelines for various reasons such as resource and time constraints, because they are 'slow adopters,' or because they use complex individual decision-making heuristics (Choudhry & Fletcher 2005; Tung 2011).

The time of day to administer insulin in Type 2 diabetes depends on the individual's blood glucose pattern, HbA_{1c}, adherence to medicines, and complication status, especially cardiovascular and renal status, and willingness to use insulin. Often a basal insulin is initiated at bedtime and the dose adjusted according to the fasting (prebreakfast) blood glucose. Prandial insulin before one or more meals is added if HbA_{1c} and blood glucose targets are not achieved. A general guide to deciding insulin requirements when initiating insulin follows, but individual needs and blood glucose pattern and frequency of hypo- and hyperglycaemia must be considered.

Indications for insulin include:

- Women with Type 2 diabetes who become pregnant and sometimes women with gestational diabetes; see Chapter 14.
- When the person actually has LADA (see Chapter 1).
- As rescue therapy in DKA, HHS, during other acute illnesses, and surgical procedures; see Chapters 7 and 9.
- Persisting hyperglycaemia indicated by elevated fasting blood glucose and/or elevated postprandial blood glucose and HbA_{1c} above the individual's target (e.g. $HbA1_c > 7\%$).
- Symptoms especially polyuria, polydipsia and weight loss.
- GLM intolerance or contraindication, for example, Metformin if creatinine is high.
- People on two GLMs and not achieving targets where insulin may be preferable to adding a third GLM, given that most people with Type 2 diabetes eventually need insulin especially if the GLMs are at maximal doses. However, there is no consensus about whether the second agent added to Metformin should be another GLM or insulin. Insulin might be preferable if the HbA_{1c} is >8.5% or the person is very symptomatic (Nathan & Buse 2006) or when there is a high tablet burden (polypharmacy). In such presentations LADA should be considered especially if the individual is thin. The National Prescribing Service advised health professionals to be '... more aggressive in their management of people with Type 2 diabetes' (NPS media release, 26 March 2008), a sentiment echoed by other experts. However, the benefits of 'insulin aggression' need to be balanced against the risks such as hypoglycaemia and its consequences (falls in older people, MI, effects on cognition).
- Recent research suggests insulin may have anti-inflammatory properties in addition to its other actions (Dandona *et al.* 2008).

The goals are to achieve optimal control without causing hypoglycaemia or excessive weight gain and with minimal impact on lifestyle. Thus, understanding the individual's perspective is essential.

For some people, commencing insulin and ceasing GLMs may represent a simpler more manageable medication regimen, for others it represents 'the end of the line' or 'the last resort.'

Insulin is often added to the GLM regimen at bedtime to reduce fasting glucose levels (Riddle *et al.* 2003; Janka *et al.* 2005). The dose is titrated according to the fasting blood glucose pattern including self-adjustment by the person with diabetes to achieve targets with minimal hypoglycaemia according to a simple algorithm (Yki-Jarvinen *et al.* 2007). Yki-Jarvinen *et al.* showed insulin could be successfully initiated in groups and achieve glycaemic targets. In addition, group insulin initiation was acceptable to patients.

The specific initiation process depends on the policies and guidelines of individual health services. Over recent years, research has demonstrated the efficacy of several processes for initiating and titrating insulin in Type 2 diabetes using various insulins and usually starting with small doses. They all used a stepwise approach and include:

- The Treat-to-Target study used basal Glargine at bedtime and titrated the dose weekly in 10 weeks (Riddle *et al.* 2003). This regimen is suitable for older people because it is associated with fewer hypoglycaemic events and is well tolerated (Janka *et al.* 2005). Isophane insulin can also be used as the basal insulin but has a higher risk of hypoglycaemia.
- The 1-2-3 study, which used daily bedtime doses of NovoMix 30 initially and subsequently added doses pre-breakfast then pre-lunch if necessary to achieve targets (Raskin *et al.* 2005).
- The INITIATE study that used BD doses of NovoMix 30 (Jain *et al.* 2005).

The stepwise approach is also used with insulin analogues such as long-acting basal lantus, Detemir and Degludec, an ultra long acting preparation currently in phase three clinical trials, and rapid acting prandial insulins such as Novorapid.

The advantage of using basal bolus insulin dose regimens is that they usually achieve better postprandial control but eating after injecting the insulin is important. BD Lispro/isophane mix and Metformin also improves pre- and postprandial blood glucose with few episodes of nocturnal hypoglycaemia (Malone *et al.* 2005).

Many researchers have compared different brands of insulin and dose regimens. Overall, the findings suggest the pharmacokinetic differences among insulin brands may not be clinically relevant and there are likely to be variations in individual patient's response to the different formulations (Zeolla 2007). The ultralong acting basal insulin in phase three testing, Degludec, appears to cause less nocturnal hypoglycaemia in Type 1 and Type 2 diabetes, and reduce fasting glucose (Wang *et al.* 2012). In reality, the choice of insulin may actually be made according to prescriber preference and local availability. Despite the similarities, indiscriminate switching between different insulin brands or using different brands together is not generally recommended.

Outpatient or community-based insulin initiation is preferable except in specific circumstances. A proforma initiation process is outlined in this chapter that can be adapted as necessary and a simple algorithm for commencing insulin in Type 2 diabetes is shown in Table 5.3 and Figure 5.2. Often, GLMs are continued with basal insulin regimens if there are no contraindications to their use. When bolus insulin doses are added, insulin secretagogue doses usually need to be reduced or the medicines discontinued.

The algorithm is based on the premise that the individual undertakes blood glucose monitoring, relevant monitoring and assessments are undertaken, relevant education is provided and the response to therapy is monitored at each step. Consider LADA if the person is not overweight, loses weight, has significant hyperglycaemia, and is very symptomatic because insulin should not be delayed in these people; see Chapter 1.

Management aims:

(1) Proactively initiate insulin. Insulin should not be delayed.
(2) Control fasting and postprandial hyperglycaemia without causing serious hyperglycaemia.
(3) Achieve HbA$_{1c}$ target relevant to the age of the individual generally <7% but maybe higher in older people.
(4) Normalise lipids to reduce cardiovascular risk.
(5) Control symptoms.

GLM = glucose lowering medicines; TZD = Thiazolidinediones.

Table 5.3 Simple decision-general guide to deciding insulin doses and dose regimen when commencing insulin (NICE 2008; DA-RACGP 2011/12), however guidelines and protocols in use should be followed. Insulin doses are adjusted by 2–4 units according to the blood glucose pattern every 3–4 days to reach the target blood glucose range and avoid hypoglycaemia.

Issues to consider	HbA_{1c} %	Insulin doses and administration times
Consider current diabetes management and glycaemic status		Insulin in units/kg depending on pre insulin treatment and weight
Decide on a safe blood glucose target range for the individual	< 7	diet alone 0.2 GLMs 0.3
Decide whether to administer insulin as a daily basal dose and/or bolus doses and when the insulin will be administered on the basis of the amount of insulin required per day and whether oral GLMs will be continued	> 7	diet alone 0.3 GLMs 0.4
Morning blood glucose high and evening blood glucose acceptable		Pre-bed basal insulin
Morning blood glucose acceptable and evening blood glucose high		Morning basal insulin
Morning blood glucose high and evening blood glucose high		Basal bolus regimen that could be with a long acting analogue before bed or before breakfast and TDS rapid acting insulin OR BD premixed insulin OR morning Isophane insulin and TDS rapid-acting insulin

Diagnosis
Diet and exercise +/– GLM
Trial for 3 months

→

Add one GLM
Metformin in overweight individuals
Trial for 3 months

Add second medicine, usually an GLM, e.g., sulphonylurea
Trial for 3 months

$HbA_{1C} \geq 6.5$–7%
Add a third GLM, e.g. a TZD
OR
Initiate insulin: preferred if $HbA_{1C} > 8\%$
Do not use GLM above maximal doses
Trial for 3 months

$HbA_{1C} \geq 7.3\%$
Add insulin e.g.,
Basal long-acting analogue at bedtime and titrate the dose weekly
OR
Isophane 6–10 units at bedtime and adjust the dose by 2–4 units every 3–4 days to gradually achieve the targets
Aim for fasting blood glucose 4.0–6.0 mmol/L
Monitor for 3 months

If the target is not achieved with 50 units of basal insulin add a second dose of insulin, e.g., premixed insulin 30/70
Give 2/3 of total dose before breakfast and 1/3 before evening meal
OR
Institute basal bolus regimen depending on the patient: rapid-short-acting before each meal and long-acting analogue of Isophane at night
Cease GLM

Figure 5.2 Algorithm for achieving blood glucose targets in Type 2 diabetes that encompasses a Quality Use of Medicines approach and adopts a proactive stepwise approach to initiating insulin.

Barriers to insulin therapy

There are many barriers to initiating insulin therapy in Type 2 diabetes: most relate to the individual with diabetes and some to health professional factors. Although patients often view insulin negatively, early explanations about the nature of Type 2 diabetes (from diagnosis), and with support and encouragement, most people usually accept they need insulin. However, their fears and concerns must be acknowledged, respected and explored. People often regard insulin as 'the last resort', and fear hypoglycaemia and weight gain (Dunning & Martin 1999). The DAWN study (Rutherford *et al.* 2004) showed that people on insulin worried about hypoglycaemia more than non-insulin users and insulin was associated with worse quality of life in people with Type 2 diabetes. This finding continues to emerge in other studies for example, (MILES 2011).

Type 2 diabetes is a silent disease with few symptoms; thus, it is often difficult for people to accept they have a serious, progressive disease. Many worry about weight gain associated with insulin use. They are often reluctant to test their blood glucose frequently and feel blood glucose monitoring and insulin interferes with their lifestyle. For some people, the stigma associated with needles is an issue.

Many doctors are reluctant to use insulin in Type 2 diabetes and often compound the patient's concerns, albeit usually unintentionally, by delaying insulin initiation. Such health professional behaviour has been referred to as 'clinical inertia' (Shah *et al.* 2005), and, like non-adherence, is a complex multifactorial issue (Tung 2011). Other health professional-related barriers include inadequate knowledge, lack of time, support and resources, worry about causing hypoglycaemia and complicating the management regimen. For example, UK practice nurses felt commencing insulin in primary care was beneficial for patients but lack of time, support, and confidence, and concerns about medico-legal implications and personal accountability made it difficult to achieve (Greaves *et al.* 2003).

Some strategies to overcome the barriers

The therapeutic relationship between the patient and the health professional has a significant effect on health outcomes and patient behaviours including adherence to medicines and improved safety (Worthington 2003; Dunning). Thus, a first step is to establish a non-judgmental, trusting relationship. Specific approaches depend on the individual and the circumstances in which insulin is required. Health professionals need to acknowledge that:

- People's previous experience of insulin and beliefs about insulin.
- Managing insulin is a complex process and is only one self-care and life task the person is expected to fulfill.
- 'Things might get worse before they get better'. For example vision often deteriorates temporarily.
- The ability to self-care changes over time due to physical and mental functional changes: normal age-related changes and changes associated with diabetes complications.
- Insulin side effects especially hypoglycaemia.
- There are usually added costs involved.

The transformational model of change can be a useful framework for addressing the need to commence insulin, especially if it is integrated with aspects of the health belief model, QUM and holistic care, where insulin is discussed as one aspect to be addressed, not an isolated event in a person's life. Research suggests timing is important when trying to initiate change. That is, it needs to be linked to an individual's stage in the change process (Prochaska & Velicer 1997) and significant life transitions, which are often also accompanied by changes in identity and behaviour (George 1993; Dunning).

Providing personalised and customised advice and written information is most useful when it is delivered in a caring relationship where the individual's concerns are acknowledged and they are invited to suggest ways they could address the issues they identify. Thus, listening, clarifying, and following up by asking about progress are essential. However, despite the focus on patient-centred care, the patient's views are often not sought and they are inadvertently placed in a passive rather than an active role particularly when communication barriers such as language, religion, culture, health literacy and numeracy, hearing impairment or other disabilities are present.

Identifying and discussing the person's concerns is essential. For example, 'needle phobia', weight gain, and hypoglycaemia. Demonstrating the various insulin delivery devices often helps reduce some concerns about needles. People on insulin gain more weight than those on diet for over 10 years (Mayfield & White 2004), partly due to better glycaemic control and losing less glucose in the urine, the fact that insulin is an anabolic hormone, lower metabolic rate and people may eat more to prevent hypoglycaemia (Birkeland *et al.* 1994). Levemir appears to cause less weight gain in both Type 1 and Type 2 diabetes (Dornhorst *et al.* 2007), whereas Glargine is associated with a modest weight increase and hypoglycaemia (ORIGIN 2012).

Strategies to avoid weight gain include selecting insulin formulations and other medicines least likely to contribute to weight gain if possible, regular exercise perhaps using a pedometer, and individualised nutrition advice. Once symptoms are controlled people often feel more active and exercise helps control weight and blood glucose.

Understanding and exploring the person's concerns about hypoglycaemia and helping them identify strategies to reduce hypoglycaemic episodes. Although the UKPD showed the frequency and severity of severe hypoglycaemia was lower in people with Type 2 diabetes than Type 1 diabetes (UKPDS 1998), more recent research suggests hypoglycaemia is a significant risk in both types of diabetes (Chapter 6). The risk increases when the HbA_{1c} is <7.4% and with insulin and oral insulin secretagogues. Carefully identifying hypoglycaemia risk factors with the individual and helping them develop strategies to minimise their individual risk, is important.

Vision can deteriorate when insulin is commenced. Sight is not usually threatened, but it is very distressing for the person with diabetes and they need a careful explanation and reassurance to help them understand. Activities of daily living such as reading and driving can be affected. Visual changes occur because the lens absorbs excess glucose in much the same way as sponge soaks up water. Changes in the amount of glucose in the lens can lead to blurred vision and can occur with high and low blood glucose levels. This phenomenon is quite different from diabetic retinopathy, which can threaten the sight.

The starting dose may not be the 'right' dose and the 'right' dose changes according to specific circumstances and individual need.

Insulin therapy

Insulin is a high risk medicine (Dooley *et al.* 2011) and is associated with significant adverse events including in hospitals and aged care facilities. For example 30% of unplanned hospital admissions for older people are associated with medicine-related adverse events (Australian Commission on Safety and Quality in Health Care 2010).

High risk medicines are likely to cause significant harm or death when given incorrectly. Even when used correctly, insulin can cause significant harm. Over one third of medical errors that result in death involve insulin use within 48 hours of the death (Anon 2005). Thus, when considering insulin the individual's risk of harm must be considered and preventative strategies used when possible.

Overview of insulin action

Insulin is a hormone secreted by the beta cells of the pancreas. Normal requirements are between 0.5 and 1.0 units/kg/day. Insulin synthesis and secretion are stimulated by an increase in the blood glucose level after meals. Insulin attaches to insulin receptors on cell membranes to facilitate the passage of glucose into the cell for utilisation as fuel or storage, and reduces hepatic glucose production. Insulin also stimulates the storage of fatty acids and amino acids, facilitates glycogen formation and storage in the liver and skeletal muscle, and limits lipolysis and proteolysis. Therefore, insulin deficiency results in altered protein, fat and carbohydrate metabolism (also refer to Chapter 1).

Insulin is vital to survival for people with Type 1 diabetes and is eventually required by most people with Type 2 diabetes.

Objectives of insulin therapy

(1) To achieve blood glucose, HbA_{1c} and lipid levels within an acceptable individual range by replacing absent insulin secretion in Type 1 and supplementing insulin production in Type 2 diabetes (see previous section).
(2) To approximate physiological insulin secretion and action.
(3) To avoid the consequences of too much insulin (hypoglycaemia) or too little insulin (hyperglycaemia).
(4) Improve quality of life and reduce the risk of long-term diabetes complications.

Types of insulin available

Insulin cannot be given orally at this stage. It is a polypeptide. Polypeptides are digested by gastric enzymes and do not reach the circulation. Research is currently underway to coat insulin in a substance that can withstand gastric juices and enable it to pass unchanged into the intestine before breaking down. Inhaled insulin is also the subject of research but is not generally used in clinical practice and some nasal insulin trials have been abandoned.

A number of different brands of insulins are available, for example, Novo Nordisk, Eli Lilly, and SanofiAventis. As indicated, the insulins are all effective and safe.

Animal insulins (bovine and porcine) are rarely used nowadays but still available in some countries often under special access schemes. 'Human' insulin (HM) is manufactured by recombinant DNA technology. The amino acid sequence of HM insulin is the same as that of insulin secreted by the beta cells of the human pancreas. Rapid acting insulin analogues (prandial insulins) have been developed that give a more physiologic response after injection and improve the blood glucose profile, for example, Humalog, Aspart, and Apidra. The advantages of these insulins are reduced postprandial hyperglycaemia and reduced risk of hypoglycaemia.

Long-acting analogues are Glargine and Levemir. Glargine has a slower onset than Isophane insulins and a smooth peakless action profile for up to 24 hours (Buse 2001). Levimir may be shorter acting than Glargine and has its maximal effect between 3 and 14 hours. Recently and ultra-long acting insulin, Degludec was introduced but clinical experience with this insulin outside research trial is limited. These insulins enable greater management flexibility and lower risk of hypoglycaemia.

Rapid-acting insulin

Rapid-acting insulin should be clear and colourless. Examples are:

- Lispro (Humalog)
- Novorapid (Aspart)
- Glulisine (Apidra).

They have a rapid onset of action, within 10–15 minutes, peak at 60 minutes and act for 2–4 hours.

They need to be given *immediately* before meals and are used in basal bolus regimes, in combination with intermediate acting insulin and long–acting analogues, or used in combination with OHAs or in insulin pumps.

Combining rapid-acting insulin with alpha-glucosidase inhibitors, which reduce glucose absorption from the gut, can increase the risk of hypoglycaemia. The first hour after injection and 2–3 hours after exercise are other peak times for hypoglycaemia.

Short-acting insulin

This should be clear and colourless. Examples are:

- Actrapid
- Humulin R
- Hypurin neutral (beef).

They begin to take effect in 20–30 minutes after injection and act between four and eight hours.

Rapid- and short-acting insulins can be used:

- Alone two to four times per day;
- In combination with intermediate- or long-acting insulins;
- For correction doses;
- As IV insulin infusions;
- In continuous subcutaneous insulin infusions via insulin pumps.

Intermediate-acting insulin

Intermediate-acting insulins must be mixed gently before use and should be milky after mixing. Examples are:

- Protophane
- Humulin NPH
- Hypurin (isophane)

They begin to act in 2–3 hours. The duration of action is between 12 and 18 hours. They can be used:

- In combination with short-acting insulin – this is the usual method.
- Alone for patients who are sensitive to short-acting insulin, or in combination with oral hypoglycaemic agents.

Long-acting insulin

- Glargine (Lantus)
- Detemir (Levemir) as described in the preceding section.

Ultra-long acting insulin

- Insulin Degludec (currently in phase 3 trials).

Biphasic insulins

Biphasic insulins are often prescribed for people with Type 2 diabetes.

These contain both short- or rapid- and intermediate-acting insulins in various combinations. They must be mixed before using. They do not enable independent adjustment of the short or intermediate components. Examples are:

- NovoMix 30 (30% Aspart /70% protamine).
- Humalog Mix 25 (Lispro 25%/Lispro protamine 75%).
- Humalog Mix 50 (Lispro 40%/ Lispro protamine 50%).
- Humalin 30/70 (Humulin 30%/Isopahane 70%).
- Mixtard 30/70 (Actrapid 30%/Isopahne 70%).

Many insulins are available in prefilled disposable insulin devices. Each insulin administration device has advantages and disadvantages and patient preference should be considered. The diabetes educator can help individuals decide which device (and therefore, to some extent which insulin) suits them best. Generally, the insulin device should be used with the insulin designed by the same manufacturer. Insulin syringes still have a role and some people with diabetes prefer to use syringes.

Storing insulin

The temperature at which insulin is stored is important to maintaining its efficacy. Insulin should be stored according to the manufacturer's directions. Unopened vials should be stored in the refrigerator at 2–8 °C. Insulin vials in use can be stored out of the refrigerator, for example, in the patient's medication drawer, provided they are not stored near a source of heat or light (Campbell *et al.* 1993; see individual product prescribing information). People with diabetes need to be educated about correct storage and handling of insulin as well as sharps disposal as part of their education about insulin therapy.

Exposure to heat and light accelerates the formation of insulin transformation products (ITP) and denatures insulin. Insulin undergoes a chemical transformation in solution and ITP are formed. The main ITPs are deanimated insulin, covalent dimmers and oligomers (Pryce 2009).

Clinical observation

Hyperglycaemia can occur when using incorrectly stored insulin and insulin that has passed the expiry date.

Practice points

(1) Long-acting analogues cannot be mixed with other insulins. Nor can they be injected in the same site.
(2) They are clear and great care must be taken to ensure they are not mistaken for rapid- or short-acting insulins. Look-alike medicine alert policies should be initiated. For example, consider storing them in a different part of the refrigerator and clearly flagging them with a 'look-alike' medication alert label.
(3) Carefully check the dose to be administered of NovoMix 30 and Humalog Mix 25 or 50 and do not mistake the numbers in the name of the insulin for the insulin dose, which has occurred and led to serious adverse medicine events.

Injection sites and administration

Administer at the appropriate time before the meal. The abdomen is the preferred site; but upper arms, thighs, and buttocks can also be used. Injection sites must be rotated to avoid lipoatrophy and lipodystrophy and should be checked on a regular basis. Injection sites should also be rotated when people use insulin pumps.

How to inject

The insulin injection technique can influence insulin absorption and, therefore, its action. Insulin should be administered subcutaneously. IM injections lead to unstable blood glucose levels (Vaag *et al.* 1990).

- Pinch up a fold of skin (dermis and subcutaneous tissue) between the thumb and index finger.
- Inject at a 90-degree angle. If the needle is long, pinch up may not be needed and a 45-degree angle can be used to avoid giving an IM injection.
- Release the skin, remove the needle, and apply gentle pressure to the site.
- Document dose and time of the injection.
- Injection sites should be regularly checked for swelling, lumps, pain or leakage of insulin.

Practice points

(1) A range of needle sizes is available. Needle size is important to people with diabetes. They usually prefer small, fine gauge needles.
(2) Injection with fine gauge needles is relatively painless.
(3) Giving the first injection is often very difficult for people with diabetes. Support and encouragement and allowing them to take their time and inject at their own pace is important.
(4) If insulin tends to leak after the injection, release the skin fold before injecting. Pressure from holding the skin fold sometimes forces the insulin back out of the needle track. Withdraw the syringe quickly to allow the skin to seal. Do not cover so that any insulin leakage can be observed.
(5) The loss of even small amounts of insulin can result in unpredictable increases in the blood glucose and inappropriate dose adjustment especially in lean

people and children. Careful observation and estimation of the amount of insulin lost is necessary to make appropriate adjustments to the individual's injection technique – this applies to both patients and nurses.

(6) The larger the volume of insulin to be injected the greater the likelihood of some insulin leaking back along the needle track. Likewise, leakage can occur if the injection is too shallow, or given intradermally.

(7) To minimise the risk of insulin loss during injection, inject slowly and leave the needle in place for 3–6 seconds after the insulin is delivered.

(8) Long-acting and pre-mixed insulins dispensed in insulin pens must be mixed gently before administration.

Instructions for teaching people how to draw up and administer insulin using a syringe appear in Chapter 16. Refer also to the manufacturer's instructions and patient information material.

Practice points

(1) Insulin syringes and pen needles are approved for single use only.

(2) Pen needles should be removed after administering an insulin dose and a new needle used for the next dose especially with premixed insulins, which can block the needle.

(3) Most insulin administration devices, except syringes, were designed to enable patients to administer their own insulin. In hospital, patients should remove the needle and place it in the sharps container after injecting to avoid needle stick injury to staff.

(4) In hospital, aged care and community settings staff should NOT recap needles.

(5) If the patient cannot remove the needle from the pen, a removal device should be used, or the insulin administered using a syringe until the patient is well enough to self-inject again.

Mixing short- and intermediate-acting insulins

General points

There is less need to 'mix insulins' now, due to the range of modern premixed insulin combinations and insulin analogues. However, it is still necessary in some settings and in some countries. Mixing short- and intermediate-acting insulins before injecting may diminish the effect of the short-acting peak, which is more marked when there is substantially more long-acting insulin in the mixture (as is usually the case), especially if the insulin is left to stand for a long time before being injected.

The clinical significance of these changes is unknown. It is more likely to apply to in home situations where home-care/domiciliary nurses or relatives draw up doses for several days in advance for people to self-administer; see Chapter 18. This practice may not be ideal, but it does enable people to retain a measure of independence where syringes are still the device of choice.

The long-acting insulin analogues cannot be mixed with other insulin or injected into the same site.

Commonly used insulin regimens

Daily injection

A combination of:

- Rapid- or short- and long-acting insulin combinations, which are usually given before breakfast. Biphasic premixed insulins such as Mixtard 30/70 are sometimes used.
- Long- or intermediate-acting insulin is often given at bedtime when it is combined with GLMs for Type 2 diabetes. Daily regimes are commonly used for:
  - older people;
  - those not willing to have more than one injection per day;
  - some situations where people require assistance to inject, are living in aged care facilities or depending on home nursing care when staff are not available to inject more than once per day.
- Daily regimens are not recommended for people with Type 1 diabetes.

It can be difficult to attain good control using biphasic insulin because the dose of the individual insulins in the mix cannot be altered, which can increase the risk of hypoglycaemia if eating is erratic, the carbohydrate intake is low, or after vigorous exercise. However, premixed insulins can reduce the medicine burden on individuals.

BD regimens

A combination of rapid- or short- and intermediate or long-acting insulin is usually given before breakfast and before the evening meal. Biphasic insulins are commonly used but do not allow a great deal of flexibility in adjusting doses. The evening dose may effectively control overnight hyperglycaemia. There is a risk of nocturnal hypoglycaemia; see Chapter 6. Usually two-thirds of the total dose is given in the morning and one-third in the evening.

Figure 5.3 depicts the action profiles of the various insulins. Understanding the action profile enables hypoglycaemia risk times to be identified so that meals, activity, and medication administration times can be planned accordingly. They also help decide which insulin to adjust when considered in conjunction with the blood glucose profile. Consideration should always be given to other factors that affect blood glucose levels; see Chapter 3.

> ### *Practice point*
> Rapid-acting insulins act very quickly. They should be given immediately before a meal, or within 15 minutes after the meal to reduce the risk of hypoglycaemia.

Basal bolus regimen

Basal bolus regimens simulate the normal pattern of insulin secretion, that is, a small amount of circulating insulin is present in the blood and restrains gluconeogenesis and glycogenolysis; this is the basal insulin. A bolus amount of insulin is stimulated by the blood glucose rise after a meal. Bolus injections of rapid- or short-acting insulin are given before each meal. The longer-acting insulin, often an analogue, is often given before bed to supply the basal insulin requirement and restrain hepatic glucose output overnight and control the pre-breakfast blood glucose (fasting) level.

Basal bolus regimens offer more flexibility to adjust insulin doses and meal times, and therefore lifestyle is not affected as much. The amount of insulin given at each dose is

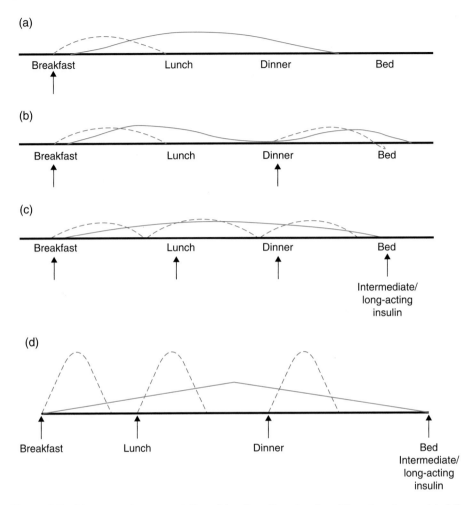

Figure 5.3 Diagrammatic representation of insulin action showing different regimens: (a) daily, (b) twice a day, (c) basal bolus using short-acting insulins and (d) basal bolus using rapid-acting insulins. *Note*: The broken line depicts short-acting insulin, the unbroken line intermediate/long-acting insulin. The arrows indicate the time of injection.

usually small; therefore, the likelihood of hypoglycaemia is reduced. Basal bolus regimens are commonly used for young people with Type 1 diabetes and increasingly for Type 2. Despite the number of injections per day, basal bolus therapy using analogues may be safer for older people, with a lower risk of hypoglycaemia and falls. Nocturnal hypoglycaemia is less frequent when long-acting analogues are used.

Interpreting morning hyperglycaemia

There are three main reasons for fasting hyperglycaemia:

(1) Insufficient basal insulin to restrain overnight hepatic glucose output. It is a common finding with daily insulin regimens when the insulin is given in the morning. A larger dose of insulin may be needed or a second dose of insulin introduced at lunch or bedtime, or if the person is on GLM and a basal anaglogue insulin, the insulin could be given at night.

(2) The Somogyi effect, which is due to the counter-regulatory response to nocturnal hypoglycaemia. The cause needs to be sought (see Chapter 6) but the basal insulin dose may need to be reduced.

(3) 'Dawn phenomenon' reflects insufficient insulin and insulin resistance. There is a normal physiological increase in many hormones early in the morning. However, elevated fasting blood glucose may indicate general hyperglycaemia. A thorough assessment is needed and the medication regimen adjusted.

Continuous subcutaneous insulin infusion (CSII)

Insulin pumps continuously deliver subcutaneous insulin, usually a rapid-acting analogue, at a pre-programmed steady basal rate or rates through a needle inserted subcutaneously, which stays in place for about three days. Bolus doses are delivered before meals or as corrective doses for hyperglycaemia. Bolus doses can be preprogrammed or delivered manually when needed. Insulin pumps enable a more physiological insulin profile to be attained and greater flexibility in meeting individual insulin requirements and lifestyle. Insulin pumps use rapid- or short-acting insulin only; therefore, if they malfunction or are removed, for example during surgery, the patient must be given insulin via another method to avoid hyperglycaemia. For example, subcutaneously or via an IV insulin infusion depending on the circumstances.

Modern insulin pumps are generally reliable and have an inbuilt alarm system that identifies a number of faults such as kinks/blockages in the tubing, tubing disconnections from the pump and low batteries, so that malfunctions can be identified early and appropriate steps taken to avoid hyperglycaemia. Some do not alarm if the tubing disconnects from the insertion site. If this occurs insulin is not delivered and can go unnoticed until the blood glucose is tested. In people with Type 1 diabetes hyperglycaemia can occur quickly and increase the risk of DKA. Reported rates vary between 2.7 and 9 episodes per 100 patient years.

Pumps are expensive and require a great deal of commitment on the part of the person with diabetes to use them safely and effectively. Health professional support and the ready availability of advice are vital. People need time to adjust to the pump regime and become accustomed to not having intermediate-acting insulin. Pumps offer a great deal of flexibility and can have significant psychological benefits. However, pumps do not suit everybody and some people dislike the thought of being constantly connected to a device.

People need to learn to count carbohydrates when they commence using an insulin pump. Structured education programmes such as Dose Adjustment for Normal Eating (DAFNE) (DAFNE Study Group 2002) are often used to help individuals learn how much insulin is required per meal (~0.5 units/10 g of carbohydrate). DAFNE is based on 10 g of carbohydrate. Recently, a blood glucose meter and smart phone apps have appeared on the market and can be useful decision-aids for people with diabetes. Combining continuous blood glucose monitoring with an insulin pump is becoming a reality and will be welcomed by people with diabetes.

Practice points

(1) Insulin pumps are not a cure for inadequate metabolic control but they can help some people achieve better control.

(2) They enable the insulin regimen and food intake to be matched to individual requirements and greater flexibility.

(3) Hypoglycaemia unawareness may be reversed and hypoglycaemia frequency and severity may be reduced.
(4) Insulin injections are not required.
(5) Blood glucose monitoring at least 4-hourly is necessary unless the person uses continuous blood glucose monitoring.
(6) Training and readily available support and advice from skilled pump experts are essential.
(7) People with existing psychological problems do worse on pumps than on other insulin regimes (DCCT 1993).
(8) Pumps are expensive to purchase and the ongoing cost of consumables is high. In Australia some health insurance funds subsidise the initial outlay for the pump according to specified guidelines. The cost of consumables is subsidised by the Commonwealth government under the National Diabetes Supply Scheme but subsidies for diabetes products is currently under review and could change in the future.

Currently there is no national Australian guideline for selecting which patients could benefit from using a pump but most diabetes centres offering pump therapy have guidelines for selecting patients and initiating pump therapy. NICE (2003) recommended that pumps be funded for people with Type 1 diabetes who suffer recurrent severe hypoglycaemia.

Continuous blood glucose sensors

Continuous glucose monitoring is a step towards a closed-loop system that links continuous blood glucose measurements to a computer-driven insulin infusion system to approximate normal glucose homeostasis. Modern sensors consist of a disposable sensor probe, which is inserted into subcutaneous tissue using an insertion device and connected to a battery-powered transmitter. The transmitter sends a signal to a receiver, which displays the blood glucose reading. The sensors last for ~3–5 days.

After the sensor is attached to the transmitter, warm-up periods between 2 and 10 hours are required and capillary blood glucose testing is required to calibrate the system. There are at least three sensors on the market and each manufacturer recommends ongoing calibration. In addition, abnormal sensor readings need to be confirmed with a

Table 5.4 Some commonly encountered factors that affect insulin absorption.

Accelerated	Delayed
Type of insulin	Type of insulin
Exercise	Low body temperature
High body temperature	Condition of injection sites
Condition of injection sites	Poor circulation
Massage round injection site	Smoking
Depth of injection	Long-acting insulins

capillary test before corrective action is taken. Thus, the current sensors are adjuncts to, rather than replacements for, capillary blood glucose testing but they enable people to have several days break from finger pricking. The cost is prohibitive for many people.

The choice of regimen and insulin delivery system depends on personal preference, management targets and the willingness and ability of the patient to monitor their blood glucose. Many factors can influence insulin absorption and consequently blood glucose; some of these factors are shown in Table 5.4.

Subcutaneous insulin sliding scales and top-up regimes

A sliding scale refers to subcutaneous insulin doses administered to reduce hyperglycemia detected on routine blood glucose monitoring. Sliding scales are reactive and retrospective rather than prospective and proactive (Hirsch *et al.* 1995). Sliding scales are not recommended, especially for older people (American Geriatrics Society Beers Criteria 2012). Sliding scales should not be confused with supplemental insulin administered at meal times based on blood glucose tests according to an algorithm (Hirsch *et al.* 1995).

Sliding scales continue to be used especially in hospital despite there being no evidence of any benefit and evidence of harm. In fact, diabetes experts have been advocating for a proactive prospective approach to managing hyperglycaemia in hospital rather than using sliding scales since 1981 (Queale *et al.* 1997).

Sliding scales treat hyperglycaemia after it occurs. They may predispose the patient to hyperglycaemia-related adverse events, particularly given the fact that insulin doses are rarely adjusted and the underlying causes and predisposing factors that lead to hyperglycaemia are not addressed (Queale *et al.* 1997). Using subcutaneous sliding scales in day-to-day management can lead to disassociation between the insulin regimen and the other parameters that affect the blood glucose such as the timing of meals, effects of illness, and medications, for example, corticosteroids and the counter-regulatory response to hypoglycaemia.

Using sliding scales to stabilise blood glucose for newly diagnosed, unstable or brittle diabetes is *not* generally recommended (Katz 1991). It is preferable to monitor the blood glucose over 24–48 hours and adjust the insulin regimen according to the emerging pattern considering the action profile of the various insulins and other factors that affect the blood glucose level.

Top-up or stat doses of insulin

Top-up or stat doses of insulin refer to temporary supplementary doses of insulin, usually rapid- or short-acting, given to correct existing hyperglycaemia found on routine blood glucose monitoring. Like traditional sliding scales, top-up dosing is reactionary and does not address the underlying causes of hyperglycaemia. When necessary, extra supplementary insulin (correction dose) is best added to the next due dose of insulin rather than being given in isolation.

Adopting a proactive problem-solving approach, considering the management regimen and nursing/medical actions occurring at the time will provide important insight into the cause/s of the hyperglycaemia, which can be appropriately treated. For example, hyperglycaemia might be a consequence of pain or fear, in which case the most effective strategy would be to manage the pain/fear. In addition, non-medicine options might be effective. Often, top-up doses continue for days before the overall blood glucose profile and medicine requirements or the underlying causes are considered.

Practice points

(1) There are no documented benefits of insulin sliding scales in people in hospital (; Gearhart *et al.* 1994; Queale *et al.* 1997) or top-up doses.
(2) Insulin sliding scales are associated with a 3-fold higher risk of hyperglycaemia especially when basal insulin is not used (Queale *et al.* 1997).
(3) Sliding scales are not recommended for older people (American Geriatrics Society Beers Criteria 2012).
(4) Sliding scales could help maintain acceptable blood glucose levels in hospital if they are used proactively according to a logical algorithm based on the action profiles of the relevant insulin regimen and delivered in relation to meals.
(5) IV insulin infusions require a sliding insulin scale and are an example of proactive hyperglycaemia management.

Intravenous insulin infusions

The IV route is preferred for very ill patients because the absorption of insulin is rapid and more reliable than from poorly perfused muscle and fat tissue. Absorption may be erratic in these patients, especially if they are hypotensive. The aims of the insulin infusion are to:

• Prevent the liver converting glycogen and fatty acids into glucose and therefore avoid hyperglycaemia, that is, restrain hepatic glucose output.
• Prevent utilisation of fatty acids and therefore limit ketone formation.
• Reduce protein catabolism and therefore limit production of glucose substrates.
• Enhance wound healing by limiting protein catabolism and normalising neutrophil function.
• Reduce peripheral resistance to insulin.
• If hyperglycaemia is present, gradually lower the blood glucose concentration to ~10 mmol/L without subjecting the patient to hypoglycaemia.

Intravenous insulin infusions are associated with lower morbidity and mortality in surgical settings (see Chapter 9), during acute illness such as MI (see Chapter 8), in patients requiring parenteral nutrition (Cheung *et al.* 2005) and in intensive care settings (Quinn *et al.* 2006). In fact, van den Berghe *et al.* (2001) demonstrated improved outcomes using insulin infusions in acutely ill non-diabetics as well as people with diabetes.

Two main insulin delivery methods are used:

(1) Insulin given via an infusion pump, and fluid administered separately.
(2) Insulin, glucose, potassium, and fluids are combined (GIK), which is efficient and safe. The glucose component is usually 5 or 10% dextrose depending on the calories required (Dagogo-Jack & Alberti 2002).

The medication order for the infusion must be clearly and legibly written on the treatment sheet. Insulin doses for IV insulin infusions are usually 0.1 unit/kg/hour. Sometimes an initial bolus of 5–10 units is given. In general, a low-dose infusion such as this has been shown to reduce the blood glucose and prevent ketosis and acidosis as effectively as high-dose regimens, without the added risk of hypoglycaemia. The rate at which the insulin is to be administered should be written in mL/hour and units to be delivered.

Several protocols exist; the following is one example only. People with insulin-treated Type 2 diabetes may require 1–2 units/hour if they are overweight and insulin resistant.

The infusion rate is adjusted according to the patient's blood glucose results (tested 1–2-hourly). For example:

Blood glucose (mmol/L)	Insulin (units/hour)
0–5.9	0
6–11.1	1
12–15.1	2
16–19	3
>19.1	4
>24	Notify doctor

The insulin order and blood glucose results should be reviewed regularly. The duration of the infusion depends on the clinical status of the patient.

Preparing the insulin solution to be infused

Two people should check and make up the solution according to the medication order and hospital protocols. In many cases it is prepared and labelled in the pharmacy.

Practice points

(1) Only clear rapid- or short-acting insulin is used for insulin infusions. Great care should be taken not to use clear long-acting insulin analogues in insulin infusions.
(2) Insulin is known to bind to plastic. Flushing the first 50 mL through the giving set tubing prevents this non-specific absorption into the infusion equipment.

Uses of insulin infusions

General use (during surgical procedures)

Insulin is added to 4% dextrose in 1/5 normal saline or 5% dextrose. The infusion is often given via burette or more commonly an infusion pump at 120 mL/hour (i.e. 8-hourly rate; see previous example scale). Monitor blood glucose 1–2-hourly and review with medical staff *regularly*.

Special needs

- Myocardial infarction. In many areas an IV insulin infusion is commenced when the patient presents to the emergency department and continues for ~24 hours, after which time subcutaneous insulin is commenced (Malmberg 1997); see Chapter 8.
- Open heart and other surgery.
- Ketoacidosis.
- Hyperosmolar states.

- Severe septicaemia or other infections
- Intensive care unit (ICU) situations.

These situations always require the use of a controlled-rate infusion pumps to ensure accurate insulin dosing. It is often necessary to limit the amount of fluid administered to avoid cerebral oedema in these situations especially in young children and the elderly. Standard regimens include:

(1) Haemaccel 100 mL +100 units rapid or fast-acting insulin = 1 unit/1 mL, used in ICU and administered via an infusion pump.
(2) Haemaccel 500 mL +100 units rapid or short-acting insulin = 1 unit/5 mL via an infusion pump.

People who are insulin-resistant, such as those who:

- have liver disease;
- are on corticosteroid therapy;
- are obese;
- have a serious infection;
- may require more insulin, that is, a high-dose infusion (more units per hour).

Practice points

- Subcutaneous insulin must be given before removing the infusion and the patient must be eating and drinking normally to avoid hyperglycaemia because of the short half-life of insulin given IV.
- Ceasing the infusion before a meal enables a smooth transition to subcutaneous insulin.

Risks associated with insulin infusions

- hypoglycaemia;
- cardiac arrhythmias;
- sepsis at the IV site;
- fluid overload and cerebral oedema especially in children, which is associated with high morbidity and mortality rates.

Factors affecting insulin delivery via IV infusions:

- accuracy of the system, including blood glucose testing;
- stability of the solution;
- circulatory insufficiency.

Mistakes associated with insulin infusions

(1) Where a burette is used and if insulin is added to the burette rather than the bag of IV fluid, refilling the burette from the bag results in no insulin being administered and hyperglycaemia results.
(2) An incorrect amount of insulin added to the bag/burette can be a result of inadequate checking, not using an insulin syringe to draw up the insulin or failing to

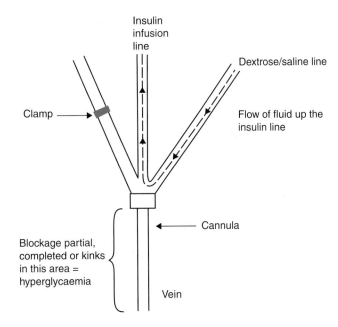

Figure 5.4 Possible results of a blockage in the IV cannula and three-way adaptor during the concurrent administration of insulin and dextrose/saline.

check illegible medical orders, especially where insulin doses are written as 'U/s' instead of 'units' and the dose is misinterpreted.

(3) Problems can arise if the insulin infusion is run at the same time through the same site as other intravenous fluids, for example, 4% dextrose in 1/5 normal saline. The most common method is to infuse the different fluids through the one IV cannula using a three-way adaptor (octopus): see Figure 5.4.

Usually, the dextrose or saline is running at a faster rate than the insulin infusion. Problems can arise if there is a complete or partial blockage of the cannula. The force of gravity pushing the fluid towards the vein can actually cause the dextrose/saline to flow back up the slower-flowing insulin line resulting in high blood glucose levels. Figure 5.6 depicts the result of a blockage in the IV cannula and three-way adaptor during the concurrent administration of insulin and dextrose/saline.

If hyperglycaemia occurs during an insulin infusion check:

- that the tubing and adaptors are patent;
- that insulin has been added to the burette/bag;
- that the amount of insulin added is correct;
- possible sources of infection, for example, UTI, the feet.

Insulin allergy

Insulin allergies are rare with modern, highly purified insulins but they do occasionally occur.

Two types of reaction have been reported:

(1) localised weal and flare with itching due to antihistamine reactions;
(2) generalised anaphylaxis, which is rare.

Clinical observation

Indicating insulin doses by writing 'U/s' still occurs despite the known association with adverse events and incorrect, in some cases fatal, insulin doses being administered. Incorrect, usually excess, insulin has been administered and can result in serious hypoglycaemia. For example, in Australia, in an aged care facility, a patient died and a court case ensued. Both the nurse who administered the insulin and the doctor who wrote the prescription were found to have contributed to the person's death. There were other issues involved with the particular patient, but the case highlights the importance of accurate documentation and the nurse's responsibility to check.

Insulin doses should always be indicated by writing or typing 'units' after the amount to be given.

Allergic reactions are most likely to occur where people have been on insulin previously, for example, during GDM, surgery or acute illness in people with Type 2 diabetes where insulin is used intermittently, for example, during surgery and with corticosteroid medications, and when injection sites are not rotated. The reaction may be due to the preservatives and other incipients in insulin rather than insulin itself.

To diagnose insulin allergy a careful case history is required. The person should be given insulin and observed where resuscitation equipment is available. Any reaction should be carefully documented. Blood test for IgG and other immune response factors can be helpful. If insulin allergy is present a desensitisation programme may be required. Local reactions can be managed by using a different insulin and antihistamine creams (Williams 1993; Dunning *et al.* 1998).

Transplants

Pancreas transplants of either the whole pancreas or islet cells or the pancreas and kidneys is available to some people with diabetes, for example, those with autonomic neuropathy causing life-threatening hypoglycaemic unawareness and end-stage renal failure. Immunosuppresive therapy is required, and if rejection does not occur, the response is good. The transplanted pancreas/beta cells secrete insulin and HbA_{1c} normalises in ~ three months.

Obtaining pancreases for transplantation or to harvest islet cells is difficult, as is actually separating the islet cells from pancreatic tissue, and other options are under study, for example, beta cell engineering and stem cell cloning. Islet cell transplants have been undertaken successfully in Canada, Australia, USA, and in the UK and an international islet cell consortium has been established to try to reproduce positive results.

Stabilising diabetes

Rationale

Optimal blood glucose control can prevent or delay the onset of long-term complications. Insulin is frequently required by people with Type 2 diabetes to achieve optimal control, as indicated.

Stabilising diabetes refers to the process of achieving an optimal blood glucose range, helping the person acquire appropriate diabetes knowledge and managing diabetic complications, either acute or chronic, but the term usually specifically refers to commencing insulin (NHMRC 1991). Stabilisation may occur at initial diagnosis of diabetes, when a change of treatment is indicated, for example, transfer from GLM to combination therapy or insulin, and for antenatal care in GDM.

In most cases, stabilising diabetes can be achieved without admitting the person to hospital. Managing diabetes in primary care settings as far as possible is a core component of both the Australian and UK diabetes management strategies (MacKinnon 1998; NDS 1998). This process is known as outpatient stabilisation. Outpatient stabilisation requires staff to have the appropriate knowledge, specific protocols and ample time if it is to be successful. It can result in considerable cost benefits, and reduces the stress and costs associated with a hospital admission.

There are considerable psychological and quality of life benefits for the person with diabetes. Home/outpatient stabilisation enables insulin to be adjusted according to the individual's usual lifestyle and reduces the risk of the person having to assume 'sick role' behaviours.

However, some patients will continue to be admitted to hospital for stabilisation of their diabetes, for example, complex issues that cannot be identified in outpatient settings, where clinical observation is necessary, or where the person is admitted with a concurrent illness or is diagnosed during an admission and commences insulin while in hospital.

Stabilising diabetes in hospital

People admitted to improve their metabolic control (stabilisation) are not generally ill and should be encouraged to:

(1) keep active;
(2) wear clothes instead of pyjamas;
(3) perform diabetes self-care tasks such as blood glucose monitoring and insulin administration.

They will require support, encouragement and consistent advice. The time spent in hospital should be kept to a minimum.

Nursing responsibilities

(1) Inform the appropriate staff about the person's admission especially the diabetes nurse specialist/diabetes educator, specialist team, and dietitian soon after they are admitted.
(2) Assess the patient carefully (refer to Chapter 2).
(3) Monitor blood glucose according to usual protocols; for example, 7 AM, 11 AM, 4 PM, and 9 PM. In some cases postprandial levels are also performed (see Chapter 3).
(4) Supervise and assess the patient's ability to test their own blood glucose and/or administer insulin, or teach these skills if the person is newly diagnosed.
(5) Ensure diabetes knowledge is assessed and updated, and select an appropriate diet: new learning may include insulin techniques, sharps disposal, hypoglycaemia and home management during illness.
(6) TPR daily, or every second day.

(7) BP, lying and standing, daily.

(8) Ensure all blood samples, urine collections and special tests are performed accurately. The opportunity is often taken to perform a comprehensive complication screen and education assessment while the person is in hospital, especially if they often miss appointments with health professionals or it has not been performed for some time. Inspection of injection sites and assessment of the person's psychological status should be included. These tests include ECG, eye referral, spot urine collection for creatinine and microalbumin and blood tests such as lipids, HbA_{1c} and kidney function.

(9) Ensure the patient has supplies, for example, test strips, lancets, insulin device, before discharge and that the appropriate follow-up appointments are made.

(10) Ensure they have a contact telephone number in case they need advice.

Community and outpatient stabilisation

The types of outpatient service provided for people with diabetes include:

- diabetes education;
- commencement on diabetes medication (GLM, insulin);
- complication screening and assessment;
- blood glucose testing;
- consultations with dietitian, diabetes nurse specialist/diabetes educator or diabetes specialist;
- clinical assessment;
- education is a key factor in a person's understanding and acceptance of diabetes. Diabetes educators often know the person well from the outpatient service and can assist ward nurses to plan appropriate nursing care and understand the person's needs.

> ### Practice point
>
> The specific protocol and policy of the relevant health care setting should be followed and all contacts including telephone advice documented. An example protocol for insulin stabilisation in the community or on an outpatient basis is shown on pages 166 and 167.

Objectives of outpatient stabilisation onto insulin

Short-term objectives:

(1) To reassure the individual and their family and allay the fear that everything about diabetes must be learned at once.

(2) Lifestyle should be modified as little as possible.

(3) To establish trust between the patient and the diabetes team.

(4) To gradually normalise blood glucose and lipids.

(5) To teach the 'survival skills' necessary for the person to be safe at home:
   - how to draw/dial up and administer insulin;
   - blood glucose monitoring;
   - recognising and treating hypoglycaemia;
   - sick day management;
   - how and when to obtain advice e.g. provide contact telephone number.

Long-term objectives

The aim in the long term is for the patient to:

(1) Develop appropriate coping and problem-solving skills and resilience to manage their diabetes and life in general.
(2) Accept diabetes as part of their life and recognise their role and responsibility in the successful management of the diabetes.
(3) Be able to make appropriate changes in insulin doses, carbohydrate intake and activity to maintain acceptable blood glucose levels.
(4) Be able to maintain an acceptable range of blood glucose, HbA_{1c}, and lipids.
(5) Be able to maintain a healthy weight range.
(6) Modify risk factors to prevent or delay the onset of the long-term complications of diabetes and therefore the need for hospital admissions.
(7) Attend regular medical/education appointments.
(8) Receive ongoing support and encouragement from the diabetes team.
(9) Maintain psychological wellbeing and quality of life.

Clinical observations

- People are often overwhelmed, unsure what to do and confused by conflicting or inaccurate advice from health professionals, family and friends and the media or obtained on the Internet.
- These issues frequently need to be addressed and clarified before commencing the insulin stabilisation process.
- The therapeutic relationship and trust between health professional and the person with diabetes is a vital aspect of their adjustment to having diabetes and changes in their diabetic management or status. Therapeutic relationships should be cultivated nurtured and treasured.

Rationale for choosing community/outpatient stabilisation

Community/outpatient stabilisation onto insulin is preferred for the following reasons:

(1) To avoid the 'sick role', which is often associated with a hospital admission.
(2) It is cost effective, that is, does not require a hospital bed.
(3) It involves less time away from work and usual activity for the patient, who can therefore be stabilised according to their usual routine, rather than hospital routines and food.
(4) To encourage self-reliance and confidence.

Patient criteria

The patient must be:

- Able to attend the service for the required period, which depends on the individual service. In some cases twice a day visits may be necessary. Telephone contact should be maintained as long as necessary.
- Physically and mentally capable of performing blood glucose monitoring and insulin administration, or have assistance to do so.

In addition, some social/family support is helpful initially for older people and is required for children.

The process of stabilisation

(1) The process should involve members of the diabetes team and relatives/carers as appropriate.
(2) Communication, especially between the doctor, practice nurses, diabetes nurse specialist/diabetes educator, dietitian and patient, is essential.
(3) Patients should be assessed on an individual basis, so that appropriate education goals and blood glucose range can be determined. The insulin regime and insulin delivery system will depend on individual requirements; follow-up advice and early assessment must be available.
(4) Formal teaching times should take account of the individual's commitments as far as is practicable.
(5) Adequate charting and documentation of progress should be recorded after each session: blood glucose results, ability to manage insulin technique, goals of management.
(6) Effective education strategies should be used. Stabilisation might be undertaken in groups (see Chapter 16).

A sample protocol for outpatient stabilisation is shown at the end of this chapter. It is included here to give nurses an overview of the kind of information required and the complex issues people with diabetes have to deal with, often when they feel vulnerable. Other protocols also exist.

> ### *Practice points*
> (1) People of all ages forget how to manage emergencies.
> (2) Health professionals and well-meaning family and friends often give inaccurate advice that either confuses the person with diabetes or causes them to ignore all advice.
> (3) People with Type 1 diabetes are at risk of ketoacidosis but often do not have ketone testing equipment at home or if they do it is out of date (Sumner *et al.* 2000; Tay *et al.* 2001).
> (4) Constant, diplomatic reminders are important. An episode in hospital represents an opportunity to remind people about diabetes self-management.

Traditionally, initiation of insulin occurred on an individual basis. Recent reports suggest that group education programmes for commencing insulin can be effective and achieve reductions in HbA_{1c} and competent insulin self-care by individuals (Almond *et al.* 2001; Yki-Jarvinen *et al.* 2007). Such programmes could be a cost effective way to manage the increasing numbers of people being commenced on insulin as a result of the DCCT and UKPDS trials, provided competent facilitation is available.

Lipid-lowering agents

Normalising the lipid profile is an essential component of diabetes management guidelines. People with diabetes, especially Type 2, are at significant risk of cardiovascular disease, which is often present at diagnosis, unless the blood glucose and lipids can be kept within normal limits. Generally, the aim is to reduce cholesterol, especially LDL-c and triglycerides, and increase HDL-c. HDL helps remove LDL cholesterol but it might also have anti-inflammatory and antithrombotic properties. HDL-c is inversely related to triglycerides in that high triglyceride levels are associated with the removal of cholesterol from HDL-c to more atherogenic lipoproteins and lipoprotein precursors. HDL-c is often low in Type 2 diabetes, partly because of the increased production of triglyceride-rich lipoproteins. LDL-c may not be elevated because of the increased level of cholesterol LDL, which suggests relying on LDL-c levels may underestimate the cardiovascular risk in people with Type 2 diabetes (Sullivan 2008).

High LDL significantly increases the risk of myocardial infarction, but other risk factors such as obesity and inflammatory processes are important and are often exacerbated by low levels of HDL (Colquhoun 2002). The cholesterol content of HDL, HDL-c, could be protective in that it reflects removal of cholesterol from atherosclerotic plaque. Low HDL-c is an independent risk factor for cardiovascular disease (Anderson *et al*. 1991). Weight loss, reducing saturated fat in the diet, exercise, and stopping smoking all effectively raise HDL-c. Alcohol increases HDL-c but excess consumption is associated with significant health risks because it causes weight gain especially around the abdomen, liver damage, contributes to malnutrition, and reduces LDL-c and triglycerides, and increases the risk of breast cancer in women. Controlling blood glucose is integral to controlling lipids (Lipid Study Group 1998). Current lipid targets aim for total cholesterol <4 and triglyceride and LDL <3 in patients with existing heart disease (National Heart Foundation 2001).

The American Diabetes Association (2007) recommended using statins to prevent cardiovascular disease in all people with Type 2 diabetes, particularly reducing LDL-c 100 mg/dL, and initiating statins in people with diabetes over 40 years without cardiovascular disease to reach the LDL-c target. Likewise, the CARDS study suggested statins are indicated in most people with Type 2 diabetes, whereas The ASPEN study (Knopp *et al*. 2006) suggested people at low risk of cardiovascular disease might receive less benefit from statin therapy. Not all people with diabetes have the same 10-year risk of cardiovascular disease, thus lipid lowering therapy needs to be commenced according to individual level of risk (Grundy 2004). However, lipid-lowering agents, including statins, must be used with an appropriate diet and exercise regimen (Ridker 2012).

Major cardiovascular prevention trials include:

- Antihypertensive and Lipid-Lowering Treatment to Prevent Heart Attack Trial (ALLHAT), which was one of the first trials to assess the efficacy of statins (Pravostatin) in people with and without diabetes. It failed to show a significant reduction in mortality but there was a trend towards a higher mortality risk in people with LDL-c >130 mg/dL. The findings were similar for those with and without diabetes.
- Heart Protection Study, which also included people with and without diabetes. The all-cause mortality and major cardiovascular event rate were significantly lower in the Simvastatin group. The outcomes were similar for those with and without diabetes in the Simvastatin group but people with diabetes in the placebo group had more vascular events than non-diabetics and the risk was additive. The researchers suggested people with diabetes have a risk equivalent to those with pre-existing cardiovascular disease and that statin therapy is beneficial for people with diabetes without cardiovascular disease and LDL-c close to the target.
- Anglo-Scandinavian Cardiac Outcomes Trial-Blood Pressure Lowering Arm (ASCOT-BPLA) compared two antihypertensive regimens in people with at least three cardiovascular risk factors. A substudy (LLA-ASCOT), compared Atorvastatin to placebo. ASCOT was stopped after an average of 3.3 years because there was no significant difference in the primary endpoints. There was an overall benefit from using Atorvastatin but it was not significant in people with diabetes. However, the

researchers recommended statin therapy should be considered in people with Type 2 diabetes and hypertension.

- CARDS included people with Type 2 diabetes, LDL-c, no history of cardiovascular disease and one additional cardiovascular risk factor and used 10 mg of Atorvastatin. There was a trend, which failed to reach significance, towards lower all-cause mortality and LDL-c was lower (<100 mg/dL) in the Atorvastatin group than in the placebo group. CARDS researchers suggested that there was no specific LDL-c threshold at which statins should be initiated in people with Type 2 diabetes. CARDS was used as the basis of American Diabetes Association (2007) recommendation that people with diabetes > age 40 and no cardiovascular diseases should be commenced on a statin regardless of their LDL-c level. The Canadian Diabetes Association (CDA) (2006) recommended the LDL-c target for people with diabetes be lowered to 2 mmol/L from 2.5 mmol/L and placed less emphasis on the LDL/HDL ratio as a primary end-point of treatment. The triglyceride level at which treatment should be commenced was also revised to >10 mmol/L from 4.5 mmol/L. The CDA suggested fenofibrate be commenced to reduce the risk of pancreatitis and a second lipid-lowering agent be added if targets were not achieved after 4–6 months.

- ASPEN included people with Type 2 diabetes and a history of cardiovascular disease and compared 10 mg Atorvastatin with placebo. The protocol was amended to include people with no history of cardiovascular disease following changes in the cardiovascular management guidelines. The results were not statistically significant but there was a trend towards clinical improvements. The researchers concluded that the level of risk (presence of multiple risk factors) affects the degree to which statins reduce the cardiovascular risk in Type 2 diabetes without cardiovascular disease.

- Veterans Affairs High-Density Lipoprotein Cholesterol Intervention Trial (VA-HIT) indicated low HDL-c is a treatable risk factor in people with and without diabetes. VA-HIT results indicate fibrates reduce cardiovascular risk by lowering LDL-c but only had a small effect on increasing HDL-c.

- FIELD study, which used fenofibrate showed reductions in the rates of macular oedema and proliferative retinopathy but did not show a significant increase in HDL-c. It lowered LDL-c and there was a reduction in major cardiovascular events in the intervention group (Field study 2005). Statins were added in the placebo group, which may have influenced the results.

- The Framingham Study indicated that low HDL-c is an independent risk factor for cardiovascular disease in people with diabetes and non-diabetics and developed a cardiovascular disease risk calculator (Anderson *et al.* 1991).

- PROSPER, which studied the effects of Pravastatin on all-cause mortality in people aged 70–82 years with cardiovascular risk factors or cardiovascular disease, but failed to show a reduction in all-cause mortality. However, a later meta-analysis that included the 4S, CARE, LIPID, HPS trials and unpublished data from PROSPER showed a reduction in all-cause mortality by 22%, as well as cardiovascular mortality by 30%, non-fatal MI by 26% and the need for revascularisation by 30% and stroke by 25% (Afilalo *et al.* 2008). Afilalo *et al.* also suggested that older people do not have higher rates of serious adverse events than younger people but they did experience higher rates of myalgia in the statin and placebo groups. Masoudi (2007) showed Ruvastatin reduced LDL-c and C-reactive protein but did not significantly reduce the combined risk of cardiovascular disease in older people (mean age 73 years), and there were fewer admissions to hospital than in the placebo group.

- Other studies such as the West Scotland Coronary Prevention Study (WESTCOPS), Air Force/Texas Coronary Athersclerosis Prevention Study (AFCAPS/TexCAPS) also showed cardiovascular benefits (Ridker 2012).

Management strategies should be based on the absolute risk rather than the lipid level alone. Individual risk assessment should include cardiovascular status, age, gender, the presence of hypertension, smoking, and family history of hyperlipidaemia, hypertension, and cardiac disease (Chapter 8). Management strategies consist of:

- Dietary modification including reducing salt, alcohol and saturated fat in the diet and increasing omega-3 fatty acids (see Chapter 4).
- Low-dose aspirin to reduce platelet aggregation.
- ACE inhibitors to control blood pressure and other antihypertensive agents as indicated.
- Stopping smoking; see Chapter 10.
- Lipid-lowering agents are recommended when the absolute cardiovascular risk is >15% in the next 5 years or when the risk is >10–15% in people with a family history of premature heart disease or who have metabolic syndrome (National heart Foundation and Cardiac Society of Australia and New Zealand 2005). Most people will be commenced on a statin unless they are contraindicated. Diet and exercise therapy must continue, even when lipid-lowering medicines are indicated. Metformin and TZDs might have some small effect on increasing HDL-c and Rimonabant is associated with significant improvements in HDL-c, possibly because of the associated weight loss.
  - Statins reduce LDL-c and have some effect on HDL. They reduce the risk of future cardiovascular disease by ~30%. However, long-term adherence to statins is poor and many older people are not commenced on these agents despite the improved cardiovascular outcomes (Diamond & Kaul 2008).
  - Nicotinic acid very effectively increases HDL-c, but is associated with side effects and non-adherence is significant. In addition, it increases blood glucose. Although the increase is not significant it contributes to overall increased cardiovascular risk.
  - Ezetimibe can be administered with a statin but it only has a modest effect on HDL-c.
  - Fibrates.
  - A new class of lipid-lowering agents, Cholesterol Ester Transfer Protein (CEPT), which block the transfer of cholesterol from HDL-c to more atherosclerotic lipoproteins, is under trial. The first agent, Torcetrapib, significantly raised HDL-c but did not prevent the progression to atherosclerosis. The trial (ILLUMINATE) was stopped early due to the rate of cardiovascular events in the treatment group (Nissen *et al.* 2007). The adverse results triggered debate about the advisability of using medicines to treat HDL. Other lipid-lowering agents under trial include Liver-X-receptor agonists, which promote cholesterol transport and reduce atherosclerosis in animal models, endothelial lipase inhibitors, which raise HDL-c and apolipoprotein A-1 mimetic peptides that improve HDL function in animal models (Zadelaar *et al.* 2007).
- Coaching.

Table 5.5 depicts the major classes of lipid-lowering agents (Colquhoun 2000 & 2002).

Side effects

The side effects of lipid-lowering agents often contribute to non-adherence to these medicines:

- Statins: tendonitis and myositis occurs in ~2% of people (Marie *et al.* 2008). Regular assessment to detect these side effects should occur, especially during the first year. Poor sleep quality has been associated with Simvastatin but not Pravastatin (Golomb 2007). Taking Simvastatin earlier in the day may reduce these effects. Simons (2002)

Table 5.5 Lipid-lowering agents.

Lipid-lowering agent and main action	Management considerations
HMG-CoA reductase inhibitors (statins): reduce LDL-c and have a modest effect on triglycerides and HDL, may increase bone mineral density, for example: Atorvastatin Simvastatin Fluvastatin Rouvastatin	Test liver function on commencing and 6 months after commencing Use caution if liver disease is present Reduce the dose if the patient commences cyclosporine. Monitor creatinine kinase (CK) and effects on muscles and tendons. Generally not recommended during pregnancy[a]
Ezetimebe reduces LDL-c by ~18% and by up to 20% if combined with a statin Ezetimebe combined with simvastatin	Prescribing authority is required in Australia and specific criteria need to be met.
Fibrates: Reduce cholesterol and triglycerides and increase HDL-c, for example: Fenofibrate Gemfibrosil	Can be combined with HMG-CoA after a trial on monotherapy but the risk of muscle toxicity is increased if used with statins or other fibrates Monitor CK and liver function 6 weeks after starting and again in 6 months
Bile acid sequestrants (Resins) Enhance LDL-c lowering effects of HMG-CoA agents – reduce triglyceride and HDL-c, for example: Cholestyramine Cholestyramine hydrochloride	Allows lower doses of the resins to be used Slows absorption of oral hypoglycaemic agents Increases hypoglycaemia risk when used with these agents. Administer 1.5 hours apart They can impair the absorption of other medicines such as statins, fat-soluble vitamins, and thyroxine Can be used with a statin
Low-dose nicotinic acid	Can be given with HMG-CoA agents

Note: The main classes of lipid-lowering medicines are depicted. Relevant prescribing information should be consulted. Combinations of statins and antihypertensive agents are also available, for example, amlopipine bensylate with Atorvastatin in eight dose combinations, which are indicated for people with hypertension and/or angina who meet the prescribing criteria for lipid-lowering agents. Educating and supporting the person to maintain a healthy lifestyle and enhance their medication self-management and improve medication adherence is essential.[a]Karamermer & Roos-Hesselink (2007).

suggested measuring creatine kinase (CK) before commencing statins and then 6-monthly when lipids are checked could help interpret minor changes in muscle enzymes especially in people at risk of muscle effects such as in women, and those with a small body frame, multisystem disease, polypharmacy, perioperative, interactions with medicines such as Cyclosporin, azole antifungals, macrolide antibiotics, some antidepressants, large amounts of grapefruit juice, and alcohol. The American College of Cardiology, American Heart Association, and National Heart Lung and Blood Institute (2002) recommended:

○ Advising people with no symptoms and raised CK to immediately report generalised muscle aches and pains.
○ Monitoring the individual if the CK is normal and the muscle effects are mild or change to another statin or another lipid-lowering agent.
○ Referring people with very high CK to a lipid specialist but continue statin therapy until the individual is assessed.
○ Carefully monitoring muscle enzymes in people with raised CK and muscle aches. Discontinue statin therapy if clinically indicated, for example, severe symptoms such as fatigue, significant pain or an interaction with statin occurs.
○ Stop statins if CK is ≥10 (upper limit of normal).
• GIT disturbances (Clofibrate).

Many people discontinue taking their lipid-lowering agents because they are unconvinced about the need, perceive that they have poor efficacy or dislike the associated side effects. Nurses can play a key role in encouraging people to adhere to their medications by explaining the reason they need them and suggesting ways to limit minor side effects. For example, Tai Chi might help reduce the muscle effects of statins.

Monitoring lipid medicines

Current lipid and other management guidelines recommend that blood lipids should be tested at diagnosis and then at least yearly. People using lipid-lowering agents should have their lipid levels measured more frequently. Lipid targets were discussed in Chapter 3. Not achieving targets is not necessarily failure: any reduction in lipid levels has a beneficial effect.

Blood glucose should also be monitored and glucose-lowering medicines adjusted as needed to reach blood glucose targets. Persistent hyperglycaemia can cause hypertriglyceridaemia, which usually falls along with cholesterol if blood glucose and weight improve. Mixed hyperlipidaemia is best treated with a statin or a fibrate initially depending on the underlying lipid abnormality. Doses are usually adjusted at four-week intervals. For example, more than 80% of the lipid-lowering effect of statins is achieved at 50% of the maximal dose (Jackowski 2008).

Liver function tests and creatine kinase (CK) should be tested before commencing lipid-lowering therapy, then in ~4–8 weeks and subsequently when doses are adjusted or if clinically indicated. For example, renal impairment, older people, severe muscle weakness. Statins may need to be temporarily ceased if the person requires macrolide antibiotics. Stopping statins is associated with an increased risk of a cardiac event, especially in the first weeks (Rossi 2007).

If the triglycerides are <4.0 mmol/L or between 2 and 4 mmol/L and HDL is <1 mmol/L, gemfibrozil may be the medicine of choice. Consider whether vitamin A, D, E, and K (the fat-soluble vitamins) supplements are needed if bile acid resins are used in high doses for long periods of time.

Omega-3 fish oils 2–5 mg/day effectively lower triglycerides (Rossi 2007) and may be a beneficial addition to other agents for hypertriglyceridaemia or mixed hyperlipidaemia. However, several products are available on the market and doses are not the same in all products or brands. It is important that people read labels and seek professional advice when using these medicines. In addition, they can interact with other medicines.

Antihypertensive agents

Hypertension is a significant risk factor for cardiovascular disease. Thus, achieving and maintaining normotension is a major therapeutic goal. There are many medicines that reduce blood pressure. Therefore the particular antihypertensive agent used depends on the underlying cardiovascular abnormality/ies and specific benefits and risks to the individual. Diabetes is associated with several cardiovascular abnormalities, thus several agents are often required. Generally, beta blockers are started at a low dose and the dose gradually increased depending on the agent used to improve left ventricular function and reduce the risk of death in patients with heart failure (Jackowski 2008). Side effects of beta blockers include:

- Fluid retention, which might be exacerbated by concomitant use of TZDs, NSAIDs, and COX –2 selective agents.
- Hypotension, which might increase the risk of falls and may be the result of an interaction with another antihypertensive agent or tricyclic antidepressants.

- Bradycardia.
- Severe fatigue; other causes should be considered such as depression, hypothyroidism and hyperglycaemia.
- Bronchospasm can occur with beta blockers in patients with asthma and COPD.
- Weight gain with some beta blockers such as atenolol, which was still apparent at the 20-year follow up of the UKPDS (Standl *et al.* 2012). Atenolol was also associated with a slight increase in tryglycerides and a mean HbA1c increase of 0.6% that required an increase in GLM doses in the UKPDS.

ACE inhibitors (ACEI) are considered first-line therapy in diabetes because they have renoprotective, cardioprotective and probably retinoprotective properties as well as reducing blood pressure. In addition, they might improve insulin sensitivity. ACEI and metabolites are predominantly excreted via the kidney and doses may need to be adjusted or another antihypertensive agent used if renal function is impaired. *Post hoc* data analysis suggests ACEI and angiotensin-11 receptor blockers reduce the risk of progression to Type 2 diabetes; however there may be different effects in different racial groups. For example, Wright *et al.* (2006) reported lower risk of progression to diabetes in African-Americans receiving Ramipril compared to Amlodipine and Metoprolol. However, in the DREAM trial Ramipril did not reduce the incidence of diabetes in non-African-Americans with impaired fasting glucose or glucose tolerance, although it did increase the regression to normoalbuminuira (Bosch *et al.* 2006).

The ACCOMPLISH trial (2008) to determine the effects of the ACE inhibitor Benazepril and a calcium channel blocker, amlodipine on morbidity and mortality was stopped early because the combination treatment was more effective than an ACE inhibitor and a diuretic (Jamerson 2008). Cardiovascular morbidity and mortality was reduced by 20%.

The main side effects of ACEI are:

- The 'ACEI cough' is a well-known side effect that is benign but often irritating to the individual and family/friends. It is less common with some of the newer agents.
- Diabetes is often associated with hyporeninaemic hypoaldosteronism syndromes particularly if renal impairment is present. The syndrome presents with unexplained hyperkalaemia, which can be exacerbated by concomitant ACEI use.
- Using an ACEI in the presence of renal artery stenosis (RAS) may critically reduce glomerular filtration. Prevalence of RAS does not appear to be higher in people with diabetes but it may be associated with, though not a cause of, hypertension. Risk factors include male gender, smoking, and peripheral vascular and coronary artery disease. Ensuring absence of RAS is important in such patients before commencing ACEI. Plasma potassium and creatinine should be regularly monitored in all patients on ACEI prior to and within one week commencing therapy (Gilbert *et al.* 1998).

Long term use of antihypertensive agents is associated with zinc loss, which may be clinically relevant if people are already at risk of low zinc, for example people with Type 2 diabetes, alcoholism, renal insufficiency and malabsorption syndromes (Braun & Rosenfeldt 2012). Antihypertensive medicines associated with zinc loss are thiasizide diuretics, ACE inhibitors angiotension-2 receptor antagonists, and is especially noticeable with Captopril.

Zinc deficiency is associated with anorexia, poor appetite, compromised immune function and changes in smell and taste and can complicate neurological diseases and age–related degenerative diseases. Improving the diet to include foods that contain zinc and supplements might be indicated and could be trialled and evaluated and continued if benefits were demonstrated.

The main types of antihypertensive medicines are shown in Table 5.6.

Table 5.6 Antihypertensive medications. Often more than one antihypertensive agent will be required in diabetes to manage the underlying cardiovascular abnormalities. Prescribing information should be followed.

Class of medicine	Generic name
Diuretics used for hypertension	
Thiazide diuretics	Hydrochlorothiazide
Sulphonamide diuretics	Chlorthalidone
	Indapamide hemihydrate
Diuretics used for heart failure	
High ceiling diuretics	Frusemide
Aryloxyacetic acid derivatives	Ethacrynic acid usually used if the person is sensitive to other oral diuretics
Potassium sparing agents:	Eplerernone
Aldosterone antagonists	Amiloride hydrochloride
Amiloride hydrochloride	
Combination potassium sparing agents and low ceiling diuretics	Hydrochlorothiazide with amiloride hydrochloride
	Hydrochlorothiazide with triamterene
Non-selective beta blockers used for hypertension	Oxyprenolol Hydrochloride
	Pindolol
	Propranolol hydrochloride
Selective beta blockers used for hypertension	Atenolol
	Metoprolol tartarate
Alpha beta blocking agents	Labetalol hydrochloride
Beta blocking agents used in heart failure	
Alpha and beta blocking agents	Carvedilol
Selective beta blocking agents	Bisoprolol fumarate
	Metropolol succinate
Beta blocking agents used as antiarhythmics	Sotalol hydrochloride
Calcium channel blockers[a]	
Selective calcium channel blockers with predominantly vascular effects – Dihydropyridine derivatives	Amlodipine bensylate
	Felodipine
	Lercanidipine hydrochloride
	Nifedipine
Selective calcium channel blockers with direct cardiac effects – phenylalkylamine derivatives	Verapamil hydrochloride
Calcium channel blockers with cardiac and vascular effects	Diltiazem hydrochloride
Agents acting on the Renin–Angiotensin System (ACE inhibitors (ACEI))[a]	
Plain ACEI	Captopril
	Enalapril maleate
	Fosinopril sodium
	Lisinopril
	Perindopril
	Quinapril hydrochloride
	Ramipril
	Tandolapril
ACEI and diuretic combinations	Enalapril maleate with Hydrocholorothiazide
	Fosinopril sodium with Hydrocholorothiazide
	Perindopril erbumine with Indapamide hemihydrate
	Quinapril hydrochloride with Hydrocholorothiazide

(Continued)

Table 5.6   (Continued)

Class of medicine	Generic name
Angiotensin-11 antagonists	Candesartan cilexetil
	Eprosartan mersylate
	Irbesartan
	Telmisartan
Angiotensin-11 antagonist combinations	Candesartan cilexetil with Hydrocholorothiazide
	Eprosartam mesylate with Hydrocholorothiazide
	Irbesartan with Hydrocholorothiazide
	Telmisartan with Hydrocholorothiazide
Centrally acting antiadrenergic agents	Methyldopa
Imidazoline receptor antagonists	Clonidine
	Moxonidine
Peripherally acting antiadrenergic agents	Prazosin hydrochloride
Hydrazinophthalazine derivatives	Hydralazine hydrochloride
Pyramidine derivatives	Minoxidil

[a]May be contraindicated in pregnancy.

Antiplatelet agents

Antiplatelet agents are indicated to reduce cardiovascular risk. Commonly used antiplatelet agents are:

- Aspirin (Salicylate). Salicylates were traditionally used to reduce inflammation, fever, and pain. They are also commonly used as antiplatelet agents to reduce the risk of cardiovascular disease particularly in people at high risk such as those who had a MI, smoke, have hypertension, and/or high cholesterol. Aspirin may be contraindicated if the individual has a bleeding disorder and sometimes asthma. Aspirin occasionally causes indigestion and a tendency to bleed freely, for example, from blood glucose testing, nosebleeds, and bruises.
- Clopidogrel hydrochloride sulphate is used if aspirin poses a significant risk of bleeding and is usually used to prevent recurrent stroke, TIA, or ischaemic event.
- Dipyridamole can be used alone or with low-dose aspirin or where aspirin represents a bleeding risk. A combination formulation is available – Dipyridamole with aspirin. These agents are used to prevent recurrent stroke, TIA, or ischaemic event.
- Warfarin and heparin. These agents are rarely combined with antiplatelet agents except when the individual is at high risk.

A recent study suggests aspirin is associated with increased risk of macular degeneration (MD) in a prospective 15 year study involving 2389 participants (Liew *et al.* 2013). Two hundred and seventy five were on aspirin, 63 of whom developed MD. Adjusting for age and other confounders suggest the cumulative risk of MD is 9.3% in aspirin users versus 3.7% risk in non-users and this is a dose–response effect. The risk of stopping aspirin must be weighed against the cardiovascular benefits and should be carefully discussed when aspirin is commenced. Caution may be required in people at risk of MD but no such warnings have been issued at the time of writing.

It is important for people to understand how their medicines work and the potential interactions with complementary medicines such St John's wort and glucosamine, which might potentiate the action of warfarin and lead to bleeding. Regular INR monitoring is essential and frequent dose adjustment may be required. Home INR monitoring systems are available but regular medical review is essential.

Medication safety, adherence and medication self-management

Factors that affect medication safety and contribute to harm are complex and can be patient-related, system/environment-related, product-related and health-professional related, therefore risks in all these categories must be considered and managed. Strategies for reducing health professional-related medicine-related errors include:

- Identifying individuals at risk.
- Using QUM as a decision-making framework.
- Considering safety standards, guidelines and advisories such as NICE, US Institute of Safe Medicine Practice, prescribing information and the Beers Criteria (AGS 2012).
- Using computerised prescribing, ALERTs, and reminders.
- Implementing automated ALERT systems e.g. to allergies, high risk medicine alerts.
- Educating health professionals. Education is more effective if it is interactive and clinically based.
- Implementing ward-based pharmacies, which enhance interprofessional communication.
- Undertaking regular comprehensive medicine reviews including home-based reviews.
- Using structured medicine validation processes in hospital.
- Ensuring practice environments are supportive. Supportive practice environments enhance nurses' ability to intercept medicine errors before they occur (Flynn *et al.* 2012).
- Improving communication among professionals, especially when the individual is discharged and during transitions among care facilities (Dooley 2011; Dunning 2013a).
- Team briefings e.g. concerning medicine alerts, high risk patients, and new medicines.

Medication self-management is an essential aspect of diabetes self-care. It becomes increasingly complex as more medicines are added to the regimen, often, as the individual grows older. Medicine non-adherence is widely documented. For example, two out of three people with diabetes adhere to <80% of their insulin doses (Donnelly *et al.* 2007). The preceding information indicates that polypharmacy is common and is probably best practice diabetes care. Polypharmacy is variously defined as using 2–10 medicines depending on the source sometimes including prescribed, over-the-counter and CAM medicines.

Polypharmacy contributes to:

- Difficulty remembering the medicine regimen, which affects medicine adherence, medication reviews and complicates prescribing.
- Increased risk of medicine interactions.
- Increased risk of non-adherence. Approximately half the medicines prescribed for people with chronic conditions are not taken. Krapek *et al.* (2004) reported people with high scores on the Moirsky Scale (denoting adherence) had lower HbA_{1c} levels. Non-adherence results in high HbA_{1c} and related health risks (Grant *et al.* 2007). Non-adherence to cardiovascular medications is high: 10–25% discontinue medicines within six months of starting, increasing to 21–47% by 24 months (Australian

Institute of Health and Welfare (AIHW) 2007). Significantly people who do not have their prescriptions filled after discharge from hospital post-MI are more likely to die within a year than those who have their prescriptions filled (Jackevicius *et al.* 2008). Non-adherence to lipid-lowering agents is also high, often because people are not sure they have any benefits, feel health professionals are not interested in the individual's input into their management plan, and the associated side effects (McGinnis *et al.* 2007). These findings suggest actually prescribing and monitoring medicines in the spirit of the newer term, 'concordance', which denotes shared decision-making and agreement might be more effective than current strategies.

- Increased likelihood of presenting to emergency or being admitted to hospital with a medication-related event. Budnitz & Knight (2007) reported one third of all presentations to emergency in the US involved older people with adverse medication events.
- Increased risk of a medication-related error in hospital. As already stated insulin, warfarin and digoxin are the top three high-risk medicines, all of which are frequently prescribed in diabetes. Adverse medicine-related events occurred in 28 500 hospital admissions in 2004–2005 predominantly in people >65 years and is probably an under estimation (AIHW 2007).
- High medicine costs.
- Increased risk of falls.
- Increased risk of driving accidents.
- Relying on medicines rather than continuing mandatory healthy lifestyle.
- Reduced quality of life and well-being.
- Health professionals not prescribing needed medicines on the basis of inadequate patient self-care (Grant *et al.* 2007) or because they do not want to complicate the regimen or for other individual decision heuristics (Tung 2011).

Other factors that contribute to patient non-adherence include:

- Low health literacy and health numeracy (Chapter 16).
- Sensory deficits such as vision and hearing loss.
- Reluctance to take medicines and a desire to minimise medicine intake (Pound *et al.* 2005).
- Cultural and other beliefs and attitudes about medicines.
- Inadequate or unclear medicines education, especially when the education is not personalised for the individual and for each medicine (Dunning 2013).
- Misinterpreting medicine labels and medicine information, which is common even when labelling requires minimal reading skills (Davis *et al.* 2008). For example instructions to take medicine twice daily (which is imprecise because 'daily' means once per day) or every 12 hours means people have to make addition decisions about what the words actually mean. 'Take medicines as directed' is even more difficult to interpret (Dunning 2013). People are more likely to understand specified medicine administration times such as 8 a.m., 6 p.m. but using time periods might suit some people better (Davis *et al.* 2008). Complex medicine regimens independently predict the likelihood people will misinterpret medicine instructions, advice or education.
- Variations in medicine colour and appearance e.g. when generic medicines are substituted for the individual's usual medicine (Kesslheim *et al.* 2012). Kesslheim *et al.*'s study concerned antiepileptic medicines but the concept is likely to apply to all medicines. Earlier studies show many people identify their medicines by the colour, size and shape.
- Medicine costs.

Medicine non-adherence is higher among people who do not attend appointments and is associated with increased rates of all-cause mortality (Currie 2012). Currie's study concerned insulin adherence, but most of the findings are likely to apply to other medicines. In addition, medicine non-adherence was common in a web-based survey of community pharmacy patients in the US (n = 2000) (Shrank *et al.* 2011). Caregivers were more likely to report they did not adhere to their medicine regimens than non-caregivers, 38% of Shrank's *et al.*'s sample described themselves as caregivers and most were women. The finding suggest health professionals may need to consider caregiver behaviours and the potential effect on their medicine adherence (and possible the adherence of the person they care for).

Enhancing medication self-care

Adherence is a complex mixture of acceptance, adherence and persistence – not merely taking a medicine. In addition, each component is itself complex. For example, acceptance involves informed-decision making that can be affected by the health professional's assessment, diagnostic, prescribing and communication skills. Significantly, agreement of all people involved in medicine adherence is essential to optimal compliance.

Barriers to appropriate medication self-care include the complexity of the regimen, the number of medicines prescribed, the dose frequency, not understanding the regimen or when or how to take the medicines, poor communication, inadequate information or information in a format the individual does not understand, beliefs and attitudes to medicines. Adherence to beneficial medicines reduces morbidity and mortality, which suggests adherence is a surrogate marker of healthy behaviour (Johnson & Shalansky 2007). Several meta-analyses have been undertaken but few show a benefit of any one strategy, which is not surprising given the complex and changing nature of managing diabetes medicines and more importantly, the fact that most strategies focus on changing patient's behaviour rather than also considering health professional's contribution to non-adherence. A truly concordant strategy would/should also address health professional- and systems-related factors that affect medicine adherence.

Nevertheless, a number of strategies for measuring and promoting patient-related medication adherence have been proposed. Some show short-term benefits, but long-term benefits are unclear. Strategies include:

- AIDES method based on a meta-analysis of 53 studies, which suggested no single strategy is more effective than any other but strategies that combine cognitive, behavioural, and affective interventions are more likely to be effective (Roter *et al.* 1998). However, the AIDES method appears complicated and there is limited evidence to support its benefit.
- Federal Study of Adherence to Medications in the Elderly (FAME) (Lee *et al.* 2006), which specifically addressed people >65 years and encompasses education, regular follow up, and customised blister packs. The strategy was based on a review of 12 interventions and was associated with improved adherence over six months from 61% at baseline to >96% and significant reductions in systolic blood pressure and LDL-c.
- Education materials such as those developed by the Australian National Prescribing Service, Consumer Medicines Information (CMI), which are available for all PBS listed medicines in Australia, Internet sites such as familydoctor.org, and the International Alliance of Patient Organisations, however, these are largely passive and their effect on medicines use is unclear. Part of medicines education is helping people understand risks and benefits and putting these into their individual context.

Woloshin & Schwartz (2007) developed a booklet designed to help people understand risks using colon cancer and medical investigations as examples. It was said to be user-friendly and used 8th grade literacy level. The booklet was tested in a high socioeconomic group and the investigators reported 'significant improvements in participants' ability to interpret risk'. It is not clear whether the information would be applicable to lower socioeconomic groups or whether behaviour changed as a consequence of enhanced ability to interpret risk.

- Education programmes for health professionals such as improving adherence to cardiovascular medicine (National Heart Foundation of Australia 2011).

From these strategies, relevant meta-analysis and the author's clinical experience using a QUM approach, the following strategies are useful. They can be used alone or in combination depending on the individual's need and agreement. That is, patient-centred medication self-management.

- Understand the health professionals' impact on patient adherence.
- Understand the individual's beliefs and attitudes towards medicines, their capabilities and their life goals.
- Understand their usual lifestyle and daily activities.
- Assess their physical and mental capability to manage medicines, whether help is available, and whether they will accept it if it is.
- Identify triggers to non-adherence, for example, on more than 5 medicines, complex dosing regimen, sound-alike medicine names, look-alike medicines, low literacy, cognitive deficits and being a carer.
- Develop strategies to address specific issues. These should be developed in consultation with the individual, for example, 'How do you think you could remember to take your insulin?' Some useful strategies include personal cues, reminders, and medicine boxes such as blister packs.
- Provide medicine information in a relevant format and language level using appropriate words suitable for the individual. Work through the information with the individual and ask them to repeat back what they learned. Explain the benefits and risks but apply them to the individual's context, that is, personalise the information. Information could include:
  ○ Why the medicines were prescribed, which will include stressing the importance of maintaining a healthy lifestyle.
  ○ The name of the medicine, the difference between generic and other medicines, and what brand names mean.
  ○ What the medicine is expected to do (outcomes) and how the person will know if it is effective.
  ○ How soon an effect will show.
  ○ The dose and dose frequency.
  ○ Special instructions such as when to take the medicine in relation to meals.
  ○ What to do if they forget a dose.
  ○ When to stop taking the medicine, if relevant.
  ○ Where and when to seek medicine advice, for example, fasting for a procedure or investigation.
  ○ Common side effects, how to recognise them and what to do about minimising or reporting them.
  ○ Storing and disposing of unused medicines or medicines that have passed their use-by date.
- How to use other self-care information to interpret the effects of medicines adherence and non-adherence on relevant outcomes, for example, their blood glucose pattern.

- How to keep their medication list up-to-date and ensure it includes over-the- counter and CAM medicines.
- Help them formulate questions to ask their doctor at the next appointment if necessary.
- Follow-up medicines self-management regularly.

Clinical observation

From the list of strategies it is clear that person-centred, individualised medicine education is complex, time consuming and probably not accomplished in the majority of people with diabetes. Reflect on how you and/or your team could improve the way you provide medicine education.

Strategies that can be used to monitor medicine adherence

In research settings, MEMs medicine containers are used. MEMs containers have microprocessors in the lid that record the date and time the container was opened. Opening the container is a proxy measure of medicines' actual use. MEMs also acts as a behavioural intervention; people are more likely to adhere if they think they are being 'watched'. However, MEMs is impractical in clinical settings. Other strategies involve:

- Providing appropriate education with behavioural support.
- Using case management and effective interprofessional communication.
- Systems approaches to reducing the cost of medicines.
- Discussing medicine use using open communication, blood glucose and other self-monitoring and laboratory results in a non-judgemental way.
- Knowing the 'right' questions to ask.
- Using open, neutral language and choose words and sentences carefully and avoid passive language and ambiguity to enhance memory and understanding.
- Using questionnaires such as the:
  - Brief Medication Questionnaire (BMQ) that measures current and potential non-adherence and can be self-completed by the individual.
  - The Morisky Scale, which measures attitudinal and behavioural factors that affect adherence. However, the language is judgemental e.g. Are you careless at times about taking your medicine? It has low internal reliability.
  - Medication Adherence report (MARS), whch views medicine use on a continuum.
  - Beliefs about Medication questionnaire (BaMQ).
  - Revised Illness Perception questionnaire (IPQ-R).

Reflecting on their own medicine-related behaviours might help them understand people with diabetes medicine-related behaviours. After all, health professionals fall into the category of carers: caring is a known risk factor for non-adherence.

Based on the preceding information about adherence, one could ask:

(1) Is adherence a patient problem?
(2) Is adherence a health professional problem?
(3) Is adherence an inter-related responsibility of the individual, the health professional, service providers and funders?
(4) Should we be promoting rights and responsibilities rather than merely adherence?

Example protocol for outpatient stabilisation onto insulin

SUGGESTED PROTOCOL

These are guidelines only and should be modified to suit individual needs.
The information can be delivered individually or in groups and over various time frames and include other information relevant to the individual.

(1) Introduce the diabetes team and area facilities.
(2) Test blood glucose; the individual should test their own blood glucose if possible.
(3) Insulin dose/frequency is determined in consultation with the doctor.
(4) The educator demonstrates insulin technique and explains the procedure to the patient and encourages the patient to practice them.
(5) It is important to encourage the patient to discuss their feelings about diabetes and to assess current diabetes knowledge, learning capacity, style, psychological status and social situation.

Education goals

(1) To give a basic explanation of what diabetes is and what an acceptable blood glucose range is.
(2) To explain the reason for instituting insulin therapy.
(3) To explain the effects of insulin on blood glucose levels, that is insulin action and the role of long- and short-acting insulin in control of blood glucose levels.
(4) To explain insulin technique:
   • preparing the dose depending on the insulin delivery system chosen
   • sites for injection
   • expiry dates of insulin bottles/cartridges
   • care and storage
   • appropriate sharps disposal.
(5) To explain why insulin must be given by injection and allow patient to handle insulin device or bottles and practice preparing the insulin dose.
(6) To explain hypoglycaemia:
   • recognising symptoms of low blood glucose levels
   • causes and prevention
   • effective management
   • patient should carry carbohydrate for 'emergencies'.
(7) Blood glucose monitoring should be encouraged, to provide feedback to the patient and enable them to telephone in the afternoon with a result if necessary. The role of monitoring should be explained as well as the timing of testing and how to record results.
(8) Basic introduction to a food plan: role of carbohydrate in blood glucose control and the need to reduce fat and the need for regular meals.
(9) Explain and enrol the patient in the National Diabetes Supply Scheme.
(10) Explain responsibilities with respect to self-care, medicine management, complication screening, and driving.[a]
(11) Ensure patient has the equipment to administer insulin and monitor blood glucose and knows how and where to obtain future supplies and knows who to contact for advice.

Other important self-care issues

(1) Discuss how to manage illness at home, in relation to:
   b. who to contact
   c. effects of illness on blood glucose
   d. emergency diet
   e. monitoring and recording of blood glucose and urine or blood ketones
   f. adjusting/continuing insulin
   g. need to rest.

(2) Discuss precautions to be taken relating to driving, work, etc.

(3) Discuss the role of exercise/activity in controlling blood glucose levels.

(6) Encourage patient to wear some form of identification.

(7) Ensure that patient has a contact telephone number and knows who to contact for advice.

(8) Provide appropriate follow-up appointments for doctor, nurse specialist/educator according to patient needs.

(9) Provide ongoing individual teaching as required.

(10) Ensure patient knows about other services available for people with diabetes, for example, diabetes associations and relevant support groups.

(11) Arrange for consultation with family if necessary.

ª*Point (10) above*: the National Diabetes Supply Scheme only applies in Australia.

References

Abraham, E., Leech, C., Lin, J., Zulewski, H. & Habener, J. (2002) Insulinotrophic hormone glucagons-like peptide-I differentiation of human pancreatic islet-derived progenitor cell into insulin producing cells. *Endocrinology*, **143**, 3152–3161.

Afilalo, J., Duque, G. & Steele, R. (2008) Statins for secondary prevention in elderly patients. *Journal of the American College of Physicians*, **51**, 37–45.

Almond, J., Cox, D., Nugent, M. *et al.* (2001) Experience of group sessions for converting to insulin. *Journal of Diabetes Nursing*, **5** (4), 102–105.

American Diabetes Association (2007) Standards of medical care in diabetes. *Diabetes Care*, **30**, S4–S41.

AGS (American Geriatrics Society) (2012) Identifying medicines that older adults should avoid or use with caution: the updated 2012 AGS Beers criteria *www.healthinaging.org* (accessed December 2012).

American Association of Clinical Endocrinologists (AACE) (2011) Guidelines for Clinical practice fro developing a diabetes mellitus comprehensive care plan. *Endocrine Practice*, **17** (2), Suppl 2 1–53.

Australian Adverse Drug Reactions Bulletin (2007) Emerging cardiovascular concerns with rosiglita-zone 26 6 *http://www.tga.gov.au/hp/aadrb-0712.htm* (accessed October 2012).

Australian Diabetes Society (ADS) (2007) *ADS Position Statement on Rosiglitzone* (AVANDIA®) May 28th, 2007. ADS, Canberra.

Australian Government Department of Health and Ageing (2001) *Smoking, Nutrition, Alcohol and Physical Activity (SNAP) Framework for General Practice. Integrated Approaches to Supporting the Management of Behavioural Risk Factors of Smoking, Nutrition, Alcohol and Physical Activity (SNAP) in General Practice*, Canberra.

Australian Institute of Health and Welfare (AIHW) (2007) *Medicines for Cardiovascular Health: Are They Used Appropriately?* Report 23rd May. AIHW, Canberra.

Bailey D. (2012) Drugs that interact with grapefruit. *Canadian Medical Association Journal* Online (accessed November 2012).

Bergman-Evans, B. (2006) AIDES to improving medication adherence in older adults. *Geriatric Nurse*, **27**, 174–182.

Birkeland K, Torjesen P, Eriksson J, et al. (1994) Hyperproinsulinemia of type II diabetes is not present before the development of hyperglycemia Diabetes Care, **17** (11), 1307–1310.

Braddon, J. (2001) Oral hypoglycaemics: A guide to selection. *Current Therapeutics*, Suppl. **13**, 42–47.

Braun, L. & Rosenfeldt, F. (2012) Pharmoco-nutrient interactions – A systematic review of zinc and antihypertensive therapy. *International Journal of Clinical Practice* DOI: 10.1111/ijcp.12040.

Budnitz, D. & Knight, S. (2007) Common drugs trigger most ER visits by seniors. www.medicinenet.com/script/main/art.asp?articlekey=85633.

Buse, J. (2001) Insulin analogues. *Current Opinion in Endocrinology*, **8** (2), 95–100.

Calabrese, A., Coley, K., Da Pos, S., Swanson, D. & Rao, H. (2002) Evaluation of prescribing practice: Risk of lactic acidosis with Metformin. *Archives of Internal Medicine*, **162**, 434–437.

Campbell, M., Anderson, D., Holcombe, J. & Massey, E. (1993) Storage of insulin: A manufacturer's view. *Practical Diabetes*, **10** (6), 218–220.

Cefalu, W., Skyler, J., Kourides, I., *et al*. (2001) Inhaled insulin treatment in patients with Type 2 diabetes. *Annals of Internal Medicine*, **134**, 242–244.

Cheung, N., Napier, B., Zaccaria, C. & Fletcher, J. (2005) Hyperglycaemia is associated with adverse outcomes in patients receiving total parenteral nutrition. *Diabetes Care*, **28**, 2367–2371.

Choudhry N, Fletcher R. (2005) Systematic review:the relationship between clinical experience and quality of health care. *Annals of Internal Medicine*, **114**, 260–273,

Colquhoun, D. (2000) Unstable angina – A definitive role for statins in secondary prevention. *International Journal of Clinical Practice*, **54**, 383–389.

Colquhoun, D. (2002) Lipid lowering agents. *Australian Family Physician*, **31** (1), 25–30.

Commonwealth Department of Health and Ageing (2000) *National Medicines Policy 2000*. http://www.health.gov.au

Currie (2012) Adherence to insulin treatment: What do surveys reveal about non-compliance? *Journal of Diabetes Nursing*, **16** (8), supplement.

Dandona, P., Topiwala, S., Chaudhuri, A. & Ghanim, S. (2008) Insulin is an antiatherogenic hormone. *International Diabetes Monitor*, **20** (1), 9–16.

DAFNE Study Group (2002) Training in flexible, intensive insulin management to enable dietary freedom in people with Type 1 diabetes: Dose Adjustment of Normal Eating (DAFNE) randomized controlled trial. *British Medical Journal*, **325**, 746.

Dagogo-Jack, S. & Alberti, G. (2002) Management of diabetes mellitus in surgical patients. *Diabetes Spectrum*, **15**, 44–48.

Davis, T., Federmann, A., Bass, P. *et al*. (2008) Improving patient understanding of prescription drug label instructions. *Journal of General Internal Medicine* **24** (1), 57–62.

DCCT (Diabetes Control and Complications Trial Research Group) (1993) Effects of intensive insulin therapy on the development and progression of long-term complications in IDDM. *New England Journal of Medicine*, **329**, 977–986.

Delafenetre, M. & Massey, N. (2008) Tendinous disorders attributed to statins: A study on ninety six spontaneous reports in the period 1990–2005 and review of the literature. *Arthritis Care Research*, **59**, 367–372.

Diabetes Australia (DA) & Royal Australian College General Practitioners (RACGP) (2011/12) *Diabetes Management in general Practice*. DA and RACGP, Canberra.

Dornhorst, T. (2001) Insulinotropic meglitinide analogues. *Lancet*, **17** (358), 1709–1716.

Dornhorst, A., Luddeke, H.J., Sreenan, S. *et al*. on behalf of the PROACTIVE Study Group (2007) Safety and efficacy of insulin determined in clinical practice: 14-week follow-up data from Type 1 and Type 2 diabetes patients in the PREDICTIVE™ European Cohort. *Clinical Practice*, **61** (3), 52–58.

DREAM (Diabetes Reduction Assessment with Ramipril and Rosiglitazone Medication Investigators (2006) Effect of Rosiglitazone on the frequency of diabetes in patients with impaired glucose tolerance or impaired fasting glucose: A randomized controlled trial. *Lancet*, **355**, 2427–2443. (correction in *Lancet* (2006) 368, 1770).

Donnelly L, Morris A, Evans J. DARTS/MEMO collaboration (2007) Adherence to insulin and its association with glycaemic control in patients with Type 2 diabetes. *Quality Journal of Medicine*, **100**, 345–350.

Dooley, M., Wiseman, M., McRae, A. *et al*. (2011) Reducing potentially fatal errors associated with high doses of insulin: A successful multifaceted multidisciplinary prevention strategy. *British Medical Journal Quality and Safety*, DOI: 10.1136/bmjqs.200.049668.

Dormandy, J., Charbonnel, B. & Eckland, D. (2005) Secondary prevention of macrovascular events in patients with Type 2 diabetes in the PRO active Study (PROspective pioglitAzoneClinical Trial in Macrovascular Events): A randomised controlled trial. *Lancet*, **366**, 1279–1289.

Dunning T. (2005) Applying a quality use of medicines framework to using essential oils in nursing practice. *Complementary Therapies in Clinical Practice*, **11**, 172–181.

Dunning T. (2013a) Medicine self-management: More than just taking pills. In Diabetes Education: Art, Science and Evidence. Dunning, T. (ed.) Wiley Blackwell, Chichester, UK, pp.177–197.

Dunning T. (2013b) Turning points and transitions. In *Diabetes Education: Art, Science and Evidence*. Dunning, T. (ed.) Wiley Blackwell, Chichester, UK, pp. 117–131.

Dunning, T. & Martin, M. (1997) Using a focus group to explore perceptions of diabetes severity. *Practical Diabetes International*, **14** (7), 185–188.

Dunning, T. & Martin, M. (1999) Health professionals' perceptions of the seriousness of diabetes. *Practical Diabetes International*, **16** (3), 73–77.

Dunning, T., Rosen, S. & Alford, F. (1998) Insulin allergy: A diagnostic dilemma. *Journal of Diabetes Nursing*, **2** (6), 188–190.

European Medicines Agency London, Press release 15 December 2005 Doc. Ref. EMEA/421484/2005 www.emea.europa.eu/docs/en_GB/document.../Press.../WC500017633.pdf (accessed October 2012).

Ekstrom, N., Schioler, L., Svensson, A.M., *et al.* (2012) Effectiveness and safety of Metformin in 51 675 patients with Type 2 diabetes and different levels of renal function: A cohort study from the Swedish National Diabetes Register. *British Medical Journal Open*, 2012:2 e001076 DOI: 10.1136/bmjopen-2012-001076.

FDA (US Federal Drug Administration) (2011) Avandia (rosiglitazone): REMS - Risk of Cardiovascular Events: includes Avandia, Avandamet, and Avandaryl. Page Last Updated: 11/04/2011 www.fda.gov/Drugs/DrugSafety/ucm241411.htm (accessed November 2012).

Field Study Investigators (2005) Effect of long term fenofibrate therapy on cardiovascular events in 9795 people with Type 2 diabetes mellitus (the Field Study) randomised controlled trial. *Lancet*, **366**, 1849–1861.

Flynn, L., Liang, Y., Dickson, G. & Xie, M. (2012) Nurses' practice environments, error interception practices, and inpatient medication errors. *Journal of Nursing Scholarship*, **44** (2), 180–186.

Gabbay, R., Hu, P., Bode, B. & Garber, A. (2005) The INITIATE Study group: Initiating insulin therapy in Type 2 diabetes: A comparison of biphasic insulin analogs. *Diabetes Care*, **28**, 254–259.

George, L. (1993) Sociological perspectives on life transitions. *Annual Review of Sociology*, **19**, 353–373.

Gilbert, R., Cooper, M. & Krum, H. (1998) Drug administration in patients with diabetes mellitus. *Drug Safety*, **1** (6), 441–456.

Golomb, B. (2007) Simvastatin but not pravastatin, may reduce sleep quality. American Heart Association Scientific Sessions. Abstract 3725, November, Orlando.

Grant, R., Adams, A., Trinacty, C. *et al.* (2007) Relationship between patient medication adherence and subsequent clinical inertia in Type 2 diabetes glycemic management. *Diabetes Care*, **30**, 807–812.

Greaves, C., Brown, P., Terry, R. *et al.* (2003) Converting to insulin in primary care: An exploration of the needs of practice nurses. *Journal of Advanced Nursing*, **42** (5), 487–496.

Goudswaard, A., Furlong, N., Valk, G., Stolk, R. & Rutten, G. (2004) Insulin monotherapy versus combinations of insulin with oral hypoglycaemic agents in patients with Type 2 diabetes mellitus. Cochrane Database of Systematic Reviews archive.library.uu.nl/.../Rutten_04_Goudswaard_Cochrane%20Syst%20Rev_2004_CD003418.pdf, The Cochrane Library, London.

Grundy, S., Cleeman, J. & Merz, C. (2004) Implications of recent clinical trials for the National Cholesterol Education Treatment Panel 111 Guidelines. *Circulation*, **110**, 227–239.

Hamilton, J., Cummings, E. & Zdravkovic, V. (2003) Metformin as an adjunct therapy in adolescents with Type 1 diabetes and insulin resistance: A randomized controlled trial. *Diabetes Care*, **26**, 138–143.

Jackevicius, C., Li, P. & Tu, J. (2008) Prevalence, predictors, and outcomes of primary non-adherence after acute myocardial infarction. *Circulation*, DOI 10.1161/CIRCULATIONAHA.107.706820.

Jackowski, L. (2008a) Lipid lowering therapy. *Australian Family Physician*, **37** (1/2), 39–41.

Jain, R., Allen, E. & Wahl, I. (2005) Premixed insulin analogues for the treatment of diabetes. *Diabetes*, **54** (Suppl. A69).

Jerrall, M. (2002) Warning over Metformin use. *Archives of Internal Medicine*, **162**, 434–437.

Hirsch, I., Paaun, D. & Brunzell, J. (1995) Inpatient management of adults with diabetes. *Diabetes Care*, **18** (6), 870–877.

Home, P., Pocock, S. & Beck-Nielsen, H. (2005) Rosaglitazone evaluated for cardiac outcomes and regulation of glycaemia in diabetes (RECORD): Study design and protocol. *Diabetologia*, **48**, 1726–1735.

Home, P., Pocock, S., Beck-Neilsen, H. *et al.* (2009) Rosiglitazone evaluated for cardiovascular outcomes in oral agent combination therapy for Type 2 diabetes (RECORD): A multicentre, randomized open-label trial. *Lancet*, **373** (681), 2125–2135.

Iedema, J. & Russell A. (2011) Optimising Metformin benefits in Type 2 diabetes. *Diabetes Management Journal*, **34**, 22–24.

Inzucchi, S. (2002) Oral antihyperglycemic therapy for Type 2 diabetes: Scientific review. *Journal of the American Medical Association*, **287**, 360–372.

Inzucchi, S., Bergenstal, R., Buse, J. *et al.* (2012) Management of hyperglycaemia in Type 2 diabetes: A patient-centred approach. *Diabetes Care*, care.diabetesjournals.org/content/35/6/1364.long (accessed May 2012).

Jackowski, L. (2008b) Beta blockers in systolic heart failure. *Australian Family Physician*, **37** (3), 137–139.

Jamerson, K. (for the ACCOMPLISH investigators) (2008) Avoiding cardiovascular events in combination therapy in patients living with systolic hypertension. American College of Cardiology Scientific Sessions, March, Chicago. www.sbm.org/meetings/2012/rapid-communication-abstracts

Janka, H., Plewe, G., Riddle, M. *et al.* (2005) Comparison of basal insulin added to oral agents versus twice daily premixed insulin as initial therapy for Type 2 diabetes. *Diabetes Care*, **28**, 254–259.

Johnson, G. & Shalansky, S. (2007) Predictors of refill non-adherence in patients with heart failure. *British Journal of Clinical Pharmacology*, **63** (4), 488–493.

Katz, C. (1991) How efficient is sliding scale insulin therapy? Problem with a 'cookbook' approach in hospital patients. *Postgraduate Medicine*, **5** (5), 46–48.

Karamermer, Y. & Roos-Hesselink, J. (2007) Coronary Heart Disease and Pregnancy *Future of Cardiology*, **3** (5) 559–567.

Keech, A., Simes, R. & Barter, P. (2005) Effects of long term fenofibrate therapy on cardiovascular events in diabetes mellitus (the FIELD study): randomized controlled trial. *Lancet*, **366**, 1649–1861.

Kesselhiem, A., Misono, A., Shrank, W. *et al.* (2012) Variations in pill acceptance of antileptic drugs and the risk of nonadherence. *Archives of Internal Medicine*, http://archive.jamanetwork.com (accessed December 2012).

Knopp, R., d'Emden, M. & Smilde, J. (2006) Efficacy and safety of Atorvastatin in the prevention of cardiovascular disease in people with Type 2 diabetes: The Atorvastatin study for the prevention of coronary heart disease endpoints in non-insulin dependent diabetes mellitus (ASPEN). *Diabetes Care*, **29**, 1478–1485.

Ko, G. T. C., Tsang, P.C.C., Wai, H. P. S., Kan, E. C. Y. & Chan, H. C. K. (2006) Rosiglitazone versus bedtime insulin in the treatment of patients with conventional oral antidiabetic drug failure: A 1-year randomized clinical trial. *Adv Ther* **23** (5), 799–808

Krapek, K., King, K., Warren, S. *et al.* (2004) Medication adherence and associated hemoglobin A_{1c} in Type 2 diabetes. *The Annals of Pharmacotherapy*, **38** (9), 1357–1362.

Kuritzky, L. (2006) Addition of basal insulin to oral antidiabetic agents: A goal directed approach to Type 2 diabetes therapy. *Medscape General Medicine*, **8** (4), 34–47.

La Rosa, J., He, J. & Vupputuri, S. (1999) Effect of statins on risk of coronary disease: A meta-analysis of randomised controlled trials. *Journal of the American Medical Association*, **282**, 2340–2346.

Lee, J., Grace, K. & Taylor, A. (2006) Effect of a pharmacy care program on medication adherence and persistence, blood pressure, and low density lipoprotein cholesterol. *Journal of the American Medical Association*, DOI:10. 100/jama.296.21.joc60162.

Leiter, L. (2006) Can thiazolidinediones delay disease progression in Type 2 diabetes? *Current Medical Research and Opinion*, **22** (6), 1193–1201.

Lewis, J., Ferrara, A., Peng, T. *et al.* (2011) Risk of bladder cancer among diabetic patients treated with pioglitazone: Interim report of a longitudinal cohort study. *Diabetes Care*, **34**, 916–922.

Liew, G., Mitchell, P., Wong, F.Y., *et al.* (2013) Aspirin association with wet macula oedema. *Journal Internal Medicine*, **213** (3), 1–7.

Lipid Study Group (1998) The long term intervention with Pravastatin in ischaemic disease. Prevention of cardiovascular events and death with Pravastatin in patients with coronary heart disease and a broad range of initial cholesterol levels. *New England Journal of Medicine*, **339**, 1349–1357.

Malone, J., Campaigne, B., Reviriego, J. & Augendre-Ferrrante, B. (2005) Twice daily pre-mixed insulin rather than basal insulin therapy alone results in better overall glycaemic control in patients with Type 2 diabetes. *Diabetic Medicine*, **22**, 374–381.

Malmberg, K. (1997) Prospective randomised study of intensive insulin treatment on long-term survival after acute myocardial infarction. *British Medical Journal*, **314**, 1512–1515.

Masoudi, F. (2007) Can statins benefit elderly patients with ischaemic heart disease? *Journal Watch Cardiology*, **6** (11), 10–16.

Mayfield, J. & White, R. (2004) Insulin therapy for Type 2 diabetes: Rescue, augmentation, and replacement of beta-call function. *American Family Physician*, **70** (3), 100–115.

MacKinnon, M. (1998) Diabetes Care in General Practice. Class Publishing, London.

McGinnis, B., Olson, K., Magid, D. *et al.* (2007) Factors related to adherence in statin therapy. *Annals of Pharmacotherapy*, **41** (11), 1805–1811.

Meier C., Kraenzlin M. , Bodmer M.et al. (2008) Use of thiazolidinediones and fracture risk. *Archives of Internal Medicine* **168**, 820–825

Montori, V. & Isley, W. (2007) Waking up from the DREAM of preventing diabetes with drugs. *British Medical Journal*, **334**, 882–884.

National Diabetes Strategy (NDS) (1998) National Diabetes Strategy and Implementation Plan. Diabetes Australia, Canberra.

National Institute for Health and Clinical Excellence (NICE) (2008) Type 2 diabetes: The Management of Type 2 Diabetes. National Health Service, London.

NHMRC (National Health and Medical Research Council) (1991a) Stabilisation of Diabetes. National Health and Medical Research Council, Canberra.

NHMRC (National Health and Medical Research Council) (1991b) The Role of Ambulatory Services in the Management of Diabetes. Document No. 1. Australia.

Nathan, D. & Buse, J. (2006) Management of hypertension in Type 2 diabetes: A consensus algorithm for the initiation and adjustment of therapy. A consensus statement from the American Diabetes Association and the Diabetes Association for the Study of Diabetes. *Diabetologia*, 49, 1711–1721.

National Institute for Clinical Excellence (NICE) (2003) Guidance on the use of continuous subcutaneous insulin infusion for diabetes. In Technology Appraisal Guidance. NICE 57, pp. 1–23.

National Heart Foundation of Australia (2001) *Lipid Management Guidelines*. National Heart Foundation, Melbourne.

National Heart Foundation of Australia (2011) *Improving adherence in cardiovascular care*. National Heart Foundation, Melbourne.

National Heart Foundation of Australia and Cardiac Society of Australia and New Zealand (2005) Position Statement on lipid management. *Heart and Lung Circulation*, 14, 275–291.

National Prescribing Service (NPS) (2000) What is Polypharmacy? *NPS News*. NPS, Canberra.

National Prescribing Service (NPS) (2008) Managing hyperglycaemia in type 2 diabetes. *NPS News*. NPS, Canberra.

National Prescribing Service (NPS) (2001) *Improving treatment of systolic heart failure*. NPS, Canberra.

National Prescribing Service (NPS) (2012) *Type 2 diabetes drug table*. www.nps.org.au (accessed November 2012).

Nichols, G., Hillier, T. & Erbey, J. (2001) Congestive heart failure in Type 2 diabetes: Prevalence, incidence, and risk factors. *Diabetes Care*, 24, 1614–1619.

Nicholson, G. (2002) Statins decrease fractures and increase bone mineral density. *Archives of Internal Medicine*, 163, 537–540.

Nisbet, J., Sturtevant, J. & Prons, J. (2004) Metformin and serious adverse events. *Medical Journal of Australia*, 180 (2), 53–54.

Nissen, S. & Wolski, K. (2007) Effect of Rosiglitazone on the risk of myocardial infarction and death from cardiovascular causes. *New England Journal of Medicine*, 10.1056/NEJMoa072761.

Nissen, S., Tardif, J. & Nicholls, S. (2007) Effect of Torcetrapib on the progression of coronary atherosclerosis. *New England Journal of Medicine*, 356, 1304–1316.

ORIGIN (2012) Basal insulin and cardiovascular and other outcomes in dysglycaemia. *New England Journal of Medicine*, 367, 319–328.

Pound, P., Britten, N., Morgan, M. *et al.* (2005) Resisting medicines: A syntheses of qualitative studies of medicine taking. *Social Science and Medicine*, 61, 133–155.

Prochaska, J. & Velicer, W. (1997) The transtheoretical model of health behaviour change. *American Journal of Health Promotion*, 12, 38–48.

Pryce R. (2009) Diabetic ketoacidosis caused by exposure of insulin pump to heat and sunlight. *British Medical Journal*, 338, 1077–1078.

Queale, W., Seidler, A. & Brancati, F. (1997) Glycaemic control and sliding scale insulin use in medical inpatients with diabetes mellitus. *Archives of Internal Medicine*, 157, 545–552.

Quinn, J., Snyder, S., Berghoff, J., Colombo, C. & Jacobi, J. (2006) A practical approach to hyperglycaemia management in the intensive care unit: Evaluation of an intensive insulin infusion protocol. *Pharmacotherapy*, 26 (10), 1410–1420.

Raskin, P., Rendell, M. & Riddle, M. (2001) A randomised trial of Rosiglitazone therapy in patients with inadequately controlled insulin treated Type 2 diabetes. *Diabetes Care*, 24 (7), 1226–1232.

Raskin, P., Allen, E., Hollander, P. *et al.* (2005) The INITIATE study group: Initiating insulin therapy in Type 2 diabetes: A comparison of biphasic and basal insulin analogues. *Diabetes Care*, 28, 260–265.

Richter, B., Bandeira-Echtler, E., Bergerhoff, K. & Lerch, C, (2008) Dipeptidyl peptidase-4 (DDP-4) inhibitors for Type 2 diabetes mellitus. Cochrane Database of Systematic Reviews, www.ncbi.nlm.nih.gov/pubmedhealth/PMH0014112/ Cochrane Library, London.

Riddle, M., Rosenstock, J. & Gerich, J. (2003) The insulin Glargine 2004 study investigators; The treat-to-target trial: Randomized addition of glargine to human NPH insulin to oral therapy in type diabetes patients. *Diabetes Care*, 26, 3080–3086.

Ridker, P. (2012) What works and in whom? A simple, easily applied, evidence-based approach to guidelines for statin therapy. *Circulation, Cardiovascular Quality Outcomes*, 5, 592–593.

Rosak, C. & Mertes, G. (2012) Critical evaluation of the role of Acarbose in the treatment of diabetes: Patient considerations. *Diabetes Metabolic Syndrome Obesity: Targets and Therapy*, 3, 357–367.

Rosenstock, J., Schwartz, S., Clark, C. *et al.* (2001) Basal insulin therapy in type 2 diabetes: 28-week comparison of insulin Glargine (HOE 901) versus NPH insulin. *Diabetes Care*, **24**, 631–636.

Rossi, S. (ed.) (2007) *Australian Medicines Handbook*. Australian Medicines Handbook Pty Ltd, Adelaide.

Roter, D., Hall, J., Mersica, R. *et al.* (1998) Effectiveness of interventions to improve patient compliance: A meta-analysis. *Medical Care*, **36**, 1138–1161.

Rutherford, E., Wright, E., Hussain, Z. & Colagiuri, R. on behalf of the DAWN Committee (2004) DAWN: *Diabetes Attitudes, Wishes and Needs. The Australian Experience*. NovoNordisk Australasia, Sydney.

Salpeter, S., Greyber, E., Pasternak, G. & Salpeter, E. (2006) *Risk of fatal and non-fatal lactic acidosis with Metformin use in Type 2 diabetes mellitus*. Cochrane Database of Systematic Reviews, www.ncbi.nlm.nih.gov/pubmed/16437448 Cochrane Library, London.

Scottish Intercollegiate Guideline Network (SIGN) (2010) *Management of Type 2 diabetes: A national Guideline*. SIGN, Edinburgh.

Shah, B., Hux, J., Laupacis, A., *et al.* (2005) Clinical Inertia in Response to Inadequate Glycemic Control. *Diabetes Care*, **28** (3), 600–606.

Shenfield, G. (2001) Drug interactions with oral hypoglycaemic agents. *Australian Prescriber*, **24** (4), 83–84.

Shrank, W., Libeman, J., Fischer, M. *et al.* (2011) Are caregivers adherent to their own medicines? *Journal of the American Pharmacists Association*, **51** (41), 492–498.

Simons, L. (2002) Test CK before starting on statins. *Medical Observer*, 30th August, 5.

Skyler, J., Cefalu, W., Kourides, I. *et al.* (2001) Efficacy of inhaled human insulin in Type 1 diabetes mellitus. *Lancet*, **357**, 331–335.

Standl, E., Erbach, M. & Schnell, O. (2012) What should be the antihypertensive drug of choice in diabetic patients and should we avoid drugs that increase glucose levels? Pros and cons. *Diabetes, Metabolism Research Reviews*, **28** (Suppl 2), 50–66.

Strowig, S., Aviles-Santa, L. & Raskin, P. (2004) Improved glycaemic control without weight gain using triple therapy in Type 2 diabetes. *Diabetes Care*, **27**, 1577–1583.

Sullivan, D. (2008) Raising HDL cholesterol in diabetes. *Diabetes Management Journal*, **22**, 16.

Sumner, J., Barber, C. & Williams, V. (2000) What do people with Type 1 diabetes know about hypoglycaemia? *Practical Diabetes International*, **17** (6), 187–190.

Tan, Y. (2006) Initiating insulin in patients with Type 2 diabetes. *Diabetes Management Journal*, **14**, 28–29.

Tay, M., Messersmith, R. & Lange, D. (2001) What do people on insulin therapy remember about safety advice? *Journal of Diabetes Nursing*, **5** (6), 188–191.

Ting, R. (2006) Metformin use increases vitamin B12 deficiency in patients with diabetes. *Archives of Internal Medicine*, **166**, 1975–1079.

Tung A. (2011) The mystery of guideline non-compliance: Why don't doctors do the right thing? *Anaesthesiology*, **503**, 3–10.

Turner, R., Cull, C., Frighi, V. & Holman, R. (1999) Control with diet, sulphonylurea, Metformin, or insulin in patients with Type 2 diabetes mellitus: Progressive requirement for multiple therapies (UKPDS 49). *Journal American Medical Association*, **281**, 2005–2012.

United Kingdom Prospective Diabetes Study (UKPDS 33) (1998) Intensive blood glucose control with sulphonylureas or insulin compared with conventional treatment and risk of complications in patients with Type 2 diabetes. *Lancet*, **352**, 837–853 (correction in *Lancet* (1999) **354**, 602).

Vaag, A., Handberg, A., Lauritzen, M. *et al.* (1990) Variation in insulin absorption of NPH insulin due to intramuscular injection. *Diabetes Care*, **13** (1), 74–76.

Victoria Medicines Advisory Committee (VMAC) (2008) *Quality Use of Medicine Alert; Subcutaneous insulin*. www.health.vic.gov.au/vmac (accessed January 2012).

Wah, C. (2008) Improved glycaemic control after surgical procedures. *Diabetes Management Journal*, **22**, 28–29.

Wang, F., Surh, J. & Kaur M. (2012) Insulin Degludec as an ultralong-acting basal insulin one a day: A systematic review. *Diabetes Metabolism and Obesity Targets and Therapy*, **5**, 191–204.

Whaley, J., Reilly, T., Poucher, S. *et al.* (2012) Targeting the kidney and glucose excretion with Dopagliflozin: Preclinical and clinical evidence for SGLT2 inhibition as a new option for treatment of Type 2 diabetes mellitus. *Diabetes Metabolic Syndrome and Obesity: Targets and Therapy*, **5**, 135–138.

Willi, C., Bodenmann, P., Ghali, W., Faris, P. & Cornuz, J. (2007) Active smoking and the risk of Type 2 diabetes: A systematic review and meta-analysis. *Journal of the American Medical Association*, **298**, 2654–2664.

Williams, G. & Pickup, J. (1992) Handbook of Diabetes. Blackwell Science, Oxford.

Williams, P. (1993) Adverse effects of exogenous insulin: Clinical features, management and prevention. *Drug Safety*, **8**, 427–444.

Wright, J., Randall, O., Miller, E. *et al.* for the African-American Study of Kidney Disease and Hypertension (2006) Differing effects of antihypertensive drugs on the incidence of diabetes mellitus among patients with hypertensive kidney disease. *Archives of Internal Medicine*, **166**, 797–805.

Woloshin, S. & Schwartz, L. (2007) The effectiveness of a primer to help people understand risk. *Annals of Internal Medicine*, **146**, 256–265.

Worthington, B. (2003) The nurses' role in patient-centred medicines management. *Professional Nurse*, **19** (3), 142–144.

Yki-Jarvinen, H., Ryysky, L., Nikkila, K. *et al.* (1999) Comparison of bedtime regimens in patients with Type 2 diabetes mellitus: A randomized controlled trial. *Archives of Internal Medicine*, **130**, 389–296.

Yki-Jarvinen, H., Juurinen, L., Alvarsson, M., *et al.* (2007) Initiate insulin by aggressive titration and educate (INITIATE). *Diabetes Care*, **30**, 1364–1369.

Zadelaar, S., Kleemann, R., Verschuren, L. *et al.* (2007) Mouse Models for Atherosclerosis and Pharmaceutical Modifiers *Arteriosclerosis Thrombosis Vascular Biology* http://www.atvbaha.org DOI:10.1161/ATVBAHA.107.142570.

Chapter 6
Hypoglycaemia

Key points

- Hypoglycaemia is one of the most common short-term complications of diabetes treatment with insulin and some oral glucose-lowering medicines.
- The brain depends on a constant supply of glucose because it is unable to synthesise or store glucose. Severe hypoglycaemia is associated with cognitive impairment that affects the person's ability to self-manage the hypoglycaemia and function normally during a hypoglycaemia and has longer term effects on various aspects of cognnotion.
- Hypoglycaemia symptoms are often atypical, especially in older people, who usually present with predominantly neurogenic symptoms.
- The glucagons response diminishes with longer duration of diabetes in both Type 1 and Type 2 diabetes but can be lost early in the course of diabetes in Type 1.
- Self-treated hypoglycaemia is associated with clinically significant effects on well-being and functioning.
- Hypoglycaemia is the most feared side effect of insulin especially in the presence of hypoglycaemic unawareness.

Rationale

Hypoglycaemia can be prevented by proactive self-care including regular blood glucose monitoring, appropriate nursing care, and recognising impending hypoglycaemia and managing it appropriately. The prevalence of hypoglycaemia is increasing due to the focus on achieving blood glucose levels as close to normal as possible and initiating insulin early in people with Type 2 diabetes. Hypoglycaemia can be a barrier to optimal control and is an independent cause of excess morbidity and increased costs (Brod &

Care of People with Diabetes: A Manual of Nursing Practice, Fourth Edition. Trisha Dunning.
© 2014 John Wiley & Sons, Ltd. Published 2014 by John Wiley & Sons, Ltd.

Barnett 2012). People who have hypoglycaemia appear to be more affected by diabetes than people who do not have hypoglycaemia and often report lower general health (Lundkvist *et al.* 2005).

Introduction

Hypoglycaemia is the most common and the most serious adverse event associated with insulin use. The prevalence of hypoglycaemia has increased since the results of the Diabetes Control and Complications Trial (DCCT) in people with Type 1 diabetes (DCCT Trial Group 1997 and DCCT/EDICT 2003) and the United Kingdom Prospective Diabetes Study (UKPDS) (UKPDS 1998) in Type 2 diabetes demonstrated that keeping blood glucose in the normal range reduced the risk of long-term diabetes complications. The blood glucose target range and HbA_{1c} indicators of 'good glycaemiac' control are now as close as possible to the normal ranges, which increases the risk of, and frequency of, hypoglycaemia.

Severe hypoglycaemia was three times more frequent in the intensive insulin treatment group compared to conventional treatment in the DCCT (61 events per 100 people). Hypoglycaemia was more common in men than women and in adolescents than adults. The risk of severe hypoglycaemia was one in three and the risk of coma one in ten (DCCT 1991). Concern about hypoglycaemia was thought to contribute to the difficulty achieving glycaemic targets. Likewise, Pramming *et al.* (1991) reported mild hypoglycaemia was 1.8 episodes per patient per week, and 1.4 episodes of severe hypoglycaemia per patient per year.

The increased rate of hypoglycaemia is largely due to the focus on achieving normoglycaemia by intensifying management in both Type 1 and Type 2 and transferring people with Type 2 diabetes onto insulin sooner since the results of these studies were released. In early reports from the UKPDS, major hypoglycaemia occurred between 0.4 and 2.3% of insulin-treated patients per year compared with 0.4% of those treated with diet or sulphonylureas (UKPDS). Later studies also show the frequency and severity of hypoglycaemia in people with Type 2 diabetes is lower than Type 1 (Yki-Jarvinen *et al.* 1999).

Wright *et al.* (2006) recorded self-reported hypoglycaemia rates and graded severity as (transient (1), temporarily incapacitated (2), requiring assistance (3), requiring medical attention (4) in various treatment groups who remained on their prescribed therapy for six years from diagnosis as part of the UKPDS). Grades 1 and 2 occurred in 0.8% in the diet and 1.7% in the Metformin groups per year and 0.1% and 0.3% respectively for grades 2–4 per year. Rates for those on sulphonylureas were 7.9% and 1.2%, 21.2% and 3.65 on basal insulin, and 32% and 5.5% on basal and pre-meal insulin.

Younger people (<45 years), women, those with HbA_{1c} <7%, and islet autoantibody-positive people were twice as likely to report hypoglycaemia. Wright *et al.* claimed the low rates of hypoglycaemia in Type 2 diabetes was unlikely to have a major negative impact on people's ability to achieve glycaemic targets. Approximately 30% of people initially recruited were lost from the study, possibly due to intensifying treatment to achieve optimal glycaemic control; thus, the numbers of people in each treatment group was small, and the overall hypoglycaemia rate was low. Not surprisingly, hypoglycaemia risk was greater in people on insulin with poorer control but lower doses of insulin were associated with a 35% lower rate of hypoglycaemia. Older people (>65) were not included in the study, thus their risk and ability to recognise hypoglycaemia is unclear from the study, but subsequent research suggests they are at high risk and often unable to recognise or treat hypoglycaemia (Chapter 12).

A number of researchers suggest the rate of mild and severe hypoglycaemia is lower in insulin-treated Type 2 diabetes than in Type 1. However, hypoglycaemia risk increases once insulin is commenced and with increasing duration of diabetes (Henderson *et al.* 2003) and the loss of counter-regulatory hormone function in Type 2 diabetes of longer duration parallels progressive beta cell loss and increases the risk of hypoglycaemia (Amiel *et al.* 2008; Unger 2012). Hypoglycaemic unawareness is uncommon in Type 2 diabetes, but when present, it is associated with a higher incidence of severe hypoglycaemia. Hypoglycaemic unawareness in adolescents with Type 1 diabetes is influenced by duration of diabetes, but can occur early after the diagnosis (Johnston *et al.* 2012).

The DARTS study in Scotland suggests the hypoglycaemia rate in people with Type 2 diabetes on insulin is the same as those with Type 1 (Leese *et al.* 2003) and that insulin treatment is a predictor of hypoglycaemia in people with Type 2 diabetes (Donnelly *et al.* 2005) and is particularly high in people treated with insulin for long periods of time (Unger 2012). Significantly, hypoglycaemia is likely to become more prevalent in people with Type 2 diabetes given the increasing prevalence of Type 2 diabetes and the trend to early initiation of insulin in Type 2 diabetes.

The cost of treating hypoglycaemia is higher for people with Type 2 than Type 1 diabetes (Farmer *et al.* 2012). Farmer collected retrospective data over 12 months (2009–2010) from the South Central Ambulance Service National Health Service Trust in the UK to estimate the incidence of severe hypoglycaemia requiring ambulance assistance. Farmer *et al.*'s findings suggest ambulance services manage a high prevalence of hypoglycaemia in younger than older age groups: 2.1% over age 15; and 7.5% in the 15–35-year age group. The prevalence was 1.9% in people over 65 years. They concluded that, despite the higher hypoglycaemia rates in young adults the absolute number of incidents was higher in older people. The authors acknowledged that ambulance services may not attend all cases of severe hypoglycaemia, thus, the study may underestimate the incidence of severe hypoglycaemia.

The rate of severe hypoglycaemia is higher in young children: 0.49 in children <6 years compared to 0.16 in children >6 (Davis *et al.* 1997). Daneman *et al.* (1989) reported 31% of children (n = 311); mean age 11.6 and mean duration of diabetes 4.6 years, had at least one coma or convulsion since diagnosis. Other researchers report rates ranging from 6.8 to 12%. In contrast, Nordfeldt & Ludvigsson (1997) stated that the incidence of hypoglycaemic coma did not increase when HbA$_{1c}$ improved from 8.1% to 6.9%, but episodes of severe hypoglycaemia increased from 1.01 to 1.26 per patient per year. Early recognition and treatment of hypoglycaemia in young children is essential because their brains are vulnerable to hypoglycaemia, which may cause permanent cognitive deficits (Tattersall 1999).

> **Practice point**
>
> People's perceptions of and beliefs about hypoglycaemia differ significantly from clinical definitions and those of health professionals. People with diabetes use different language and explanatory models to explain hypogylycaemia and its severity. It is essential to understand people's perceptions of hypoglycaemia to help them develop suitable hypoglycaemia prevention/management strategies.

The counter-regulatory response

Normal glucose homeostasis was discussed in Chapter 1. Counter-regulatory hormones, especially glucagon, the catecholamines, growth hormone, and cortisol are released when the blood glucose falls below the normal range to maintain the blood glucose level and ensure a constant supply of energy to the brain. Glucagon and the catecholamines stimulate gluconeogenesis and reduce glucose utilisation. The severity and duration of hypoglycaemia determines the magnitude of the counter-regulatory response and begins as the blood glucose falls to ~3.5–3.7 mmol/L before cognitive function is impaired around 3.0 mmol/L (Heller & Macdonald 1996).

The counter-regulatory hormones are largely responsible for the signs and symptoms of hypoglycaemia through activating the autonomic nervous system. Several researchers have compiled lists of hypoglycaemic symptoms and most diabetes-related text books and chapters list the signs and symptoms of diabetes. Recognising the signs enables early treatment to be initiated. Significantly, symptoms are specific to the individual and are interpreted differently from health professionals. For example, people report symptoms differently if they are asked to indicate the relevance of each symptom to themselves (Tattersall 1999, p. 57; Unger 2012).

In the author's experience, some people think 'a hypo means you go into a coma' and do not associate mild symptoms with hypoglycaemia, other people and their relatives associate trembling, vagueness and aggressive behaviour as 'having a fit', which suggests some information included in hypoglycaemia education programmes may not be appropriate to everybody, and that hypoglycaemia education should be individualised taking account of the person's hypoglycaemia risk profile. Worryingly, a US national survey (n = 2530) found many people reported they are not informed about hypoglycaemia risk factors and often experience hypoglycaemia in their daily lives while they are working and driving (Moghissi 2011).

When the blood glucose is <3.0 mmol/L, fine motor coordination, mental speed and concentration, and some memory functions become impaired. Reaction times are slower, especially when the individual needs to make decisions, do mental arithmetic, and short-term verbal memory and working memory are impaired (Sommerfield *et al.* 2003). McAuley *et al.* (2001) also demonstrated significant impairment of attentional ability during hypoglycaemia but found fluid intelligence (problem-solving ability) was not impaired. Thus, many everyday tasks appear to be impaired during hypoglycaemic events, including the individual's ability to manage the hypoglycaemic episode.

Factors associated with increased cognitive deficits include male gender, hypoglycaemic unawareness, Type 1 diabetes, and high IQ. These findings have implications for effective hypoglycaemia self-management and safety. For example, people drive slowly, swerve more, steer inappropriately, spend more time driving off the road and position the car badly on the road when the blood glucose is <2.6 mmol/L (Chapter 10). The counter-regulatory response to recurrent hypoglycaemia may be blunted in subsequent hypoglycaemia and the individual may not recognise hypoglycaemia signs and symptoms. Often, people do not recall severe hypoglycaemic episodes.

Results from continuous glucose monitoring systems (CSII) suggest people taking four insulin injections per day have at least one blood glucose level <2.8 mmol/L of varying duration per day, which may not cause symptoms (Thorsteinsson *et al.* 1986). The hypoglycaemia frequency and severity is affected by a number of factors including the number of injections per day, the type of insulin, and variations in food absorption within individuals and among injection sites.

Emotions are also affected and mood changes in the three basic mood types: energetic arousal (feel active), tense arousal (feel anxious), and hedonic state (feel happy) occur during or in anticipation of hypoglycaemia. Many people with diabetes fear hypoglycaemia, which can lead them to inappropriately lower their insulin doses to reduce the risk of hypoglycaemia; see Chapter 15. Thus, the effects of hypoglycaemia are complex and multifactorial. Education and strategies to prevent/manage hypoglycaemia should be individualised and accompany changes in medication management and include family and significant others.

Definition of hypoglycaemia

Hypoglycaemia is defined in various ways using different parameters by various organisations and many differ in the threshold set for hypoglycaemia, which range form < 3.9 to < 3 mmol/L. The 2012 American Diabetes Association (ADA, 2013) *Standards of Medical Care in Diabetes* defined hypoglycaemia as a fasting blood glucose < 3.9 mmol/L, which is higher than the threshold often used in clinical trials. However, The ADA set the threshold at a higher level because the aim of treatment is to avoid hypoglycaemia. Thus, hypoglycaemia is often defined biochemically as blood glucose below a specific level.

It is also defined according to severity as:

- Mild: symptomatic where the individual is able to self-treat. The symptoms are often vague and may not be related to the actual blood glucose level. The most commonly reported initial symptoms that closely reflect the actual blood glucose level are trembling, sweating, tiredness, difficulty concentrating and hunger.
- Severe: symptomas associated with neuroglycopaenia where help is required to treat the episode. People do not always remember a severe hypoglycaemic episode because of retrograde amnesia or denial. Severe hypoglycaemia can occur without coma.
- Profound: associated with coma and sometimes convulsions (Tattersall 1999, pp. 55–87).

In addition, a grading system is sometimes used, especially in research, as follows:

- Grade 1 – mild: the person recognises and self-treats.
- Grade 2 – moderate: the person requires assistance but oral treatment normalises the blood glucose.
- Grade 3 – severe: the person is semiconscious and requires assistance, and glucagon or IV glucose may be needed.

None of the definitions appear to state the important fact that hypoglycaemia occurs in people with diabetes treated with insulin or oral glucose-lowering medicines (GLMs). Hypoglycaemia can occur as a consequence of rare endocrine conditions such as insulinoma, but concomitant insulinoma and diabetes is rare. Significantly, part of the diagnostic process for suspected insulinoma includes screening for surreptitious insulin of GLM use.

> ### Practice points
>
> (1) People with diabetes managed on diet alone do not usually have hypoglycaemia and do not require treatment of low blood glucose levels.
> (2) People treated with insulin are at the greatest risk of hypoglycaemia.
> (3) Hypoglycaemia is the most significant side effect of insulin, including the newer insulin analogues. Although hypoglycaemia is lower with insulin analogues, particularly nocturnal hypoglycaemia in clinical trials, 'real world' data is lacking (Brod & Barnett 2012).

In addition to insulin and/or GLM treatment, age, gender, and associated medical conditions such as liver disease, cerebrovascular disease, autonomic neuropathy, and the rate at which the blood glucose falls influences the development and recognition of

Table 6.1   Signs and symptoms of hypoglycaemia. These symptoms are so common that they are used in the Edinburgh Hypoglycaemia Scale (Deary 1993). Symptoms are different in young children and older people and may vary between episodes in the same individual. Some people may not experience any of the symptoms listed; therefore it is important for people to learn to recognise their own hypoglycaemic cues.

Sympathetic or adrenergic[a]	*Neuroglycopaenic*[b]
Weakness	Headache
Pale skin	Tiredness
Sweating	Hypothermia
Tachycardia	Visual disturbances
Palpitations	Difficulty concentrating
Shaking	Difficulty speaking
Tremor	Confusion
Nervousness or feeling anxious	Amnesia
Irritability	Seizures
Tingling of the mouth and fingers	Coma
Hunger	Inappropriate behaviour

[a] Caused by increased activity of the autonomic nervous system triggered by a rapid fall in blood glucose. Also referred to as sympathetic and sympathomedullary.

[b] Caused by decreased activity of the central nervous system because of very low blood glucose. Psychomotor function deteriorates. Some people appear withdrawn, others become restless and irritable. They may refuse treatment. Recovery can be slow, or rarely the person may die if they do not have help.
Nausea and vomiting may occur but are unusual.

hypoglycaemic symptoms. In general, a rapid fall in blood glucose results in the development of the classic symptoms of hypoglycaemia described in Table 6.1. The classic presentation is more likely to occur in insulin-treated patients.

The onset of hypoglycaemia is usually slower with sulphonylureas especially in older people and hypoglycaemia can be prolonged and recur for >24 hours, despite treatment. Mortality rates between 4 and 10% are reported and permanent neurological damage is present in 5% of those who survive (Salas & Caro2002). Long-acting sulphonylureas increase the risk because of their long duration of action, active metabolites, and the reduced ability to mount a counter-regulatory response that occurs with increasing duration of diabetes and increasing age. Presenting symptoms may be neuroglycopaenic, often confusion, dizziness, and altered behaviour, rather than sympathetic and the hypoglycaemia can be mistaken for stroke, transient ischaemia, or early dementia and lead to unnecessary investigations and delayed treatment (Dunning 2005 Sinclair 2006).

Risk factors for hypoglycaemia in older people include:

- Treatment with sulphonylureas or insulin, especially long-acting agents, although long-acting insulin analogues have significantly lower risk, hypoglycaemia can still occur with such analogues; see Chapters 5 and 12.
- Recent discharge from hospital especially if the GLM was changed in hospital and documentation and/or discharge planning is inadequate and the person lives alone.
- Erratic eating or malnutrition.
- Renal or liver disease.

- Excess alcohol consumption.
- Inadequate knowledge of the signs and symptoms of hypoglycaemia (people with diabetes, their carers and health professionals).
- Inability to self-treat the hypoglycaemia, for example, due to confusion, delirium or concomitant geriatric syndromes.
- On multiple medicines.
- Using glucose-lowering conventional and complementary medicines together.

Many recent management guidelines recommend individualising diabetes management, including blood glucose and HbA_{1c} targets, to ensure patient safety (Del Prato *et al.* 2010).

Recognising hypoglycaemia

Some, or all, of the signs and symptoms listed in Table 6.1 can be present. A number of factors affect the individual's ability to recognise hypoglycaemia, as indicated. In addition, some commonly consumed substances such as caffeine, which can increase the intensity of the symptoms, and alcohol, which clouds judgement, can make it difficult for people to recognise hypoglycaemia.

Symptoms are more varied in children than adults and between hypoglycaemic episodes in the same child, and they have more difficulty recognising the symptoms. Young children may become naughty, aggressive, complain of abdominal pain, feeling 'awful', yawning, daydreaming, and warm to the touch (Ross *et al.* 1998). As indicated, older people with Type 2 diabetes commonly present with neurological symptoms. Many emergency departments now have a policy of testing the blood glucose in all unconscious patients to detect hypoglycamia.

Gonder-Frederick *et al.* (1997) described a number of factors that affect the individual's ability to detect and treat hypoglycaemia including:

- The blood glucose level.
- Usual metabolic control.
- Recent hypoglycaemia.
- Chronic hypoglycaemia, which can occur 'acutely' in older people as a result of repeated unrecognised hypoglycaemia or as a result of hypoglycaemic unawareness; see Chapter 8.
- Counter-regulatory response and amount of adrenaline secreted. The counter-regulatory response, especially glucagon release, diminishes over time in Type 1 diabetes.
- Medications such as beta blockers can mask the sympathetic warning signs, and caffeine can cause trembling and sweating that can be mistaken for hypoglycaemia. Smoking confers a 2.6 times greater risk of severe hypoglycaemia in Type 1 diabetes (Klein .2007) as well as contributing to the long-term complications of diabetes and other diseases.
- Distractions such as concentrating on work, when anxious and stressed, which also activates the autonomic nervous system ('fight or flight' response).
- Knowledge such as not recognising the symptoms.
- Hypoglycaemic unawareness or impaired mental function, which inhibits appropriate management.
- Cognitive impairment.

Other research shows older people, especially those living alone, young children who depend on their parents (McCrimmon *et al.* 1995), adolescents (DCCT 1997), those

Table 6.2 The counter-regulatory hormonal response to hypoglycaemia.

Hormone	Action
Glucagon	Increases glucose output from liver and muscle (glycogenolysis)
Adrenaline and noradrenaline	Enhances glycogenolysis in liver and muscle Enhances gluconeogenesis Reduces insulin secretion Causes many of the signs and symptoms of hypoglycaemia (autonomic response; [see Table 6.1])
Cortisol	Mobilises the substrates for gluconeogenesis
Growth hormone	Acts with cortisol and adrenaline to inhibit peripheral glucose utilisation

determined to achieve strict glycaemic control, lower social class (Muhlhauser *et al.* 1998), and pregnant women with Type 1 diabetes, experience more hypoglycaemia. For example, 45% of pregnant women with Type 1 diabetes experience severe hypoglycaemia during pregnancy, particularly in the first trimester and 3–5 mild hypoglycaemic events per patient-week especially in the presence of previous severe hypoglycaemia and impaired or hypoglycaemia unawareness (Ringholm & Nielsen 2008).

Counter-regulatory hormonal response to hypoglycaemia

The brain requires 120–140 g glucose per day to function normally and has limited capacity to manufacture its own glucose. Therefore, it depends on adequate levels of circulating blood glucose. When the blood glucose falls below normal the body releases hormones to counteract the effects of hypoglycaemia. This is known as the counter-regulatory response. Glycogen stores are liberated and new glucose is formed in the liver from precursors, for example, fatty acids and protein. The hormones released are shown in Table 6.2, along with their resultant action, the net result being an increase in blood glucose.

Causes of hypoglycaemia

Although hypoglycaemia is associated with insulin and GLM use, the relationship among these agents and food intake, exercise, and a range of other contributory factors is not straightforward. Some episodes can be explained by altered awareness or mismatch between food intake and/or food absorption and insulin. It should be noted that serum insulin levels and glucose clearance following insulin injections varies in the same individual even when the same dose is injected at the same time, dose and approximate site each day (Galloway & Chance 1994), even with modern purified insulins (Del Prato *et al.* 2010).

Exercise is also a contributing factor in many cases but the effect of exercise is also difficult to predict and depends on exercise intensity and duration, planned or spontaneous, time of the day, previous food intake, when it occurred in relation to insulin/ GLM dose, and the insulin injection site. For example, absorption is enhanced if exercise commences immediately after injecting insulin but not if exercise commences >35 minutes after injecting.

As indicated, sulphonylureas cause hypoglycaemia but less often than insulin; however, when sulphonylurea-induced hypoglycaemia does occur, it causes significant morbidity and mortality, may be prolonged and may accompany or precipitate a stroke or myocardial infarction. Interactions with other medicines including complementary medicines should be considered especially in the setting of compromised renal function; see Chapters 8 and 19. Alcohol may be a contributing factor. Frequent hypoglycaemia might indicate changing renal function and insulin doses may need to be reduced. GLMs may be contraindicated. Lowered appetite and nausea accompanying renal disease may contribute to hypoglycaemia risk.

If no reasonable common contributing factor can be identified, less common causes such as endocrine disorders, gastroparesis, and coeliac disease should be considered (Chapter 10). Psychological factors also need to be considered; see Chapter 15. However, a specific reason for the episode cannot always be found, which makes prevention difficult:the number of hypoglycaemic events where a cause cannot be identified ranges between 19 and 38%.

Various authors attribute hypoglycaemia to 'patient non-compliance' such as manipulating insulin doses, reducing intake, or omitting meals. While these behaviours do occur, especially in adolescents (Chapter 13) health professionals need to understand the reason for the behaviour rather than attaching a label to the individual. They need to appreciate the complexity of achieving diabetes balance and the frustration it causes many people with diabetes and the fear associated with hyppoglycaemia (Jones 2011; Bernard *et al.* 2012). The view that achieving blood glucose balance is an equation where:

$$insulin/GLMs + appropriate\ diet + appropriate\ exercise = target\ glucose\ levels$$

is simplistic, and ignores significant individual factors not included in the equation.

Preventing and managing hypoglycaemia

Preventing hypoglycaemia is challenging and may be impossible to achieve. It is possible to help people understand hypoglycaemia and recognise their unique symptoms and signs and limit the severity and frequency of hypoglycaemia. Key management strategies include:

- Undertaking a personalsied hypoglycaemia risk profile especially with vulnerable people such as older people, children, those with recurrent severe hypoglycaemia, those with hypoglycaemic unawareness, those with cognitive impairment, those with renal and liver disease and people who consume excess alcohol. The assessment should include helping people identify situations that increase the risk of hypoglycaemia. In hospital settings people at high risk of hypoglycaemia include those on insulin infusions.
- Using the information to determine safe blood glucose and HbA_{1c} targets for the individual.
- Appreciating the emotional and psychological components of hypoglycaemia and the associated fear and impacts on self-care. These aspects should be part of an individualised, comprehensive assessment when people commence insulin and at regular intervals especially when the person experiences an hypoglycaemic event.
- Appropriate prescribing and medicine reviews and dose adjustment.
- Including medicine reviews in annual complication screening programmes.
- Educating the person about insulin action, hypoglycaemia symptoms, and food intake and exercise in relation to insulin action, and managing hypoglycaemic episodes. The education might include insulin dose adjustment and carbohydrate counting especially for people using insulin pumps and those on basal bolus regimens. Regular education revision is advisable.

- Regular blood glucose-self-monitoring and using the information to tailor food, exercise and medicine doses.
- Wearing appropriate identification and carrying hypogycaemic treatment at all times.
- Using new technologies such as blood glucose meters and algorithms embedded in insulin pumps and glucose sensor systems that can be programmed to identify high and low blood glucose. Systems are available that suspend insulin for two hours when hypoglycaemia is detected. Continuous glucose monitoring can be used as part of a risk assessment and a range of mobile phone apps are available to help people manage their diabetes.
- Having back up and support systems in place if the individual is unable to manage the hypoglycaemic episode themselves.
- Helping people with hypoglycaemia unawreness recognise changed body signs of hypoglycaemia including structured programmes such as BGATT (Cox *et al.* 2001).

Hypoglycaemic unawareness

The ability to recognise hypogycaemia warning signs is essential to prevention of severe hypoglycaemia and associated risk of injury, falls and coma. People's experience of hypoglycaemia varies considerably from each other and between hypoglycaemic episodes (Speight 2011). Hypoglycaemic unawareness may encompass reduced intensityof the symptoms and/or a change in the type of symptoms the individual experiences (Speight 2011). Hypoglycaemic unawareness means people no longer recognise the early autonomic hypoglycaemic signs and do not recognise hypoglycaemia; thus, they do not treat it and are at risk of severe hypoglycaemia and coma.

Recurrent episodes of hypoglycaemia reduce the counter-regulatory response, associated symptoms and cognitive responses, which affects the individual's ability to recognise and treat the episode. People with both Type 1 and Type 2 diabetes have compromised counter-regulatory response, and a cycle of recurrent hypoglycaemia where each episode becomes increasingly severe may develop. If counter-regulation is compromised endogenous insulin secretion is not inhibited. Significantly, glucagon release in response to hypoglycaemia is impaired soon after diagnosis of diabetes and becomes progressively defective in people with diabetes. Adrenaline release is also reduced, which ultimately contributes to hypoglycaemic unawareness (DCCT Research Trial Group 1991; Unger 2012).

Hypoglycaemic unawareness may develop when the usual blood glucose is in the low/normal range and people may begin to recognise the symptoms again if the blood glucose targets are raised. Chronic hypoglycaemic unawareness develops with long duration of diabetes usually as a result of autonomic neuropathy and diminished counter-regulatory response. Both acute and chronic hypoglycaemic unawareness can be aggravated by medicines such as beta blockers, alcohol, and stimulants such as caffeine. Hypoglycaemic unawareness increases the risk of severe and profound hypoglycaemia and is one criterion for islet cell transplants.

Prevalence of hypoglycaemic unawareness

Determining the prevalence of hypoglycaemic unawareness is difficult because experts use different definitions and assessment methods. An estimated 19.5–25% of adults with Type 1 diabetes have hypoglycaemic unawareness and are older than people who recognise hypoglycaemic symptoms (Geddes *et al.* 2008). Rates for people with Type 2 diabetes are more difficult to determine because fewer data are available, but increasing age and duration of diabetes contribute to hypoglycaemic unawareness, which may be present in 8% of people with Type 2 diabetes (Speight 2011). However, hypoglycaemic unawareness in people with Type 2 diabetes could be under-recognised and under-reported.

Indicators that chronic hypoglycaemia might be present in older people, especially those on GLMs, include confusion, changes in cognition, personality changes, and disordered behaviour and must be distinguished from other less easily reversible causes of these signs. Accurately monitoring the blood glucose levels is important to detect chronic hypoglycaemia and CGMS can be useful. Management consists of revising the care plan and checking:

- That carbohydrate intake is adequate and evenly distributed.
- The individual is able to accurately prepare and administer their insulin.
- Whether any new medications or complementary therapies were commenced and reviewing the individual's medication self-management practices.
- Teeth/dentures to ensure there is no infection or mouth ulcers and that false teeth fit and are worn;
- Presence of diabetic complications or comorbidities that can affect self-care ability.
- Knowledge, which might mean relatives and friends need information about managing hypoglycaemia including how and when to use. People may benefit from education programmes such as BGATT (see this book, Chapter 16) and some regain the ability to recognise hypoglycaemia or new body cues after a period free from hypoglycaemia.

Several methods are used to assess hypoglycaemic unawareness and include careful questioning when hypoglycaemic unawareness is suspected, for example changed hypoglycaemic symptoms over time, combined with appropriate use of the individuals blood glucose monitoring pattern and serial HbA_{1c} levels, frequent presentations to emergency for hypoglycaemia, and continuous blood glucose monitoring (CGM). Clinical trial methods include the:

- Clarke method assesses people's threshold for and symptomatic response to hypoglycaemia but is limited by out-dated definition of severe hypoglycaemia and lack of consensus about the glycaemic thresholds for hypoglycaemic severity.
- Gold Method is a single item measure of hypoglycaemic unawareness and is the most frequently used method but it is limited by the difficulty of interpreting scores between 1 (awareness) and 4 (unawareness).
- Pederson-Bjergaad method could overestimate the prevalence of hypoglycaemic unawareness.
- Functional neuroimaging to measure regional brain metabolism, which is a proxy measure of neuronal activation, during hypoglycaemic episodes (Dunn *et al.* 2007).
- Hypoglycaemicia Awareness Questionnaire (HYPOA-Q) is a new tool that consists of 18 items that assess a range of issues related to hypoglycaemic unawareness. In future the HYPOA-Q could enable earlier diagnosis and evaluation of hypoglycaemic unawareness and proactive management and might be the most clinically relevant measure.

Nocturnal hypoglycaemia

Nocturnal hypogycaemia is defined as blood glucose, 3.3 mmol/L occurring during the night and mainly occurs in Type 1 diabetes, usually as a consequence of relative insulin excess and impaired glucose production overnight. Increased insulin sensitivity overnight plays a role. More than 80% of people treated with insulin experience nocturnal hypoglycaemia; 40% of these episodes are severe and are associated with significant morbidity and rarely, death. CGSM suggests the prevalence of nocturnal hypoglycaemia is 10–56%, lasts for ~6 hours, the time of the lowest level (nadir) depends on the insulin type and regimen (Raju *et al.* 2006). Raju *et al.* (2006) did not find differences in mean nocturnal blood glucose or mean nadir using CGSM to compare four insulin regimens in people with Type 1 diabetes with HbA$_{1c}$ <7.1%, but detected high rates of under- and overestimation of the glucose level.

Pramming *et al.* (1985) tried to identify predictors of early morning hypoglycaemia. They suggested if the blood glucose was <6 mmol/L at 11 p.m. there was an 80% chance of nocturnal hypoglycaemia compared to 12% risk if the blood glucose was >5 mmol/L. Other researchers report similar predictive blood glucose levels but the likelihood of nocturnal hypoglycaemia increases if multiple injections are used compared to CSII (Whincup & Milner 1987; Bendtson *et al.* 1988). Vervoort *et al.* (1996) found the bedtime blood glucose level predicted hypoglycaemia in the early part of the night but not hypoglycaemia occurring in the early morning and that a fasting blood glucose (before breakfast) <5.5 mmol/L indicated early morning hypoglycaemia.

However, the only risk factor Cooperberg *et al.* (2008) identified in a study to determine the amount of glucose needed to prevent exercise-induced hypoglycaemia, was frequent exercise. In Young *et al.*'s study, nocturnal hypoglycaemia occurred on both exercise and sedentary nights. Blood glucose 7.2 mmol/L at 9 p.m. predicted overnight hypoglycaemia on sedentary days. Exercise has multiple effects on fuel utilisation and mobilisation. Initially, in the first 5–10 minutes muscle glycogen is the primary fuel source, followed by circulating glucose and then fuel derived from gluconeogenesis and fatty acid oxidation (Silverstein 2008). When the counter- regulatory response is abnormal, people are unable to effectively mobilise glucose stores for gluconeogenesis.

In many cases the individual does not recognise the signs of nocturnal hypoglycaemia and does not wake up. Repeated episodes of nocturnal hypoglycaemia reduce the counter-regulatory response to hypoglycaemia. Undetected autonomic dysfunction and nocturnal hypoglycaemia can increase the risk of fatal cardiac ventricular dysrrhythmias ('dead in bed' syndrome).

Indicators of nocturnal hypoglycaemia

- Night sweats.
- Nightmares or vivid dreams.
- Unaccustomed snoring.
- Morning lethargy or chronic fatigue.
- Headaches or 'hung over' feeling.
- Mood change, particularly depression.
- High blood glucose before breakfast (Somogyi effect).
- Morning ketouria.
- Relatives notice unusual behavior such as snoring or 'sleep walking.'

Factors that contribute to nocturnal hypoglycaemia include preceding physical activity that may have occurred many hours previously, insufficient carbohydrate in meals, excess insulin as a result of these factors, enhanced sensitivity to insulin and/or inappropriate insulin dose, and alcohol consumption.

The Somogyi effect refers to pre-breakfast hyperglycaemia following an overnight hypoglycaemic episode. If any of the above symptoms occur, the blood glucose should be measured at 2 to 3 a.m. over several nights to establish whether nocturnal hypoglycaemia is occurring. The insulin is then adjusted accordingly by decreasing the morning long-acting dose for those on a daily insulin, the afternoon long-acting dose for those on BD insulin or the pre-evening meal or bedtime dose for basal bolus regimes.

Clinical observations

(1) Sometimes the evening short-acting insulin, rather than the intermediate or long-acting insulin, causes nocturnal hypoglycaemia, depending on the time the insulin was administered.
(2) Rapid-acting insulins have a shorter duration of action and are less likely to cause nocturnal hypoglycaemia.
(3) Stress and illness are usually associated with hyperglycaemia; however, they can induce hypoglycaemia in some people with Type 1 diabetes.

Practice point

The Somogyi effect should be distinguished from another condition that results in morning hyperglycaemia, the 'dawn phenomenon'. The dawn phenomenon refers to a situation where insulin requirements and blood glucose concentration increase between 5 a.m. and 8 a.m., which occurs in up to 75% of people with diabetes. Treatment consists of *increasing* the insulin dose.

Many other hormones have a normal physiological rise in the early morning, for example, testosterone, which causes early morning erections.

Managing nocturnal hypoglycaemia

Not surprisingly, people with diabetes and their relatives are very fearful of hypoglycaemia at any time, but particularly at night, and careful explanations about the possible causes and suggestions of ways to prevent nocturnal hypoglycaemia are essential. Families/significant others need to know how to manage the hypoglycaemia by maintaining the person's airway and calling an ambulance. If they have glucagon at home, they should give the injection.

Various methods have been used to prevent nocturnal hypoglycaemia, these include providing carbohydrate snacks at bedtime, although there is no real evidence to support the practice (Allen & Frier 2003) or demonstrate efficacy (Raju *et al.* 2006), and adjusting the insulin regimen. The long-acting insulin analogues, with their more predictable action profile, are associated with significantly lower rates of nocturnal hypoglycaemia. Helping the individual and their family/carers recognise cues to hypoglycaemia through hypoglycaemia training programmes such as HYATT and BGATT may be effective (Cox *et al.* 2004). CGSM may provide important clues to assist in such training.

More recently, antihypoglycaemic agents such as β_2-adrenergic agonists (Terbutaline) were trialled and a significant reduction in the frequency and severity of nocturnal hypoglycaemia was demonstrated (Raju *et al.* 2006). The morning blood glucose was significantly higher after Terbutaline and the pulse rate was elevated. Acarbose with a carbohydrate bedtime snack also reduced the mean blood glucose nadir but did not prevent nocturnal hypoglycaemia.

Relative hypoglycaemia

People who are accustomed to high blood glucose levels for long periods of time may experience the symptoms of hypoglycaemia when blood glucose control improves and blood glucose levels normalise. In general, it is not necessary to treat the symptoms once the blood glucose is recorded, but reassurance, support, and education are necessary until the person adapts to the new blood glucose range.

Medicine interactions

Some commonly prescribed medicines can interact with sulphonylureas and increase the possibility of hypoglycaemia (see Table 6.3).

Practice points

- Consider whether the person is using complementary medicines such as herbs, supplements and other complementary therapies (CAM) such as massage and relaxation therapies. These therapies can exert hypoglycaemic effects themselves, interact with conventional medicines or cause liver or renal damage that alters the pharmacokinetics and pharmacodynamics of medicines and predisposes the person to hypoglycaemia, or indirectly affect the blood glucose by reducing stress (see Chapter 19).
- People with diabetes are high CAM users.

Table 6.3 Commonly prescribed medicines that can increase the hypoglycaemic effect of sulphonylurea medicines.

Medicines	Means of potentiation
Sulphonamides	Displaces sulphonylureas from protein binding sites
Salicylates	
Warfarin	
Clofibrate	
Phenylbutazone	
Coumarin derivatives	Inhibits/decreases hepatic metabolism of the sulphonylurea
Chloramphenicol	
Phenylbutazone	
Probenecid	Delays urinary excretion of the sulphonylurea
Salicylates	
Tuberculostatics	
Tetracyclines	
MAO inhibitors	Increases action by an unknown mechanism

Objectives of care

In hospital settings staff need to be alert to the possibility of hypoglycaemia in all patients on insulin or GLMs, and should hypoglycaemia occur to:

(1) Supply quick-acting carbohydrate to immediately raise blood glucose levels if the person is conscious and able to eat.
(2) Maintain blood glucose levels within the acceptable range of 4–8 mmol/L most of the time for most people but the range may vary in specific situations such as surgical procedures.
(3) Ascertain the cause of the hypoglycaemic episode.
(4) Limit further episodes of hypoglycaemia.
(5) Allay fear and anxiety including that of relatives.
(6) Prevent trauma occurring as a result of hypoglycaemia; for example, falls.
(7) Assess the individual's knowledge about managing hypoglycaemia and educate or refer to a diabetes educator if necessary. In particular people should be assisted to recognise their personal risk of hypoglycaemia and learn to recognise their individual 'hypo symptoms' rather then being provided with a list of textbook signs and symptoms.
(8) Consider including an alert in the individual's medical record if they are at high risk of hypoglycaemia.
(9) Consider safety issues related to hypoglycaemia such as falls and associated fractures in older people and plan care and organise the environment to reduce such risks. Johnston *et al.* (2012) examined hypoglycaemic events and fall-related fractures in people with Type 2 diabetes over 65 years over two consecutive 12-month periods. They also collected data about the presence other falls risk factors such as vascular disease, medicines including TZDs. Johnston *et al.* found hypoglycaemia was independently associated with increased risk of falls-related fractucres. Common fractures included hip, spine, pelvis, leg and upper arm. The findings suggest hypoglycaemia should be included on falls risk assessment tools when the individual has GLM-treated diabetes (Dunning 2005).

Treatment

Rapid treatment is important to prevent mild hypoglycaemia progressing to severe hypoglycaemia and limit the potential adverse risks associated with severe episodes. The following management refers to people in hospital but can be applied in other settings.

Mild hypoglycaemia

Test and record the blood glucose level.
   Provide 10–15 g of carbohydrate as quick-acting glucose or other high glycaemic index carbohydrate to raise the blood glucose immediately, for example:
   3 level teaspoons sugar in 1/2 cup water
   or   1/2 regular sugary/soft drink (*not low calorie* (joule))
   or   proprietary glucose preparation such as glucose gels/tablets or person's usual hypoglycaemia treatment, for example, jelly beans.
   Traditional treatment advice is to follow the initial glucose treatment with long-acting carbohydrate to maintain blood glucose until the next meal. However, the extra carbohydrate may not always be necessery if the hypoglycaemia is due to rapid-acting

insulins with short duration of action. The person's experience and clinical judgement are important determinants of the need for extra carbohydrate, but remember many people over treat hypoglycaemia. If follow up carbohydrate is required provide:

1/2 sandwich

or   2 to 4 dry biscuits (unsweetened)

or   1 piece of fruit.

Check blood glucose in one hour and then as necessary. The next dose of insulin or GLM is not usually withheld following a mild hypoglycaemic episode. However, if hypoglycaemia occurs frequently, the management regimen might need to be adjusted, for example, extra carbohydrate in the diet, reduced medication dose.

Severe hypoglycaemia with impaired conscious state

Note: Do not give anything by mouth if the person is unconscious. Confused patients often spit fluids out or refuse to swallow. Gels are preferable and can be smeared onto the buccal mucosa but the dose may not be sufficient to reverse the hypoglycaemia.

(1) Place the person on their side.
(2) Clear airway.
(3) Notify the doctor in hospital settings or call an ambulance.
(4) Test the blood glucose level and confirm with the laboratory (i.e. urgent glucose).
(5) Give IM glucagons. Instructions for glucagon administration are shown at the end of the chapter. Prepare an IV tray containing 50% dextrose. Fifty per cent glucose should be given into an antecubital vein because injection into hand veins often results in extravasation and thrombophlebitis. Ten per cent glucose is recommended for children to reduce the risk of hyperosmolality. Dose: adult 20–30 mL 50% glucose; child 2–5 mL/kg bolus 10% glucose then 0.1 mL/kg/minute until the child regains consciousness. Consciousness usually returns within five minutes (Therapeutic Guidelines (TG) 2004).
(6) Monitor blood glucose 1–2 hourly until blood glucose level is stable above 5 mmol/L and then revert to the usual testing regimen.
(7) Give complex carbohydrate low glycaemic index food to maintain the blood glucose level when consciousness returns. The patient may still be confused and may need to be reminded to chew and swallow.

The patient should be monitored for at least 36 hours. Ascertain the time and dose for the next insulin injection/OHA dose. Provide education, counselling and support to the individual and their family/carers.

Prolonged hypoglycaemia

Recovery from hypoglycaemia can be prolonged if the episode is severe, prolonged, and/or associated with coma and/or seizures. Other causes of impaired consciousness should be considered such as stroke and insulin overdose. Insulin overdose should be excluded when high doses of IV glucose are needed to maintain the blood glucose >5 mmol/L.

Hypoglycaemia related to long-acting sulphonylureas is a medical emergency and the person should be managed in hospital. Prolonged infusion of 10% IV and 1–2 hourly blood glucose monitoring is often necessary. Some experts recommend using 50 mg of subcutaneous octreotide 8 hourly for three doses (TG 2004). In some cases a brain scan will be indicated, and if cerebral oedema is present, IV mannitol is administered. Shorr *et al.* (1996) suggested the crude rate of prolonged hypoglycaemia associated with long-acting sulphonylureas is 16.6% per 1000 person years compared to 1.9% in second-generation agents. However, long-acting sulphonylureas are no longer used in most countries. Significantly, recent discharge from hospital is a significant predictor of serious medicine-associated hypoglycaemia in older people (days 1–30), especially the very old, frail, those on more than 5 medicines (Shorr *et al.* 1997).

Recovery should be rapid. If recovery does not occur in 10–15 minutes, exclude other causes of unconsciousness.

(1) Record episode and blood glucose level on the appropriate chart/s and in patient's medical record. Consider whether an 'alert sticker' should be included in their medical record.
(2) Monitor progress/recovery from the episode.
(3) Look for the cause of hypoglycaemia, for example, meal delayed or missed, inadequate intake of carbohydrate, unaccustomed activity, excessive medication, medication/medication, medication/herb or herb/herb interactions.
(4) Reassure the patient and relatives.
(5) Ensure patient has an understanding of causes and management of hypoglycaemia (refer to diabetes nurse specialist/diabetes educator).
(6) See Chapter 12 for information about managing hypoglycaemia in older people.

Patients most at risk of hypoglycaemia

A number of factors significantly increase the risk of hypoglycaemia. These include:

- Those taking insulin or GLM, especially long-acting formulations and intensive insulin therapy; see Chapter 12. However, the long-acting insulin analogues have lower hypoglycaemia risk than the other long-acting and biphasic insulins.
- Medicine doses not adjusted for changes such as weight loss, increased activity, following acute illness, and when reducing oral corticosteroid doses.
- Beginning an exercise/diet regimen or prolonged aerobic exercise. Hypoglycaemia can occur many hours after exercise, often during the night. Unaccustomed activity such as rehabilitation programmes should be considered 'exercise'.
- People on insulin achieving blood glucose within the normal range.
- History of hypoglycaemia.
- People with an irregular lifestyle and irregular meal and exercise patterns and when carbohydrate content of the meal is low.
- Eating disorders.
- Young children. It is difficult to predict their activity levels and food intake and the presenting signs may be difficult to distinguish from other causes such as tiredness and misbehaving. It is important to support and educate the family.
- Adolescents, possibly because of their erratic eating patterns and experimentation with alcohol and striving for 'good control'.
- Older people especially those who live alone.
- Insulin-treated pregnant women and newborn babies of women with GDM or on insulin.
- Those with renal or hepatic disease. Severe hypoglycaemia is independently associated with microalbuminuria in people with Type 2 diabetes (Jae-Seung *et al.* (2013).
- Those with long-standing diabetes who may have autonomic neuropathy are at risk of hypoglycaemic unawareness, and effects on the gastrointestinal tract that may delay gastric emptying and food absorption.

- People with brittle diabetes (Chapter 10).
- People fasting for a procedure/surgery or religious reasons, for example, Ramadan and Buddhist Lent.
- People with diarrhoea and vomiting where food absorption is impaired. Hypoglycaemia may impair gastric emptying (Russo *et al.* 2005).
- Those with an impaired conscious state.
- Those sedated or on narcotic infusions.
- Endocrine diseases such as insulinoma, hypothyroidism and hypoadrenalism.
- Alcohol may also cause hypoglycaemia particularly if food is not eaten at the same time. The hypoglycaemia can occur hours after consuming alcohol.
- People taking a lot of medications and/or complementary medicines, especially those that lower blood glucose.
- Social class where people may not be able to afford appropriate food or hypoglycaemia treatment and prevention.

Practice points

(1) The signs of alcohol intoxication can make hypoglycaemia difficult to recognise. Alcohol impairs cognitive function and reduces the ability to recognise and effectively treat hypoglycaemia. Self-care and diet are often inadequate. In addition, chronic alcohol abuse leads to malnutrition and limited glucose stores to mount an effective counter-regulatory response.

(2) People with chronic alcohol addiction are very difficult to manage because OHAs are often contraindicated and insulin puts them at high risk of hypoglycaemia.

Psychological effects of hypoglycaemia

Hypoglycaemia is feared and hated by many people with diabetes and the effects are often under-rated by health professionals. The importance of recognising and accepting these concerns cannot be overemphasised. Hypoglycaemia has profound effects on people's quality of life, social activities, for example, driving and work, and they fear brain damage and death from hypoglycaemia. It is not unusual for people to deliberately run their blood glucose levels high to avoid hypoglycaemia (Dunning 1994) (see Chapter 15). They can then be termed 'non-compliant' and placed in a conflict situation. Commonly expressed concerns about hypoglycaemia are:

- loss of control of the situation;
- reminder that they have diabetes;
- losing face and making a fool of themselves;
- blood glucose rising too high after treatment;
- sustaining brain damage; however, the DCCT and EDIC studies did not show a relationship between hypoglycaemia and declining cognitive function (DCCT Trial Group/ EDICT 1993). The DCCT is not relevant to older people. Hershey *et al.* (2005) found impaired spatial long-term memory performance and repeated episodes of severe hypoglycaemia, particularly when the hypoglycaemia commenced before five years of age. Severe, repeated hypoglycaemia has also been associated with a lower volume of grey matter in the left superior temporal region of the brain, which is associated with episodic memory, in young people with Type 1 diabetes (Perantie *et al.* 2007).

- recovery can take days following serious hypoglycaemia and leave residual headache and tiredness;
- death.

Hypoglycaemia can affect the individual's confidence in their ability to cope. Support and understanding, and exploring all of the issues, physical, mental, and social that affect coping is an important part of management.

Clinical observation

Pet dogs sometimes recognise their owner's hypoglycaemia and alert them in time for them to be able to treat the hypoglycaemia or rouse another family member.

Consequences of hypoglycaemia

There are a number of physical sequels to hypoglycaemia in addition to the psychological consequences that include:

- *Neurological impairment*. Two main areas of the brain function are affected: cognitive ability, most commonly hippocampal functions such as memory, and affective ability, which affects mood and anxiety level. Blood glucose <1 mmol/L is referred to as neurogycopaenia and usually results in coma, loss of consciousness, seizures and death or permanent brain damage (Mc Nay & Cotero 2010). Less profound hypoglycaemia, blood glucose < 2 mmol/L, can interfere with the individual's ability to perform usual activities and lead to irritability, drowsiness, vision changes, difficulty speaking and confusion (Unger & Parkin 2011). These neurological changes are particularly dangerous in older people and contribute to or accelerate dementia. Zhang *et al.* (2010) suggested that the risk of dementia attributable to hypoglycaemia is 2.9% per year. However, the longer term neurological effects are controversial. Interestingly, Dunn *et al.* (2007) suggested that, although hypoglycaemia is distressing, it might also be weakly rewarding because the brain regional networks serving hedonic responses are relatively unaffected in hypoglycaemic people. Amiel, one of the coauthors, used the term 'hypo junkies' in a presentation in Melbourne to refer to a very small group of people who derived pleasure from hypoglycaemia.
- *Cardiovascular outcomes*. Symptomatic mild and severe hypoglycaemia is associated with increased cardiovascular events, hospital admissions from all causes and mortality from all causes (Pai-Feng *et al.* 2012). Likewise Zoungas (2010) found a significant increase in risk of major macrovascular events (hazard ratio (HR) 2.88; 95% confidence interval (CI), microvascular events (HR1.81, 95% CI 1.19–2.74, death from macrovascular events (HR 2.68 95% CI 1.72–4.19) and death from any cause(HR 2.69, 95% CI 1.97–3.67) (p all < 0.001) associated with severe hypoglycaemia. The presence of macroalbuminuria predicts severe hypoglycaemia (Jae-Seung *et al.* 2013).
- Non-*vascular outcomes* are also affected (Zoungas 2010). Associations between severe hypoglycaemia and outcomes such as respiratory, digestive and skin conditions.
- Falls and fall-related fractures (Johnston *et al.* 2012), which compromise self-care, mobility, increase anxiety and could mean admission to an aged care facility.

Guidelines for administering glucagon

Glucagon is a hormone produced by the alpha cells of the pancreas. Glucagon stimulates glycogenolysis and hepatic glucose output. Glucagon is available in a single dose pack containing one vial of glucagon hydrochloride powder (1 mg) and a glass syringe prefilled with sterile water (for injection).

Indication

Glucagon is used to treat severe hypoglycaemia in people with diabetes treated with insulin or GLMs, primarily people who are unable to take glucose orally, for whom oral glucose is ineffective, who are unconscious or uncooperative or having a seizure. Glucagon can be administered by relatives.

Instructions for use

(1) Individual patients must be assessed to determine the appropriate dose and route of administration. Glucagon is given according to body weight and muscle bulk (intramuscularly or subcutaneously). The buttock is the ideal injection site.
(2) The intravenous route may be the preferred route in hospital in profound hypoglycaemia to ensure rapid absorption and reversal of the hypoglycaemia. DCCT data suggest unconscious patients recover within ~6 minutes of the glucagon injection. Glucagon may be ineffective in people with low glycogen stores such as thin frail older people, and those with liver disease including alcoholics.
(3) Check the expiry date. Do not reconstitute the glucagon until just before it is administered (prepare and administer). Glucagon should be used soon after reconstitution. Do not use if reconstituted solution is not clear and colourless.
(4) Follow the instructions in the package to prepare the injection and the medical order for the dose.
(5) Record the time and route of administration, the dose, and the patient's response.

Dosage

- Adults and children of weight >25 kg full dose (1 mg).
- Children of weight <25 kg half dose (0.5 mg).

Practice points

(1) A second dose of Glucagon can be given; however, repeated injections can cause nausea, making subsequent food intake difficult, thus, repeat dosing is not recommended.
(2) If recovery does not occur within 10–15 minutes, IV glucose might be required. Slow recovery could indicate limited glucose stores but other causes of unconsciousness should be considered.
(3) Glucagon may be contraindicated where glycogen stores are low, for example, in fasting states, chronic hypoglycaemia, chronic adrenal insufficiency and malnutrition where the individual is unable to mount an effective counterregulatory response.

Adverse reactions

Adverse reactions are rare. Occasionally transient nausea occurs that can make it difficult to consume sufficient oral carbohydrate, which is necessary to avoid the blood glucose dropping again. Vomiting occurs occasionally, usually only after a second dose.

Glucagon is a peptide, so theoretically hypersensitivity is possible and is more likely in atopic patients. In reality hypersensitivity is rare.

Clinical observations

- Hypothermia can prolong recovery from hypoglycaemia especially in the elderly in winter. Management of the hypothermia as well as the hypoglycaemia is usually required.
- Hypothermia represents a poor prognosis.

References

Accord Study Group (2008) Effects of intensive glucose lowering in Type 2 diabetes. *New England Journal of Medicine*, **358** (24), 2545–2559.

Allen, K. & Frier, B. (2003) Nocturnal hypoglycaemia: Clinical manifestations and therapeutic strategies towards prevention. *Endocrine Practice*, **9**, 530–543.

American Diabetes Association (2013) Standards of Medical Care in Diabetes – 2013. *Diabetes Care* January 2013 36:S4-S10; DOI: 10.2337/dc13-S004.

Amiel, S., Dixon, T., Mann, R., Jameson, K. (2008) Hypogycaemia in Type 2 diabetes. *Diabetic Medicine*, **25** (3), 245–254.

Bernard, K., Cavan, D., Ziegler, R. *et al.* (2012) The ticking time bomb: Fear of hypoglycaemia and its impact on diabetes control: Baseline results from ABACUS. Poster presented at the European Association for the Study of Diabetes, Berlin.

Bendtson, I., Kverneland, A., Pramming, S. & Binder, C. (1998) Incidence of nocturnal hypoglycaemia in insulin-dependent diabetic patients on intensive therapy. *Acta Medica Scandinavica*, **223**, 543–548.

Brod, M. & Barnett, A. (2012) Impact of self-treated hypoglycaemia in Type 2 diabetes: A multinational survey in patients and physicians. *Current Medical Research and Opinion*, **28** (12), 1947–1958.

Cooperberg B, Breckenridge S, Arbelaez A, et al. (2008) Terbutaline and the prevention of nocturnal hypoglycemia in type 1 diabetes. *Diabetes Care*, **31**, 2271–2272.

Cox, D., Clarke, W., Gonder-Frederick, L. *et al.* (1985) Accuracy of perceiving blood glucose in IDDM. *Diabetes Care*, **8**, 529–536.

Cox, D. & Gonder-Frederick, W. (2001) Blood glucose awareness training (BGAT 3) long term benefits. *Diabetes Care*, **24** (4), 637–642.

Cox, D., Kovatchev, B. & Koev, D. (2004) Hypoglycaemia anticipation, awareness training (HYATT) reduces occurrences of severe hypoglycaemia among adults with Type 1 diabetes. *International Journal Behavioural Medicine*, **11**, 212–218.

Davis, E., Keating, B., Byrne, G., Russell, M. & Jones, T. (1997) Hypoglycaemic incidence and clinical predictors in a large population based sample of children and adolescents with IDDM *Diabetes Care*, **20**, 22–25.

Daneman, T., Frank, M., Perlman, K., Tamm, J. & Ehrlich, R. (1989) Severe hypoglycaemia in children with insulin dependent diabetes: Frequency and predisposing factors. *Journal of Paediatrics*, **115**, 681–685.

Deary, I. (1993) Effects of hypoglycaemia on cognitive function, in *Hypoglycaemia and Diabetes: Clinical and Pyysiological Aspects* (eds B. Frier and B. Fisher), Edward Arnold, London, pp. 80–92.

Del Prato, S., LaSalle, J., Mattheai S. & Bailey, C. (2010) Tailoring treatment to the individual in Type 2 diabetes practical guidance from the Global Partnership for Effective Diabetes Management. *International Journal of Clinical Practice*, **64** (3), 295–304.

DCCT (Diabetes Control and Complication Trial Research Group) (1991) Epidemiology of severe hypoglycaemia in the Diabetes Control and Complications Trial. *American Journal of Medicine*, **90**, 450–459.

DCCT (Diabetes Control and Complication Trial Research Group) (1997) Hypoglycaemia in the Diabetes Control and Complications Trial. *Diabetes*, **46**, 271–286.

Diabetes Control and ComplicationsTrial (DCCT)/Epidemiology of Diabetes Interventions and Complications Research Group (DCCT) (1993) The effect of intensivetreatment of diabetes on the development and progression of long-term complications in insulin dependent diabetes mellitus. *New England Journal Medicine*, **329**, 977–986.

Diabetes Control and ComplicationsTrial (DCCT)/Epidemiology of Diabetes Interventions and Complications Research Group (2003). Intensive diabetes therapy and carotid intima-media thickness in type 1 diabetes mellitus. *New England Journal Medicine* **348**, 2294–2903.

Dunn, J., Cranston, I., Marsden, P., Amiel, S. & Reed, L. (2007) Attenuation of amydgala and frontal cortical responses to low blood glucose concentration in asymptomatic hypoglycaemia in Type 1 diabetes: A new player in hypoglycaemic unawareness. *Diabetes*, **36**, 2706–2773.

Dunning, P. (1994) Having diabetes: Young adult perspectives. *The Diabetes Educator*, **21** (1), 58–65.

Dunning, T. (2005) *Managing Diabetes in Older People*. Wiley Blackwell, Chichester.

Donnelly, L., Morris, A. & Frier, D. (2005) Frequency and predictors of hypoglycaemia in Type 1 diabetes and insulin treated Type 2 diabetes: A population based study. *Diabetic Medicine*, **22** (6), 749–755.

Farmer A, Brockbank K, Keech M, et al. (2012) Incidence and costs of severe hypoglycaemia requiring attendance by the emergency medical services in South Central England. *Diabetic Medicine* Mar 21. DOI: 10.1111/j.1464-5491.2012.03657.x.

Galloway, J. & Chance, R. (1994) Improving insulin therapy: Achievements and challenges. *Hormone and Metabolic Research*, **26**, 591–598.

Geddes, J., Schopman, J., Zammitt, M. & Frier, B. (2008) Prevalence of impaired awareness of hypoglycaemia in adults with Type 1 diabetes. *Diabetic Medicine*, **24** (4), 501–504.

Gonder-Frederick, L., Cox, D., Driesen, N., Ryan, C. & Clarke, W. (1994) Individual differences in neurobehavioural disruption during mild to moderate hypoglycaemia in adults with IDDM. *Diabetes*, **43**, 1407–1312.

Henderson, J., Allen, K., Deary, I. & Frie, H. (2003) Hypoglycaemia in insulin-treated Type 2 diabetes: Frequency, symptoms and impaired awareness. *Diabetic Medicine*, **20** (12), 1016–1021.The measurement of cognitive function during acute hypoglycaemia: experimental limitations and their effect on the study of hypoglycaemia unawareness.

Heller, S. & Macdonald, I. (1996) *Diabetic Medicine* **13** (7), 607–15.

Hepburn, D. (1993) Symptoms of hypoglycaemia, in *Hypoglycaemia and Diabetes: Clinical and Physiological Aspects* (eds B. Frier and B. Fisher), Edward Arnold, London, pp. 93–103.

Hershey, T., Perantie, D. & Warren, S. (2005) Frequency and timing of severe hypoglycaemia affects spatial memory in children with Type 1 diabetes. *Diabetes Care*, **28**, 2372–2377.

Jae-Seung Y, Sun-Hye K, Sun-Hee K (2013) resence of Macroalbuminuria Predicts Severe Hypoglycemia in Patients With Type 2 Diabetes Mellitus: A 10-year follow-up study. *Diabetes Care*, December 17, 2012, DOI: 10.2337/dc12-1408.

Jones, T. (2011) Strategies for preventing hypoglycaemia in intensively managed Type 1 diabetes patients. *Diabetes Management*, **37**, 30–34.

Jones, T., Porter, P. & Sherwin, R. (1998) Decreased epinephrine responses to hypoglycaemia during sleep. *New England Journal of Medicine*, **338**, 1657–1662.

Johnston, S., Conner, C., Aagren, M., Ruiz, K. & Bouchard, J. (2012) Association between hypoglycaemic events and fall-related fractures in Medicare-covered patients with Type 2 diabetes. *Diabetes, Obesity and Metabolism*, **14**, 634–643.

Klein, R. (2007) Smoking is linked to hypoglycaemia in Type 1 diabetes. *Diabetes Care*, **30**, 1437–1441.

Laing, S., Swerdlow, A. & Slater, S. (1999) The British Diabetic Cohort Study 1. All-cause mortality in patients with insulin-treated diabetes mellitus. *Diabetic Medicine*, **16**, 459–465.

Leese, G., Wang, J. & Broomhall, J. (2003) Frequency of severe hypoglycaemia requiring emergency treatment in Type 1 and Type 2 diabetes: A population based study of health service resource use. *Diabetes Care*, **26** (4), 1176–1180.

Lundkvist, J., Bolinder, C. & Johnson, L. (2005) The economic and quality of life impact of hypoglycaemia. *European Journal of Health Economics*, **6**, 197–202.

McAuley, V., Deary, I., Ferguson, S. & Frier, B. (2001) Acute hypoglycaemia in humans causes attentional dysfunction while nonverbal intelligence is preserved. *Diabetes Care*, **24**, 1745–1750.

McCrimmon, R., Gold, A., Deary, I., Kelnar, C. & Frier, B. (1995) Symptoms of hypoglycaemia in children with IDDM. *Diabetes Care*, **18**, 851–861.

McNay, E. & Cotero, V. (2010) Mini-review: Impact of recurrent hypoglycaemia on cognitive and brain function. *Physiology Behaviour*, **100** (3), 234–238.

Muhlhauser, I., Overmann, H., Bender, R., Bott, U. & Berger, M. (1998) Risk factors of severe hypoglycaemia in adult patients with Type 1 diabetes – A prospective population based study. *Diabetologia*, **14**, 1274–1282.

Morris, A. DARTS/MEMO Collaboration (2003) Frequency of severe hypoglycaemia requiring emergency treatment in Type 1 and Type 2 diabetes: A population-based study of health service resource use. *Diabetes Care*, **26**, 1176–1180.

Moghissi E. (2011) Patients with diabetes lack knowledge about hypoglycaemia. Presented at the 20th Annual Meting and Clinical Congress of the American Association of Clinical Endocrinologists, San Diego California.

National Health and Medical Research Council (1991) *Hypoglycaemia and Diabetes*. Australian Government Printers, Canberra.

Nordfeldt, S. & Ludvigsson, J. (1997) Severe hypoglycaemia in children with IDDM. A prospective study, 1992–1994. *Diabetes Care*, **20**, 497–503.

Pai-Feng, H., Shih-Hsien, S., Hao-Min, C. *et al.* (2012) Association of clinical symptomatic hypoglycaemia with cardiovascular events and total mortality in Type 2 diabetes mellitus: A nationwide population-based study. *Diabetes Care* DOI: 10.2337/dc12-0916.

Perantie, D., Wu, J. & Koller, J. (2007) Regional brain volume differences associated with hyperglycaemia and severe hypoglycaemia in youth with Type 1 diabetes. *Diabetes Care*, **30**, 2331–2337.

Pramming, S., Thorsteinsson, B., Ronn, B. & Binder, C. (1985) Nocturnal hypoglycaemia in patients receiving conventional treatment with insulin. *British Medical Journal*, **291**, 376–379.

Pramming, S., Thorsteinsson, B., Bendtson, I. & Binder, C. (1991) Symptomatic hypoglycaemia in 411 Type 1 diabetic patients. *Diabetic Medicine*, **8**, 217–222.

Raju, B., Arbelaez, A., Breckenridge, S. & Cryer, P. (2006) Nocturnal hypoglycaemia in Type 1 diabetes: An assessment of preventative bedtime treatments. *Journal Clinical Endocrinology and Metabolism*, **91**, 2087–2092.

Ringholm, N. & Nielsen, L. (2008) Hypoglycaemia most common in early pregnancy in women with Type 1 diabetes. *Diabetes Care*, **31**, 9–14.

Ross, L., McCrimmon, R., Frier, B., Kelnar, C. & Deary, I. (1998) Hypoglycaemic symptoms reported by children with Type 1 diabetes mellitus and by their parents. *Diabetic Medicine*, **15**, 836–843.

Russo, A., Stevens, J., Chen, R. *et al.* (2005) Insulin-induced hypoglycaemia accelerates gastric emptying of solids and liquids in long standing Type 1 diabetes. *Journal of Clinical Endocrinology and Metabolism*, **90**, 4489–4495.

Salas, M. & Caro, J. (2002) Are hypoglycaemia and other adverse effects similar among sulphonylureas? *Adverse Drug Reactions Toxicology Review*, **21**, 205–217.

Silverstein, J. (2008) The lows of exercise: Another piece of the puzzle. *International Diabetes Monitor*, **20** (1), 44–46.

Shorr, R., Daugherty, W. & Griffin, M. (1996) Individual sulfonylureas and serious hypoglycaemia in older people. *Journal of the American Geriatric Society*, **44** (7), 751–755.

Shorr, R., Ray, W., Daugherty, J. & Griffin, M. (1997) Incidence and risk factors for serious hypoglycaemia in older persons using insulin or sulphonylureas. *Archives of Internal Medicine*, **157** (15), 1681–1686.

Sinclair, A. (2006) Special considerations in older adults with diabetes: Meeting the challenge. *Diabetes Spectrum*, **19**, 229–233.

Sommerfield, A., Deary, I., McAuley, V. & Frier, B. (2003) Short-term delayed, and working memory are impaired during hypoglycaemia in individuals with Type 1 diabetes. *Diabetes Care*, **26**, 390–396.

Speight J. (2011) Assessing impaired awareness of hypoglycaemia. *Diabetes Management* **34**, 36–37.

Siafarikas, A., Johnston, R., Bulsara, M. *et al.* (2012) Early loss of the glucagons response to hypoglycaemia in adolescents with Type 1 diabetes. *Diabetes Care*, **35**, 1757–1762.

Tattersall, R. (1999) Frequency, causes, and treatment of hypoglycemia, in Frier, B. and Fisher, B. (eds), *Hypoglycemia in Clinical Diabetes*, Wiley, Chichester, UK, pp. 55–87.

Therapeutic Guidelines (TG) (2004) *Hypoglycaemia*. http://www.tg.com.au/etg_demo/tcg/edg/1473.htm (accessed December 2007).

Thorsteinsson, B., Pramming, S., Lauritzen, T. & Binder, C. (1986) Frequency of daytime biochemical hypoglycaemia in insulin-treated diabetic patients: Relation to daily median blood glucose concentrations. *Diabetic Medicine*, **3**, 147–151.

UKPDS (1998) Intensive blood glucose control with sulphonylureas or insulin compared with conventional treatment and risk of complications in patients with Type 2 diabetes (UKPDS 33). *Lancet*, **352**, 837–853 (correction *Lancet* (1999) **354**, 602).

Unger J. (2012) Uncovering undetected hypoglycaemic events. *Diabetes Metabolic Syndrome and Obesity*, **5**, 57–74.

Unger, J. & Parkin, C. (2011) Hypoglycaemia in insulin-treated diabetes: A case for increased vigilance. *Postgraduate Medical Journal*, **123** (4), 81–91.

Vervoort, G., Goldschmodt, H. & van Doorn, L. (1996) Nocturnal blood glucose profiles in patients with Type 1 diabetes on multiple (>4) daily insulin injection regimens. *Diabetic Medicine*, **13**, 794–799.

Veneman, T., Mitrakou, A., Mokan, M., Cryer, P. & Gerich, J. (1993) Induction of hypoglycaemia unawareness in asymptomatic nocturnal hypoglycaemia. *Diabetes*, **42**, 1233–1237.

Whincup, G. & Milner, R. (1987) Prediction and management of nocturnal hypoglycaemia in diabetes. *Archives of Diseases in Childhood*, **62** (4), 333–337.

Wright, A., Cull, C., Macleod, K. & Holman, R. (2006) Hypoglycaemia in Type 2 diabetic patients randomized to and maintained on monotherapy with diet, sulphonylurea, Metformin, or insulin for six years from diagnosis. UKPDS 73. *Journal of Diabetes Complications*, **20**, 395–401.

Yki-Jarvinen, H., Ryysy, L., Nikkila, K., *et al.* (1999) Comparison of bedtime insulin regimens in patients with Type 2 diabetes mellitus. A randomised, controlled trial. *Archives of Internal Medicine*, **130**, 399–396.

Yogev, Y., Chen, R. & Ben-Haroush, A. (2003) Continuous glucose monitoring for the evaluation of gravid women with Type 1 diabetes mellitus. *Obstetrics and Gynaecology*, **101**, 633–638.

Zhang, Y., Wieffer, H., Modha, R., *et al.* (2010)The burden of hypoglycaemia in Type 2 diabetes: A systematic review of patient and economic perspectives. *Journal of Clinical Outcomes Management*, **17** (12), 547–557.

Zoungas, S. (2010) Severe hypoglycaemia and risks of vascular events and death. *Results in Diabetes*, **3** (1), 3.

Chapter 7

Hyperglycaemia, Acute Illness, Diabetic Ketoacidosis (DKA), Hyperosmolar Hyperglycaemic States (HHS), and Lactic Acidosis

Key points

- Acute illness most commonly causes hyperglycaemia and less commonly hypoglycaemia.
- Untreated hyperglycaemia can precipitate ketoacidosis and hyperosmolar states, which are serious short-term complications of diabetes, even if they are managed competently.
- Meticulous attention to detail and proactive insulin use reduces morbidity and mortality.
- Monitor hydration status closely especially in children and older people.
- *Gradually* lower the blood glucose level to avoid hypoglycaemia.
- Monitor ketone clearance in blood.
- Consider whether infection could be an underlying cause, but note the white cell count is often elevated in hyperglycaemic states and may not indicate infection.
- Hyperglycaemia-related abnormalities favour thrombosis, inflammatory changes and impair ischaemic preconditioning, which is a protective mechanism and predisposes the individual to cardiac events, and the formation of superoxide anion (oxidative stress) that cause tissue damage.
- Hyperglycaemia is associated with cerebral neuronal damage possibly due to elevated tissue acidosis and lactate levels that occur in hyperglycaemia.
- Insulin is the most effective way to manage hyperglycaemia-induced abnormalities and reduce the associated complications.
- Educate the person with diabetes and their family about how to manage future intercurrent illnesses.
- Consider psychological and social issues especially if there are repeated admissions for DKA.

Care of People with Diabetes: A Manual of Nursing Practice, Fourth Edition. Trisha Dunning.
© 2014 John Wiley & Sons, Ltd. Published 2014 by John Wiley & Sons, Ltd.

Rationale

This chapter primarily concerns managing hyperglycaemia associated with illnesses in hospital settings, but preventative self-care is included. Hyperglycaemia, DKA, and HHS are preventable short-term complications of diabetes. When hyperglycaemia does occur, effective proactive management can reduce the progression to DKA or HHHS and limit the attendant metabolic derangements should these conditions occur. Hyperglycaemia induces a range of metabolic abnormalities that predispose the individual to cardiovascular, cerebrovascular and cognitive complications and other adverse events.

People with well-controlled diabetes do not usually experience higher rates of intercurrent illness than non-diabetics. However, those with persistent hyperglycaemia may have lower immunity, delayed wound healing, and are at increased risk of infections including infections, including infections caused by organisms that are not normally pathogenic such as tuberculosis, and have a poorer response to antibiotics (Australasian Paediatric Endocrine Group (APEG) 2005; Australian Diabetes Society (ADS) 2012). Infection is the most common cause of DKA and HHS. Thus, optimal blood glucose targets, and the most appropriate method to achieve the target for people in hospital need to be decided. Maintaining the blood glucose range between 5 and 10 mmol/L is appropriate for most patients (ADS 2012) including those on corticosteroid medicines (Chapter 10) (Clement *et al.* 2004).

However, a number of factors affect clinical decisions, and where possible decisions should be made with the individual concerned and their relatives and carers, or according to their advanced care plan (ACP) (Chapter 18). Key factors that affect clinical decisions are:

- duration and acuity of the presenting problem;
- risks associated with hyperglycaemia and/or ketosis;
- duration of diabetes: long standing diabetes or new diagnosis;
- presence of existing diabetes complications and/or other comorbidities;
- nutritional status;
- medicine regimen and risk of hypoglycaemia and consequent adverse events (Chapter 6);
- life expectancy;
- available resources and expertise (Ismail-Beigi *et al.* 2011).

Prevention: proactively managing intercurrent illness

Prevention strategies consist of educating the person with diabetes and their family about how to prevent intercurrent illness or proactively manage intercurrent illnesses to limit the metabolic consequences. Illness prevention/management strategies should be individualised and based on a thorough physical, psychological, and social assessment using a risk management and quality use of medicines (QUM) approach (Chapter 5). General health care should be considered as well as diabetes-related issues and encompass risk screening for breast and other forms of cancer such as bowel and prostate disease, and preventative vaccinations in children, adults and older people.

Illness prevention education should encompass:

- Proactive health care such as identifying key illness risk times, for example, colds and flu during winter, having an individualised documented plan for managing illness, and a kit containing essential equipment and information such as ketone test strips and relative's and health professional's telephone numbers.

- Recognising and managing the signs and symptoms of DKA and HHS, which includes the importance of monitoring blood glucose and ketones and using the information to adjust glucose-lowering medicine (GLM) doses or to seek medical advice, and how to maintain fluid intake.
- How to adjust insulin/GLMs and dietary intake to control blood glucose levels.
- When to seek assistance.

In addition, health professionals should regularly reassess the individual's illness self-care capability including:

- Knowledge, according to the factors outlined in the preceding list.
- Physical ability to manage such as mobility, sight, manual dexterity, and other activities of daily living, bearing in mind these may all be compromised by hyperglycaemia. This is an important aspect of long-term complication screening programmes. Groups likely to need assistance are children, pregnant women, frail older people who live alone, people with disabilities, those who are acutely ill and those who are depressed. The most effective management strategy for these people may be to seek health professional advice quickly.
- Psychosocial factors such as mental health and coping skills, cognitive function, and available support from family or other carers, considering the carer's state of health and coping ability, especially older people.
- Preventative health care strategies such as vaccinations, mammograms, prostate checks, bowel screening, usual metabolic control, and their sick day management plan and kit. Annual influenza and pneumococcal vaccinations are recommended for people with diabetes, COPD and cardiovascular disease, including children with these conditions (National Asthma Council 2005). Mortality increases by 5–15% in people with diabetes during influenza epidemics especially those with cardiovascular and renal complications (Smith & Poland 2004). The increased risk may be due to older age cardiovascular disease or to the diabetes itself due to the impaired immune function due to DKA/HHS (Diepersloot *et al.* 1990). Kornum (2007) suggested that Type 2 diabetes predicted mortality associated with pneumonia and further, hyperglycaemia on admission, >11 mmol/L in people with diabetes and >6 mmol/L in non-diabetics, predicts pneumonia-related mortality.
- Observational data suggest influenza vaccination prior to and during an influenza epidemic reduces the associated hospital admissions and mortality in people with diabetes (Wang *et al.* 2004). Thus, all people with diabetes aged 6 months and older should receive annual influenza vaccination unless contraindicated. Contraindications include allergy/anaphylactic reaction to eggs and/or the vaccine, intercurrent illness with fever >38 °C.
- Regular medicine reviews including complementary and over-the-counter medicines. In particular, assessing the continued need for diabetogenic medicines such as atypical antipsychotic medications, glucocorticoids and thiazide diuretics. If these medicines are necessary and there are no alternatives, the lowest effective dose should be used for the shortest possible time.
- Early recognition of new presentations of diabetes.
- Good access to competent medical and nursing care and ongoing education.
- Good knowledge on the part of people with diabetes and health professionals.
- Good communication/therapeutic relationship between the person with diabetes and their health professionals (Munro *et al.* 1973: this is an old reference but it is still pertinent in the light of the frequent presentations to hospital with hyperglycaemia-associated conditions).
- Psychological screening should be incorporated into routine complication assessment programmes (Ciechanowski *et al.* 2000; Dunning 2001).

Self-care during illness

People with Type 1 diabetes are at greatest risk of DKA, but DKA can occur in seriously ill people with Type 2 diabetes and HHS is associated with significant morbidity and mortality. A suggested plan for monitoring blood glucose and ketones is shown in Table 7.1 (International Society for Paediatric and Adolescent Diabetes (ISPAD) 2000; Kitabchi *et al.* 2006; American Diabetes Association 2002; Laffel *et al.* 2005; Australian Diabetes Educators Association (ADEA) 2006; Dunning 2007). In the early stages of the illness people may be able to be managed at home if they are capable of performing self-care, have support and can telephone their doctor at least every 1–2 hours. Admission to hospital is advised in the following situations:

- children especially younger than 2 years;
- persistent vomiting and/or bile-stained vomitus;
- persistent diarrhoea;
- blood glucose persistently ≤ 4 mmol/L or >15 mmol/L and ketones present;
- severe localised abdominal pain;
- hyperventilation (Kussmaul's respirations);
- dehydration;
- coexisting serious illness;
- impaired conscious state;
- the individual, parent or care providers are unable to cope.

Hyperglycaemia

Hyperglycaemia refers to an elevated blood glucose level (>10 mmol/L) due to a relative or absolute insulin deficiency. The symptoms of hyperglycaemia usually occur when the blood glucose is persistently above 15 mmol/L. The cause of the hyperglycaemia should be sought in people with an established diagnosis of diabetes and corrected to avoid the development of diabetic ketoacidosis (DKA) or HHS. Hyperglycaemia, DKA and HHS are often referred to as short-term complications of diabetes. DKA develops relatively quickly. HHS is often insidious and usually evolves over several days to weeks.

Hyperglycaemia disrupts multiple organ systems and needs to be treated to reduce the morbidity and mortality associated with the illness and its metabolic consequences (American Association of Clinical Endocrinologists (AACE) 2011; ADS 2012; Inzucchi *et al.* 2012). Fluid resuscitation corrects dehydration, improves microcirculation, and reduces tissue damage during acute sepsis, which helps correct hyperglycaemia, but increased insulin doses and/or dose frequency or rescue insulin therapy in Type 2 diabetes is usually required.

Many researchers have demonstrated that hyperglycaemia is associated with adverse outcomes in hospitalised people both people with diabetes and non-diabetics, and that controlling the blood glucose improves outcomes (Abourzik *et al.* 2004; Clement *et al.* 2004; ACE Taskforce 2006; ACE/ADA Taskforce 2006; Inzucchi et al. 2012). However, higher rates of hypoglycaemia are associated with stringent control of blood glucose below 5 mmol/L, and hypoglyacaemia, especially severe hypoglycaemia, is associated with significant adverse events (Unger 2011); Chapter 6. There is still debate about whether continuous IV insulin infusion is the safest way to manage hyperglycaemia in hospital despite the well described benefits in people with and without diabetes (van den Berghe *et al.* 2001; AACE 2011). Intensive insulin therapy protects renal function in critically ill patients and reduces the incidence of oliguria and the need for renal replacement therapy in surgical patients and improves lipid and endothelial profile (Schetz 2008).

Table 7.1   Self-management advice for managing blood glucose, ketones and fluid during illness. These recommendations should be tailored to the individual's self-care capabilities, available assistance, and their physical condition. Ketosis can develop rapidly in people using insulin pumps. The underlying cause needs to be ascertained and treated.

	Type 1	Type 2
Blood glucose (BG)	Monitor 2 hourly Monitor ketones 2 hourly if >15 mmol on two consecutive occasions in a 2–6 hour period	Monitor 2 hourly If >15 mmol on two consecutive occasions in an 8–12 hour period increase monitoring frequency to 2–4 hourly QID testing may be adequate in people managed with diet and exercise
Blood ketones		
<1 mmol/L	BG 4–15 mmol/L recheck in 2 hours	Follow the same test procedure as described for Type 1 diabetes
1–1.4 mmol/L:	BG, <8 mmol/L extra sweet fluids: >8 mmol/L extra 5% insulin	Ketones are less common in Type 2 diabetes but do occur in serious illness such as septicaemia and myocardial infarction
>1.5 mmol/L: <1 mmol/L	BG, <8 mmol/L extra sweet fluids: >8 mmol/L extra 5–10% insulin BG 15–22 mmol/L 5% extra insulin	
1–1.4 mmol/L	10% extra insulin	
>1.5 mmol/L	15–20% extra insulin and hospitalise if ketones persist	
<1 mmol/L	BG >22 mmol/L 10% extra insulin	
1 –1.4 mmol/L	15% extra insulin	
>5 mol/L	20% extra insulin and hospitalise if ketones persist	
Medicines	Give supplemental doses of quick/rapid acting insulin 2–4 hourly	*GLMs* Consider ceasing Metformin Increase sulphonylurea dose unless on maximal doses or on a slow release preparation when insulin is preferred[1] *GLM and insulin* Supplemental doses of quick/rapid-acting insulin *Insulin treated* Supplemental doses of quick/rapid-acting insulin
Refer to hospital	Unable to maintain fluid intake Blood glucose and ketones not falling despite supplemental insulin Unable to self-care and no support available Condition deteriorating	Unable to maintain fluid intake Blood glucose and ketones not falling despite supplemental insulin Unable to self-care and no support available Condition deteriorating
Fluids	BG <4 mmol/L usual meals and extra sweet fluids if tolerated ~10–12 mmol/L and able to tolerate food 150 ml easily digested fluid every 1–2 hours, for example soup, fruit juice, ice cream BG >12 mmol/L and unable to tolerate food, 100–300 ml low calorie fluids every hour, for example, gastrolyte, low calorie soft drink, mineral water, water Unable to tolerate fluids at any BG level, refer to hospital	BG <4 mmol/L usual meals and extra sweet fluids if tolerated ~10–12 mmol/L and able to tolerate food 150 ml easily digested fluid every 1–2 hours, for example, soup, fruit juice, ice cream BG >12 mmol and unable to tolerate food 100–300 ml low calorie fluids every hour, for example, gastrolyte, low calorie soft drink, mineral water, water Unable to tolerate fluids at any BG level, refer to hospital

[a]If the person has no experience of insulin they will need reassurance and a careful explanation about why insulin is needed. If they are not able to manage or do not have assistance and home nursing is not available they may need to be managed in hospital.

Laboratory or capillary blood glucose tests are used to monitor blood glucose during hospitalisation. Capillary tests are undertaken more frequently than laboratory tests except in intensive care situations, and may give better insight into the blood glucose pattern (Cook *et al.* 2007). The trend of the blood glucose pattern over time (up or down) is important information on which to base management decisions, including about medicines.

Quality management organisations in the US are currently developing hospital outcome measures for managing hyperglycaemia in hospitalised patients (Joint Commission on Accreditation of Healthcare Organisations 2006). Despite the evidence that insulin requirements increase during illness, insulin doses are often reduced, even in the presence of significant hyperglycaemia, because health professionals are concerned about causing hypoglycaemia, whereas the factors contributing to hypoglycaemia are only rarely investigated and addressed (Cook *et al.* 2007). Coughlin (2012) suggested that hospitals need to focus on patients' views of their hospital experience, which should be measured using appropriate tools rather than the ubiquitous 'patient satisfaction' questionnaires.

Diabetic ketoacidosis (DKA)

Diabetic ketoacidosis is a life-threatening complication of diabetes. In the absence of sufficient insulin glucose is unable to enter the cells and accumulates in the blood. Insulin deficiency leads to catecholamine release, lipolysis and the mobilisation of free fatty acids and subsequently the formation of ketone bodies, B-hydroxybutyrate, acetoacetate, and acetone, resulting in metabolic acidosis (ADA 2002). Protein catabolism also occurs and forms the substrate for gluconeogenesis, which further increases the blood glucose. At the same time, glucose utilisation in tissues is impaired. DKA usually only occurs in people with Type 1 diabetes, but can occur in people with Type 2 people in the presence of severe infections or metabolic stress. The mortality rate in expert centres is <5% but is higher at the extremes of age and if coma and/or hypotension are present (Chiasson *et al.* 2003).

Diabetic ketoacidosis is characterised by hyperglycaemia, osmotic diuresis, metabolic acidosis, glycosuria, ketonuria and dehydration. The definition by laboratory results is blood glucose >17 mmol/L; ketonaemia (ketone bodies) >3 mmol/L; acidosis, pH <7.30 and bicarbonate <15 mEq/L. The signs, symptoms of, and precipitating factors for DKA are shown in Table 7.2, and Figure 7.1 outlines the physiology and the signs and symptoms that occur as a result of impaired glucose utilisation, and the biochemical manifestations found on blood testing.

Late signs of severe DKA

The initial signs and symptoms of DKA (polyuria, polydipsia, lethargy, and Kussmaul's respirations) are compensatory mechanisms to overcome the acidosis. If treatment is delayed the body eventually decompensates. Signs of decompensation (late signs) include:

- peripheral vasodilation with warm, dry skin;
- hypothermia;
- hypoxia and reduced conscious state;
- oliguria;

Table 7.2 Early signs, symptoms, and precipitating factors of diabetic ketoacidosis (DKA).

Symptoms and signs	Precipitating factors

Thirst
Polyuria
Fatigue
Weight loss
Nausea and vomiting
Abdominal pain
Muscle cramps
Tachycardia
Kussmaul's respirations (early sign)
	(1) Newly diagnosed Type 1 (5–30%)
	(2) Omission of insulin therapy/GLMs (33%)
	(3) Inappropriate insulin/GLM dose reduction. DKA has also been associated with inaccurate use of insulin delivery devices after changing devices in both older people and adolescents (Bhardwaj & Metcalfe 2006).
	(4) Eating disorders
	(5) Severe emotional distress, either directly or by insulin manipulation
	(6) Relative insulin deficiency due to:
	(7) Insulin pump failure
	(8) Severe morning sickness during pregnancy
	  (a) Acute illness:
	    Infection (10–20% of cases)
	    Myocardial infarction
	    Trauma, burns
	    Cerebrovascular accident
	    Surgical procedures
	  (b) Endocrine disorders (rare):
	    Hyperthyroidism
	    Pheochromocytoma
	    Acromegaly
	    Cushing's disease
	  (c) Medications:
	    Glucocorticoids
	    Thiazide diuretics
	    Sympathomimetic agents
	    Alcohol
	    Illicit drugs
	Brittle diabetes: life-disrupting blood glucose lability associated with frequent admission to hospital (Benbow *et al.* 2001) (Chapter 10)

- slow respiratory rate and absence of Kussmaul's respirations;
- bradycardia.

The signs and symptoms can be masked by intercurrent illness. For example, pneumonia can cause tachyapnoea, dry mouth and dehydration; abdominal pain and vomiting are symptoms of gastrointestinal disease; likewise, abdominal pain is usual in appendicitis and in labour. Polyuria and polydipsia can be difficult to detect in toddlers not yet toilet trained, bedwetters, and incontinent older people. Unexplained bedwetting in these groups needs to be investigated and DKA considered when the onset of incontinence and bedwetting is sudden. Hypothermia as a result of peripheral vasodilation can mask fever due to underlying infection and is associated with poor prognosis.

Differential diagnosis

- Starvation ketosis, which can be determined by taking a careful clinical history of the presentation.
- Alcoholic ketosis where the blood glucose is usually only mildly elevated or low.

The implications of the metabolic and physiological changes associated with DKA are shown in Table 7.3.

PRECIPITATING FACTORS

INSULIN DEFICIENCY

Decreased glucose uptake
Increased Counter-regulatory Hormone Response
(glucagon, epinephrine, cortisol, growth hormone)

Metabolic ⟶	*Blood Chemistry* ⟶	*Signs and Symptoms*
Increased glycogenolysis	Electrolyte loss	Polydipsia
Increased gluconeogenesis	(Na+, Cl−, K+, Mg+, P)	Osmotic diuresis
Increased lipolysis	Increased urea	Glycosuria
Increased ketogenesis	Increased creatinine	Ketonuria
(betahydroxybuterate, acetone,	Increased serum osmolarity	Dehydration
acetoacetate)		Nausea
Increased blood glucose		Vomiting
		Abdominal pain
		Tachycardia
		Impaired conscious state
Ketoacids link with sodium for excretion	Decreased pH	Warm dry skin
Decreased total body sodium	Decreased bicarbonate	Decreased circulating blood
Increased hydrogen	Decreased CO_2	Volume (hypotension)
	Decreased Na	Increased respirations
	Increased K	(Kussmaul's respirations)
		Acetone breath

ACIDOSIS

Late signs: coma, absence of Kussmaul's respirations, death

Figure 7.1   An outline of the physiology, signs, and symptoms and biochemical changes occurring in the development of diabetic ketoacidosis (DKA).

Assessment

The following factors should be established:

- whether the person has known diabetes;
- usual insulin/GLM dose, dose interval and type/s of insulin/GM;
- the time the last dose was taken and dose administered;
- presence of fever, which can be a sign of myocardial infarction as well as infection;
- duration of the deteriorating control/illness;
- remedial action taken by the patient (sick day self-care);
- whether the person has taken any other medications, complementary medicines, alcohol or illegal drugs;
- conscious state.

A thorough physical assessment should be undertaken and blood taken to:

- Establish the severity of the DKA: glucose, urea and electrolytes, pH and blood gases, degree of ketonaemia. If severe acidosis is present, pH <7.1, and the blood glucose is not significantly elevated, alcohol, aspirin overdose or lactic acidosis need to be excluded especially in older people. Ketones in the presence of low blood glucose can indicate starvation, malnutrition or cachexia.
- Assess the cause: full blood count, cardiac enzymes, blood cultures, ECG, chest X-ray, urine culture.

Table 7.3　The metabolic consequences of diabetic ketoacidosis and associated risks. Many of these changes increase the risk of falls in older people.

Metabolic consequences of ketoacidosis	Associated risk
Metabolic acidosis	Nausea and vomiting Cardiac arrest Coagulopathies Increased white cell count, which may not be a sign of infection. The white cell function is changed in hyperglycaemic states.
Hyperlipidaemia	Thrombosis/embolism Substrate for ketone formation if insulin is not replaced
Haemoconcentration and coagulation changes	Myocardial infarction, stroke, thrombosis
Dehydration	Volume depletion Renal hypoperfusion Can cause acute tubular necrosis
Gastric stasis	Inhalation of vomitus, aspiration pneumonia Delayed absorption of food and fluids given via the oral route Abdominal discomfort
Hyperkalaemia but overall deficit in total potassium due to loss in osmotic diuresis.	Cardiac arrhythmias
Hyperglycaemia, which is exacerbated by glycogenolysis and gluconeogenesis	Plasma hyperosmolality Cellular dehydration Osmotic diuresis Compromised immune function leading to infection and delayed wound healing, also thrombosis, low mood, vision changes
Glycosuria	Hyponatraemia and ketonaemia, which contributes to sodium, potassium, and chlorine loss Hyponatraemia is common but if sodium is <120 mmol/L may indicate hypertriglyceridaemia
Abdominal pain	Unnecessary surgery, inappropriate pain relief causing further respiratory distress, missed labour
	Death

Aims of treatment of DKA

Treatment aims to:
(1) Correct:
 • Dehydration;
 • electrolyte imbalance;
 • ketoacidosis;
 • hyperglycaemia by slowly reducing the blood glucose to 7–10 mmol/L. Hyperglycaemia, relative insulin deficiency, or both, predispose people with and without diabetes to complications such as severe infection, polyneuropathy, multiorgan failure and death (van den Bergh *et al.* 2001; Clement *et al.* 2004).
(2) Reverse shock.
(3) Ascertain the cause of DKA and treat appropriately.
(4) Prevent complications of treatment.
(5) Educate/re-educate the patient and their family/carers.

Objectives of nursing care

To support the medical team to:
(1) Restore normal hydration, euglycaemia and metabolism.
(2) Prevent complications of DKA including complications occurring as a result of management.
(3) Pay meticulous attention to detail.
(4) Document progress of recovery e.g. blood glucose levels, medicines administered, vital signs.
(5) Re-educate/educate the patient and their family/carers about the management of illness at home or general diabetes education if the person is newly diagnosed. Patient education about managing diabetes during illness can be found in this chapter.
(6) Ensure follow-up care is arranged after discharge, in particular: review of diabetes knowledge, nutritional assessment and physical and psychological assessment.

Preparing the unit to receive the patient

Assemble:
(1) Oxygen and suction (tested to ensure they are in working order).
(2) Intravenous trolley (IV) containing:
   • dressing tray and antiseptic solution
   • local anaesthetic
   • selection of intravenous cannulae
   • IV fluids: normal saline, SPPS, dextrose/saline
   • IV giving sets, burette
   • IMED pump or syringe pump
   • clear short- or rapid-acting insulin, preferably administered as an IV infusion
   • blood gas syringe
   • blood culture bottles.
(3) Cot sides and IV pole.
(4) Blood glucose testing equipment (cleaned, calibrated).
(5) Blood ketone testing equipment.
(6) Appropriate charts:
   • fluid balance
   • blood glucose monitoring
   • medication
   • conscious state.
(7) Urinary catheterisation equipment.
(8) Nasogastric tubes may or may not be used. Some experts recommend passing a nasogastric tube to prevent gastric dilatation and aspiration.
(9) Initial care in the intensive care unit is preferable for moderate to severe ketoacidosis. If the patient is admitted to the intensive care unit, central venous pressures, continuous blood gas, and electrocardiogram monitoring is usually performed.

Practice point

Rapid-acting insulin and quickly promotes transport of glucose into the cells. Intravenous administration is preferred because absorption is more predictable than by the subcutaneous route.

Nursing care/observations

The nursing management of DKA involves traditional nursing actions as well as monitoring the response to medical therapy.

Initial patient care
Initial patient care is often given in the intensive care unit. The procedure is:

- Maintain the airway.
- Nurse the patient on their side, even if the patient is conscious, because gastric stasis and inhalation of vomitus is a possible and preventable complication of DKA.
- Ensure strict aseptic technique.

Nursing observations (1–2 hourly)
(1) Observe 'nil orally'. Provide pressure care especially in older people.
(2) Provide mouth care to protect oral mucous membranes and relieve the discomfort of a dry mouth.
(3) Administer IV fluid according to the treatment sheet usually initially isotonic saline until the blood glucose is <12 mmol/L then 10% dextrose. However, the first litre of saline may be 0.45% in the presence of hypernatraemia (sodium >150 mmol/L).
(4) Administer insulin according to the treatment sheet; it is usually given via an insulin infusion and the dose adjusted according to blood glucose tests, see Chapter 7. Intensive insulin therapy maintains the blood glucose within a narrow range and thereby reduces the morbidity and mortality associated with critical illness (van den Berghe *et al.* 2001). In some cases rapid- or short-acting insulin is given intramuscularly, usually in remote areas where ICU units are not available.
(5) Replace serum potassium. If the initial biochemical result is >5.0 mmol/L, potassium is not required initially. It should be added to the second or third litres of IV fluid or when levels fall to <4.5 mmol/L depending on expected potassium loss, for example, from vomiting. Initially potassium levels should be monitored on an hourly basis.
(6) There is general agreement that bicarbonate replacement is not required if the pH is >7.0. There is no consensus about pH <7.0. Some experts state that bicarbonate should be given to minimise respiratory decompensation. Others believe bicarbonate automatically corrects as the acidosis resolves with fluid and insulin (Hamblin 1995). Some experts use bicarbonate if the pH is <7.1, if the patient presents with a cardiac arrest, or cardiac arrest is imminent.
(7) Estimate blood glucose levels 1–2 hourly and confirm biochemically in the early stages.
(8) Observe strict fluid balance. Record second hourly subtotals of input/output *from admission*. Urine output should be >30 mL per hour measured hourly in a calibrated collecting device. Report a urine output of <30 mL per hour. Measure specific gravity (SG). Be aware that some creatinine assays cross react with ketones and creatinine may not reflect renal function in DKA.
    - *Heavy* glycosuria invalidates SG readings.
    - Record fluid loss, for example, vomitus.
(9) Monitor central venous pressure.
(10) Monitor conscious state. In children with DKA the level of consciousness initially, is significantly associated with pH as well as age but not blood glucose or sodium levels (Edge *et al.* 2006). Therefore, cerebral function in DKA is related to the severity of the acidosis in children even when cerebral oedema is not present. Cerebral oedema is a serious complication of DKA and has a high morbidity rate in children and older people. If coma is prolonged heparin might be indicated to prevent thrombosis and pulmonary embolism.

(11) Record pulse, respiration, and blood pressure. Fever associated with DKA indicates sepsis. But it should be noted that an elevated white cell count can be due to metabolic abnormalities and does not necessarily indicate the presence of infection.
(12) Administer oxygen via face mask or nasal catheter.
(13) Monitor and report all laboratory results (electrolytes and blood gases).
(14) Report any deterioration of condition immediately.
(15) Physiotherapy may be helpful to prevent pneumonia and emboli due to venous stasis, and to provide passive mobilisation.
(16) Administer other medications as ordered (potassium, calciparine, broad-spectrum antibiotics to treat underlying infections, Mannitol to reduce cerebral oedema).
(17) Reposition and provide skin care to avoid pressure areas and/or venous stasis.

Subsequent care
As the patient's condition improves:

- Review the frequency of blood glucose testing, decreasing to 4-hourly including the night time.
- Allow a light diet and ensure the patient is eating and drinking before the IV is removed.
- Administer subcutaneous insulin before the IV is removed. Often the infusion is turned off before a meal but the IV line left *in situ* until the person can eat and drink normally and the blood glucose level is stable within the normal range.
- Continue to monitor temperature, pulse and respiration every 4 hours.
- Provide support and comfort for the patient.
- Establish the duration of deteriorating control and identify any precipitating factor such as infection.

Plan for:

- Medical follow-up appointment after discharge.
- Nutrition review.
- Education/re-education about appropriate management (for days when the patient is unwell); see Chapter 16.
- Review medication dosage, especially insulin. DKA can occur as a result of incorrect use of insulin delivery devices, which highlights the importance of checking insulin administration technique particularly given hospital staff do not consider incorrect technique as a potential cause (Bhardwaj & Metcalfe 2006).
- Consider psychological review. For example, sexual assault is an uncommon but important cause of DKA and should be considered when repeated admissions occur. This is a difficult area to assess and should be undertaken by people with the appropriate skills and with consideration of the legal implications and the effect on the individual and their family.

Practice points
- Psychiatric consultation should be considered if a patient repeatedly presents in DKA. Eating disorders complicate 20% of recurrent cases of DKA (Polonsky et al. 1994).
- People, especially young women, reduce their insulin doses to avoid weight gain and hypoglycaemia. Reducing or stopping insulin is also a form of risk taking and rebellion at having diabetes (Dunning et al. 1994).

Brittle diabetes and hyperglycaemia

Brittle diabetes is difficult to understand and manage for people with diabetes and their carers and health professionals. Brittle diabetes most commonly occurs between 15 and 30 years of age and often leads to frequent hospital admissions for DKA or hypoglycaemia. However, brittle diabetes also occurs in older people. Criteria for brittle diabetes in older people are >60 years, treated with insulin, experiencing unstable blood glucose associated with frequent, often prolonged admissions to hospital (Gill *et al.* 1996; Benbow *et al.* 2001). In the older group, women are more likely to present with brittle diabetes than men but the preponderance of women may reflect the proportion of older men and women in the population. There does not appear to be consistent underlying causative factors but cognitive behavioural factors appear to play a role (Benbow *et al.* 2001). See also Chapter 10.

Complications that can occur as a result of DKA

Most complications of DKA are due to complications of treatment and most are avoidable:

(1) hypoglycaemia due to over-zealous treatment;
(2) inhalation of vomitus causing aspiration pneumonia;
(3) hypokalaemia, which may lead to cardiac arrhythmias;
(4) cerebral oedema is rare and can be fatal. It occurs in 0.7–10% of children especially on the first presentation of diabetes and any morbidity that occurs is permanent (Rosenbloom 1990);
(5) myocardial infarction;
(6) deep venous thrombosis;
(7) adult respiratory distress syndrome.

Be extra vigilant with:

(1) Older people, especially those with established vascular and coronary disease. Risks include myocardial infarction and deep venous thrombosis.
(2) Children are at increased risk of cerebral oedema, which has a high mortality rate in this group of patients.

Euglycaemic DKA

Munro *et al.* originally documented euglycaemic DKA in 1973 (Munro *et al.*1973). Euglycaemic DKA refers to ketoacidosis in the setting of near normal blood glucose levels. Euglycaemia indicates that the blood glucose level and development of DKA do not necessarily correlate. De & Child (2001) postulated that heavy glycosuria triggered by counter-regulatory hormone activity or reduced hepatic glucose production could result in lower than expected blood glucose levels. Although euglycaemic DKA is a rare condition, it highlights the importance of monitoring serum ketones and blood gases and using low-dose IV insulin infusions in all people with diabetes during illness.

Ketosis without hyperglycaemia occasionally occurs postoperatively in the presence of repeated vomiting. Rehydration with dextrose/saline and controlling the vomiting are required to restore depleted hepatic glycogen stores.

Hyperosmolar Hyperglycaemic States

HHS is a serious metabolic disturbance characterised by a marked increase in serum osmolality, the absence of ketones, hyperglycaemia (usually >40 mmol/L) and extreme dehydration caused by a concomitant illness (often infection) that leads to inadequate fluid intake. It most commonly occurs in people with Type 2 diabetes, usually in older people >65, however, HHS has been reported in a 9-month-old baby, toddlers (Goldman 1979; Sagarin *et al.* 2005) and children (Kershaw *et al.* 2005). People with Type 2 diabetes usually secrete enough endogenous insulin to prevent lipolysis and ketoacidosis (Kitabchi *et al.* 1994) but not sufficient to prevent hyperglycaemia and hepatic glucose output. HHS has a higher mortality rate than DKA, an estimated 10–20%, although mortality rates as high as 58% are reported. The severity of the metabolic derangements, especially delay establishing the diagnosis, inadequate treatment and the degree of dehydration contribute to the high mortality rate (Hemphill & Schraga 2012).

In addition, the hyperosmolality may limit ketogenesis and the level of free fatty acids available for ketogenesis (Sagarin *et al.* 2005). Type 2 diabetes is associated with progressive beta cell loss so the risk of DKA and HHS may be higher with long duration of Type 2 diabetes or people with LADA; see Chapter 1. Approximately one third of cases occur in people with no previous diagnosis of diabetes. Dehydration is usually severe. The patient is often confused, and focal and general neurological signs are usually present, however, despite the name, coma is rare, occurring in < 10% of cases (Sagarin *et al.* 2005; Hemphill & Schraga 2012). Once HHS develops it can be difficult to differentiate it from the precipitating illness (Hemphill & Schraga 2012).

> ### *Practice point*
>
> People with Type 2 diabetes usually still have sufficient endogenous insulin production to prevent the formation of ketones.

HHS occurs in ~17.5 cases per 1 000 000 in the US and has a mortality rate of 10–20% with a slightly higher prevalence in women (Sagarin *et al.* 2005). The onset is associated with severe stress such as acute febrile illnesses including infection, for example, pneumonia and UTI, extensive burns, myocardial infarction, stroke and/or reduced fluid intake. People in aged care facilities are at the highest risk of HHS because they are often unaware of thirst and are not always offered fluids in hot weather. However, the cause is not identifiable in many people.

Other precipitating factors include an acute illness that increases the counter-regulatory hormone response in the setting of insulin deficiency such as:

- stroke;
- intracranial haemorrhage;
- silent myocardial infarct, which should be considered in all presentations of HHS until it is excluded;
- pulmonary embolism;
- underlying congestive heart failure and/or renal disease, although hyperosmolality can trigger rhabdomyolysis and cause acute renal failure;
- surgery, especially cardiac surgery; some endocrine conditions such as Cushings syndrome;

- some medications such as diuretics, for example IV diazoxide and furosemide in the surgical setting, corticosteroids, atypical antipsychotice, beta blockers, Histamine$_2$ blockers immunosuppressant agents;
- dialysis;
- parenteral nutrition solutions that contain dextrose;
- IV fluids that contain dextrose;
- non-adherence with GLMs and other diabetes self-care.

There is a high mortality rate associated with HHS. The mortality rate has decreased since the 1960s but is still 10–20% (ADA 2002; Sagarin *et al.* 2005).

Presenting signs and symptoms

HHS usually develops over days to weeks. People may complain of thirst, polyuria (or increased incontinence or new onset of incontinence in people with dementia), weight loss (primarily due to fluid loss), and lethargy. Oral hydration may be compromised by lack of thirst, dementia, vomiting, and mobility deficits.

A thorough physical examination should be carried out to detect sources of infection and include eyes, ears, nose, throat and teeth and gums, pneumonia, UTI, skin, meningitis, pelvic infection, and triggers such as CCF, and acute respiratory distress syndrome. HHS is the initial presentation in 30–40% of presentations (Kitabchi *et al.* 2006).

- Neurological signs such as drowsiness and lethargy, delirium, seizures, visual disturbances, hemiparesis, diminished reflexes, unsteady gait, and sensory deficits.
- Dehydration indicated by: reduced skin turgor, sunken eyes, and dry mouth.
- Tachycardia is an early sign; hypotension is a late sign and indicates profound dehydration. Tachycardia could also indicate thyrotoxicosis.
- Tachypnoea as a consequence of respiratory compensation for the metabolic acidosis.
- Hypoxaemia, which may compound the effects of dehydration on mental function.
- Signs of infection such as enlarged lymph nodes. Warm moist skin is an early indication of infection whereas cool dry skin indicates late sepsis.
- Vision changes and other sensory and speech deficits.
- Focal or generalized seizures.

Specific investigations depend on the results of the physical assessment. Laboratory investigations include blood glucose, ketones, electrolytes, renal function (BUN and creatinine, which can be elevated due to the dehydration), osmolality ($\geq$320 mOsm/kg), creatine phosphokinase (CPK), blood cultures, coagulation studies, arterial blood gases (pH is usually >7.30), bicarbonate ($\geq$15 mEq/L) and urine cultures. Other investigations such as ECG, cardiac enzymes and troponins, lumbar puncture and CSF studies, chest X-ray, head and abdominal CT, and HbA$_{1c}$ as an indication of preceding metabolic control may be useful to plan future management (Kitabchi *et al.* 2006).

The nursing care and objectives are similar to those for DKA, but extra vigilance and close monitoring is needed because of the age of most people presenting with HHS.

- Record strict fluid balance.
- IV fluid rate. Central venous access may be used. In some cases a Swan-Ganz catheter is inserted to monitor intravascular volume. There is usually a large fluid deficit (~10 L). Replacement: in the first 2 hours 1–2 L isotonic saline but the rate depends on the degree of dehydration, if severe a higher volume may be indicated; lower volumes may be used if there is no urine output. Half normal saline is used once the blood pressure and urine output are normalised and stable.

- An arterial line may be inserted in ICU settings to monitor blood gases.
- Blood glucose may fall with rehydration alone over the first 1–3 hours but usually insulin is indicated to correct the hyperglycaemia and is usually given as an IV insulin infusion adjusted according to the blood glucose level (tested 1–2 hourly).
- ECG.
- Urine output. A urinary catheter may be indicated to accurately measure output and obtain a clean urine specimen to detect infection but can introduce infection.
- Neurological observations.
- Manage the airway.
- Maintain skin integrity including the feet. Compromised peripheral circulation and peripheral neuropathy increases the risk of foot ulcers, which are slow to heal and increase length of stay and the risk of amputation. Nursing on air mattresses may be indicated.
- Observe for deep venous thrombosis or embolism.
- Administer medications as indicated, which might include antibiotics, which might be administered IV. Subsequent care as for DKA.

Education may be more difficult initially because of the mental confusion associated with HHS and the age of these patients. Ensuring that the family/caregivers understand how to care for the patient and ensuring follow-up education occurs in 2–3 weeks is important.

Figure 7.2 outlines the factors involved in the development of hyperosmolar coma. There are similarities with DKA, and some important differences. Ketone production is absent or minimal because the patient is usually producing enough endogenous insulin to allow the ketone bodies to be metabolised and utilised. The degree of dehydration is often greater in HONK and the serum and urine osmolality is increased.

Lactic acidosis

Lactic acidosis is another uncommon condition that sometimes occurs in people with diabetes. Lactic acidosis occurs in 0.06 cases per 1000 patient years, usually those with predisposing factors (Pillans 1998). Lactate is a product of anaerobic glucose metabolism. Disordered lactate metabolism frequently occurs in critically ill people who are at risk of multiorgan failure and the mortality rate is ~70% if the serum lactate remains >2 mmol/L for >24 hours (Nicks 2006). Lactate is primarily cleared from the blood by the liver, kidneys, and skeletal muscles.

Lactic acidosis is defined as metabolic acidosis associated with serum lactate >5 mmol/L. It occurs due to either an increase in hydrogen ions or reduction in bicarbonate with increased acid production, loss of alkali and reduced renal clearance of acids. Lactic acidosis should be considered during acute illness in patients with vasoconstriction, hypotension and with underlying diseases associated with poor tissue perfusion and hypoxia such as:

- recent myocardial infarction;
- cardiac failure and cardiogenic shock;
- pulmonary disease;
- cirrhosis;
- sepsis;
- renal impairment;
- medicines and toxins such as isoniazid, salicylates, beta-adrenergic agents, alcohol and biguanides especially in older people with hypoxic diseases and/or dehydration;
- surgery;
- inborn errors of metabolism such as fructose 1, 6-diphosphatase deficiency.

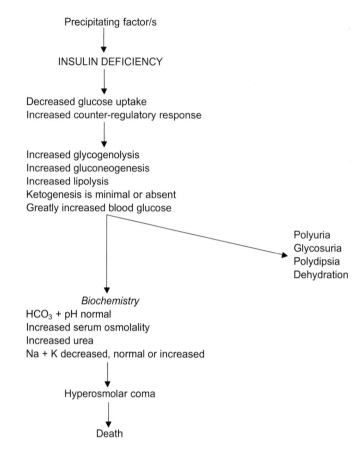

Precipitating factor/s

↓

INSULIN DEFICIENCY

↓

Decreased glucose uptake
Increased counter-regulatory response

↓

Increased glycogenolysis
Increased gluconeogenesis
Increased lipolysis
Ketogenesis is minimal or absent
Greatly increased blood glucose

→ Polyuria
Glycosuria
Polydipsia
Dehydration

↓

Biochemistry
HCO_3 + pH normal
Increased serum osmolality
Increased urea
Na + K decreased, normal or increased

↓

Hyperosmolar coma

↓

Death

Figure 7.2   An outline of the development of hyperosmolar Hyperglycaemic States (HHS).

Excess lactate is produced in ischaemic skeletal muscle and to a lesser extent in the intestine and erythrocytes and accumulates due to a fall in lactate consumption in the liver, which overwhelms the buffering system (Nicks 2006). Lactate levels correlate with tissue hypoperfusion and mortality and the duration and degree of lactic acidosis predicts morbidity and mortality. Lactate >4 mmol/L for >24 hours carries an 11% mortality rate in critically ill patients. After 48 hours, only 14% survive.

Signs and symptoms

- signs that the cardiovascular system is compromised, for example, cyanosis, cold extremities, tachycardia, hypotension, dyspnea;
- lethargy, confusion, stupor;
- dry mucous membranes.

Biochemistry shows an anion gap, lactate 4–5 mmol/L (normal ~1 mmol/L) low pH, usually <7.1 but only moderate, if any ketones, and mildly elevated blood glucose, usually <20 mmol/L. Lactic acidosis should be managed in ICU settings.

Lactic acidosis associated with Metformin

Ninety per cent of metformin is excreted unchanged via the kidneys and the half-life is prolonged and renal clearance reduced in patients with renal impairment where creatinine clearance is reduced. Renal impairment may develop slowly as a complication of diabetes or acutely. Metformin is contraindicated when the creatinine >0.16 mmol/L, hepatic disease, and conditions associated with hypoxia (Pillans 1998). Some experts suggest 0.15 mmol/L (Nesbit *et al.* 2004) and that age, muscle mass, and protein turnover influence the creatinine clearance rate. Although Metformin-associated lactic acidosis is rare, it remains the most frequently reported cause of medicine-associated mortality (Pillans 1998). It may present as respiratory failure and shock, cardiac arrhythmias, hypothermia and hypoglycaemia (Cohen 2008).

In Australia, 48 cases of metformin-induced lactic acidosis were reported to the Australian Adverse Drug Reactions Advisory Committee (ADRAC) between 1985 and 2001 (ADRAC 2001). Thirty-five had known risk factors for lactic acidosis. An average of six Metformin-related adverse events are reported to ADRAC per year. Nisbet *et al.* (2004) calculated the prevalence of lactic acidosis in Australia to be 1 in 30 000 based on ~200 000 metformin prescriptions per year and the reported adverse event rate. They caution that the actual rate may be higher due to under-reporting.

In the US 204 of 263 patients admitted to hospital were taking Metformin; 27% had at least one contraindication and Metformin was continued in 41% of these despite the contraindication (Calabrese & Turner 2002). Emslie-Smith *et al.* (2001) identified contraindications to Metformin in 24.5% of 1847 of people taking the medicine. Regular physical assessment to identify patients at risk of lactic acidosis including monitoring renal function, structured medication reviews, adhering to Metformin prescribing guidelines, and reporting medicine adverse events are important aspects of care.

Management

Management consists of:

- IV fluid replacement with normal saline to maintain the circulating volume and tissue perfusion;
- Oxygen therapy;
- Bicarbonate given early to correct the acidosis and should be administered slowly to avoid causing metabolic alkalosis and ventilatory failure.

Thiamine 50–100 mg IV followed by 50 mg orally for 1–2 weeks in some cases where thiamine deficiency is likely such as malnourished older people and alcoholics.

- IV insulin at a rate of 10–12 units/hour in dextrose solution;
- Monitoring renal and cardiac status;
- The mental status should be monitored as well as monitoring the physical status;
- Withdrawing precipitating medicines or toxins, which might include haemodialysis in some cases;
- Antibiotics if sepsis is present;
- Medication review and discontinuing medication or reducing the dose if contraindications exist. Metformin is the medicine of choice in overweight Type 2 patients but doses >500 mg per day should be used with caution in older people with renal, liver, and cardiac disease or other hypoxic diseases (Nisbet *et al.* 2004).

References

Abourzik N, Vora C, Verma P. (2004) Inpatient diabetology: the new frontier. *Journal General Internal Medicine* **19**: 466-471

American College of Endocrinology and American Diabetes Association (ACE & ADA) (2006) Consensus statement on inpatient diabetes and glycemic control *Ace/ada task force on inpatient diabetes Endocrine Practice* **12** (4):458–468.

American Diabetes Association (ADA) (2002) *Hyperglycaemic Crisis in Patients with Diabetes Mellitus*. American Diabetes Association, USA.

American Association of Clinical Endocrinologists (AACE) (2011) Medical guidelines for clinical practice for developing a diabetes mellitus comprehensive care plan. *Endocrine Practice*, **17** (Suppl 2):1–53.

Australian Diabetes Educators Association (ADEA) (2006) *Guidelines for Sick Day Management for People with Diabetes*. ADEA, Canberra.

Australian Diabetes Society (ADS) (2012) Guidelines for routine glucose control in hospital ADS, Canberra **ADSGuidelinesforRoutineGlucoseControlinHospital**Final2012_000.pdf (accessed November 2012).

Australian Drug Reactions Bulletin (ADRAC) (2001) *Incidence of lactic acidosis between 1985–2001*. ADRA 20 (1) http://.www.tga.gov.au/aarb/aadr9505/htm (accessed December 2007).

Australian Paediatric Endocrien Group (APEG) (2005) The Australian Clinical Practice Guidelines on the Management of Type 1 Diabetes in Children and Adolescents http//:www.chw.edu.au/prof/services/endocrine/apeg/ (accessed January 2013)

Benbow, S., Walsh, A. & Gill, G. (2001) Brittle diabetes in the elderly. *Journal of the Royal Society of Medicine*, **94**, 578–580.

van den Berghe, M., Wouters, P., Weekers, F. *et al.* (2001) Intensive insulin in critically ill patients. *New England Journal of Medicine*, **345**, 1359–1367.

Bhardwaj, V. & Metcalfe, N. (2006) Diabetic ketoacidosis after changing insulin pens: Check technique to avoid complications. *British Medical Journal*, **332**, 1259–1260.

Brunkhurst, F. (2008) Intensive insulin therapy, Pentastarch may be harmful for patients with severe sepsis. *New England Journal of Medicine*, **358**, 125–139.

Calabrese, A. & Turner, R. (2002) Evaluation of prescribing practices: Risk of lactic acidosis with Metformin therapy. *Archives of Internal Medicine*, **162**, 434–437.

Chiasson J. Josse R, Gomis. et al. (2002)STOP-NIDDM Trial Research Group. Acarbose treatment and the risk of cardiovascular disease and hypertension in patients with impaired glucose tolerance: the STOP-NIDDM Trial *Lancet* **359**: 2072–2077

Ciechanowski, P., Katon, W. & Russo, J. (2000) Depression and diabetes. Impact of depressive symptoms on adherence, function and costs. *Archives of Internal Medicine*, **160**, 3278–3285.

Clement S, Braithwaite S, Magee M, *et al.* (2004) Management of diabetes and hyperglycaemia in Hospitals. *Diabetes Care*, **27** (2), 553–591.

Cohen, Z. (2008) *Lactic acidosis*. American Thoracic Society. http://www.thoracic.org/sections/clinical-information/critical-care/critical-care-cases/ (accessed 9 February 2008).

Cook, C., Castro, J., Schmidt, R. *et al.* (2007) *Journal of Hospital Medicine*, **2** (4), 203–211.

Coughlin C. (2012) An ethnographic study of main events during hospitalization: Perceptions of nurses and patients. *Journal of Clinical Nursing*, DOI: 10.111/j.1365-2702.2012.04083.x.

De, P. & Child, D. (2001) Euglycaemic ketoacidosis – Is it on the rise? *Practical Diabetes International*, **18** (7), 239–240.

Diepersloot, R., Bouter, K. & Hoekstra, J. (1990) Influenza infection and diabetes mellitus. Case for annual vaccination. *Diabetes Care*, **13**, 876–882.

Dunning, P., Ward, G. & Rantzau, C. (1994) Effect of alcohol swabbing on capillary blood glucose measurements. *Practical Diabetes*, **11** (4), 251–254.

Dunning, T. (2001) Depression and diabetes, summary and comment. *International Diabetes Monitor*, **13** (5), 9–11.

Dunning, T. (2007) Diabetes: Managing sick days, a patient-centred approach. *General Practice Continuing Education Conference Proceedings*. Exhibition Centre, Royal Australian College of General Practitioners (RACGP) Melbourne.

Edge, J., Roy, Y., Bergomi, A. *et al.* (2006) Conscious level in children with diabetic ketoacidosis is related to severity of acidosis and not to blood glucose concentration. *Pediatric Diabetes*, **7**, 11.

Emslie-Smith, A., Boyle, D. & Evans, J. (2001) Contraindications to Metformin therapy in patients with Type 2 diabetes – A population based study of adherence to prescribing guidelines. *Diabetic Medicine*, **18**, 483–488.

Gill, G., Lucas, S. & Kent, L. (1996) Prevalence and characteristics of brittle diabetes in Britain. *Quarterly Journal of Medicine*, **89**, 839–843.

Goldman, S. (1979) Hyperglycaemic hyperosmolar coma in a 9-month-old child. *Archives of Paediatrics and Adolescent Medicine*, **133** (2), 30.

Hamblin, S. (1995) *Diabetic ketoacidosis*. Australian Diabetes Educator's Association Journal, Spring, 17.

Hemphill R. & Schraga E. (2012) Hyperosmolar Hyperglycaemic State http://emedicine.medscape.com. article/1914705 (accessed October 2012).

Inzucchi, S., Bergenstal, R., Buse, J.*et al.* (2012) Management of hyperglycaemia in type 2 diabetes: a patient-centered approach. Position Statement of the American Diabetes Association (ADA) and the European Association fo the Study of Diabetes (EASD) *Diabetologia*, DOI: 10.1007/s00125-012-2534-0.

Ismail-Beigi, F., Moghissi, A., Tiktin, M., *et al.* (2011) Individualising glycaemic targets in Type 2 diabetes mellitus: Implications of recent clinical trials. *Annals of Internal Medicine* **54**, 554–559.

Joint Commission on Accreditation of Health Care Organisations (2006) www.irmi.com/.../joint-commission-on-accreditation-of-healthcare-organizations-jcaho.aspx -(accessed January 2013)

Kershaw, M., Newton, T., Barrett, T., Berry, K. & Kirk, J. (2005) Childhood diabetes presenting with hyperosmolar dehydration but without ketoacidosis. *Diabetic Medicine*, **22** (5), 645–647.

Kitabchi, A., Fisher, J., Murphy, M. & Rumbak, M. (1994) Diabetic ketoacidosis and the hyperglycaemic hyperosmolar nonketotic state, in *Joslin's Diabetes Mellitus* (eds C. Kahn & G. Weir), Lea & Febiger, Philadelphia, pp. 738–770.

Kitabchi, A., Umpierrez, G., Murphy M., & Kreisberg, R. (2006) Hyperglycaemic crises in adult patients with diabetes: A consensus statement from the American Diabetes Association. *Diabetes Care*, **29** (12), 2739–2748.

Kornum, J. (2007) Type 2 diabetes linked to higher pneumonia-related mortality. *Diabetes Care*, **30**, 2251–2257.

Laffel L, Wentzell K, Loughlin C, et al. (2005): Sick day management using blood 3-hydroxybutyrate (3-OHB) compared with urine ketone monitoring reduces hospital *Diabetes Care* , 28:1277–1281.

Malone, M., Gennis, V. & Goodwin, J. (1992) Characteristics of diabetic ketoacidosis in older versus younger adults. *Journal of the American Geriatric Society*, **40**, 1100–1104.

Munro, J., Campbell, I., McCuish, A. & Duncan, L. (1973) Euglycaemic ketoacidosis. *British Medical Journal*, **2**: 578–580.

National Asthma Council Australia (2005) *Roles of Influenza and Pneumococcal Vaccinations in Subgroups with Asthma, COPD, Diabetes or Heart Disease*. CSL Pharmaceuticals, Canberra.

Nicks, B. (2006) Lactic acidosis. *E medicine* http://www.emedicine.com/emerg/topic291.htm (accessed January 2008).

Nisbet, J., Sturtevant, M. & Prins, J. (2004) Metformin serious adverse effects. *Medical Journal of Australia*, **180** (2), 53–54.

Pillans, P. (1998) Metformin and fatal lactic acidosis. Center for Adverse Reactions Monitoring (CARM) http://www.medsafe.govt.nz/profs/Puarticles/5.htm (accessed January 2008).

Polonsky, W., Anderson, B., Lohrer, P. *et al.* (1994) Insulin omission in women with IDDM. *Diabetes Care*, **17**, 1178–1185.

Rosenbloom, A. (1990) Intracerebral crises during treatment of diabetic ketoacidosis. *Diabetes Care*, **13**, 22–33.

Sagarin, M., McAfee, A., Sachter, J., *et al.* (2005) Hyperosmolar Hyperglycaemic Coma. *E medicine* http://www.emedicine.com/emerg/topic24.htm (accessed January 2008).

Schetz, M. (2008) Intensive insulin therapy may protect renal function in critically ill patients. *Journal of the American Society of Nephrologists Online*, January 30 (accessed January 2008).

Shulman, R., Finney, J., O'sullivan, C., Glynne, P. & Greene, R. (2007) Tight glycaemic control: A prospective observational study of computerized decision-supported intensive insulin therapy. *Critical Care*, **11** (4), R75 (DOI:10.1186/cc5964).

Smith, S. & Poland, G. (2004) American Diabetes Association: Influenza and pneumococcal immunisation in diabetes. *Diabetes Care*, **27** (Suppl. 1) S111–S113.

Unger R, Cherrington A (2011) Glucagonocentric restructuring of diabetes: a pathophysiologic and therapeutic makeover *Journal of Clinical Investigation* **122** (1):4-12.

Unger J. (2012) Uncovering undetected hypoglycaemic events. *Diabetes,Metabolic Syndrome, Obesity Targets and Therapy* **5**, 57–74.

Wang, C., Wang, S. & Lai, C. (2004) Reducing major cause-specific hospitalization rates and shortening hospital stays after influenza vaccination. *Clinical Infectious Diseases*, **39**, 1322–1332.

Chapter 8
Long-Term Complications of Diabetes

Key points

- Diabetes is associated with devastating long-term complications that are psychologically, physically and financially costly to the person with diabetes.
- Diabetes complications cause a great deal of morbidity and represent a significant cost to the health system.
- Maintaining euglycaemia reduces the likelihood of complications developing, however, in Type 2 diabetes complications are often present at diagnosis and/or trigger the diagnosis.
- People with diabetes, especially older people, often require assistance to perform diabetes self-care and other activities of daily living as a consequence of complications.
- People with diabetes worry about developing complications and the worry and/or actuality of complications affects their emotional well-being and can lead to depression.
- People with diabetes often have other comorbidities in addition to diabetes complications, which increases the risk of less than best practice care, frequent hospitalisations and polypharmacy.
- Proactive, preventative complication screening and assessment is essential and should encompass assessing the individual' risk profile to plan holistic, personalised care.
- Focusing on improving the individual's self-care skills and detecting and managing diabetes-related distress and improving the patient-health professional relationship and communication is as essential as the medical aspect of care.

Introduction

The physical long-term complications of diabetes are generally classified as:

- Macrovascular disease: cardiovascular disease, cerebrovascular disease, and peripheral vascular disease. These are common in Type 2 diabetes and are often present at diagnosis. Type 2 diabetes is often preceded by the metabolic syndrome, which confers a high level of cardiovascular risk. Significantly, myocardial infarction is often 'silent' and sudden.
- Microvascular disease: nephropathy and retinopathy. These are a major concern in both Type 1 and Type 2 diabetes. Type 2 diabetes-related nephropathy is one of most common reasons for commencing dialysis.
- Neuropathy: peripheral, which predominantly affects the feet and legs and autonomic, which can lead to gastroparesis, erectile dysfunction (ED), and hypoglycaemic unawareness.

These conditions are inter-related and often occur concomitantly. For example, ED has vascular and nerve components. In the long term in the presence of persistent hyperglycaemia, diabetes can affect almost all body systems and is associated with a number of other disease processes, especially Type 2 diabetes where there is an association between obesity, some cancers, and sleep apnoea. Diabetes is also associated with a range of musculoskeletal diseases, osteoporosis, depression, and dementia although the causal links are not clear in all cases (Chapter 10). The presence of other concomitant and age-related diseases such as arthritis contribute to reduced quality of life and depression and inhibit self-care, thus, psychological issues are also complications of diabetes.

The simultaneous occurrence of two or more chronic conditions (multimorbidity) (Bayliss *et al.* 2008) increases the risk that the individual will not receive best practice care, will be hospitalised more frequently and for longer length of stay, use a greater range of health services at increased cost, and be prescribed more medicines (polypharmacy) (Taylor *et al.* 2010). Prevalence estimates for multimorbidity range from 35% to 80% (Fortin *et al.* 2005; Nagel *et al.* 2008; Britt *et al.* 2008), although the prevalence is difficult to determine because different data collection methods and definitions are used and many studies focus on older people. The prevalence of multimorbidity increases with age but it is also an issue in younger age groups: more than 40% of people <60 years have several comorbidities (Taylor *et al.* 2010).

Multimorbidity often coexists with smoking and obesity, which increase the risk the person will develop more morbidities. Multimorbidites affect self-care and can represent a significant carer burden for relatives. Thus, a multifactorial approach to managing diabetes complications and other concomitant morbidities is needed and encompasses regular systematic, individualised risk assessment processes, effective self-care, optimising physical and mental health and diabetes education to prevent/reduce the morbidity and mortality and reduce the health costs associated with diabetes.

Pathophysiology of diabetes complications

The pathophysiology of diabetes complications is complex but glycaemic control is the most important determinant of optimal mitochondrial function and therefore, long-term diabetic complications (Brownlee 2000). Changes in mitochondrial function result in oxidative stress and play a key role in the development and progression of both micro and macrovascular complications associated with diabetes. Thus, maintaining normoglycaemia to preserve normal oxidative mitochondrial function is needed to delay or prevent the progression of complications (Forbes & Cooper 2007).

Increases in HbA$_{1c}$ from normal to 9.5% confer a 10-fold increased risk of microvascular disease. The relationship between macrovascular disease and hyperglycaemia is not as clear; for example, only a twofold increase in macrovascular disease risk at the same HbA$_{1c}$ was noted in the UKPDS (UKPDS 1998). This finding might be partly explained by the fact that free fatty acids can also be utilised as fuel for oxidative processes in the mitochrondria.

Hyperglycaemia initiates a cascade of pathological changes that underlie diabetes complications. Glucose is the major source of fuel for energy production by oxidative phosphorylation. Hyperglycaemia has significant effects on metabolic pathways concerned with generating cellular energy especially in the mitochondria. Most cells have the capacity to reduce glucose transport across the plasma membrane into the cytosol to maintain glucose homeostasis in the presence of hyperglycaemia. However, some cells are not able to adapt and reduce glucose transport sufficiently to prevent intercellular changes in glucose concentration. Cells are at particular risk include capillary endothelial cells in the retina, mesangial cells in renal glomeruli, and neuronal and Schwann cells in peripheral nerves (Forbes & Cooper 2007).

An increasing body of research suggests that reactive oxygen species (ROS) initiate the development of diabetic complications (Nishikawa *et al.* 2000). ROS are generated by damaged or dysfunctional mitochondria. The antioxidant chain is a complex pathway involving the metabolism of oxygen and the transfer of electrons from glucose and other fuels through the respiratory chain via a complex series of reactions. When excess fuel enters the respiratory chain, the mitochondrial membrane potential is overwhelmed and leaks electrons to oxygen to form superoxide (Nishikawa *et al.* 2000). However, despite the increasing evidence that ROS plays a role in the pathogenesis of diabetes complications the exact mechanisms are still being determined. Maintaining optimal mitochondrial function appears to be important to reduce the progression of diabetes complications. More recent research suggests preventing glucose variability might also be important (Weber & Schnell 2009; Wen *et al.* 2012; Picconne *et al.* 2012).

The role of antioxidant agents in managing diabetes complications and reducing oxidative damage is controversial, although is widely promoted by complementary practitioners. Folic acid has been shown to reduce oxidative damage in Type 2 diabetes (Lazalde-Ramos *et al.* 2012). Likewise, Coenzyme Q10 (CQ-10) is essential for all energy-dependent processes in the heart, consequently the heart is very sensitive to CQ-10 deficiencies (Kumar *et al.* 2009). CQ-10 is often deficient in diabetes and cardiac disease. CQ-10 is available in foods such as beef, poultry and broccoli, fish oils and peanuts, but dietary intake is inadequate to achieve optimal CQ-10 levels in the blood. Supplements reduce the progression of atherosclerosis, proinflammatory cytokines and blood viscosity (Kumar *et al.* 2009).

Hyperglycaemia contributes to cell death, thickened basement membranes in blood vessels, stiffened vessels and reduces the functionality and structure of resistance vessels (proximal vessels before the blood flows into the capillaries). Calcium-regulated potassium channels are disrupted, which affects smooth muscle cell contraction, which contributes to hypertension. As a result, both under-perfusion and over-perfusion occur. The myogenic response is lost, so the resistance vessels no longer have the capacity to cope with the increased blood flow. Increased basement membrane dysfunction and reduced nerve fibre density is apparent in impaired glucose tolerance. Micro- and macrovascular and endothelial cell damage and reduced lumenal size also occur.

Brownlee (2000) suggested that no 'unifying hypothesis' links the four main hypotheses proposed to explain the pathogenesis of diabetic complications shown below, but suggested either redox changes in the polyol pathway, or hyperglycaemia-induced formation of ROS, might account for all the underlying biochemical changes.

(1) Formation of advanced glycation endproducts (AGE). Products of glucose metabolism from glycolysis and the tricarboxylic acid cycle initiate protein glycosylation more

rapidly than glucose. The protein–glucose complex is broken down by proteosomes or form AGE that become cross-linked and resistant to proteosome activity. Tissues become stiffened and function is compromised. AGE formation may be due to the effects of glucose metabolites rather then glucose itself (Wells-Knecht *et al*. 1995; Dantas *et al*. 2012). The interaction of AGEs with their receptor (RAGE) triggers a variety of cellular signaling processes that mediate gene expression and enhance the release of proinflammatory molecules and oxidative stress (Farmer & Kennedy. 2009).

(2) Activation of protein kinase C (PKC) isoforms. Hyperglycaemia stimulates diacylglycerol, the lipid second messenger, which activates isoforms of PKC and alters gene and protein expression in organs prone to complications. Inhibiting PKC prevents renal and retinal damage in animal models and a number of clinical trials are in progress involving ruboxisataurin (Forbes & Cooper 2007).

(3) Increased flux through the polyol pathway. In the polyol pathway glucose is converted into sorbitol via aldose reductase and subsequently oxidised to fructose, which eventually contributes to the mitochondrial respiratory chain. Intracellular hyperglycaemia results in increased production of sorbitol and reduces the level of other important enzymes involved in detoxifying toxic aldehydes such as glutathione and adenine dinucleotide phosphate, and compounds oxidative stress. Sorbitol does not cross cell membranes and causes osmotic stress. Inhibiting aldose reductase delays or prevents diabetes complications especially neuropathy (Kaiser *et al*. 1993). To date, aldose reductase inhibitor medications have been disappointing despite improvements in nerve physiology and nerve fibre density, largely due to poor tissue penetration and side effects (Hotta *et al*. 2001).

(4) Increased flux through the hexosamine pathway. When intracellular glucose is high, the normal glucose-6-phosphate metabolic cascade is disrupted and a series of moieties are produced that bind to transcription factors and increase the synthesis of some proteins such as transforming growth factor-b_1 and plasminogen activator inhibitor type 1, both of which have adverse effects on blood vessels (Du *et al*. 2000). The role of the hexosamine pathway in the pathogenesis of diabetic complications is still evolving.

CARDIOVASCULAR DISEASE AND DIABETES

Key points

- Cardiovascular disease is a leading cause of death in people with diabetes.
- Excess mortality from cardiovascular disease is evident in all age groups but especially in young people with Type 1 diabetes.
- People with diabetes and no heart disease need to be treated as if they have heart disease, especially people with Type 2 diabetes.
- Chest pain may be atypical in people with diabetes, and may present as weakness, fatigue, hyperglycaemia or congestive cardiac failure (CCF).
- Women with diabetes have a higher relative risk of death from cardiovascular disease than men but the absolute risk is lower.
- Primary prevention by managing dyslipidaemia, hypertension and hyperglycaemia is imperative to lower the risk of heart disease and stroke.
- Smoking increases micro- and macrovascular damage. Smoking cessation is imperative.
- Depression is common in people with diabetes and cardiac disease.
- Transient ischaemic attacks (TIA) may indicate impending stroke.

Rationale

Diabetes is a significant risk factor for cardiovascular disease, for example, coronary heart disease, cardiomyopathy, peripheral vascular disease and stroke (Australian Institute of Health and Welfare (AIHW) 2007; Dantas *et al.* 2012). Cardiovascular disease contributes to 54% of all male deaths and 59% of all female deaths in Australia (AIHW 2011) and is a major cause of hospital admissions and mortality in people with diabetes. It is often associated with other vascular disease and depression. Complex metabolic abnormalities are present and the need for surgical intervention is high. Autonomic neuropathy can give rise to atypical presentations of cardiovascular disease and heart attack and lead to delayed treatment. The major clinical manifestations of cardiovascular disease involve:

- the heart and coronary circulation;
- the brain and cerebral circulation;
- the lower limbs: peripheral vascular disease.

Cardiac disease is a common complication of diabetes, and carries a higher mortality rate than for people without diabetes. The World Health Organization (WHO) (2003) estimated ~16.7 million people die from cardiovascular disease each year. Cardiac disease accounts for >50% of deaths in Type 2 diabetes (Standl & Schnell 2000; Huang *et al.* 2001) and half of these people die before they reach hospital. The mortality rate has not been reduced despite new therapeutic measures and preventative health programmes. Myocardial infarction may be a diabetes risk equivalent in non-diabetics. Diabetes often occurs within 3.5 years of an infarct particularly in older people, those with a high BMI, hypertension and smokers. The risk is lower in people consuming a Mediterranean diet and those on lipid-lowering medicines (Mozaffarian 2007).

There is an association among increasing age, duration of diabetes, the presence of other complications and mortality. Cardiac disease is associated with diffuse atherosclerosis, coexisting cardiomyopathy, autonomic neuropathy, hyperglycaemia and hyperlipidaemia, the metabolic consequences being hypercoagulability, elevated catecholamines and insulin resistance. Atherosclerosis is more frequent and more severe in people with diabetes. It occurs at a younger age than in people without diabetes and is more prevalent in women, especially after menopause. Female sex hormones, especially oestrogen has many haemodynamic, vascular and metabolic effects, which are associated with cardiovascular protection in women (Dantas *et al.* 2012).

The protective effects of oestrogen include:

- Influencing the metabolism of lipoproteins.
- Controlling blood pressure.
- Reducing formation of atheromatous plaques.
- Increasing NO bioavailability.
- Regulating the production of endothelium-derived relaxing factors and endothelium-derived hyperpolarizing factors, which affect vascular relaxation and resistance. Oestrogen also has an effect on vascular constrictor factors.
- Suppressing vascular inflammation by down regulating proinflammatory molecules including cytokines and adhesion molecules.
- Regulating energy balance, fat distribution and insulin sensitivity, which is largely lost after the menopause. Oestrogen replacement therapy in postmenopausal women has beneficial effects on diabetes and cardiovascular risk (Margolis *et al.* 2004) but the benefits must be weighed against the risks for each individual woman.

A number of clinical trials and guidelines emphasise the importance of reducing lipids, blood pressure, and blood glucose to reduce the risk of cardiovascular disease (Hansson *et al*. 1998; UKPDS 1998; NICE 2009; SIGN 2010; ADA 2013). Hypertension leads to thicker, less elastic blood vessel walls and increases the strain on the heart. There is a linear relationship between the diastolic blood pressure and the eventual outcome of Type 2 diabetes. Reducing the blood pressure below 90 mmHg significantly improves the outcome (UKPDS 1998).

Subtle changes occur in the heart as a result of ischaemia-induced remodelling and the effects of hyperglycaemia on the endothelium of large blood vessels that predispose the individual to heart failure (Standl & Schnell 2000). Heart muscle metabolism is critically dependent on glucose during ischaemia, and heart muscle performance is improved in the presence of insulin, which stimulates glucose uptake, which support the use of IV insulin in acute myocardial infarction (Malmberg *et al*. 1995). However, impaired heart performance is multifactorial and blood pressure, lipids, and prothrombin imbalance all play a part. Table 8.1 outlines some of the diabetes-specific abnormalities linked to the development of cardiovascular disease.

Myocardial infarction is 'silent' in 32% of people with diabetes, which leads to delay in seeking medical attention and may be a factor in the increased mortality rate. 'Silent' infarct means that the classic pain across the chest, down the arm and into the jaw is absent. Only mild discomfort, often mistaken for heartburn, may be present. The atypical nature of the chest pain may make it difficult for people to accept that they have had a heart attack. Risk factor modification may not be seen as essential. The person may present with hypertension, heart failure, cardiogenic shock or, in older people with diabetes, ketoacidosis or hyperosmolar states.

Diabetes may be diagnosed at the time an infarct occurs or during cardiac surgery. Emotional stress, and the associated catecholamine response, leads to increased blood glucose levels in 5% of patients admitted to coronary care units (CCU). The blood glucose may normalise during convalescence; however, counselling about diabetes and its management is important, especially if other diabetes risk factors are present. Tact and sympathy are necessary when informing the patient about the diagnosis of diabetes in these situations.

Women with cardiovascular disease have poorer outcomes than men, regardless of other comorbidities and management (Davidson *et al*. 2011). As discussed earlier, low female sex hormone levels after menopause, especially oestrogen, may play a role in cardiovascular disease in women. Atrial fibrillation in women confers a greater risk of stroke than in men and anticoagulation therapy is associated with a higher risk of bleeding problems (Davidson *et al*. 2011)

Medicines and cardiovascular disease

Many types of medicines may be needed to prevent and/or manage cardiovascular disease (Chapter 5). The choice of medicines depends on the clinical indications, patient factors such as cardiovascular risk, contraindications/precautions, risk of medicine interactions, availability, and cost.

Generally, management targets address hypertension, hyperglycaemia, coagulopathies and hyperlipidaemia. Most modern guidelines recommend individualising targets and commonly recommend:

- Blood pressure 130/80 mm Hg including in people with albuminuria.
- LDL cholesterol <2 mmol/L.

Table 8.1 Some diabetes-specific cardiovascular abnormalities that predispose an individual to heart disease.

Abnormality	Relevance to cardiovascular disease
Insulin resistance	Increases cardiovascular mortality
Chronic hyperglycaemia	Every 1% (11 mmol/mol) increase in HbA1c is associated with a 15% increase in hazard of all-cause mortality, 25% for cardiovascular mortality and 17% fatal coronary heart disease (Zhang *et al.* 2012) In the UKPDS each 1% (11 mmol/mol) reduction in HbA$_{1c}$ was associated with a 21% lower risk of diabetes-related death and 14% lower risk of MI over 10 years Contributes to microvascular disease
Microvascular disease with microalbuminuria	May be detected earlier than macrovascular disease and often occurs concomitantly with macrovascular disease Affects nutrient and oxygen exchange Nephropathy, frequently in association with retinopathy Nephropathy doubles the risk cardiac disease in people with Type 1 diabetes (Lehto *et al.* 1999) but it is not clear whether reducing microalbuminuria reduces cardiovascular risk
Autonomic neuropathy	Postural hypotension Abnormal cardiovascular reflexes Loss of sinus rhythm Resting sinus tachycardia Painless myocardial ischaemia and infarction 'silent MI' Delayed recognition and treatment Increased anaesthetic risk Increased risk in critical care situations Sudden death
Endothelial damage in basement membrane or outer lining of large blood vessels	Weak vessel walls, stiffened vessels contributing to hypertension Impaired blood flow Reduced tissue oxygenation and nourishment
Hypertension	Thickening of blood vessel walls Increased strain on the heart Risk of cardiovascular disease increases progressively with increasing systolic blood pressure Each 10 mm Hg reduction in systolic blood pressure is associated with 15% reduction in risk of cardiovascular death over 10 years
Hyperlipidaemia Obesity predisposes the individual to insulin resistance, dyslipidaemia and high circulating free fatty acids (FFA) but does not appear to be an independent risk factor for cardiovascular disease Ethnicity needs to be considered when determining obesity	Increased LDL cholesterol or total cholesterol is an independent risk factor for cardiovascular death Type 2 diabetes is associated with high triglycerides, low HDL and small dense LDL A 1 mmol/L reduction in LDL represents a 21% reduction in risk Hypertriglyceridaemia is an independent marker of increased cardiovascular risk in Type 2 diabetes Increased lipolysis as FFA are liberated from adipose tissue Increased mediators of vascular function such as angiotensinogen, adiponectin, IL-6, prostaglandins and TNF∂
Adiponectin and adipocyte-derived protein	Associated with metabolic derangements including type 2 diabetes via their role in glucose regulation and catabolism of fatty acids Adiponectin levels correlate with the development of insulin resistance, progression of Type 2 diabetes and hypertension. High adiponectin is related to higher all-cause mortality after controlling for other confounders (Singer *et al.* 2012)

- HbA_{1c}:
  - Diabetes short duration and no cardiovascular risk <6% (<42 mmol/mol);
  - Lifestyle management with or without Metformin <6.5% (<48 mmol/mol);
  - Requiring any glucose lowering medicine besides Metformin or insulin <7% (<53 mmol/mol);
  - Requiring insulin <7% (< 53 mmol/mol);
  - Diabetes of long duration and/or presence of cardiovascular disease because these people do not benefit from tight blood glucose control <7% (<53 mol Mol) (Accord Study Group 2011);
  - If the person has severe hypoglycaemia or hypoglycaemic unawareness and older people <8% (<64 mmol/mol) (National Prescribing Service (NPS) 2012).

The Accord Study Group (2011) found that tight blood glucose control (<6 % <42 mmol/mol) resulted in 10 extra deaths per 1000 people over 3.5 years. Likewise, severe hypoglycaemia is associated with increased morbidity and mortality (Chapter 6). It is also associated with long duration of diabetes and microalbuminuria (Yun *et al.* 2012). These significant adverse events highlight the importance of determining individual risk for cardiovascular disease and the risks associated with treatment.

Estimating cardiovascular risk in people with diabetes is complicated: currently available risk calculators such as the Framingham and UKPDS risk calculator are inaccurate in people with diabetes (Coleman *et al.* 2007) and people should be informed that the risk calculation is only an estimate of their actual risk (NICE 2009). However, the likelihood of error is reduced if the person has several cardiovascular risk factors (NICE 2009). Risk calculators can underestimate risk in South Asian, Maori, Pacific Islanders and Middle Eastern peoples (NPS 2012).

In addition to medicines, stopping smoking, a healthy diet and regular exercise and effective self-care are essential to achieving optimal control. Sedentary time is associated with increased risk of Type 2 diabetes (112% increased relative risk (RR)), cardiovascular disease (90% RR) and all cause mortality (40% RR) (NPS 2012; Wilmot *et al.* 2012). Sedentary time includes occupational sitting and watching TV. Medicines may be required to manage cardiovascular risk or treat cardiovascular disease.

Medicine commonly used to manage cardiovascular disease include:

- Antithrombotic medicines to prevent thromboembolism generally and during coronary procedures and surgery, prevent stroke in patients with atrial fibrillation, prevent thromboembolism in patients with prosthetic heart valves, and treat acute MI. Types of medicines include Vitamin K antagonists (warfarin), heparin (enoxaparin), platelet aggregation inhibitors (aspirin), and thrombolytic enzymes (alteplase). These medicines require frequent monitoring and interact with many other medicines including complementary medicines (CAM). The benefits of low dose aspirin (75–150 mg/day) outweigh the risks in adults with diabetes and existing cardiovascular disease. However, evidence for the benefits for people without existing cardiovascular disease, including people with diabetes, is weak (NPS 2012). Thus aspirin is not recommended for primary prevention (SIGN 2010). The risk of major bleeds and macular degeneration are significant. Consequently the NPS the National Vascular Disease Prevention Alliance Guidelines and SIGN 2010 do not recommend routine use of low dose aspirin in people without existing cardiovascular disease. (NICE 2009) recommends offering 75 mg aspirin/day to anybody with blood pressure <145/90 mmHg, and the American Diabetes Association (ADA) (2012) recommends people with 10-year cardiovascular disease risk 10% should take

75 mg aspirin/day. ADA does not advocate using aspirin for people whose cardio-vascular risk is <5% and that clinical judgement should be used for people whose 10 year risk is 5%–10%.

- Cardiac medicines to treat arrhythmias (cardiac glycosides such as digoxin), heart failure antiarrythmics such as amiodarone), relieve cardiac symptoms such as angina (vasodilators such as isorbide), treat high and low blood pressure, cardiogenic shock and MI (cardiac stimulants such as adrenaline).
- Antihypertensive agents often used as primary prevention to reduce the risk of micro-vascular disease. These include low dose diuretics as first-line treatment (frusemide), peripheral vasodilators (oxpentifylline), calcium channel blockers (amlodipine). Antihypertensive therapy is usually selected according to the comorbidities present to achieve blood pressure 130/80 in people with cardiovascular disease. The first-line medicine for people with diabetes and hypertension is an ACEI or an ARB; the most appropriate choice in an older person following a MI is a calcium channel blocker to reduce the risk of stroke, however, most people require several antihypertensive medi-cines (European Society of Hypertension 2007).
- Beta blocking agents (Atenolol, Metorpolol, Propanolol), which can be used with a diuretic and an ACE inhibitor. Beta blockers confer benefit in the medium- to long-term but can cause decompensation and worsen heart failure and hypotension in the short term. They should be started at a low dose and gradually increased. Contraindications include asthma, heart block and symptomatic hypotension.
- Medicines acting on the renin–angiotensin system such as ACEI, which are first-line treatment in heart failure, left ventricular dysfunction following MI, and diabetes in the presence of microalbuminuria (Ramipril); angiotensin 11 antagonists (Irbesartin), which are used if the person cannot tolerate ACE. For example, ACE inhibitors are associated with a three times higher rate of cough. SIGN (2010) recommends ACEI be considered in people with all New York Heart Association (NYHA) functional classes of heart failure due to left ventricular systolic dysfunction.
- Lipid-lowering agents such as HMG-CoA reductase inhibitors (statins, e.g. Atorvastatin), which reduces LDL cholesterol, fibrates, which are first choice if tri-glycerides are elevated, nicotinic acid, which lowers both cholesterol and triglycerides but is not tolerated very well (*Australian Medicines Handbook* 2006). However, there is not enough evidence to recommend fibrates, Ezetimibe or nicotinic acid for primary prevention (SIGN 2010).
- Glucose-lowering medicines are discussed in Chapter 5.

However, these medicines are not always prescribed optimally. For example, antithrom-botic medicines, ACE inhibitors, ACE, and beta blocker combinations, and antihyper-tensive agents are under-utilised (National Institute of Clinical Studies 2005). Patient non-adherence with many medicines is high and is a significant limiting factor in achiev-ing optimal outcomes.

Complementary medicines (CAM)

Recently, WS 1442, a formula of *Crataegus monogyna* (hawthorn) was shown to increase intracellular calcium concentration, contractile force, action potential and the refractory period, improve coronary blood flow and reduce preload and after load (Pittler *et al.* 2008). Animal studies have also demonstrated a smaller area of infarction after induced MI using *Crataegus monogyna*. These findings suggest WS

1442 might have a place in managing cardiovascular disease, but that place is not yet defined.

Coenzyme Q_{10} (CQ_{10}) lowers systolic and diastolic blood pressure and reduces inflammation. Individuals with mild-to-moderate hypertension and cardiac disease might benefit from CQ_{10} supplements (Rosenfeldt *et al.* 2007), but like W1442, its place is under-researched. CQ_{10} is an antioxidant and is present in LDL-c where it reduces the potential for LDL-c to be oxidised and become atherogenic. Some experts suggested CQ_{10} might be a useful addition to statins to reduce myotoxicity. However, while it may have a place, at present there is no recommendation to use CQ_{10} in people taking statins (Barenholtz & Kohlhaas 2006). If people do elect to use CQ_{10} the effects on their conventional medicines need to be monitored.

Other complementary therapies such as massage, meditation, and Tai Chi can help reduce stress, improve quality of life and manage pain but should be used within a Quality Use of Medicine framework (Chapter 19).

Other management considerations

Hyperglycaemia is common in MI and there is an association between initial blood glucose level and outcomes including mortality even if the blood glucose is only mildly elevated (ADS 2012). However, hyperglycaemia is also associated with adverse outcomes (Chapter 6). Various guidelines suggest different blood glucose targets in acute MI; generally the aims should be blood glucose <10 mmol/L and IV infusions are recommended when resources permit (ADS 2012). The International Diabetes federation (IDF) (2011) suggested a two-hour postprandial blood glucose >7.8 mmol/L is a stronger predictor of cardiovascular events than fasting blood glucose and recommended monitoring postprandial blood glucose and to aim for <7.5 mmol/L.

Patients with an acute cardiovascular event are usually cared for in CCUs but patients in other wards and in the community may develop cardiovascular problems, including silent MI. A longer stay in CCU may be indicated for people with diabetes, because 35% of patients die, often in the second week after the infarct (Karlson *et al.* 1993). People with diabetes and unstable angina, MI without ST elevation or STEMI have a higher mortality risk within one year of the onset of acute coronary syndrome than non-diabetics (Donahoe *et al.* 2007).

Silent MI may be relatively common in common critical care settings, the diagnosis can be difficult to establish and the MI is often missed due to analgesia controlling chest pain, intubation, sedation, and coma (Lim *et al.* 2008). Lim *et al.* (2008) suggested screening for elevated troponin levels in critically ill patients and performing an ECG could reduce mortality and that elevated troponins might be predicative of mortality. Although more research is needed, these findings might be particularly relevant to people with diabetes where the risk of cardiovascular disease is likely to be high.

Short- and long-term morbidity and mortality can be improved by IV insulin/glucose infusion followed by multidose subcutaneous insulin injections (Malmberg *et al.* 1995). Acute myocardial infarction causes a rapid increase in catecholamines, cortisol, and glucagon. Insulin levels fall in the ischaemic myocardium and tissue sensitivity to insulin falls and impairs glucose utilisation by cardiac muscle. Free fatty acids are mobilised as fuel substrates and potentiate ischaemic injury by direct toxicity or by increasing the demand for oxygen and inhibiting glucose oxidation. IV insulin during acute episodes and subcutaneous insulin for three months after the infarct may restore platelet function, correct lipoprotein imbalance, reduce plasminogen activator inhibitor-1 activity and improve metabolism in non-infarcted areas of the heart.

The need for invasive procedures depends on the severity at presentation and the results of relevant investigations. Pfisterer (2004) showed that invasive treatment provided short-term symptomatic relief reduced the rate of revascularisation and hospitalisation and less frequent use of antianginal medicines, compared to medicine treatment. In the longer term, both strategies were effective in older patients with angina. Mortality risk factors included age >80 years, prior heart failure, left ventricular ejection <45%, and the presence of two or more comorbidities.

Mental health and cardiovascular disease

Anxiety is common among people with cardiac disease and can have serious consequences for self-care and long-term outcomes if it is not recognised and managed to prevent depression. However, anxiety can be life-saving if it prompts the person to seek help early (Moser 2007). Significantly depression is an independent risk factor for cardiovascular disease and its prognosis. Both depression and heart disease are associated with social isolation and lack of social support (Bunker *et al.* 2003). These factors need to be considered when estimating cardiovascular risk.

Several trials have investigated the cardiovascular benefit of treating depression. These include ENRICH (cognitive behaviour therapy and SSRI medicines), which is difficult to interpret but which showed no significant difference between treatment and usual care. SADHART (SSRI), showed improvements in mild-to-moderate depression but no significant differences in cardiac events. The results of CREATE (SSRI (Citalopram) and interpersonal psychotherapy) are not yet available but suggest depression improves but HbA_{1c} does not significantly improve (Reddy 2008).

The effects on mental health may change; for example, Gudjhar & Dunning (2003) found that people with diabetes were most concerned about the implications of the MI immediately after the event and less concerned about the impact of diabetes on their long-term physical health, mental health, and quality of life. Patient generated quality-of-life tools were used. As people recovered and realised they would survive, about four months after the MI, concern about the MI began to diminish and pre-MI worry about diabetes and its complications re-emerged.

Depression may increase cardiovascular risk and vice versa via several mechanisms:

- Risk behaviours such as inadequate diet and inactivity, smoking and non-compliance with medicines.
- Effects on autonomic function by enhancing sympathetic nervous system activity and heart rate variability.
- Consequence model: inflammatory processes with sub-chronic elevation of cytokines activate the stress response and inhibit serotonin. MI might also induce physical changes in the brain that are mediated by the inflammatory response and cause depression.
- Coincidence model: autonomic dysregulation decreased heart rate variability and increased risk of ventricular arrhythmias, changes in platelets, inflammation and changes in endothelial function, some of which might be linked to dietary factors. For example, increasing omega-3 fatty acids improves cardiac function (Lesperance & Frasure-Smith 2007).

Objectives of care in hospital

Nursing care should be planned to avoid constantly disturbing the patient and allow adequate rest and sleep. The objectives of care are to:

- treat the acute attack according to medical orders, guidelines and standard protocols;
- stabilise cardiac status and relieve symptoms;
- prevent extension of the cardiac abnormality and limit further episodes;
- retain independence as far as possible;
- achieve and maintain euglycaemia but prevent hypoglycaemic events, thus blood glucose monitoring is important;
- provide psychological support;
- prevent complications while in hospital;
- counsel about risk factor modification;
- educate/re-educate about diabetes.

Nursing responsibilities

(1) To be aware that myocardial infarction can present atypically in people with diabetes and may present as CCF, syncope, vomiting, abdominal pain, and fatigue that improves with rest. An ECG should be performed urgently if any of these symptoms are present. A high resting heart rate is associated with mortality in people with diabetes. Sanchis (2007) developed a risk assessment process for patients without an increase in troponins or ST deviation that was able to identify patients with a similar prognosis to patients with elevated troponins and ST depression that might be useful in people with diabetes.

(2) To provide psychological, educational, and physical care.

(3) To monitor blood glucose, 2–4 hourly depending on stability and route of insulin administration.

(4) To provide adequate pain relief, and to control vomiting, which contribute to/exacerbate high blood glucose levels.

(5) To deliver care according to the medical orders for the specific cardiac abnormality.

(6) To administer insulin:
- Many patients on GLMs are changed to insulin during the acute phase to improve blood glucose control.
- Insulin is usually administered via an infusion at least for the first 48 hours. Only clear insulin is used. Insulin infusions are discussed in Chapter 7. The patient should be eating and drinking normally before the infusion is removed, and a dose of subcutaneous insulin given to prevent hyperglycaemia developing.

Some endocrinologist/cardiologist teams have adopted Malmberg *et al.*'s recommendations, the so-called DIGAMI protocol, or some variation of it, which usually involves commencing an IV insulin infusion for people with diabetes presenting with MI from the time of presentation in the emergency room. IV insulin is usually continued for 24 hours after which time subcutaneous insulin is commenced and maintained for three months.

The aim of the IV insulin is to normalise glucose utilisation in the myocardium, achieve normoglycaemia and reduce morbidity and mortality.

(7) Other medications: GLMs should be stopped while the patient is having IV insulin to reduce the risk of hypoglycaemia. Thiazide diuretics can:
- Increase blood glucose levels.
- Cause hypokalaemia.

- Beta blockers reduce mortality by >30%. Ace inhibitors improve blood pressure and cardiac remodelling and stabilise the rate of progression of renal disease. There is a close association between cardiac and renal disease in diabetes.

Non-cardiac-specific beta-blocking agents may mask the signs of hypoglycaemia. Patients who are normally on oral GLMs will require support and education about the use of insulin. It should be explained that insulin is being given to increase the glucose available to the myocardium and decrease free fatty acids in the blood. Units where IV insulin infusions are used often discharge the patient on subcutaneous insulin, which is continued for three months then reassessed the individual's medicine needs are reassessed.

(8) Physical status:
- Monitor fluid balance and maintain accurate documentation to help assess kidney function.
- Monitor blood pressure, lying, and standing. Some antihypertensive medications can cause orthostatic hypotension. Counsel the patient to change position gradually, especially on getting out of bed or out of a chair. Postural hypotension is a risk factor for falls especially in older people.
- Monitor ECG.
- Observe for weakness, fatigue, CCF or unexplained hyperglycaemia, which could indicate another infarct or extension of the original infarct.
- Provide appropriate skin care to prevent dryness and pressure areas.

(9) Investigative procedures:
- Monitor serum electrolytes, cardiac enzymes, blood gases and potassium levels. Report abnormalities to the doctor promptly. Fluctuating potassium levels can cause or exacerbate cardiac arrhythmias.
- Prevent hypoglycaemia by carefully monitoring the blood glucose and carbohydrate intake.
- Prepare the individual for investigative procedures appropriately, and inform them what to expect (Chapter 9).

(10) Thrombolytics are beneficial to reduce plaque. Low-dose aspirin reduces emboli and reduces the risk of cardiac disease and stroke in people with existing cardiovascular disease; see the previous section.

(11) If relevant, consider end-of-life care (Chapter 18) and support the family to cope with the crisis.

In many cases metabolic control prior to the MI was suboptimal and insulin therapy indicated for some time before the infarct occurred.

Some OHAs are contraindicated if cardiac, renal, and/or liver disease is present (see Chapter 5).

Practice points

(1) The person may not recognise the signs of hypoglycaemia if:
- Autonomic neuropathy is present.
- Non-selective beta-blocking agents are used.
(2) Neuroglycopenic signs of hypoglycaemia (confusion, slurred speech or behaviour change) may predominate. Alternatively, these signs may indicate a cardiovascular event.

Medical tests/procedures (see Chapter 9)

(1) The eyes should be assessed *before* thrombolytic medications are commenced. If proliferative retinopathy is present, bleeding into the back of the eye may occur, requiring urgent treatment.

(2) Diagnostic procedures that require the use of contrast dyes, for example, angiograms, have been associated with renal complications. Ensure adequate hydration before and after procedures and monitor urine output, especially in older people and people with renal disease.

(3) There is a high prevalence of cardiovascular disease in people with renal disease (Levin 2000).

Rehabilitation

Structured rehabilitation after an acute cardiovascular event and heart failure improves long-term outcomes, reduces social isolation, and improves function and quality of life.

(1) Encourage activity within tolerance limits. Refer for physiotherapy/occupational therapy.

(2) Encourage independence.

(3) Counsel about resumption of normal activity, including sexual intercourse, after discharge home.

(4) Explain restrictions on driving after cardiac surgery.

(5) Ensure diabetes education/re-education is available. Refer to diabetes nurse specialist/ diabetes educator, dietitian, and physiotherapist. Education should include the need to protect kidney function and also address the risk factors involved in the development of cardiac disease. Particular areas of concern are:
   - recognise hypoglycaemia;
   - correct insulin technique;
   - correct blood glucose monitoring technique;
   - possible indicators of further cardiac problems;
   - dietary assessment and advice;
   - risk factor modification;

(6) explain the need for multi-medicine therapy and the importance of adhering to the medicine regimen;

(7) monitor to detect anxiety and depression and treat early.

Modifying risk factors associated with the development of cardiac disease

Current cardiovascular management guidelines focus on reducing global cardiovascular risk, which requires a proactive approach and attention to multiple risk factors taking age into account: cardiovascular risk, which can be stratified and individualised to enable personalised teaching using tools such as the QRISK and ASSIGN in the UK and the Framingham algorithm, which is sex-specific and is based on the presence of hypertension, dyslipidaemia, and smoking. The Systematic Coronary Risk Evaluation (SCORE) based on cholesterol, blood pressure, and age was developed for European countries (Zannad 2008). Note the discussion about the limitations of risk scores in a previous section of this chapter.

Significantly, research suggests that doctors do not adequately assess cardiovascular risk and this contributes to patients not achieving management targets (Bohm 2008; Mulnier 2012). Other researchers found general practitioners overestimate the risk of diabetes complications but the impact on patient care and service utilisation or outcomes was not reported (Haussler *et al*. 2007).

People with diabetes require both information and support to manage diabetes and reduce the risk of adverse health outcomes. Personalised information is more effective than generalised information. Management targets are described in this chapter and Chapter 2. As indicated in Chapter 16, helping people determine their cardiovascular age could be a useful way to help people understand their cardiovascular risk and help them adhere to their risk reduction strategies.

Key messages are to:

- Stop smoking.
- Avoid high calorie foods and high fat intake especially trans fats to achieve sensible weight reduction. Include omega-3 fatty acids in the diet. Reduce salt intake. Suitable diets are described in Chapter 4 and include the DASH and Mediterranean diets.
- Limit alcohol intake.
- Maintain a healthy weight range suitable to age and developmental stage. In particular reduce abdominal obesity.
- Increase regular exercise/activities.
- Achieve acceptable blood glucose levels.
- Reduce blood lipids. If this is not achieved by diet and exercise, lipid-lowering agents are needed; see Chapter 5. High LDL-c, low HDL-c, and mixed hyperlipidaemia significantly increase the risk of developing cardiovascular disease (Hansel 2004).
- Reduce blood pressure by appropriate diet, exercise and stopping smoking. Optimal blood pressure control is important and people are often prescribed three or more antihypertensive agents. The choice of medication is individualised and includes reducing blood glucose as part of a comprehensive cardiovascular risk management plan (Lowe 2002). Hypertension is also a risk factor for poorer performance on verbal and concept formation tests in Type 2 diabetes (Elias *et al*. 1997), which has implications for self-care and activities of daily living.
- Manage hypertension and monitor the day-night dip. A blunted day-night dip is associated with a blunted morning BP surge and vice versa. A blunted morning BP surge could be an independent predictor of cardiovascular events (Verdecchia *et al*. 2012).
- Secondary prevention programmes such as cardiac rehabilitation are important to help individuals regain the best possible functioning.
- Manage stress. Long-term stress is associated with increased risk of cardiovascular disease in both men and women, and a high level of trait anger in middle aged men with hypertension is associated with increased risk of hypertension progression to a cardiovascular event (Player *et al*. 2007).
- Seek treatment for depression.
- People with known cardiac disease should have a written action to plan to follow if they experience chest pain. They should know early management is important and not to delay presenting to hospital. The plan might include using short-acting nitrate medicines, resting, taking aspirin if they are not already prescribed this medicine, calling an ambulance, notifying their doctor, and wearing medic alert information.

Telephone coaching

Telephone coaching for people with coronary heart disease and suboptimal lipid levels improves adherence to medication therapy and dietary advice. It contributes to an improved lipid profile and could be an important aspect of cardiac rehabilitation programmes (Vale *et al.* 2003). The COACH protocol is currently under investigation in a general practice setting with practice nurses providing coaching with support from the COACH investigators (Young *et al.* 2007).

Cerebrovascular disease

The incidence of stroke associated with diabetes is high and mortality following a stroke is higher in people with diabetes than non-diabetics. The brain is supplied with blood by four main arteries: two carotids and two vertebral arteries. The clinical consequences of cerebrovascular disease depend on the vessels or combination of vessels involved. Transient ischaemic attacks (TIAs) arise when the blood supply to a part of the brain is temporarily interrupted without permanent damage. Recovery from a TIA usually occurs within 24 hours. If TIAs occur frequently they can indicate impending stroke. Small repeated strokes that cause progressive brain damage can lead to multi-infarct dementia, which is common in diabetes. Signs of multi-infarct dementia include:

- gradual memory loss;
- diminished intellectual capacity;
- loss of motor function;
- incontinence.

Strokes are classified as thrombotic or haemorrhagic and occur when a major vessel is blocked. They frequently cause permanent damage requiring prolonged rehabilitation and often significantly reduced self-care potential and quality of life. In these cases diabetes management should be discussed with the family or carers who will be responsible for assisting the person with diabetes.

The risk factors for cerebrovascular disease are similar to those for cardiovascular disease. High BMI >25 kg/m² and systolic hypertension increase risk of death after a stroke among men (Chen 2008). However, there appear to be some significant differences between men and women. Women may have worse outcomes after acute stroke than men if they do not receive thrombolytic therapy, and women are more likely to benefit from thrombolytic therapy than men (Lutsep 2008). Likewise, healthy women over age 65 benefit from alternate day aspirin (100 mg) to prevent stroke but aspirin has not been shown to prevent strokes in healthy men (Ridker *et al.* 2005). However, the NPS, SIGN. NICE and ADA guidelines regarding aspirin use should be considered.

There are also gender differences in response to treatment and outcome following acute stroke. Women with carotid artery stenosis have a lower risk of recurrent stroke than men and receive less benefit from surgical treatment of moderate carotid artery stenosis than men (Alamowitch *et al.* 2005). Women with intracranial stenosis are at higher risk of recurrent stroke than men (Williams *et al.* 2007).

Poor sleep quality is linked to increased risk of vascular events including stroke; and daytime sleepiness could be an independent risk factor for stroke conferring a 4.5-fold increased risk (Boden-Albala 2008) (Chapter 10).

Signs and symptoms

- A careful history will elicit failing mental function.
- Carotid bruits are usually present and can be evaluated using Doppler studies.
- Angiography is required in symptomatic cases.

Management

There is limited evidence concerning managing stroke in people with diabetes. The preventative measures outlined for cardiovascular disease apply to cerebrovascular disease. Acute stroke is managed the way as for people without diabetes, but hyperglycaemia and hyoglycaemia should be avoided Blood glucose monitoring will aid decisions about titrating GLM medicine doses and the dose regimen.

Carotid endarterectomy is indicated if the carotid arteries are significantly narrowed. Low-dose aspirin may be beneficial considering the risks and benefits.

Management in a stroke unit improves outcomes and optimal collaboration among care providers in the emergency department and stroke unit is essential. Nursing responsibilities include care during investigative procedures (see Chapter 9). Rehabilitation focuses on returning the person to optimal functioning and independence within their capabilities. Observational data suggests there is an association between blood glucose in the first 24-hours and mortality and infarct size. ADS (2012) recommends maintaining blood glucose ~ 10 mmol/L and avoiding hypoglycaemia <5 mmol/L.

Middleton *et al.* (2011) developed a treatment protocol, Fever, Hyperglycaemia Swallowing (FeSS), for managing stroke in the first 72 hours following an acute stroke. The protocol involves:

- Monitoring and documenting fever every 4 hours and treating fever >37.5 with paracetamol, IV, rectally or orally unless contraindicated.
- Monitoring venous blood glucose on admission and capillary glucose every 1–6 hours.
- Commencing an IV saline infusion and deliver for 6 hours when blood glucose is between 8 and 11 mmol/L in people with diabetes or 8 and 16 mmol/L in people without diabetes.
- Commencing an IV insulin infusion if the blood glucose is >11 mmol/L in people with diabetes and if the blood glucose is >16 mmol/L in non-diabetics.
- Screening for dysphagia and clearly documenting the findings in the person's medical record. Middleton *et al.* developed an education program to train nurses to undertake dysphagia screening. Speech therapists usually undertake such assessments. People who were managed using the FeSS protocl had better outcomes after discharge.

Middleton *et al.* like other stroke researchers, used a combination of strategies and it is difficult to separate the different contribution of the IV insulin infusion. The *combination* may be the important element. However ADS (2012) choose not to include the FeSS study in their review when developing guidelines for managing hyperglycaemia in hospital.

Other important assessments after the acute phase include functional ability and mental health as well as social support and whether the home environment requires modification. Rehabilitation programmes can help people improve physical functioning and independence. Driving assessment needs to be undertaken following a stroke and assessed regularly; see Chapter 10.

DIABETES AND EYE DISEASE

Key points

- Encourage independence. People with visual loss are capable of caring for themselves if they are provided with appropriate sight aids and information. However, vision impairment has a profound impact on an individual's ability to learn diabetes self-care tasks and on their psychological well-being.
- Becoming blind is a significant fear for people with diabetes.
- Maintain a safe environment.
- Orient patient to the environment and staff.
- Explain procedures carefully, fully recognising that the person is probably not a visual learner.
- Return belongings to the same place.
- Use appropriate teaching style to the individual's learning style.

Rationale

Retinopathy is a significant complication of diabetes. Prevention and early identification of people at risk are essential. Nurses need to be aware of the impact of visual loss on the self-care and psychological well-being of people with diabetes and their role in preventative care. Other vision changes occur in people with diabetes in addition to diabetic retinopathy, for example macular degeneration is common in older people. Age-related macular degeneration might be related to elevated levels of high-sensitivity CRP. Cataracts and glaucoma are common in people with diabetes but also occur in non-diabetics.

Introduction

Vision impairment and blindness are significant complications of diabetes. Blindness occurs in 50–60 people/100 000 people with diabetes (Cormack *et al.* 2001). Most people with diabetes do not have sight-threatening retinopathy but if they have macular oedema and/or proliferative retinopathy it must be treated to reduce the progression to vision impairment. Screening programmes have enabled early identification and treatment of early retinal changes and reduced the progression to sight-threatening retinopathy.

The specific cellular mechanisms that lead to reduced visual acuity have not been defined. (Antonetti *et al.* 2006) proposed a combined nerve and vascular mechanism that causes loss of neurons, which compromises neurotransmission and altered structure and function of retinal cells types. Macular cysts could scatter light and reduce the quality of the image and/or visual function could decline as a result of fluid accumulation in the retina. The neurons are susceptible to circulating amino acids, antibodies and/or inflammatory cells that reach the retina through leaking capillaries. The vascular leakage can affect vision even when macular oedema is not present (Antonetti *et al.* 2006).

Kim et al. (2012) found an association between 1,5-anhydroglucitol (1,5-AG), a marker of postprandial hyperglycaemia, and diabetic retinopathy especially in people with 'moderate' glucose control but not albuminuria. The authors suggested 1,5-AG could be used as a marker to target people at risk of retinopathy. There is also evidence that cognitive ability declines over time in people with diabetes and may be linked to complications such as proliferative retinopathy (Ryan *et al.* 2003).

Key changes in the eye include:

- Maculopathy: macular oedema and macular ischaemia. The macular may be distorted or elevated or vitreous haemorrhages may occur and distort the ocular media (Antonetti *et al.* 2006).
- Retinopathy: stages of retinopathy have been described based on a system of photographic grading that requires comparison with a standard set of photographs showing different features and stages of retinopathy (DRS 1981; EDTRS 1991).
- Generalised ocular oedema.
- Lens opacity: cataract.
- Papillopathy: optic disc swelling that occurs in Type 1 diabetes.

Some degree of retinopathy occurs in almost all people with Type 1 diabetes after 20 years duration of diabetes and 70% of people with Type 2 diabetes (DRS 1981; DCCT 1993). Retinopathy occurs as a result of microvascular disease that manifests as increased capillary permeability and closure of the retinal capillaries, which causes vascular leakage, retinal oedema, and accumulation of lipids that is seen as hard exudates in the retina and retinal ischaemia.

Risk factors for retinopathy

The factors that lead to an increased risk of retinopathy are similar to the risk factors for other complications and include:

- long duration of diabetes;
- poor metabolic control;
- renal disease with microalbuminuria and proteinuria;
- hyperlipidaemia, especially hypertriglyceridaemia, which contribute to macular exudates and oedema;
- low haematocrit;
- pregnancy in people with diagnosed diabetes. Pregnancy may exacerbate existing retinopathy (see Chapter 14) but it does not usually develop in women with gestational diabetes;
- smoking, although the effect of smoking on the development and progression of retinopathy is unclear;
- hypertension.

People with diabetic eye disease are at greater risk of developing other diabetes-related complications unless they are screened regularly, take appropriate preventative action and treatment is commenced early.

Vision impairment from non-diabetic causes can coexist with diabetes. People with diabetes also have an increased incidence of glaucoma and cataracts and there is an increasing correlation with age-related macular degeneration. Many of the underlying causes that lead to macular degeneration are also associated with diabetes; see Table 8.2, which depicts risk factors for age-related macular degeneration (Lim 2006). Many of these risk factors are similar to the risk factors for diabetic retinopathy and the same risk reduction strategies apply to both conditions. The table shows modifiable and non-modifiable factors. Sun exposure, and iris and hair colour do not appear to be associated with AMD (Khan *et al.* 2006).

Table 8.2 Risk factors for age-related macular degeneration (Data from Lim [2006]).

Modifiable factors	Non-modifiable factors
Cigarette smoking, the risk increases with long duration of smoking	Increasing age: for both exudative and non-exudative AMD[1]
Diet high in fats especially monounsaturated and polyunsaturated fats. Linoleic acid increases the risk for advanced AMD	Ethnicity. AMD is more prevalent in Whites. Especially for the components of late AMD, increased retinal pigmentation and retinal pigment
Omega-3 fatty acids are associated with lower risk High GI[2] food is related to the development of retinal pigmentation abnormalities (Chui *et al.* 2006). Emerging research suggests a diet rich in fruit and vegetables especially carotenoids may help prevent AMD. Vitamins C and E and zinc (van Leeuwen *et al.* 2005)	epithelial depigmentationCataracts and glaucoma are more common in Blacks
High BMI[3]. The risk of developing AMD increases with increasing BMI and geographic atrophy could be associated with high BMI, low education and antacid use (Clemons *et al.* 2005)	Genetic inheritance
Hypertension is associated with exudative AMD but not non-exudative AMD Hypercholesteraemia is also associated with exudative AMD	
Inflammation. Recent studies suggest C-reactive protein is associated with intermediate and advanced AMD (Seddon *et al.* 2004)	

AMD: age-related macular degeneration.
GI: glycaemic index.
BMI: body mass index.

Poor vision can be a significant disadvantage during diabetes education and general living because most diabetic and general health information contains essential visual components .

Practice points

(1) The shape of the lens changes with changes in blood glucose concentrations, leading to refractive changes and blurred vision. This usually corrects as the blood glucose is normalised, but may take some time if the blood glucose has been high for a long time.

(2) Vision can worsen in the short term when blood glucose control begins to improve, for example, when commencing insulin and during pregnancy.

(3) The temporary vision disturbance creates significant stress for the person with diabetes and a careful explanation is needed.

Eye problems associated with diabetes

(1) One-third of people with diabetes have retinopathy as a result of microvascular disease. The incidence is related to the duration of diabetes. Sixty per cent of people with diabetes and duration of more than 15 years have some degree of retinopathy,

especially women. Up to 30% people with Type 2 diabetes have retinopathy at diagnosis (4%–8% is sight-threatening). There is increasing evidence that ACE inhibitors can reduce the risk of microvascular disease (see Chapter 5).

(2) People can have severe eye damage without being aware of it. Vision is not always affected and there is usually no pain or discomfort.

(3) Cataracts are more common in people with diabetes.

(4) Maculopathy is the most common cause of visual loss in people with diabetes.

(5) Sudden loss of vision is normally an emergency. It may be due to:
   • vitreous haemorrhage;
   • retinal detachment;
   • retinal artery occlusion.
   Reassurance, avoidance of stress and sudden movement, and urgent ophthalmo-logical assessment are required.

(6) Prevention and early detection are important aspects in the management of visual impairment. It involves:
   • Good blood glucose control can slow the rate of progression in Type 1 diabetes (DCCT 1993).
   • Regular eye examinations commencing at diagnosis in Type 2 and from age 12 in Type 1. Screening should be undertaken annually if retinopathy is present of every two years it there is no retinopathy (SIGN 2010).
   • Using an ophthalmoscope opportunistically during regular appointments.
   • 7-field stereoscopic photography with the pupils dilated to investigate macula oedema and proliferative retiopathy
   • Retinal photography or slit lamp biomicroscopy
   • Confocal microscopy is increasingly being applied to diabetes complication screening, especially to detect eye changes and neuropathy. Confocal micros-copy enables greater contrast to be achieved and three-dimensional images to be created that show great detail. The technique uses a spatial pinhole to elimi-nate out of focus light and flare. It enables faster diagnosis, is non-invasive and painless.
   • Fluorescein angiography is still sometimes used.

(7) Laser treatment is very effective in preventing further visual loss. Vitrectomy if there is evidence of persistent vitreous haemorrhage. Cataract extraction should not be delayed when indicated. Advanced cataracts need to be removed or stabilised prior to surgery and reviewed closely in the postoperative period (SIGN 2010).

(8) Medicines include intravitreal Triamcinolone, which reduces retinal thickness in the short term and improves visual acuity but may not have long-term benefits. Small studies suggest Simvaststin reduces oedema and improves visual acuity (Sen et al. 2002) and Atorvastation reduced the severity of hard exudates after laser treatment in people with Type 2 diabetes and high lipids (Gupta et al.2004). Although there is some befefits using antivascular endothelia growth factor (VEGF) in combination with laser therapy, there is insufficient evidence recommend using VEGF routinely (SIGN 2010).

Clinical observation

Eye drops occasionally cause pain and increased pressure in the eye some hours after they were instilled. If this occurs the patient should be advised to call the doctor.

Resources for people with visual impairment

People with significant visual loss often require assistance to perform blood glucose monitoring and to administer their own insulin. It is important to encourage independence as far as possible. Careful assessment is important and should include assessment of the home situation.

Vision Australia and the Royal National Institute for the Blind in the UK and similar organisations in other countries offer a variety of services for people who have degrees of visual loss. These services include:

- assessing the home situation to determine whether modifications are necessary to ensure safety at home;
- low vision clinics;
- talking library and books in Braille;
- training on how to cope in the community with deteriorating vision.
- Guide dogs. It takes time to train a dog to guide a blind person and time for a person to learn to work with a guide dog, usually through a harness, and for the person to recognise tactile and sound clues to complement their knowledge of the environment. Several factors can affect the individual's ability to work with a guide dog including loss of sensitivity in hands or feet, hypoglycaemia, which affects concentration and sometimes behaviour (Stanway 2012). Interestingly, dogs can perform more than one kind of medical assistance and actually enjoy the extra work (medical detection dogs). For example, they can be trained to become familiar with chemical markers associated with diabetes and can detect hypoglycaemia and fetch the person's hypo kit or alert another person. A recent report in the author's local newspaper described a how a blue heeler dog, which was deaf, was learning to recognise sign language.

Other help includes:

- Services such as pensions, which may be available from the government.
- A range of diabetes products are available that can help vision impaired people remain independent (see next section).

The community nurses and home-based services play a major role in maintaining vision-impaired people in their own homes, especially when they are older.

Aids for people with low vision

Various magnifying devices are available to help people continue to care for themselves. They can be obtained from diabetes associations and some pharmacies specialising in diabetes products. Other aids include:
(1) Insulin administration:
- Instaject devices, clicking insulin pens;
- chest magnifying glass (available from some opticians); Magniguide – fits both 50 and 100 unit syringes and enlarges the markings;
- location tray for drawing up insulin if syringes are used.
(2) Blood glucose monitoring:
- strip guides for accurate placement of the blood on to the strips;
- talking blood glucose meters, blood pressure monitors, and talking weight scales;
- meters with large result display areas.

(3) Medications:
  • dosette boxes, which can be prefilled with the correct medication;

Nursing care of visually impaired patients

Aims of care
• To encourage independence as far as possible.
• To ensure the environment is safe when the patient is mobile.

People confined to bed
(1) Introduce yourself and address the patient by name, so the patient is aware that you are talking to them.
(2) Ascertain how much the patient is able to see. (Few people are totally blind.) Assess whether the blood glucose fluctuates at certain times. High and low levels can interfere with clear vision. Plan education to avoid these times and determine measures that can avoid such fluctuations, for example, appropriate timing of meals and medications. Dexterity and cognitive function may also be impaired especially in the elderly and hamper diabetes education. Visual impairment increases the risk of falls in elderly patients (see Chapter 12).
(3) Some people prefer a corner bed because it makes location easier, avoids confusion with equipment belonging to other patients and enables greater ease in setting up personal belongings.
(4) Introduce the patient to other people in their ward or close by.
(5) If you move the patient's belongings they must be returned to the same place.
(6) Explain all procedures carefully and fully before commencing. (An injection when you can't see it and don't expect it can be very unnerving.)
(7) If eye bandages are required, make sure the ears and other sensory organs are not covered as well.
(8) Consider extra adjustable lighting for those patients with useful residual vision.
(9) Mark the person's medication with large print labels or use a dosette.
(10) A radio, talking clock, talking watch, Braille watch, or a large figured watch, helps the patient keep orientated to time and place.
(11) Indicate when you are leaving the room and concluding a conversation.

People who are mobile
(1) A central point like the person's bed helps them orient around the room.
(2) When orientating a person to a new area, walk with them until they become familiar with the route.
(3) Keep obstacles (trolleys, etc.) clear of pathways where possible.

Meal times
(1) Describe the menu and let the person make a choice.
(2) Ensure the person knows their meal has been delivered.
(3) Ask 'Do you need assistance with your meal?' rather than say, 'I will cut your meat for you.'
(4) Colour contrast is important for some patients. A white plate on a red tray-cloth may assist with location of place setting.
  When the person has a guide dog, provide water in hot weather bur remember the dog is doing a job. Ask the owner's permission before patting the dog or offering treats, which can distract the dog and confuse it.

DIABETES AND RENAL DISEASE

Key points

- Diabetes is the most common cause of renal disease.
- Measuring microalbuminuria is a useful method of detecting abnormal renal function. Microalbuminuria indicates early renal disease and predicts cardiovascular disease in people with diabetes.
- Microalbuminuria predicts severe hypoglycaemia in people with Type 2 diabetes.
- Hypertension is an early indicator of renal disease.
- There is a strong association between retinopathy and renal disease. Women with diabetes have greater prevalence of advanced kidney disease than men with diabetes, especially among older people.
- People with diabetes and nephropathy are at increased risk of cardiovascular disease.

Introduction

Diabetic nephropathy is a significant microvascular complication of diabetes and diabetes is the second most common cause of end-stage renal disease in Australia and the UK (ANZDATA 2000; Department of Health 2001). There is a similar initial disease progression in both Type 1 and Type 2 diabetes. Eventually, microalbuminuria occurs in up to 20% of people with Type 1 diabetes and in a similar percentage of people with Type 2. Some cultural groups are at significant risk, for example, Aboriginal and Torres Strait Islander Peoples and Afro-Caribbeans.

Stages of chronic kidney disease

Kidney disease is progressive unless it can be prevented and is usually classified according to the following stages:

	GFR ml/min/1.73 m²
(1) Kidney damage with normal glomerular filtration rate (GFR)	>90
(2) Kidney damage with mild reduction in GFR	60–89
(3) Moderately reduced GFR:	
a. 3A	45–59
b. 3B	30-44
(4) Severe reduced GFR	15–29
(5) End stage renal failure	<15

Proteinuria must be present to diagnose stages 1 and 2. People on dialysis are classified as stage 5D and people with a functioning renal transplant are denoted by the suffix 'T.'

Proteinuria is an important marker for cardiovascular disease in Type 2 diabetes.

Prediction equations that improve the inverse correlation between serum creatinine and GFR have been developed and take account of variables that affect the relationship, for example:

- Cockcroft-Gault equation, which estimates creatinine clearance, which encompasses age, gender, weight and creatinine.
- Four variable formula used in the Modification of Diet in Renal Disease (MDRD) study, which encompasses age, gender and ethnicity.

Risk factors for renal disease

There is a strong link between hypertension and the progression of renal disease. The risk of end-stage renal failure increases as the diastolic blood pressure increases to >90–120 mmHg . Other risk factors include:

- Smoking, which represents a significant and dose-dependent risk.
- Hyperglycaemia, predialysis control is an independent predictor of the outcome in people with Type 2 diabetes on haemodialysis (Wu *et al.* 1997). The Diabetes Control and Complications Trial (DCCT) demonstrated that good control of blood glucose delayed the rate and progression of microvascular disease including renal disease (DCCT 1993).
- The presence of microalbuminuria and proteinuria are independent risk factors for the development and progression of renal disease in people with diabetes (Keane 2001). People with diabetes are at risk of renal disease if they have any of the following. The more of these factors present the greater the risk:
  - A urine albumin excretion rate in the upper range of normal (20–30 mg/day).
  - Systolic blood pressure >130 mmHg.
  - HbA_{1c} >9%. Preventing and managing hyperglycaemia reduces the development of renal disease.
  - Total cholesterol >5.2 mmol/L (Sheldon *et al.* 2002). Duration of diabetes exceeding 5 years (Kerr 2008). Treatment includes minimising proteinuria using ACEIs and ARBs, often in combination. Hyperkalaemia is a risk when ACEI and ARBs are combined but may not be significant.
  - Tests for microalbuminuria include timed urine collections (12- or 24-hour collections) usually on an outpatient basis, but compliance is poor. The spot albumin–creatinine urine test, which corrects the albumin level for the urine concentration, is the optimal screening test for early renal disease. A level >3.5 mg/mmol most likely indicates early renal disease (Kerr 2008). However, alternative causes of proteinuria such as nephrosclerosis and hypertensive renal disease should be considered: The estimated GFR (eGFR), which approximates the GFR rate and is based primarily on serum creatinine as well as age and gender, gives a reasonable approximation of the GFR (Kerr 2008). However, renal function declines with age by approximately one mL/min/year after age 25. Thus, approximately 60% of people over age 65 will have an eGR in the normal range (60–90 mL/min).
  - Hypertension, which is a risk factor for cardiovascular disease and kidney disease, and the risk is continuous and independent of other cardiovascular risk factors (Committee on the Prevention, Detection, Evaluation, and Treatment of High Blood Pressure: Chobanian *et al.* 2003). Most people with advanced renal disease develop hypertension. If not controlled, hypertension can accelerate the rate of decline in renal function. If the cycle from hypertension to renal impairment can be halted, fewer people would require dialysis(Nurko 2004). Thus, good blood pressure control is important and is the single most effective measure to slow the progression of renal disease. The Australian and New Zealand Society of Nephrology and Diabetes recommend that everybody with diabetes and microalbuminuria or nephropathy should be treated with an ACE- inhibitor and recommend a target blood pressure of 130/85 in people over 50 years and 120/70–75 in people younger than 50 years. The Guidelines also advise that multiple antihypertensive agents might be needed.
- presence of retinopathy (Gilbert *et al.* 1998);
- long duration of diabetes;
- male gender, although a recent study suggests women are more at risk of diabetes-related renal disease than men with diabetes, especially in the older age group (Yu *et al.* 2012).
- increasing age.

However, people with Type 2 diabetes often have microalbuminuria at diagnosis, which is consistent with the fact that impaired glucose tolerance or diabetes is often present for many years before it is diagnosed. Thus screening should begin at diagnosis in Type 2 diabetes. Microalbuminuria is rarely present in Type 1 diabetes at diagnosis so screening usually begins at ~5 years duration of diabetes. However, people with LADA may present differently and screening might need to be commenced earlier in these patients.

Practice points

(1) False-positive results can occur after heavy exercise or if the person has an UTI.
(2) Women with diabetes may develop proteinuria during pregnancy and the cause should be investigated to ensure the protein is not an early sign or preeclampsia especially if they also present with hypertension.
(3) If a person develops heavy proteinuria in a short period of time other cause should be investigated.
(4) Serum creatinine alone is a poor indicator of renal status in older people. Underweight and overweight are risk factors for misclassifying the degree of renal dysfunction (Giannelli *et al.* 2007).

Renal failure

Early referral to a nephrologist is imperative to improve the long-term outcomes especially when dialysis or transplantation may be needed. However, collaboration with diabetes and other relevant experts must still occur. Late referral is associated with higher morbidity and mortality rates in people on dialysis even when they survive the first year on dialysis (Cass *et al.* 2002). Nephrologists can advise about managing issues associated with renal failures such as:

• Calcium and phosphate abnormalities
• Calcific medial stenosis, which contributes to cardiovascular disease. Phosphate binders might be prescribed to manage the problem if the phosphate is >1.6 mmol/L.
• Managing anaemia, which might include erythropoietin as well as iron, vitamin B12.
• Preparing the person for dialysis.

Renal failure, often requiring dialysis, occurs in 25% of people diagnosed with diabetes before the age of 30. The presence of mild renal disease increases the risk of cardiovascular disease even with only small elevations of urinary protein, but the relationship is not clear. The presence of other cardiovascular risk factors increases the risk, and endothelial cell dysfunction may play a part. Angiotensin converting enzyme (ACE) inhibitors have been shown to delay or stabilise the rate of progression of renal disease and to decrease cardiac events (Keane 2001; Kerr 2008).

The development of renal problems is insidious and frank proteinuria may not be present for 7–10 years after the onset of renal disease. Microalbuminuria, on the other hand, is detectable up to 5–10 years before protein is found in the urine. Regular urine collections to screen for microalbuminuria are still used in some places controlling blood glucose and blood pressure, the use of ACE inhibitors (Type 1) and angiotensin receptor blockers (Type 2) and avoiding nephrotoxic agents can attenuate renal and cardiac disease (Gilbert & Kelly 2001).

ACE inhibitors have been shown to be more effective than other antihypertensive agents in reducing the time-related increase in urinary albumin excretion and plasma creatinine in Type 2 diabetes and in people with other cardiovascular risk factors, heart failure and myocardial infarction (Ravid *et al.* 1993). Likewise, the HOPE and MICRO-HOPE studies demonstrated that ACE inhibitors reduced cardiovascular events and overt nephropathy whether or not microalbuminuria was present (HOPE 2000). An ARB can be used in people with Type 1 diabetes do not tolerate ACE and people with Type 2 should be treated with ACE and/or ARB (SIGN 2010). However ACE and ARBs are more effective in Caucasians than Blacks of African descent and the benefits need to be assessed in these people.

Great care should be taken if IV contrast media are required for diagnostic purposes; see Chapter 9. Contrast-induced nephropathy (CIN) is defined as renal dysfunction following any investigative procedure where radi-opaque contrast media were used (Rudnick *et al.* 2006). Most episodes of CIN do not cause oliguria but result in a rise in serum creatinine ~2 days after the procedure, which usually returns to pre-procedure levels within a week. CIN occurs in 7–15% of patients and up to 50% in high risk groups such as people with diabetes, with a mortality rate of 14% (Rudnick *et al.* 2006).

Risk factors for CIN are:

- pre-existing renal disease;
- increasing age;
- congestive heart failure;
- hypotension;
- using large volumes of contrast media;
- the type of contrast media used;
- presence of anaemia;
- diabetes.

In addition to diabetes *per se*, people with diabetes are likely to have greater than two other risk factors for CIN, which puts them in a very high-risk group. A rise in serum creatinine by 25% is an indicator of CIN but the inaccuracy of creatinine in various states has been outlined. Therefore, eGFR may be a better marker.

The Australian Adverse Drug Reactions Bulletin (2008) issued a warning about using gadolinium-containing contrast agents in people with renal impairment because of the risk of nephrogenic systemic fibrosis (NSF). The incidence of NSF may vary between the different gadolinium agents available. Renal function should be assessed in all patients before using gadolinium, especially if they are in a high-risk category and the risks and benefits of using gadolinium carefully considered.

Using as low a volume of contrast media as possible and ensuring the person is well hydrated are important preventative measures (Meschi *et al.* 2006). However, recent research suggests IV sodium bicarbonate administered seven hours before procedures involving radio contrast media reduces the incidence of CIN from 15% to 2% (Briguori 2007). Research is currently underway to determine whether oral sodium bicarbonate will be effective.

Renal function can decline in critically ill patients especially people with diabetes and is associated with high morbidity and mortality (Schetz *et al.* 2008). For example, hyperglycaemia and insulin resistance are common in critically ill patients with and without diabetes. Associations between interoperative hyperglycaemia during cardiac surgery, cardiac catherisation, total parenteral nutrition, and acute kidney injury have been noted. Intensive insulin therapy in these settings is renoprotective. The incidence of oliguria, and the need for renal replacement therapies (dialysis) is reduced (Schetz *et al.* 2008). The authors suggested insulin improves the lipid profile and reduces nitric oxide levels and oxidative damage, as well as controlling hyperglycaemia.

Over 50% of patients on GLMs with significant renal disease require insulin therapy. Insulin requirements often reduce in people already on insulin because insulin, like many other medicines, is degraded and excreted by the kidney. Kidney damage can delay degradation and excretion of many medicines and prolong their half-life, increasing the risk of unwanted side effects and medicine interactions. The medicine/s dose, or dose interval may need to be altered.

The American Society of Nephrology (2012) released new recommendations to avoid unnecessary testing and reduce costs as part of the 'Choosing Wisely' campaign. The recommendations are not specific for diabetes and stress the need for close collaboration between the patient and their doctors and the following key recommendations:

- Avoid cancer screening in people receiving dialysis who have limited life expectancy unless they have signs and symptoms of cancer.
- Do not administer erthropoiesis-stimulating medicines if the person had haemoglobin >10 g/dl unless they have symptoms of anaemia.
- Avoid nonsteroidal anti-inflammatory agents in people with hypertension, heart failure or chronic kidney disease from all causes including diabetes.
- Avoid placing peripherally inserted central catheters in people with stages 3–5 renal disease without consulting a nephrologist.
- Avoid initiating chronic dialysis without discussing all the issues with the person concerned and their carers and other health professionals.

Renal disease and anaemia

Anaemia occurs as a consequence of chronic renal insufficiency. Renal anaemia occurs earlier in people with diabetes than in people without diabetes. It is more severe and is associated with other factors such as erythrocyte abnormalities and increased osmotic stress that are associated with decreased erythropoietin production (Bosman *et al.* 2001; Ritz 2001). As renal function declines the anaemia becomes more marked. Anaemia is associated with fatigue, decreased quality of life, depression, left ventricular hypertrophy, decreased exercise capacity, malaise, and malnutrition. Annual testing is recommended on people with renal disease stages 3–5. Anaemia is treated with recombinant human erythropoietin (rhEPO) in conjunction with intravenous iron.

Clinical observation

To date there has been little, if any, focus on monitoring haemoglobin (Hb) as part of routine biochemical monitoring or diabetes complication screening in patients with renal impairment. Dunning *et al.* (2012) demonstrated Hb can be determined in point of care testing at the same time as blood glucose tests are performed, provided staff are trained to use the equipment.

Diet and renal disease

Improving nutritional status can delay end-stage renal failure (Chan 2001 & 2008). Nutritional needs are individual and depend on the stage and type of renal disease. The aim is to maintain homeostasis and electrolyte balance, decrease uraemic symptoms and regularly reassess dietary requirements to ensure changing needs are addressed

(National Kidney Foundation 2002). The nutritional goals for people with renal disease need to be individualised and assessed regularly to ensure they are appropriate for the degree of renal damage. The goals focus on:

- Maintaining a desirable body weight, body composition and nutritional status and prevent protein loss (Protein Energy Wasting).
- Control accumulation of uraemic toxins.
- Control uraemic symptoms and its consequences such as nausea.
- Manage blood glucose and lipids.
- Maintain fluid and electrolyte balance, which may involve fluid restriction.
- Manage comorbidities such as blood glucose, reducing salt intake or omitting salt (hypertension), maintaining calcium, phosphate and vitamin D balance (bone disease and hyperparathyroidism, calcific medial arteriosclerosis), reducing lipids (cardiovascular disease), maintaining iron, folate, and vitamin B12 (anaemia).
- Improve graft survival if the person receives a transplant.

Specific goals apply to the stages of CK:

- Stages 1–4: the predialysis stages: the aim is to slow the progression of renal disease and preserve remaining renal function.
- Stage 5 end stage renal disease: conservative management, control symptoms and provide nutritional support. Stage 5 on dialysis: replace dialysis nutrient losses, which include protein and water-soluble vitamins.
- Stage 5 transplant: manage side effects of immunosuppressant medicines, manage. Monitor dietary needs (Chan 2012).

Conversations about management options, preparing for end-of-life care and preparing advanced care directive may be appropriate in any of these stages but especially stage 5. The diet generally comprises:

- 15–20% of protein in daily intake but low protein diet, 0.6 g/kg/day, might be required to slow the declining eGFR. 0.8 g/kg/day is recommended to alleviate uraemic symptoms. Protein requirements increase once dialysis is implemented. Protein sources should supply all the essential vitamins and minerals.
- Carbohydrates should contribute 50%–60% of the total daily energy. When protein requirements change in advanced renal disease, extra carbohydrates are sometimes needed.
- Fat intake should be about 30% of daily total energy and where possible should come from unsaturated fat, but the proportion may increase in advanced kidney disease. Mono- and polyunsaturated fats are preferred. People on dialysis and those who have a renal transplant require a low fat diet.
- Vitamin and mineral supplements may be required, especially when dialysis commences, for example iron, and water-soluble vitamins e.g. B12 and C as well as vitamin D.

Protein and energy malnutrition are common and need to be corrected to prevent catabolism, lipid metabolism, and anaemia. Sodium restriction is often recommended, but salt substitutes should not be used because they are usually high in potassium and can increase the serum potassium, usually already elevated in renal disease.

Anorexia is often a feature of renal disease and food smells can further reduce appetite and predispose the patient to malnutrition. Small frequent meals may be more appealing. Malnutrition has implications for the individual's immune status and phagocyte function and increases the risk of infection (Churchill 1996). Referral to a dietitian is essential.

Malnutrition is prevalent in haemodialysis patients and has a high mortality rate (Lopes *et al.* 2007). Lack of appetite is a significant predictor of malnutrition and is related to inflammation and may link protein-energy malnutrition in these patients. However, appetite varies and is often lower on haemodialysis days. This predisposes the person to hypoglycaemia in the short term and malnutrition in the long term. Lopes *et al.* (2007) suggested asking people with diabetes on haemodialysis about their appetite in the past four weeks or asking them to keep a food and appetite diary for 3–4 days is helpful. The Kidney Disease Quality of Life-Short Form (KDQOL-SF) (Hays *et al.* 1994) includes questions about appetite.

Depression, the presence of several coexisting comorbidites, cachexia, using oral medicines, being older, and women on haemodialysis are particularly at risk of malnutrition. As anorexia increases markers of malnutrition decreases (serum albumin, creatinine, nPCR, and BMI) (Lopes *et al.* 2007) (see also Chapters 4 and 12).

Renal disease and older people

Older people with renal disease are at increased risk of adverse medicine events. A wide range of medicines are used in older people and some may need dose adjustments especially digoxin, ACE inhibitors, narcotics, antimicrobials, and GLMs (Howes 2001). Long-acting agents are contraindicated because of the risk of hypoglycaemia (see Chapters 5 and 6). Medicine therapy needs to be closely monitored along with monitoring renal function and nutritional status and non-medicine alternatives used where possible.

Practice points

(1) Lower rates of creatinine are produced by older people and creatinine clearance rates can be misleading especially in people with low muscle mass.
(2) Renal disease is an important cause of medicine toxicity in older people, necessitating a hospital admission.

Kidney biopsy

See Chapter 9. Extra care is required for people with renal disease undergoing renal biopsy. A pressure dressing should be applied to the site and the patient should lie supine after the procedure for six hours. The blood pressure should be monitored and fluids encouraged to maintain urine output unless fluid is restricted. Activity should be reduced for two weeks.

Renal dialysis

Dialysis can be used in the management of diabetic kidney disease. Dialysis is a filtering process, which removes excess fluid and accumulated waste products from the blood. It may be required on a temporary basis or for extended periods of time. Some patients may eventually receive a kidney transplant. Several forms of dialysis are in use.

Haemodialysis

Blood is pumped through an artificial membrane then returned to the circulation. Good venous access is required and special training in management. Haemodialysis is usually

administered three times per week. A recent Canadian study suggests frequent nocturnal haemodialysis (six times per week) is associated with improved left ventricular
mass, fewer antihypertensive agents, improved mineral metabolism and improvements
in some aspects of quality of life (Culleton 2007).

Hypotension is common when haemodialysis therapy is first commenced. Management
consists of:

- An appropriate haemodialysis prescription.
- Minimising interdialytic fluid gains by setting limits on fluid intake.
- Elevating the foot of the bed.
- Differentiating between disequilibrium syndrome and hypoglycaemia.
- Advising the patient to sit on the edge of the bed or chair to allow the blood pressure
  to stabilise before standing (Terrill 2002).
- Maintaining good glycaemic control. Significantly, >50% of people with diabetes on
  haemodialysis have HbA_{1c} >7%, especially those with long duration of diabetes,
  microvascular disease and on insulin (Iliescu 2007). These findings probably reflect
  advanced diabetes and may not be due to haemodialysis. However, given the amount
  of glucose in dialysate it is imperative that HbA_{1c} be as close to normal as possible
  without causing excess hypoglycaemia to reduce the risk of infection and other complications. Iliescu (2007) suggested it may not be possible to achieve good control
  with medicines and suggested insulin pumps might be a useful strategy. Significantly
  poor glycaemic control is linked to lower survival rates in patients on haemodialysis
  (Oomichi *et al.* 2007).

Strict aseptic technique and careful patient education are essential when managing dialysis therapies. Patients with CKD are susceptible to infections due to abnormal immune
function, which is likely to be worse in people with diabetes and hyperglycaemia where
neurophil function is abnormal and malignancies (Choudhury & Luna-Salazar 2008).
Mucocutaneous barriers are often disrupted secondary to skin excoriation from pruri-
tis, xerosi and sweat gland atrophy. Common bacterial infections include *Staphylococcus
species, Escherichia coli, Klebsiella* and *Mycobacterium tuberculosis*. Viral infections
are also common. Strict aseptic technique and careful patient education are essential
when managing dialysis therapies.

Peritoneal dialysis

The filtering occurs across the peritoneum. This form of dialysis is an excellent method
of treating kidney failure, in people with and without diabetes. The uraemia, hypertension, and blood glucose can be well controlled without increasing the risk of infection,
if aseptic techniques are adhered to. However, infection is a significant risk and is often
the reason people change to haemodialysis.

Continuous ambulatory peritoneal dialysis (CAPD)

CAPD is a form of peritoneal dialysis in which dialysate is continually present in the
abdominal cavity. The fluid is drained and replaced 4–5 times each day or overnight if
the patient is on automated peritoneal dialysis (APD). The person can be managed at
home, which has psychological advantages, once the care of equipment is understood
and the person is metabolically stable. CAPD can also be used postoperatively to control uraemia related to acute tubular necrosis or early transplant rejection.

Insulin added to the dialysate bags achieves smoother blood glucose control because
the insulin is delivered directly into the portal circulation and is absorbed in the dwell

phase, which is closer to the way insulin is normally secreted after a glucose load. However, it also has disadvantages and is an infection risk and is not always recommended.

The usual insulin dose may need to be increased because of glucose absorption from the dialysate fluid (and to account for insulin binding to the plastic of the dialysate bags and tubing if it is added to the dialyslate bag). The continuous supply of glucose and lactate in the dialysate fluid are calorie-rich energy sources and can lead to weight gain and hyperglycaemia. The art is to calculate insulin requirements to avoid hyperinsulinaemia, which carries its own complication risks. Glucose-free solutions such as Nutrimeal and glucose polymers may help reduce complications associated with high insulin and glucose levels (Rutecki & Whittier 1993). Insulin is usually administered subcutaneously if the person is on APD. Many renal dialysis units do not advocate adding insulin to dialysate bags due to the increased risk of infection.

Priorities of dialysis treatment

(1) remove waste products and excess fluids from the blood (urea and creatinine);
(2) to provide adequate nutrition and safe serum electrolytes, and to prevent acidosis;
(3) patient comfort;
(4) to prevent complications of treatment;
(5) to provide information and support to the patient;
(6) to ensure privacy.

Objectives of care

The individual's ability to carry out self-care tasks needs to be assessed early when considering renal replacement therapies. Changed joint structure due to oedema and tissue glycosylation (e.g. carpel tunnel syndrome) can limit the fine motor skills required to manage CAPD. Visual impairment due to retinopathy frequently accompanies renal disease and if present, can limit self-care abilities.

(1) To assess the patient carefully in relation to:
   • knowledge of diabetes;
   • preventative healthcare practices;
   • ability to use aseptic technique;
   • usual diabetic control;
   • presence of other diabetic complications;
   • support available (family, relatives);
   • motivation for self-care;
   • uraemic state.
(2) To ensure thorough instruction about administration of dialysate and intraperitoneal medication (insulin).
(3) To ensure a regular meal pattern with appropriate carbohydrate in relation to dialysate fluid.
(4) To maintain skin integrity by ensuring technique is aseptic especially in relation to catheter exit site and skin care.
(5) To monitor urea, creatinine, and electrolytes carefully.
(6) To provide psychological support.
(7) To encourage simple appropriate exercise.
(8) To ensure adequate dental care and regular dental assessments. Poor oral health causes chronic inflammation and is a site of infection. Untreated uraemia is

associated with stomatitis and patients on dialysis are prone to gingivitis and peridontitis. Prophylactic antibiotics for dental procedure may be advisable (Choudhury & Luna-Salazar 2008).

(9) To prevent pain and discomfort, especially associated with the weight of the dialysate.
(10) To ensure the patient reports illness or high temperatures immediately.
(11) Monitor for infections and advise people to have preventative vaccines such as influenza and pneumococcal vaccination and an annual screen for tuberculosis. Regular screening for nasal *staphylococcal* infections, certain types of malignancy may also be indicated, for example, renal cell carcinoma, prostate cancer, breast, and cervical cancer.

Nursing responsibilities

(1) Meticulous skin care.
(2) Inspect catheter exit site daily, report any redness, swelling, pain or discharge.
(3) Monitor fluid balance carefully:
  • measure all drainage;
  • maintain progressive total of input and output;
  • report a positive balance of more than 1 litre: the aim generally is to achieve a negative balance to maintain the dry weight.
(4) Monitor blood glucose.
(5) Monitor temperature, pulse, and respiration, and report abnormalities.
(6) Monitor nutritional status – intake and biochemistry results.
(7) Weigh daily to monitor fluid intake and nutritional status.
(8) Ensure patency of tubes and monitor colour of outflow. Report if:
  • cloudy;
  • faecal contamination;
  • very little outflow (tube blocked).
(9) Report lethargy and malaise that can be due to uraemia or high blood glucose levels.
(10) Warm dialysate before the addition of prescribed drugs and before administration to decrease the possibility of abdominal cramps.
(11) Oral fluid intake may be restricted – provide mouth care and ice to suck.
(12) Assess self-care potential:
  • blood glucose testing;
  • adding medication to bags;
  • aseptic technique;
  • psychological ability to cope.
(13) Protect the kidney during routine tests and procedures by avoiding dehydration and infection (Chapter 9).

Commencing CAPD in patients on insulin

A 24-hour blood glucose profile is often undertaken prior to commencing intraperitoneal insulin to assess the degree of glycaemia and calculate insulin requirements. The glucose profile should be carried out following catheter implantation, with the patient stabilised on a CAPD regimen. One method consists of:

(1) Obtaining venous access for drawing blood samples.
(2) Obtaining hourly blood glucose levels for 24 hours.

(3) Sending at each bag change:
- 10 mL new dianeal fluid for glucose analysis;
- 10 mL drained dianeal fluid for glucose and insulin analysis to the appropriate laboratory.

One protocol for administering insulin to people with diabetes on CAPD based on four bag changes each day is:

(1) Calculate usual daily requirement of insulin and double it.
(2) Divide this amount between the four bag changes.
(3) The overnight bag should contain half the daytime dose. Some centres only administer 10% of the total daily dose at night.

Example

usual total insulin units	= 60 units
multiply this amount by 2	= 120 units
divide 120 units by 4 exchanges	= 30 units
3 daily exchanges	= 30 units/bag
overnight exchange	= 15 units/bag

Adjustments for the dextrose concentration of the dialysate may be necessary. Intraperitoneal insulin requirements are usually one-third higher than the amount needed before CAPD.

Practice point

Many renal units no longer recommend adding insulin to dialysis bags because of the risk of infection.

Subcutaneous insulin via an insulin pump using a basal bolous regimen could be an effective way of administering insulin to people receiving dialysis providing absorption was affected and the individual has the knowledge and skills to manage the insulin pump.

Educating the patient about CAPD

The patient should be instructed to:

(1) Not have a shower or bath for the first 5 days after the catheter is inserted.
(2) Always carefully wash hands prior to changing the bags.
(3) Wear loose fitting clothes over exit site.
(4) Examine feet daily for signs of bruising, blisters, cuts or swelling.
(5) Wear gloves when gardening or using caustic cleaners.
(6) Avoid hot water bottles and electric blankets because sensory neuropathy can diminish pain perception and result in burns.
(7) Avoid constrictive stockings or wearing new shoes for a long period of time.
(8) Wash cuts or scratches immediately with soap and water and apply a mild antiseptic (e.g., betadine ointment). Any wound that does not improve within 24–36 hours or shows signs of infection (redness, pain, tenderness) must be reported promptly.

(9) Bag exchanges should be carried out 4–6 hours apart. The person may be on APD having overnight exchanges.
(10) Only short-acting clear insulin must be used in bags.
(11) Adjust insulin doses according to diet, activity, and blood glucose levels and at the physician's discretion.
(12) Accurately monitor blood glucose 4-hourly. A blood glucose meter may be required.
(13) Provide written information.

Immediate help should be sought if any of the following occur:

- decreased appetite;
- bad breath/taste in mouth;
- muscle cramps;
- generalised itch;
- nausea and vomiting, especially in the morning;
- decreased urine output;
- signs of urinary infection such as burning or scalding.

Supportive care

Some people, especially older people, may require supportive care if they are not suitable for or choose not to have dialysis or a renal transplant. Supportive care is generally conservative (Moustakas *et al.* 2012). Although some experts differentiate supportive care from palliative care, they have similar goals and encompass shared decision-making, promoting autonomy, optimal functioning within the person's capabilities, maintaining quality of life and comfort. End of life care should be part of shared decision-making and documented in an Advanced Care Plan (Chapter 18).

Renal disease and herbal medicine (see also Chapter 19)

People with end-stage renal failure often try complementary therapies to alleviate the unpleasant symptoms of their disease. Some therapies, for example, aromatherapy to reduce stress and maintain skin condition, or counselling for depression, are beneficial and usually safe. Herbal medicines are popular with the general public but they may not be appropriate for people with renal disease (Myhre 2000).

The kidneys play a key role in eliminating medicines and herbal products from the system. Some of these medicines and herbs can cause kidney damage that may be irreversible and put already compromised renal function at great risk. In addition, some herbal products, particularly those used in traditional Chinese medicine (TCM) are often contaminated with drugs, heavy metals and other potentially nephrotoxic products (Ko 1998). Frequently these contaminants are not recorded in the list of ingredients in the product. As well as the direct effect of the herbs on the kidney, the intended action of particular herbs can complicate conventional treatment.

An herb, *Taxus celebica*, used in TCM to treat diabetes, contains a potentially harmful flavonoid and has been associated with acute renal failure and other vascular and hepatic effects (Ernst 1998). Kidney damage can be present with few specific overt renal symptoms; therefore, it is vital that kidney and liver function is closely monitored in people taking herbs, especially if kidney function is already compromised by diabetes.

Potentially adverse renal effects include:

- electrolyte imbalances, for example, *Aloe barbedensis*;
- fluid imbalances, for example, *liquorice root*;
- hypokalaemia, for example, *Aloe, Senna*;
- kidney damage, for example, *Aristolochia*.

In addition, herbal and conventional medicine interactions may occur; see Chapter 19.

Practice points

(1) Nurses must know when their renal patients are taking herbal medicines so that their kidney function can be closely monitored. People should be asked about the use of complementary therapies periodically.
(2) Conventional medicines can also cause significant renal damage and dose adjustments may be needed or alternative medicines used, for example, NSAID, statins, OHA.

PERIPHERAL AND AUTONOMIC NEUROPATHY

Key points

- Lower limb problems represent a significant physical, psychological, social, and economic burden for people with diabetes and the health system.
- Forty to seventy per cent of lower limb amputations occur in people with diabetes.
- Peripheral neuropathy, vascular disease, infection, foot deformity, and inappropriate footwear predispose people to foot disease.
- Screening for foot disease and preventative self-care practices is essential.
- Foot complications are common in older people.
- A multidisciplinary team approach and good communication are essential to optimal management.
- Many subgroups of neuropathy occur, including mononeuropathy, peripheral, and autonomic neuropathy. The two most common forms are discussed in this chapter are: peripheral and autonomic neuropathy.

Introduction

Peripheral neuropathy is present in >20% of people with Type 1 diabetes after 20 years duration of diabetes and is already present at diagnosis in 10% of people with Type 2 at diagnosis and 50% by 20 years duration of diabetes. Peripheral neuropathy leads to inability to sense pressure and pain in the feet, dry skin, reduced joint mobility, bony deformity, and problems with balance, which increases the risk of falling. Common foot deformities associated with diabetes are claw toes, hammer toes, *hallus valgus, haalus rigidus* callus, flattened or high foot arches, Charcot's feet and amputation sites. These changes mean the normal cushioning that protects the feet during usual activities are deficient and the foot is at high risk of injury.

Foot ulcers occur in ~25% of people with diabetes: ~25% develop an infection, 20–60% of ulcers involve bone (osteomyelitis) and 34% present with a recurrent ulcer/ year. Careful assessment, consideration of the causative factors, and managing the existing problems can limit further exacerbation of diabetic foot disease. Appropriate nursing care can prevent foot problems occurring as a result of hospitalisation or placement in an aged care facility.

Diabetic foot disease is a common cause of hospital admissions and is associated with long length of stay: 59% longer than for non-foot admissions, and significant morbidity and mortality. Significantly, foot ulcers also occur during hospital admissions. Diabetic foot disease is a heterogeneous disease entity, defined as a group of syndromes that lead to tissue breakdown. Infection, neuropathy, and ischaemia are usually present and increase the risk of infection (Apelqvist & Larsson 2000).

Foot disease and its management have an adverse impact on the well-being and quality of life of people with diabetes (Brod 1998). The disease itself and some management practices, for example, non-weight-bearing regimes restrict physical activity and social interaction and often result in non-adherence.

Foot care self-care and foot care in hospital is an extremely important aspect of the nursing care of people with diabetes in any setting. Significantly, preventative foot care is often neglected in acute care settings. The combination of mechanical factors and vascular and nerve damage as a complication of diabetes leads to an increased risk of ulceration, infection, and amputation. In older people, these factors increase the risk of falling. An estimated 40% of people with diabetes have peripheral neuropathy but it occurs in up to 50% of older people (Boulton 2005) and 20% of hospital admissions are for foot-related problems. Not surprisingly, peripheral neuropathy is associated with significantly impaired quality of life and effects on energy, pain, mobility, and sleep (Papas *et al.* 2103).

Forty to seventy per cent of lower limb amputations occur in people with diabetes and most begin with an ulcer. The amputation rate can be reduced by preventative foot care. The spectrum of diabetic foot disease varies globally depending on socioeconomic circumstances, but the basic underlying pathophysiology is the same (Bakker 2000). Charcot's deformity is a severe form of diabetic foot disease that is often missed through misdiagnosis in the early stages and delay in appropriate management. The possibility of Charcot's deformity should be considered in any person with long-standing diabetes, neuropathy, and foot disease.

Vascular changes

People with diabetes and peripheral vascular disease are predisposed to atherosclerosis, which is exacerbated by chronic hyperglycaemia, endothelial damage, nonenzymatic tissue glycosylation, and polyneuropathy. These conditions impair vascular remodelling. The risk increases when the individual smokes, has hypertension and hypelipidaemia.

(1) *Macrovascular* (major vessel) disease may lead to:
   • intermittent claudication and rest pain;
   • poor circulation to the lower limbs which leads to malnutrition, tissue hypoxia, and delayed healing if any trauma occurs in this area. The injured tissue is prone to infection and gangrene can result.
(2) *Microvascular* (small vessel) disease leads to thickening of capillary basement membranes, poor blood supply to the skin and tissue hypoxia, predisposing the feet to infection and slow healing.

Infection

Foot infections are a common and serious problem in people with diabetes. They are prone to infections and non-healing wounds. Foot infection occurs as a result of skin ulceration or deep penetrating injuries, for example, standing on a drawing pin. These injuries can go unnoticed for days because the person does not feel pain if they have peripheral neuropathy. They act as a portal for infection that can involve tissues at all levels and foot structures including bone. The diagnosis of an infected wound is based on clinical signs. These include purulent discharge or two or more of erythemia, swelling, local heat, and pain. These signs may also indicate the presence of Charcot's foot rather than infection and alkaline phosphatase, ESR, X-ray, and/or MRI may be indicated (Papas *et al* 2013), samples should also be collected to determine what organisms are present in the wound. The samples need to be collected from deep within the wound after the wound has been debrided or biopsy samples from the base of the wound rather than superficial swabs.

Acute infections are usually due to aerobic Gram-positive cocci such as *Staphylococcus aureus* or β-*haemolytic streptococci* especially if the individual has limited exposure to antibiotics previously. Chronic ulcers and deep infections are often due to Gram-negative bacilli and anaerobic organisms such as *Escherichia coli, Klebsiella, Proteus, Bacteroides*, and *Peptostreptococcus* with *Staphylococcus aureus* is also likely to be present, sometimes as the only pathogen but usually in combination with other pathogens (Lipsky & Berendt 2000; Papas *et al* 2013).

Charcot's foot is a relatively common, under-diagnosed condition that complicates management of the neuropathic foot and can lead to significant pain, mobility deficits, and amputation (Piaggesi *et al*. 2005). Charcot's foot is due to the progressive destruction of the bones and joints in neuropathic diabetic feet secondary to inflammation following trauma, which is usually not recognised by the person with diabetes. Inflammation is followed by sclerosis, which leads to changes in the bony architecture of the foot and reduces the capacity to reduce subsequent everyday stress such as walking. Reactivation of the inflammatory process increases bone reabsorption and increases the risk of further trauma. Higher rates of foot fractures and Charcot's feet have been observed in patients following successful pancreas transplants and those on long-term corticosteroid therapy, possibly because these medicines reduce bone resistance to minor trauma (Jeffcoate *et al*. 2000). Regular assessment of bone densitometry may be indicated in people on long-term corticosteroids.

Managing diabetic foot pathology requires a collaborative team approach and includes:

- Admission to hospital for a thorough foot and clinical assessment including self-care ability, bed rest, administration of broad-spectrum antibiotics, which needs to be continued after the acute phase resolves and surgical procedures if indicated.
- Broad-spectrum antibiotics are usually commenced initially until the results of the wound swabs are known and may be given IV for severe infections. Antibiotic therapy may be required for 1–2 weeks and up to 6 weeks if osteomyelitis is present. The risk of the person developing antibiotic resistance must be considered and every effort made help them to prevent recurrent foot infections. The person should be asked whether they are allergic to penicillin before commencing antibiotic therapy. Flucloxacillin can be used for superficial infections and cellulitis if the person is not allergic to penicillin. Cephalexin can be used for minor infections and Clindamycin for severe infections. If the infection is deep, Augmentin or a combination of ciprofloxacin and Clindamycin may be indicated.
- X-ray (although the classical finding of osteomyelitis are not usually seen on plain X-ray until 10–21 days after the onset of bone infection), MRI bone scans to determine

Table 8.3 Medicines used to manage diabetic peripheral neuropathy. Usually medicines are started at a low dose and titrated up to maximal doses over a few weeks depending on symptoms (Data from Semla et al. 2002; Boulton 2005).

Medicine	Dose range and frequency	Side effects	Cautions and contraindications
Antidepressants **Tricyclic** Amitriptylline[a] Desipramine[b] Doxepin[a] Impramine[a] Nortriptyline[b]	10–25 mg QID maximum dose 300 mg/day When ceasing these medicines the dose should be reduced slowly over 2–4 weeks to prevent withdrawal syndrome	Constipation, dry mouth, blurred vision, cognitive changes, tachycardia, urinary hesitation, sedation Secondary amines have fewer effects. Older people are more likely to experience side effects and lower doses and slower titration is recommended	**Caution**: angle-closure glaucoma, benign prostatic hyperplasia, urinary retention, constipation, cardiovascular disease, impaired liver function **Contraindications**: second- or third-degree heart block, arrhythmias, prolonged QT interval, severe liver disease, recent acute MI
Venlafaxine	75 mg	Nausea	
Anticonvulsants Carbamazepine Gabapentin Approved for people over 18 years Lamotrigine	100 mg BD or QID maximum 1200 mg/day 300 mg QID maximum 3600 mg/day pain relief may only occur at higher doses 50 mg QID maximum 700 mg/day	Somnolence, dizziness, ataxia, fatigue, occasionally tremor, diplopia, nystagmus Ataxia, blurred vision, incoordination, diplopia Rarely Stevens–Johnson syndrome, angioedema	**Caution**: liver function tests and full blood count before commencing and repeat 2-monthly for 2 months then annually **Contraindication**: bone marrow depression **Caution**: renal dysfunction
Miscellaneous medicines Clonidine Oral or Weekly transdermal patch Mexiletine	0.1 mg maximum 2.4 mg/day Usually a last resort 200 mg 8 hourly maximum 1200 mg/day An IV 'lidocaine test' may be performed to predict the response to Mexiletine (an oral congener of Lidocaine). It targets superficial pain: allodynia, burning and tingling	Hypotension, dry mouth, dizziness, sedation, constipation, sexual dysfunction Local skin irritation with patches Gastrointestinal symptoms, dizziness, tremor, irritability, nervousness and headache, seizures at high doses	**Cautions**: cardiac abnormalities, cardiac symptoms should be evaluated before commencing **Contraindicated**: second- or third-degree heart block
Topical agents Lidocaine patch Topical nitrate to the feet may relieve burning Capsaicin	5% maximum 4 patches/day Depletes substance P and may be most effective for localised pain Wear gloves to apply		
Opioid analgesics Recent trials support some efficacy and they may have a role as add-on therapy Tramadol Controlled release oxycodone	Sustained relief for up to 6 months	Somnolence, nausea, constipation, dependence	

PN: peripheral neuropathy; QID: four times per day; BD: twice per day.

[a] Secondary amines.

[b] Tertiary amines.

whether osteomyelitis is present and determine the extent of the soft-tissue injury. If it is a long course of antibiotics and/or amputation is indicated. Alkaline phosphatase 135U/L, ESR >70 mm/hour and/or being able to feel bone when probing the base of the wound are suggestive of osteomyelitis.

- Bone densitometry or ultrasound may be indicated.
- Surgical débridement to clean the wound and appropriate dressings. Referral to the wound care nurse and/or infectious disease team may be warranted.
- Revascularisation, for example, femoral/popliteal bypass, or amputation if indicated.
- Selection and application of appropriate wound dressings (Edmonds *et al.* 2000; Harding *et al.* 2000).
- Pressure off-loading to improve blood supply to the foot. Biomechanical measures such as total contact casts to relieve pressure in high-pressure ulcers and Charcot's foot deformity. Casts enable the person to remain mobile thus improving their social and psychological wellbeing. Infection and subsequent oedema must be managed because they aggravate the pressure on muscles and can lead to muscle necrosis. In hospital settings high specification foam mattresses make a significant difference in preventing neuropathic foot ulcers. Prefabricated walkers are also used but must be correctly fitted.
- Improving blood glucose control and diet to ensure optimal neutrophil functioning and nutrition to promote wound healing.
- Dietetic assessment.
- Counselling to stop smoking if relevant.
- Rehabilitation including regular podiatric assessment. Footwear and orthotics may need to be modified.

Practice points

(1) Swabs need to be taken from deep in the ulcer cavity, which can be painful and analgesia may be required. Superficial swabs often do not identify all the organisms present, particularly anaerobes.

(2) Hyperglycaemia inhibits wound healing. Thus, people undergoing amputations and other surgical procedures are at high risk of post-operative infections. Good metabolic control, optimal nutrition and aseptic technique reduce the risk.

Diabetes-related peripheral neuropathy

Diabetic neuropathy is defined as the presence of clinical or subclinical evidence of peripheral nerve damage, which cannot be attributed to any other disease process (Boulton *et al.* 1998). Neuropathy can affect the sensory nerves resulting in pain, tingling, pins and needles, or numbness. These symptoms are often worse at night. The sensory loss results in insensitivity to pain, cold, heat, touch, and vibration. The patient may not detect trauma, pressure areas, sores, blisters, cuts, and burns. Callous formation, ulceration and bone involvement can occur.

The motor nerves can also be affected, resulting in weakness, loss of muscle fibres and diminished reflexes. Both types of nerves can be affected at the same time. Medications may not be effective in the treatment of neuropathic pain, but some commonly used medicines prescribed to manage the discomfort are shown in Table 8.3.

Differentiating between the different types of nerve fibres involved allows a more targeted approach to pain management. Where unmyelinated C-fibres are affected, characterised by burning, dysthetic pain, capsaicin or Clonidine may be effective. Where the alpha fibres are involved the pain is often deep and boring and insulin infusion, lignocaine or gabapentin may be effective (Vinik *et al.* 2000). Often both types of fibres are affected.

Medicines under study include a-Lipoic acid, an antioxidant that scavenges free radicals and has been shown to reduce pain when administered parenterally (Ziegler *et al.* 2004). Preliminary studies suggest the protein kinase C inhibitor (LY33531) improves allodynia, and prickling pain (Litchy *et al.* 2002). C-peptide has recently been shown to improve early neurological abnormalities in people with Type 1 diabetes with established clinical neuropathy (Brismar *et al.* 2007). It is given subcutaneously QID and appears to be most effective when baseline neuropathy is mild. Aldose reductase inhibitors have been under study for many years with various degrees of success. Recent research suggests Epalrestat improves objective and subjective measures of peripheral neuropathy and might slow the progression of retinopathy (Hotta 2006).

Other pain management strategies

Other non-medicine options with varying degrees of evidence to support their benefits include:

- Physiotherapy and exercise such as Tai Chi to maintain muscle tone and strength.
- Percutaneous nerve stimulation, static magnetic field therapy, low intensive laser therapy, bodyflow technology, and monochromatic infrared light. These techniques might improve peripheral circulation, and reduce local oedema, which reduces some of the local pressure and relieves local pain.
- Acupuncture, which has benefits up to six months (Abusaisha *et al.* 1998).
- Other non-medicine measures include improving blood glucose control, stopping smoking, reducing alcohol intake, and eating a healthy diet.

The autonomic nervous system may also be affected by diabetes. Autonomic nervous system involvement may lead to an absence of sweating, which causes dry, cracked skin, and increases the risk of infection. Other effects of autonomic neuropathy include gastric stasis, erectile dysfunction, hypoglycaemic unawareness, and incontinence. The small muscle wasting secondary to longstanding neuropathy can lead to abnormal foot shapes, for example, clawing of the toes, making the purchase of well-fitting shoes difficult.

Vascular disease, neuropathy, and infection are more likely to develop if there is longstanding hyperglycaemia, which contributes to the accumulation of sorbitol through the polyol pathway, leading to damage to the nerves and small blood vessels. Figure 8.1 illustrates the inter-related factors that lead to foot problems in people with diabetes.

Table 8.4 lists changes in feet due to the normal ageing process. These factors should all be incorporated in the nursing assessment to ensure that appropriate foot care is part of the overall management of the patient.

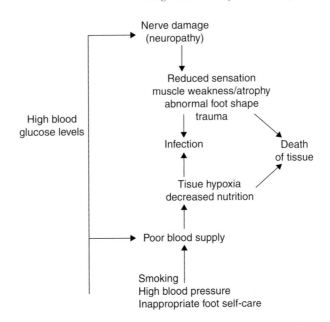

Figure 8.1 Diagrammatic representation of the factors leading to foot problems in people with diabetes.

Table 8.4 Changes in feet due to normal ageing.

(1) Skin becomes thin, fragile
(2) Nails thick and often deformed
(3) Blood supply is reduced
(4) Nerve function often impaired
(5) Muscle weakness and wasting
(6) Arthritis, may lead to pain and deformity

Stages of peripheral neuropathy

- Chronic and painful – improve metabolic control.
- Acute and painful – analgesia.
- Painless – education, orthoses, regular assessment.
- Late complications (Vinik *et al.* 2000).

Risk factors for developing foot problems

(1) Diabetes, especially if blood glucose is continually high.
(2) Smoking: people with chronic neuropathic pain are twice as likely to smoke as those with chronic nociceptive pain but this might not represent a causative effect (Todd *et al.* 2008). Some studies suggest nicotine has a mild analgesic effect.
(3) Obesity.
(4) High blood pressure.
(5) Cardiovascular disease.
(6) Lack of or inadequate foot care, which is likely to be multifactorial including inability to reach the feet and lack of knowledge.
(7) Vision impairment.
(8) Inappropriate footwear.

(9) Delay in seeking help.
(10) Previous foot problems and amputation.
(11) Depression.

These factors should be part of the nursing assessment. The more risk factors present the greater the likelihood of amputation (Pecorara 1990). Routine assessment to detect neuropathy and associated foot changes should be part of regular health assessment in primary care.

Objectives of care

(1) To assess the individual's risk of developing a foot ulcer by screening at least annually. The result of a structured foot examination can be entered into online screening tools such as the SCI-DC, which automatically stratifies the risk and recommends a management plan. Risk stages and key factors entered into the SCI-DC are:
  - high risk: active ulcer, infection, ischaemia, and/or gangrene;
  - moderate risk: previous ulcer and/or amputation, more than one risk factor such as reduced sensation, callous;
  - moderate risk: one risk factor such as peripheral vascular disease;
  - high risk: no risk factors present.
(2) Identify feet most at risk of trauma, ulceration and infection in aged care, rehabilitation, and hospital settings by assessing vascular, nerve, and diabetic status:
  - *Sensation* using 10 g Semmes–Weinstein monofilaments, 128 Hz tuning forks and disposable pin prickers (Apelqvist and Larson 2000); recently, a new non-invasive test that can be undertaken by the person with diabetes was developed and is said to have 87% sensitivity and 66% specificity (Papas *et al.* 2013)). The test, the indicator plaster neuropad (IPN) can be performed in 10 minutes and might be a useful screening tool to incorporate into the individual's foot self-care regimen.
  - *Presence of vascular insufficiency* by checking capillary return and the presence of foot and peripheral pulses; Doppler ultrasound, toe pressures, and transcutaneous oxygen measurement are used in some centres.
  - *Foot deformity.*
(3) To assess patient knowledge of foot care.
(4) To reinforce appropriate preventative foot care.
(5) To prevent trauma, infection, and pressure ulcers.
(6) To treat any problem detected.
(7) To refer to podiatry, orthotics, physiotherapy, rehabilitation, diabetes nurse specialist/diabetes educator or specialist foot clinic as necessary.
(8) To control or eliminate any factors which predispose the patient to the risk of foot problems in hospital.
(9) Risk of falls in the elderly (see Chapter 12).
(10) Pain management.

Nursing responsibilities

(1) Prevent neuropathic ulcers occurring in people with diabetes and peripheral neuropathy during a hospital admission.
(2) To assess the feet carefully on admission. Assess self-care potential (can the patient reach the feet, see clearly?). When assessing the feet, obtain information about:
  (a) Past medical history:

- glycaemic control;
- previous foot-related problems/deformities;
- smoking habits;
- nerve and vascular related risk factors;
- claudication, rest pain;
- previous foot ulcer/amputation;
- alcohol intake.

(b) Type of footwear (socks, shoes):
- hygiene;
- activity level.

(c) Social factors:
- living alone;
- older.

(3) When examining the feet:
- *Check both feet*;
- check pulses, dorsalis pedis, posterior tibial;
- assess toenails: thick, layered, curved, ingrowing toenails will need attention;
- note foot structure; overlapping toes, prominent metatarsal heads on the sole of the foot;
- check for callous, cracks and fungal infections that can indicate inadequate foot care and poor hygiene.

(4) Note also:
- pallor on elevation of leg;
- capillary return (normally 1–2 seconds);
- any discoloration of legs;
- hair loss on the feet.

(5) To ensure appropriate foot hygiene:
- wash in lukewarm water – use pH-neutral soap products that do not dry the skin especially in older people or people on steroid medications and those with atopic skin;
- check water temperature with wrist before putting the patient into a bath;
- dry thoroughly, including between toes;
- apply cream to prevent dryness and cracks (urea cream, sorbelene).

(6) Ensure Elastoplast/Band Aids, bandages do *not* encircle toes as they can act like tourniquets and reduce the circulation, which could result in gangrene. Apply elastic support stockings correctly.

(7) Maintain a safe environment:
- use a bed cradle;
- ensure shoes are worn if walking around the ward;
- strict bed rest may be necessary while the ulcer is healing;
- maintain aseptic technique.

(8) Check feet daily and report any changes or the development of any callus, abrasion or trauma.

(9) Monitor blood glucose control.

(10) Attend to dressings and administer antibiotics according to treatment order. Antibiotics are often given intravenously if foot infection is present.

(11) Take the opportunity to ensure self-care knowledge is current and that complication screening has been attended to. Ensure preventative foot care education is provided, to give the patient with diabetes:
- an understanding of effects of diabetes on the feet;
- a knowledge of appropriate footwear;
- the ability to identify foot risk factors;

- an understanding of the principal effects of poor control (continual hyperglycaemia) on foot health;
- knowledge about the services available for assistance with their diabetes care and how to obtain advice about foot care;
- knowledge about appropriate foot care practices, in particular that they must inspect their feet daily and seek help early if any problems are found;
- odour control can be an issue when infection and gangrene are present. Some wound dressings have an absorbent layer that eliminates odour by absorbing bacteria. Good foot hygiene helps reduce the odour.

Classification of foot ulcers

A number of ulcer classification systems are in existence and nurses are advised to follow the system in their place of employment. In 2002 an international working party was established to develop an international consensus foot ulcer classification system. Foot ulcers can be loosely classified as:

(1) clean, superficial ulcer;
(2) deep ulcer, possibly infected, but no bone involvement;
(3) deep ulcer, tracking infection and bone involvement;
(4) localised gangrene and necrosis (usually forefoot, heel);
(5) extensive gangrene of foot.

The depth and width of the ulcer should be recorded regularly; a plastic template, dated and filed in the patient's history, aids in the assessment of changes in ulcer size. The presence, amount, and type of exudate must be recorded.

Clinical observation

Aromatherapy essential oils on the *surface of the secondary dressing* can help reduce wound odour. They should not be applied directly to the wound. They can be used in a vapouriser for environmental fragrancing. Some essential oils can help improve mood.

Wound management

Dressings may be needed to absorb the exudate and protect the foot. No dressing is appropriate for all wound types. Surgical débridement, amputation or an occlusive dressing may be required. It is important to keep the temperature at 37 °C, the dressing moist and the pH acidic to promote healing. Choose a dressing that does not cause tissue damage when it is removed, that is, does not stick to the wound and

Practice point

Painting the area with a betadine or other skin antiseptic is of little value. Coloured antiseptics can obscure some of the signs of infection.

protects the wound from infection. The moisture aids in pain relief, decreases the healing time and gives a better cosmetic result. An acidic environment promotes granulation tissue. The management of ulcers in hospital and other specific foot problems are listed in Table 8.5.

Diabetic foot ulcers heal slowly and bed rest is important. The patient may be otherwise well. Encourage independence with blood glucose testing and insulin administration. Refer for occupational therapy. The person may benefit from counselling if they are depressed.

Careful discharge planning is imperative:

- To ensure mobilisation and rehabilitation and that there is a safe environment at home.
- Interim placement in an extended care facility may be necessary.
- Assess the physical and social support available after discharge.

Table 8.5 Managing of specific foot problems while the person is in hospital or community settings.

Problem	Treatment
Burning, paraesthesia, aching	Assess neuropathic status Encourage person to walk Maintain euglycaemia Appropriate analgesia Manage depression if present
Pain	Foot cradle, sheepskin Analgesia
Dry skin, cracks	Clean, dry carefully, apply moisturiser, for example, urea cream, sorbelene A duromet can be used to evaluate skin hardness and identify areas of where plantar hyperkeratosis is likely to develop Plantar pressures, which can indicate force and workload
Claudication	Medications as ordered Rest Elevate feet Cardiovascular assessment; peripheral pulses, ankle/brachial pressure index (APBI), transcutaneous oxygen tension (Tcp O$_2$) Angiography
Foot deformity	Clinically evaluate and describe Estimate joint mobility Refer to podiatrist Physiotherapy Orthotist
Charcot's deformity	
Ulcers, infection	The presence of a lesion transforms an at-risk foot into an acute clinical emergency. Grade the ulcer, for example, University of Texas Staging System for Diabetic foot ulcers X-ray and MRI may be indicated to assess the depth Record the width and depth, for example, using a polyurethane sheet Refer to specific medical order Assess daily Make template to note change in size of ulcer Antibiotics Débridement, amputation

ABPI >0.9 normal; 0.9–0.5 indicates peripheral vascular disease is present; <0.5 indicates critical limb ischaemia. ABPI >1.3 usually indicates medial artery calcification (Monckerberg sclerosis), an indirect sign of autonomic neuropathy (Piaggesi *et al.* 2005).
TcpO$_2$ pressure <60 mmHg indicates local ischaemia; <40 mmHg indicates critical ischaemia. (Piaggesi *et al.* 2005).

> **Practice point**
>
> Orthopaedic patients with diabetes and foot or leg plasters should be encouraged *not* to scratch under the plaster, especially if they have 'at risk' feet. Damage can occur and remain undetected until the plaster is removed.

Wound management techniques under study

Several new wound management products for hard-to-heal ulcers are under study:

- platelet-derived growth factor applied topically to increase granulation;
- Hyaff;
- Dermagraft;
- Apilgraf;
- granulocyte-colony stimulating factor (Edmonds *et al.* 2000).

Hyperbaric oxygen may be beneficial in some serious ulcers. Oxygen is necessary for wound healing and hyperbaric oxygen can increase tissue oxygen levels and improves the killing power of phagocytes (Bakker 2000).

Rehabilitation

Despite the best care, amputations are required in 5–15% of people with diabetes presenting with a foot problem particularly in the presence of gangrene, non-healing ulcers, which may be associated with osteomyelitis and severe foot infection. A rehabilitation process is necessary once the acute stage has settled. Below-knee amputations give a favourable result even if the popliteal pulses are diminished (Steinberg 1991). The goals of rehabilitation are:

- Appropriate stump care. In the early stages this may involve bandaging to reduce oedema. Circular bandages should be avoided because they tend to act like tourniquets and reduce the blood supply to the stump. Analgesia should be available. Later, correctly fitting the stump into the socket of the prosthesis and regular inspection for the presence of infection or pressure areas.
- Prevent muscle contracture with regular physiotherapy.
- Help the person be as independent and active as possible.
- Ambulation with a prosthesis or wheelchair depending on the individual assessment. However, not all people with diabetes benefit from having a prosthesis, people who have advanced neurological disease such as stroke, Parkinson's disease, CCF, obstructive pulmonary disease, unstable angina, knee and hip contractures may not be suitable for a prosthesis. These people often have limited ability to mobilise even before an amputation. High risk of gangrene or infection in the other limb may warrant delaying an amputation.
- Early mobilisation in whatever capacity is usually desirable after amputation to reduce postoperative complications. The person will need to learn how to manage whatever mobilisation method is appropriate.
- Care of the stump is important to prevent wound contractures.

Practice points

(1) Amputation should not always be seen as treatment failure. It can relieve pain, enable the person to return home and enjoy an improved quality of life. Amputation is distressing for the person with diabetes and their family and careful explanation, support, and counselling are essential. The patient should be included in the decision-making process and make the final decision. Their social and psychological situation should be considered as well as their physical needs.

(2) Amputation increases the risk of a second amputation.

Autonomic neuropathy

Key points

- Often several organs are involved.
- Signs and symptoms are often non-specific.
- Autonomic neuropathy is often undiagnosed.
- Postural hypotension is the most significant sign of autonomic neuropathy.
- People with postural hypotension and nocturnal diarrhoea should be investigated for autonomic neuropathy.
- The progression to autonomic neuropathy is related to poor metabolic control.
- It is more common in people over 65 but it can occur in the first year after diagnosis.

Introduction

Autonomic neuropathy is a distressing condition for people with diabetes. It can cause erratic blood glucose readings. People are often accused of manipulating their food and/or diabetic medications, which causes stress and anxiety. The symptoms associated with the various manifestations of autonomic neuropathy can be uncomfortable, painful and have an adverse impact on the individual's quality of life. The autonomic nervous system plays an important role in the regulation of carbohydrate metabolism. Many processes are affected by autonomic neuropathy, for example it both facilitates and inhibits insulin secretion.

(1) Stimulates the right vagus nerve, which innervates the pancreatic islet cells, or the beta-adrenergic receptors in the islet cells, stimulates insulin secretion.
(2) Stimulates the alpha-adrenergic receptors in the islet cells decreases insulin secretion, which is an essential aspect of blood glucose regulation and to maintaining glucose homeostasis.

The autonomic nervous system also has a role in the conversion of glycogen into glucose in the liver where free fatty acids undergo further metabolism to ketones. Neurogenic stimulation of the hypo-pituitary axis results in cortisol secretion, one of the counter-regulatory hormones that have a role in correcting hypoglycaemia. In stress situations, especially prolonged stress, hyperglycaemia results.

Diabetes is the commonest cause of autonomic neuropathy but it also occurs in association with other diseases such as advanced Parkinson's disease and Guillain–Barre syndrome. Autonomic neuropathy is a common, under-diagnosed condition associated with a range of signs and symptoms, depending on the specific nerves and organs affected (Vinik *et al.* 2000; Aly & Weston 2002). It has a slow onset and affects up to 30–40% of people with diabetes, and although many people only have mild, often subclinical features, significant functional abnormalities can be present.

Rarely, in <5% of cases, overt clinical features develop. Autonomic neuropathy can involve any system, but commonly affects the heart, GIT, and genitourinary systems (Spallone & Menzinger 1997). The GIT is one of the most frequently affected systems but GIT problems, not associated with autonomic neuropathy, occur in 50% of the general population and are more common in people with diabetes (Lock *et al.* 2000). Older people are at risk of having many neuropathic GIT changes but some GIT changes are age-related or associated with the use of vasoconstrictive drugs (Aly & Weston 2002).

Delayed gastric emptying is present in 25%–55% of people with Type 1 and 30% with Type 2 (Wegener *et al.* 1990). Consequences of gastrointestinal autonomic neuropathy include early satiety, abdominal distension, reflux, stomach spasm, postprandial nausea, vomiting, altered medicine absorption and food absorption, malnutrition and glucose variability. In addition, it causes significant diabetes-related distress and reduces quality of life.

Practice points

(1) Autonomic neuropathy is physically uncomfortable and treatment options are limited. Where the GIT is involved, frequent adjustment to the food and medication regimen is often needed. Blood glucose monitoring is important to allow such changes to be made appropriately.

(2) Psychological distress is common. Support and understanding are important aspects of management.

The commonly affected systems and associated clinical manifestations are shown in Table 8.6.

Table 8.6 Organs commonly affected by diabetic autonomic neuropathy and the resultant clinical features.

Affected organ	Main clinical features	Consequences
Gastrointestinal tract (gastroparesis)	Decreased peristalsis Abdominal distension and feeling of fullness Early satiety Postprandial nausea Vomiting undigested food Diarrhoea, especially at night Depression	Weight loss Erratic blood glucose control Stomach may not be empty even after fasting, for example, for procedures
Urinary tract	Distended bladder Urine overflow Feeling of incomplete bladder emptying Stress incontinence Nocturia Vaginal mucous membrane excoriation in women	Silent urinary tract infection Falls in elderly people Sleep disturbance Uncomfortable sexual intercourse

Table 8.6 Continued.

Affected organ	Main clinical features	Consequences
Genitals	Erectile dysfunction in men. Indeterminate, if any effect in women Possibly vaginal dryness in older women	Psychological sequelae including depression Negative impact on sexual health
Cardiovascular system	Blood pressure: Postural hypotension Loss of diurnal variation Dizziness when standing Resting tachycardia Reduced sympathetic tone Decreased beta-adrenergic responsiveness	Silent myocardial infarction Stroke Falls
Lower limbs	Reduced sweating Reduced blood flow Reduced pain Redness Defective thermoregulation	Foot ulcers and infection Sleep disturbance
Brain	Cognitive impairment	Reduced self-care ability
General	Excessive sweating, especially of the upper body, resembling a hot flush and sometimes mistaken for hypoglycaemia Slow pupillary reaction Heat intolerance	Trauma Depression

Note: Many of these conditions predispose elderly people to falls (see Chapter 12).

Diagnosis and management

Special tests are required to make a definitive diagnosis. The particular test depends on which organs are being tested, for example, gastric emptying times for the GIT, Valsalva manoeuvre for the cardiovascular system and voiding cystourethrogram to determine the effects on the bladder. In many cases specific treatment is commenced on the basis of the clinical history and assessment.

Management consists of:

(1) Adopting preventative strategies early by:
  - improving blood glucose control and lipid levels;
  - treating hypertension;
  - regular complication screening;
  - adequate self-care;
  - being aware that antioxidants may have a role in preventing oxidative tissue damage and pre- and probiotics may have a role in maintaining normal gut flora and reducing inflammation, although evidence specify to gastric autonomic neuropathy is limited (Chapter 1).
(2) Direction when present.

Treatment is often by trial and error and is aimed at alleviating the unpleasant symptoms. Preventative measures should be continued. Treatment for specific autonomic neuropathic conditions consists of:

(a) Gastrointestinal tract
  - Dietary management depends on the degree of malnutrition present and the symptoms. Frequent small, light, easily digested or fluid meals that are low in fat

and fibre and contain a consistent proportion of carbohydrate place less burden on the gastrointestinal tract and reduce glucose variability (Sadiya 2012). Large meals and fat delay gastric emptying and exacerbates the already slow gastric emptying time. It is imperative to ensure essential protein, vitamins and minerals are consumed; thus, people with severe malnutrition might need supplements and/or enteral feeding (Chapter 4). Consuming a liquid diet when the symptoms are worse sometimes helps.
- Manage distress and depression.
- GLM medicine dose usually need to be adjusted frequently, thus a basal bolous or insulin pump provides the greatest flexibility
- Stimulants such as caffeine, alcohol and tobacco should be avoided. Likewise chewing gum increases air swallowing and contributes to bloating, and foods that contain mint, chocolate, fat and caffeine lower oesophagal sphincter pressure.
- Medications such as Metoclopramide and Cisapride may give some relief but should not be used continuously.
- Antibiotics such as Tetracycline or Trimethoprim, may be required to treat bacterial overgrowth that occurs as a consequence of gastric stasis.
- Cholestyramine can be used to chelate bile salts, which immobilise the gut.
- Treating constipation, nausea, and vomiting as they occur.
- Elevating the head of the bed to use gravity to assist gastric emptying.
- Anecdotally gentle abdominal massage and compresses help reduce spasm and relieve bloating and constipation.
- Jejunostomy is a last resort.

(b) Cardiovascular system
- Support garments such as stockings or a body stocking to support venous return and relieve stress on the heart. They should be put on while the person is lying down.
- Managing postural hypotension – finding a balance between increasing the pressure on standing and preventing hypertension when lying. Fludrocortisone or Midodrine can be used. Medications should be reviewed to exclude drugs that precipitate postural hypotension.

(c) Genitourinary
- Urinary catheterisation and self-catheterisation. Sometimes parasympathomimetic drugs are also used.
- Managing erectile dysfunction with drugs such as Sildenafil, intracavernosal injections or mechanical and implanted devices and counselling (see Chapter 17).

(d) General measures
- Adjusting insulin or OHAs and diet to cater for the erratic blood glucose profile.
- Topical glycopyrrolate to alleviate gustatory sweating.
- Stopping smoking.
- Careful explanations about autonomic neuropathy and counselling to address the psychological consequences and treatment options.
- Encouraging activity.

Nursing care

Nursing care is palliative and supportive in nature. Providing a safe environment and reducing the risk of falls is essential, especially in older people, to prevent trauma, for example, fractures. This could involve ensuring the home environment is safe before discharging patients.

Nurses can have a role in the early identification of autonomic neuropathy by having a level of suspicion and taking a careful history.

Important nursing responsibilities are:

(1) The prevention, early recognition, and management of hypoglycaemia.
(2) Taking care when moving the patient from a lying to a sitting position, and from sitting to standing. Give them time for the blood pressure to adjust. Ensure their footwear will not contribute to the risk of falling.
(3) Providing adequate foot care and appropriate advice to minimise the risk of ulcers, including advice about footwear.
(4) Arranging counselling if indicated.
(5) Using aseptic technique.
(6) Being alert to the possibility of silent pathology – myocardial infarction, urinary tract infection.
(7) Encouraging people to remain physically active within their individual limits. Physical activity aids many body systems and improves mental outlook.

Clinical observation

Gentle abdominal massage and warm compresses can help alleviate the discomfort of gastroparesis. Aromatherapy essential oils can be added to the compress. The abdomen is a vulnerable part of the body and this needs to be taken into consideration when offering an abdominal massage (see Chapter 19).

References

Pathophysiology of diabetes complications & Cardiovascular disease and diabetes

American Diabetes Association (ADA) (2012) Standards of Medical care in diabetes 2012. *Diabetes Care*, 35 Suppl 1) 11–63.

American Diabetes Association (ADA) (2013) Standards of Medical Care in Diabetes, *Diabetes Care* care.diabetesjournals.org/content/36/Supplement_1/S11.full.pdf+html (accessed February 2013). Australian Diabetes Society (ADS) (2102) Guidelines for routine glucose control in hospital. ADS, Canberra.

AIHW (2011) Cardiovascular disease: Australian facts. AIHW, Canberra.

ACCORD Trial Study Group (2008) Intensive glucose control group of ACCORD Trial halted for excess deaths. National Heart, Lung and Blood Institute. February 2008.

ACCORD Study Group (2011) Long term effects of intensive glucose lowering on cardiovascular outcomes. *New England Journal of Medicine* 364, 11–63.

Alamowitch, S., Eliasziw, M. & Barnett, H. (2005) The risk and benefit of endarterectomy in women with symptomatic internal carotid artery disease. *Stroke*, 36, 27–31.

Australian Institute Health and Welfare (AIHW) (2007) *Medicines for Cardiovascular Health*. AIHW Cardiovascular Series No. 27. AIHW, Canberra.

Australian Medicines Handbook (2006) Australian Medicines Handbook PTY Ltd, Adelaide.

Barenholtz, H. & Kohlhaas, H. (2006) Considerations for supplementing with coenzyme Q_{10} during satin therapy. *Annals of Pharmacotherapy*, 40, 290–294.

Bayliss E, Edwards A, Steiner J, Main D. (2008) Processes of care desired by elderly patients with multimorbidities *Family Practice*, 25 (4), 287–293.

Boden-Albala, B. (2008) Daytime sleepiness is an independent risk factor for stroke. *Proceedings of the American Stroke Association International Stroke Conference*. Abstract 94. New Orleans.

Bohm, M. (2008) Treating to protect: Current cardiovascular treatment approaches and remaining needs. *Medscape Journal Medicine*, **10** (Suppl. 3), 1–13.

Brownlee, M. (2000) Mechanisms of Hyperglycaemic damage in diabetes, in *Atlas of Diabetes* (ed. R. Kahn), Science Press, London.

Bruckert, E. & Hansel, B. (2007) HDL-c is a powerful lipid predictor of cardiovascular disease. *International Journal of Clinical Practice*, **61** (11), 1905–1913.

Bunker, S., Colquhoun, D., Esler, M. *et al.* (2003) 'Stress' and coronary heart disease: Psychosocial risk factors. *Medical Journal of Australia*, **178**, 271–276.

Chen, Z. (2008) High BMI linked with stroke mortality in obese, overweight men. *Stroke Online* January 31. http://www.medscape.com/viewarticle/569864?src=mp (accessed February 2008).

Chiu, C., Hubbard, I., & Armstrong, J. (2006) Dietary glycaemic index and carbohydrate in relation to early age-related macular degeneration. *American Journal of Nutrition* **63**, 880–886.

Coleman, R., Stevens, R., Retnakaran, R. & Holman, R. (2007) Framingham SCORE and DECODE risk equations do not provide reliable cardiovascular risk estimates in type 2 diabetes. *Diabetes Care*, **30**, 1292–1293.

Cormack, T., Grant, B., Macdonald, M., Steel, J. & Campbell, I. (2001) Incidence of blindness due to diabetic eye disease in Fife 1990–9. *British Journal of Ophthalmology* **85** (3), 354–356.

Dantas, P., Fortes, B., Catelli de Carvalho H. (2012) Vascular disease in diabetic women: Why do they miss the female protection? *Experimental Diabetes Research*, DOI: 10.1155/2012/570598 (accessed September 2012).

Davidson, P., Mitchell, J., DiGiacomo, M. *et al.* (2011) Cardiovascular disease in women: Implications for improving cardiovascular health outcomes. *Collegian*, **19**, 5–13.

Donahoe, S., Stewart G., McCabe C. *et al.* (2007) Diabetes mortality following acute coronary syndromes. *Journal American Medical Association*, **298** (7), 765–775.

Du, X., Edelstein, D. & Rossetti, L. (2000) Hyperglycaemia induced mitochondrial superoxide overproduction activates the hexosamine pathway and induces plasminogen activator inhibitor-1 expression by increasing Sp1 glycosylation. *Proceedings of the National Academy of Science USA*, **97**, 1222–1226.

Elias, P., Elias, M., D'sgostino, R. *et al.* (1997) NIDDM and blood pressure as risk factors for poor cognitive performance. The Framingham Study. *Diabetes Care*, **20** (9), 138–139.

European Society of Hypertension (2007) Guidelines on treatment of hypertension. *Journal of Hypertension*, **25**, 1105–1187.

Farmer, D. & Kennedy, S. (2009) RAGE vascular changes tone ans vascular diseaase. *Pharmacology and Therapeutics*, **124** (2) 185–194.

Faerch, K., Bergman, B. & Perreault, L. (2012) Does insulin resistance drive the association between hyperglycaemia and cardiovascular risk? *PloS one*, **75**, e39260.

Forbes, J. & Cooper, M. (2007) The role of mitochondrial dysfunction in diabetic complications. *International Diabetes Monitor*, **19** (6), 9–15.

Fortin, M., Lapointe, L., Hudon, C., & Vanasse, A. (2005) Multimorbidity is common to family practice: Is it commonly researched? *Can Fam Physician*, **51**, 244–245.

Giannelli, S., Patel, K., Windham, G., Ferrucci, F. & Guralnik, J. (2007) magnitude of undr-ascertainment of impaired kidney function in old: normal serum creatine *Journal America Geriatric Society* **55** (6), 816–823.

Gudjhar, A., Dunning, T. & Alford, F. (2003) Metabolic and cardiac outcomes after acute myocardial infarction. *Journal of Diabetes Nursing*, **7** (6), 208–212.

Hansel B, Giral P, Nobecourt E. (2004). Metabolic syndrome is associated with elevated oxidative stress and dysfunctional dense high-density lipoprotein particles displaying impaired antioxidative activity. *Journal Clinical Endocrinology and Metabolism.* **89** (10), 4963–4971.

Hansson, L., Zanchetti, A., Carruthers, S. *et al.* (1998) Effects of intensive blood pressure lowering and low dose aspirin in patients with hypertension: principal results of the Hypertension Optimal Treatment (HOT) randomised trial. *Lancet*, **351** (9118), 1755–1762.

Haussler, B., Fischer, G., Meyer, S. & Sturm, D. (2007) Risk assessment in diabetes management: How do general practitioners estimate risks due to diabetes? *Quality and Safety in Health Care*, **16**, 208–212.

Hotta, N., Toyota, T. & Matsuoka, K. (2001) Clinical efficacy of fidarestat, a novel aldose reductase inhibitor, for diabetic peripheral neuropathy: A 52-week multicenter placebo-controlled double blind parallel group study. *Diabetes Care*, **24**, 1176–1182.

International Diabetes Federation (IDF) (2011) *Guidline for Management of Post Meal Glucose in Diabetes*. IDF, Brussels.

Kaiser, N., Sasson, S. & Feener, E. (1993) Differential regulation of glucose transports by glucose in vascular endothelial and smooth muscle cells. *Diabetes*, **42**, 80–89.

Kim, C-Y., Lee, K-B., Park, S-E. *et al.* (2012) Serum 1,5-Anhydroglucitol Concentrations Are a Reliable Index of Glycemic Control in Type 2 Diabetes With Mild or Moderate Renal Dysfunction. *Diabetes Care*, **35**(2): 281–286.

Kumar, A., Kuar, H., Devi, P. & Mohan V. (2009) Role of coenzyme Q10 (coQ10) in cardiac disease, hypertension and Meniere-like syndrome. *Pharmacology and Therapeutics*, **124**, 259–268.

Laukkanen, J., Makikallio, T., Ronkainen, K., Karppi, J. & Kurl S. (2013) Impaired fasting plasma glucose and type 2 diabetes are related to the risk of out-of-hospital sudden cardiac death and all-cause mortality. http://care.diabetesjournals.org/content/early/2012/12/14/dc12-0110-short (accessed January 2013).

Lazalde-Ramos, B., Zanoura-Perez, A., Sosa-Macia, M., Guerrero-Velazquez, C. & Mises-Zunkia-Gonzalez, G. (2012) DNA and oxidative damages decrease after ingestion of folic acid in patients with type 2 diabetes *Archives of Medical Research*, **43** (6), 476–481.

Leite-Moreira, A. & Castro-Chaves, P. (2008) Heart failure: Statins for all? *British Medical Journal*, www.heartjnl.com (accessed February 2008).

Lesperance, F. & Frasure-Smith, N. (2007) Depression and heart disease. *Cleveland Clinic Journal of Medicine*, **74** (Suppl. 1), S63–S66.

Lim, W., Holinski, H., Devereaux, P. *et al.* (2008) Detecting myocardial infarction in critical illness using screening troponin measurements and ECG recordings. *Critical Care*, **12**, R36DOI:10.1186/cc6815.

Lutsep, H. (2008) Stroke treatment and prevention are not the same in men and women. *Medscape Medical Journal*, **10** (2), 26–27.

Margolis, K., Bonds, D. & Rodnbough, R. (2004) Effect of oestrogen plus progestin on the incidence of diabetes in postmenopausal women: Results of the women's health initiative hormone trial. *Diabetologia*, **47** (7),1175–1187.

Middleton, S., Ward, J., Grimshaw, M. *et al.* (2011) Implementation of evidence-based treatment protocols to manage fever, hyperglycaemia, and swallowing dysfunction in acute stroke (QASC): A cluster randomized trial. *The Lancet*, DOI: 10.1016/s0140-6736(11)51485-2 (accessed June 2012).

Moser, D., Kimble, L. & Alberts, M. (2007). Reducing delay in seeking treatment by patients with acute coronary syndrome and stroke: a scientific statement from the American Heart Association Council on Cardiovascular Nursing and Stroke Council. *Journal of Cardiovascular Nursing*. **22**, 326–343.

Mozaffarian, D. (2007) Acute myocardial infarction: A prediabetes risk equivalent? *The Lancet*, **25**, 667–675.

Mulnier, H. (2012) Macrovascular disease and diabetes. *Journal of Diabetes Nursing*, **16** (8), 307–313.

Nakao, N., Yoshimura, A., Morita, H. *et al.* Combination treatment of angiotensin-II receptor blocker and angiotensinconverting-enzyme inhibitor in non-diabetic renal disease (COOPERATE): arandomised controlled trial. *Lancet*, **361** (9352):117-24.

National Institute of Clinical Studies (NICS) (2005) *Evidence-Practice Gaps Report*, Vol. **2**. NICS, Melbourne.

National Prescribing Service (NPS) (2012) Cardiovascular disease risk in type 2 diabetes. www.nps.org.au (accessed September 2012).

National Institute of Clinical Care Excellence (NICE) (2009) Guidelines for Managing Diabetes. www.nice.org.uk/- (accessed march 2012).

National Institute of Health and Clinical Excellence (NICE) (2008) Nice clinical guideline 66, The management of type 2 diabetes London NICE (www.nice.org.uk)

Nagel, G., Peter, R., Braig, S. *et al.* (2008) The impact of education on risk factors and the occurrence of multimorbidity in the EPIC-Heidelberg cohort. BMC Public Health 8 (384). DOI: 10.1186/1471-2458-8-384

Ning, F., Tumilehto, J., Pyorala, K. & Sodeberg, S. (2011) Cardiovascular disease mortality in Europeans in relation to fasting and 3-h plasma glucose. *Diabetes Care*, **33**, 2211–2216.

Nishikawa, T., Edelstein, D. & Du, X. (2000) Normalising superoxide production blocks three pathways of hyperglycaemic damage. *Nature*, **404**, 787–790.

Pfisterer, M. (2004) In elderly patients with chronic angina, drugs offer outcomes equal to invasive treatment. *Circulation on line*, http://www.medscape.com/viewarticle/488214 (accessed August 2007).

Picconi, F., Flaviani, A., Malandruccio, I., Giordani, L. & Frontoni, S. (2012) Impact of glycaemic variability on cardiovascular outcomes beyond glycated haemoglobin. Evidence and clinical perspectives. *Nutrition, Metabolism and Cardiovascular Diseases*, DOI: 10. 1016/jnumecd.2012.03.006 (accessed July 2012).

Pittler, M., Guo, R. & Ernst, E. (2008) Hawthorn extract for treating chronic heart failure. *Cochrane Database of Systematic Reviews*, Issue 1, Art No. CD005312 DOI: 10. 1002/14651858.CD005312. pub2.

Player, M., King, D., Mainous, A. & Geesey, M. (2007) Psychosocial factors and progression from pre-hypertension to hypertension or coronary heart disease. *Annals of Family Medicine*, 5 (5), 403–411.

Reddy, P. (2008) Diabetes and depression. Practical tools for the diabetes educator. Sanofi-Aventis Diabetes Partnership Seminar 12 April 2008. Novotel, Melbourne.

Ridker, P., Cook, N. & Lee, I. (2005) A randomized trial of low dose aspirin in the primary prevention of cardiovascular disease in women. *New England Journal of Medicine*, 352, 1293–1304.

Rosenfeldt, F., Haas, S. & Krum, H. (2007) Coenzyme Q$_{10}$ in the treatment of hypertension: A meta-analysis of the clinical trials. *Journal of Human Hypertension*, 21, 297–306.

Sanchis, J. (2007) Risk score useful in assessing chest pain with normal troponin levels. *American Journal of Cardiology*, 99, 797–801.

Singer, J., Palmas, W., Teresi, J. *et al.* (2012) Adiponectin and all-cause mortality in elderly people with type 2 diabetes. *Diabetes Care* DOI: 10.2337/dc11-2215 (accessed August 2012).

SIGN (2010) *Management of Diabetes: A National Clinical Guideline*. SIGN, Edinburgh.

Taylor, A., Price, K., Gill, T., *et al.* (2010) Morbidity – not just an older person's issue. Results from an Australian biomedical study. *BMC Public Health*, 10, 718.

United Kingdom Prospective Study (UKPDS) Group (1998) Effect of intensive blood glucose control with metformin on complications in overweight patients with type 2 diabetes. *Lancet*, 352, 854–865.

Wilmot, E., Edwardson, C., Achana, F. *et al.* (2012) Sedentary time in adults and the association with diabetes, cardiovascular disease and death: A systematic review and meta-analysis. *Diabetologia*, DOI: 10.1007/s00125-012-2677-z (accessed October 2012).

Vale, M., Jelinek, M., Best, J. *et al.* (2003) Coaching patients on achieving cardiovascular health (COACH): A multicenter randomized trial in patients with coronary heart disease. *Archives of Internal Medicine*, 163, 2775–2783.

Verdecchia, P., Angeli, F., Mazzotta, G. & Carofe, M. (2012) Ambulatory blood pressure monitoring: Day-night dip and early-morning surge in blood pressure in hypertension. *Hypertension*, 60, 34–42.

Wen, Y., Hung, L., Te, L. *et al.* (2012) Variability in hemoglobin A1c predicts all-cause mortality in patients with type 2 diabetes. *Journal of Diabetes and its Complications*, DOI: 1016/jda-comp.2012.03.029 (accessed August 2012).

Wells-Knecht, K., Zyzak, D. & Litchfield, J. (1995) Mechanism of autoxidative glycosylation: Identification of glyoxal and arabinose as intermediates in the autooxidative modification of proteins by glucose. *Biochemistry*, 34, 3702–3709.

Williams, J., Chimowitz, M., Cotsonis, G., Lunn, M. & Waddy, S. (2007) WASID Investigators. Gender differences in outcomes among patients with symptomatic intracranial arterial stenosis. *Stroke*, 38, 2055–2062.

WHO (2003) Cardiovascular Diseases (CV) fact sheet 317 updated March 2013, Geneva WHO www.who.int/mediacentre/factsheets/fs317/ (accessed January 2013).

Young, D., Furler, J., Vale, M. *et al.* (2007) Patient engagement and coaching for health: The PEACH study – A cluster randomised controlled trial using the telephone to coach people with type 2 diabetes to engage with their GPs to improve diabetes care. *BMC Family Practice*, 8 (20), 8–13.

Zhang, Y., Hu, G., Yuan, Z. & Chen, L. (2012) Glycosylated haemoglobin in relation to cardiovascular outcomes and death in patients with type 2 diabetes: A systematic review and meta-analysis. *PloS One 2012*; 7 (8): e42551.

Zannad, F. (2008) Cardiovascular high risk patients – Treat to protect, but whom? *Medscape Journal of Medicine*, 10 (Suppl. 2), 1–11.

Diabetes and eye disease

Antonetti, D., Barber, A., Bronson, S. *et al.* (2006) Diabetic retinopathy: Seeing beyond glucose-induced microvascular disease. *Diabetes*, 55 (9), 401–411.

Chui, C., Hubbard, L. & Armstrong, J. (2006) Dietary glycaemic index and carbohydrate in relation to early age-related macular degeneration. *American Journal of Nutrition*, 63, 880–886.

Clemons, T., Milton, R., Klein, R., Seddon, J. & Ferris, F. Age-Related Eye Disease Study Research Group. (2005) Risk factors for the incidence of advance age-related macular degeneration in the Age-Related Eye Disease Study (AREDS). *AREDS report no. 19. Ophthalmology*, 112, 533–539.

Gupta, A., Gupta, V., Thapar, S. & Bhansali, A. (2004) Lipid-lowering drug atorastatin as an adjunct in the management of diabetic macular oedema. *American Journal of Ophthalmology*, **137** (4), 675–682.

Khan, J., Shahid, H. & Thurlby, D. (2006) Age-related macular degeneration and sun exposure, iris colour, and skin sensitivity to sunlight. *British Journal of Ophthalmology*, **90**, 29–32.

van Leeuwen, R., Boekhoorn, S. & Vingerling, J. (2005) Dietary intake of antioxidants and risk of age-related macular degeneration. *Journal American Medical Association*, **294**, 3101–3107.

Lim, J. (2006) Risk factors for age-related macular degeneration. *eMedicine*. http://www.medscape.com/viewarticle/532642 1–5 (accessed November 2007).

Park, H., Kim, Y., Song, S. & Ahn, H. (2012) Serum 1,5-anhydroglucitol is associated with diabetic retinopathy in type 2 diabetes. *Diabetic Medicine*, **29**, 1184–1190.

Ryan, C., Geckle, M. & Orchard, T. (2003) Cognitive efficiency declines over time in adults with Type 1 diabetes: Effect of micro- and macrovascular complications. *Diabetologia*, DOI: 10.1007/soo125-003-1128-2, 940–948.

Seddon, J., Gensler, G., Milton, R., Klein, M. & Rifai, N. (2004) Association between C-reactive protein and age-related macular degeneration. *Journal American Medical Association*, **292**, 704–710.

Sen, K., Misra, A., Kumar, A. & Pandey, R. (2002) Simvastatin retards progression of retinopathy in diabetic patients with hypercholeserolaemia. *Diabetes Research and Clinical Practice*, **56** (1), 1–11.

SIGN (2010) *Management of Diabetes: A National Guideline*. SIGN, Edinburgh.

Stanway, L. (2012) Multi-ability alert dogs for people with diabetes and visual impairment. *Diabetes Voice*, **57** (1), 39–42.

Diabetes and renal disease

American Society of Nephrology (ASN) (2012) Kidney disease recommendations. *Clinical Journal of the American Society Nephrology*. www.asnonline.org/publications/kidneynews/.../2012/KN_2012_07_jul.pdf -

ANZDATA Registry (2000) *Australian and New Zealand Dialysis Transplant Registry*. Adelaide, South Australia.

Bosman, D., Winkler, A., Marsden, J., MacDougall, I. & Watkins, P. (2001) Anemia with erythropoietin deficiency occurs early in diabetic nephropathy. *Diabetes Care*, **24** (3), 495–499.

Briguori, C. (2007) Renal insufficiency following contrast media administration trial (REMEDIAL): A randomized comparison of 3 preventative strategies. *Circulation*, **115**, 1211–1217.

Cass, A., Cunningham, J., Arnold, P., Snelling, P., Wang, Z. & Hoy, W. (2002) Delayed referral to a nephrologist: outcomes among patients who survive at least one year. *Medical Journal of Australia*, **177** (3), 135–138.

Chadban, S. & Lerino, F. (2005) Welcome to the era of CKD and the eGFR. *Medical Journal of Australia*, **183** (3), 117–118.

Chan, M. (2001) Nutritional management in progressive renal failure. *Current Therapeutics*, **42** (7), 23–27.

Chan M. (2008) Nutrition, diabetes and chronic kidney disease. *Diabetes Management Journal*, **25**, 6–7.

Chan M. (2012) Nutrition, diabetes and chronic kidney disease. *Australian Diabetes Educator*, **15** (3), 18–23.

Chobanian, A., Bakris, G. & Black, H., (2003) National Heart, Lung, and Blood Institute Joint National Committee on Prevention, Detection, Evaluation, and Treatment of High Blood Pressure National High Blood Pressure Education Program Coordinating Committee. The Seventh Report of the Joint National Committee on Prevention, Detection, Evaluation, and Treatment of High Blood Pressure: the JNC 7 report. *Journal of the American Medical Association*, **289**, 2560–2572.

Choudhury, D. & Luna-Salazar, C. (2008) Preventive health care in chronic kidney disease and end stage renal failure. *Clinical Practice Nephrology*, **4** (4), 3–16.

Churchill, D. (1996) Results and limitations of peritoneal dialysis, in *Replacement of Renal Function by Dialysis* (eds C. Jacobs, C. Kjellstrand, K. Koch & F. Winchester). Kluwer Academic Publishers, Boston.

Culleton, B. (2007) Frequent nocturnal hemodialysis may have better outcomes than conventional hemodialysis. *Journal of the American Medical Association*, **298**, 1291–1299.

DCCT (Diabetes Control and Complications Trial Research Group) (1993) Effects of intensive insulin therapy on the development and progression of long-term complications in IDDM. *New England Journal of Medicine*, **329**, 977–986.

Department of Health (2001) *Diabetes National Service Framework: Standards for Diabetes Services.* Department of Health, London.

Duncan, H., Pittman, S., Govil, A. *et al.* (2007) Alternative medicine use in dialysis patients: Potential for good and bad. *Nephrology and Clinical Practice*, **105** (3), 108–113.

Dunning, T., MacGinley, R. & Ward, G. (2012) Is point of care testing for anaemia (Hb) and microalbumin feasible in people with type 2 diabetes attending diabetic outpatient clinics? *Renal Society of Australasia Journal* **8** (2), 76–81.

Ernst, E. (1998) Harmless herbs? A review of the recent literature. *American Journal of Medicine*, **104** (2), 170–178.

Giannelli, S., Patel, K., Windham, G., Ferrucci, F. & Guralnik, J. (2007) Magnitude of underascertainment of impaired kidney function in old normal serum creatine. *Journal of the American Geriatric Society*, **55** (6), 816–823.

Gilbert, R., Akdeniz, A. & Jerums, G. (1992) Semi-quantitative determination of microalbuminuria by urinary dipstick. *Australian New Zealand Journal of Medicine*, **22**, 334–337.

Gilbert, R., Akdeniz, A. & Jerums, G. (1997) Detection of microalbuminuria in diabetic patients by urinary dipstick. *Diabetes Research in Clinical Practice*, **35**, 57–60.

Gilbert, R., Tsalamandris, C., Allen, T., Colville, D. & Jerums, G. (1998) Early nephropathy predicts vision-threatening retinal disease in patients with Type I diabetes mellitus. *Journal of the American Society of Nephrology*, **9**, 85–89.

Hays, R., Kallich, J., Mapes, D., Coons, S. & Carter, W. (1994) Development of the kidney disease quality of life instrument (KDQOL-SF). *Quality of Life Research*, **3**, 329–338.

HOPE (Heart Outcomes Prevention Evaluation Study Investigators) (2000) Effects of ramipril on cardiovascular and microvascular outcomes in people with diabetes mellitus: Results of the HOPE study and MICRO-HOPE substudy. *Lancet*, **355**, 253–259.

Howes, L. (2001) Dosage alterations in the elderly: Importance of mild renal impairment. *Current Therapeutics*, **42** (7), 33–35.

Iliescu E. (2006) Glycaemic control often poor among hemodialysis patients. *Diabetes Care*, **29**, 2247–2251.

Keane, W. (2001) Metabolic pathogenesis of cardiorenal disease. *American Journal of Kidney Disease*, **38** (6), 1372–1375.

Kerr P. (2008) Diabetic nephropathy: Who to refer and when. *Diabetes Management Journal*, **25**, 4–5.

Ko, R. (1998) Adulterants in Asian patent medicines. *New England Journal of Medicine*, **339**, 847.

Lehto, S., Ronnemaa, T., Pyorala, K. & Laakso, M. (1999) Poor glycaemic control predicts coronary heart disease events in patients with type 1 diabetes without nephropathy. *Arteriosclerosis Thrombosis Vascular Biology*, **19**, 1014–1019.

Levin, S., Coburn, J., Henderson, W., Colwell, J. & Emanuele, N. (2000) Effect of intensive glycaemic control on microalbuminuria in type 2 diabetes. Veterans Affairs Cooperative Study on Glycaemic Control and Complications in type 2 diabetes. *Diabetes Care*, **23** (910), 1478–1485.

Lopes, A., Elder, S., Ginsberg, N., *et al.* (2007) Lack of appetite in haemodialysis patients: Associations with patient characteristics, indicators of nutritional status and outcomes in the international DOPPS. *Nephrology Dialysis Transplant*, **22** (12), 3538–3546.

Meschi, M., Detrenis, S., Musini, S., Strada, E. & Savazzi, G. (2006) Facts and fallacies concerning the prevention of contrast medium-induced nephropathy. *Critical Care Medicine*, **34** (8), 2060–2068.

Moustakas, J., Bennett, P., Nicholson, J. & Tranter, S. (2012) The needs of older people with advanced chronic kidney disease choosing supportive care: A review. *Renal Society of Australasia Journal*, **8** (2), 70–75.

Myhre, M. (2000) Herbal remedies, nephropathies and renal disease. *Nephrology Nursing Journal*, **27** (5), 473–480.

National Kidney Foundation (2002) Clinical practice guidelines for nutrition in chronic renal failure. Kidney Outcome Quality Initiative, *American Journal of Kidney Disease*, **35** (6), Supp. 2.

Oomichi, T., Emoto, M., Tabata, E. *et al.* (2007) Impact of glycemic control on survival of diabetic patients on chronic regular hemodialysis: A 7-year observational study. *Diabetes Care*, **29**, 1496–1500.

Oyibo, S., Prichard, G., Mclay, L. *et al.* (2002) Blood glucose overestimation in diabetic patients on continuous ambulatory peritoneal dialysis for end-stage renal disease. *Diabetic Medicine*, **19**, 693–696.

Quellhorst, E. (2002) Insulin therapy during peritoneal dialysis: Pros and cons of various forms of administration. *Journal of the American Society of Nephrology*, **13**, S92–S96.

Ravid, M., Savin, H. & Jutrin, I. (1993) Long-term stabilising effect of angiotensin-converting enzyme on plasma creatinine and on proteinuria in normotensive Type II diabetic patients. *Annals of Internal Medicine*, **118**, 577–581.

Ritz, E. (2001) Advances in nephrology: Success and lessons learnt from diabetes. *Nephrology Dialysis Transplant*, **16** (Suppl. 7), 46–50.

Rudnick, M., Kesselheim, A. & Goldfarb, S. (2006) Contrast-induced nephropathy: How it develops, how to prevent it. *Cleveland Clinic Journal of Medicine*, **73** (1), 75–87.

Rutecki, G. & Whittier, F. (1993) Intraperitoneal insulin in diabetic patients on peritoneal dialysis, in *Dialysis Therapy* (eds A. Nissenson & R. Fine). Hanley & Belfus, Philadelphia.

Schetz, M., Vanhorebeck, I., Wouters, P., Wilmer, A. & van der Berghe, G. (2008) Tight blood glucose control is renoprotective in critically ill patients. *Journal American Society of Nephrology*, DOI:10.1681/asn2006101091.

Terrill, B. (2002) *Renal Nursing: A Practical Approach*. Ausmed Publications, Melbourne.

Wu, M., Yu, C. & Yang, C. (1997) Poor pre-dialysis glycaemic control is a predictor of mortality in Type II diabetic patients on maintenance haemodialysis. *Nephrology Dialysis Transplant*, **12**, 2105–2110.

Yu, M., Rees-Lyles, C., Bent-Shaw, L. & Young, B. (2012) Risk factor, age and sex differences in chronic kidney disease prevalence in a diabetic cohort: The Pathways Study. *Nephrology*, **36** (3), 245–251.

Peripheral and autonomic neuropathy

Abusaisha, B., Constanzi, J. & Boulton, A. (1998) Acupuncture for treatment of chronic painful diabetic neuropathy: A long-term study. *Diabetes Research Clinical Practice*, **39**, 115–121.

Aly, N. & Weston, P. (2002) Autonomic neuropathy in older people with diabetes. *Journal of Diabetes Nursing*, **6** (1), 10–14.

Apelqvist, J. & Larsson, J. (2000) What is the most effective way to reduce incidence of amputation in the diabetic foot? *Diabetes/Metabolism Research and Reviews*, **16** (Suppl. 1), s75–s83.

Apelqvist, J., Bakker, K., van Houtum, W., Nabuurs-Franssen, M. & Schaper, N. (2000) The international consensus and practical guidelines on the management and prevention of the diabetic foot. *Diabetes/Metabolism Research and Reviews*, **16** (Suppl. 1), s84–s92.

Bakker, D. (2000) Hyperbaric oxygen therapy and the diabetic foot. *Diabetes/Metabolism Research and Reviews*, **16** (Suppl. 1), s55–s58.

Boulton, A. (2000) The diabetic foot: A global view. *Diabetes/Metabolism Research and Reviews*, **16** (Suppl. 1), s2–s5.

Boulton, A. & Jervell, J. (1998) International guidelines for the management of diabetic peripheral neuropathy. *Diabetic Medicine*, **15** (6), 508–514.

Boulton, A., Gries, F. & Jervell, J. (1998) Guidelines for the diagnosis and outpatient management of diabetic peripheral neuropathy. *Diabetes Medicine*, **15**, 508–514.

Brismar, K., Johansson, T., Lindström, B., et al. (2007) C-Peptide replacement therapy and sensory nerve function in type 1 diabetic neuropathy *Diabetes Care*, **30** (1), 71-6.

Brod, M. (1998) Quality of life issues in patients with diabetes and lower limb extremity ulcers: Patients and caregivers. *Quality Life Research*, **7**, 365–372.

DCCT (1993) The effect of intensive treatment of diabetes on the development and progression of long-term complications in insulin-dependent diabetes mellitus. *New England Journal of Medicine*, **329**, 977–986.

DRS (1981) Photocoagulation treatment of proliferative diabetic retinopathy: Clinical implications of DRS findings. DRS Report No. 8. *Ophthalmology*, **88**, 583–600.

Edmonds, M., Bates, M., Doxford, M., Gough, A. & Foster, A. (2000) New treatments in ulcer healing and wound infection. *Diabetes/Metabolism Research and Reviews*, **16** (Suppl. 1), s51–s54.

EDTRS (1991) Early photocoagulation for diabetic retinopathy: EDTRS Report No. 9. *Ophthalmology*, **98** (Suppl.), 767–785.

Foster, A., Eaton, C., McConville, D. & Edmonds, M. (1994) Application of Op-cite film: A new effective treatment for painful diabetic neuropathy. *Diabetic Medicine*, **11**, 768–772.

Harding, K., Jones, V. & Price, P. (2000) Topical treatment: Which dressing to choose. *Diabetes/Metabolism Research and Reviews*, **16** (Suppl. 1), s47–s50.

Hemstreet, B. & Lapointe, M. (2001) Evidence for the use of gabapentin in the treatment of diabetic peripheral neuropathy. *Clinical Therapeutics*, **23** (4), 520–531.

Hotta, N. (2006) Epalrestat may delay progression and reduce symptoms of diabetic neuropathy. *Diabetes Care*, **29**, 1538–1544.

Huang, E., Meigs, J. & Singer, D. (2001) The effect of interventions to prevent cardiovascular disease in patients with Type 2 diabetes. *American Medical Journal*, **11** (8), 663–642.

International Diabetes Federation Consultative Section on Diabetes (2000) *Diabetes Education for People who are Blind or Visually Impaired*. Position Statement. International Diabetes Federation, Brussells, pp. 62–72.

Karlson, B., Herlitz, J. & Hjalmarson, A. (1993) Prognosis of acute myocardial infarction in diabetic and non-diabetic patients. *Diabetic Medicine*, **10**, 449–454.

Larkins, R. (1995) Aspirin: The effects are complex. *Diabetic Communication*, **10** (3), 5–6.

Lipsky, B. & Berendt, A. (2000) Principles and practice of antibiotic therapy of diabetic foot infections. *Diabetes/Metabolism Research and Reviews*, **16** (Suppl. 1), s42–s46.

Litchy, W., Dyck, P., Tesfaye, S. for the MBBQ Study Group (2002) Diabetic peripheral neuropathy (DPN) assessed by neurological examination and composite scores is improved with LY333531 treatment. *Diabetes*, **45**, A197.

Locke, D., Ill, G. & Camileri, M. (2000) Gastrointestinal symptoms among persons with diabetes in the community. *Archives of Internal Medicine*, **160**, 2808–2816.

Lowe, J. (2002) Hypertension in diabetes. *Australian Prescriber*, **25** (1), 8–10.

Malmberg, K., Ryden, L., Efendic, S. *et al.* (1995) Randomised trial of insulin–glucose infusion followed by subcutaneous insulin treatment in diabetic patients with acute myocardial infarction (DIGAMI study): Effects on mortality at 1 year. *Journal of the American College of Cardiology*, **26**, 57–65.

Papas, N., Boulton, A., Malik, R. *et al.* (2013) A simple new non-invasive sweat indicator test for the diagnosis of diabetic neuropathy. *Diabetic Medicine*, **30**, 525–534.

Pecorara, R. (1990) Pathways to diabetic limb amputation. *Diabetes Care*, **13** (5), 513–530.

Ponchilla, S., Richardson, K. & Turner-Barry, M. (1990) The effectiveness of six insulin measurement devices for blind persons. *Journal of Visual Impairment and Blindness*, **84**, 364–370.

Sadiya, A. (2012) Nutritional therapy for the management of gastric paresis: A clinical review. *Diabetes, Metabolic Syndrome and Obesity Targets and Therapy*, **5**, 329–335.

Semla, T., Beizer, J. & Higbee M. (2002) (eds.) *Geriatric Dosage Handbook*. Hudson, Ohio: Lexi-Company.

Spallone, V. & Menzinger, G. (1997) Autonomic neuropathy: Clinical and instrumental findings. *Clinical Neuroscience*, **4** (96), 346–358.

Standl, E. & Schnell, O. (2000) A new look at the heart in diabetes: From ailing to failing. *Diabetologia*, **43**, 1455–1469.

Steinberg, F. (1991) Rehabilitation after amputation. *Diabetes Spectrum*, **4** (1), 5–9.

Surwit, R. & Feinglos, M. (1988) Stress and autonomic nervous system in Type 2 diabetes. A hypothesis. *Diabetes Care*, **11**, 83–85.

Sutton, M., McGrath, C., Brady, L. & Wood, J. (2000) Diabetic foot care: Assessing the impact of foot care on the whole patient. *Practical Diabetes International*, **17** (5), 365–372.

Todd, M., Welsh, J., Key, M., *et al.* (2008) Survey of Doppler use in lymphoedema practitioners in the UK. *British Journal Community Nursing*, **13** (4), S11–2, S14, S16–17.

UKPDS Group (1998) Intensive blood glucose control with sulphonylureas or insulin compared with conventional treatment and risk of complications in patients with Type 2 diabetes (UKPDS 33). *Lancet*, **352**, 837–853.

Vale, M., Jelinek, M., Best, J. & Santamaria, J. (2002) Coaching patients with coronary heart disease to achieve cholesterol targets: A method to bridge the gap between evidence-based medicine and the 'real world' – randomized controlled trial. *Journal of Clinical Epidemiology*, **55**, 245–252.

Vinik, A., Park, T., Stansberry, K. & Henger, P. (2000) Diabetic neuropathy. *Diabetologia*, **43**, 957–973.

Wegener, M., Borsch, G., Schaffsten, J., Luerweg, C. & Leverkus, F. (1990) Gastrointestinal transit disorders in patients with insulin-treated diabetes. *Digestive Disorders*, **8** (1), 23–26.

Zhang, W., Kamiya, H. & Ekberg, K. (2007) C-peptide improves neuropathy in Type 1 diabetic BB/Wor-rats. *Diabetes Metabolism Reviews*, **12**, 1471–1488.

Ziegler, D., Nowak, H., Kempler, P., Vargha, P. & Low, P. (2004) Treatment of symptomatic diabetic neuropathy with antioxidant alpha-lipoicacid: A meta-analysis. *Diabetic Medicine*, **21**, 114–121.

Chapter 9

Management During Surgical and Investigative Procedures

SURGICAL PROCEDURES

Key points

- Surgery induces the counter-regulatory response that can increase the blood glucose 6–8 times higher than normal in people with and without diabetes. Optimal control before, during, and after surgery reduces morbidity and mortality and length of stay.
- Preventing hyperglycaemia reduces the risk of adverse outcomes in people with diabetes.
- Morning procedures are desirable.
- Insulin should never be omitted in people with Type 1 diabetes.
- Complications should be stabilised before, during, and after surgery.
- Cease oral glucose lowering medicines 24–36 hours before the procedure depending on the particular medicine and their duration of action; but note some experts recommend continuing oral agents until the day of surgery if the blood glucose is high.
- Ascertain whether the person is using any complementary therapies especially herbal medicines with a high risk of interacting with conventional medicines and/or causing bleeding.
- An insulin-glucose infusion is the most effective way to manage hyperglycaemia in the operative period.

Rationale

Diabetes is associated with an increased need for surgical procedures and invasive investigations and higher morbidity than non-diabetics. Anaesthesia and surgery are associated with a complex metabolic and neuroendocrine response that involves the release of counter-regulatory hormones and glucagon leading to insulin resistance, gluconeogenesis, hyperglycaemia and neutrophil dysfunction, which impairs wound healing. The stress response also occurs in people without diabetes but is more pronounced and difficult to manage in people with diabetes due to the underlying metabolic abnormalities. Advances in diabetes management, surgical techniques, anaesthetic medicines and intensive care medicine have significantly improved surgical outcomes for people with diabetes.

Introduction

People with diabetes undergo surgery for similar reasons to those without diabetes; however, because of the long-term complications of diabetes they are more likely to require:

- cardiac procedures such as:
  - ○ angioplasty or stents
  - ○ bypass surgery
- ulcer debridement, amputations (toes, feet);
- eye surgery such as cataract removal, repair retinal detachment, vitrectory;
- carpal tunnel decompression.

Surgical-induced stress results in endocrine, metabolic and long-term effects that have implications for the management of people with diabetes undergoing surgery (see Table 9.1). Stress induces hyperglycaemia, which causes osmotic diuresis, increased

Table 9.1 Hormonal, metabolic, and long-term effects of surgery.

Hormonal	Metabolic	Long-term effects if optimal blood glucose control is not achieved
↑ Secretion of[a] epinephrine, norepinephrine, ACTH, cortisol and growth hormone ↓ secretion of insulin due to impaired beta cell responsiveness Insulin resistance	Catabolic state and ↑ metabolic rate Hyperglycaemia Insulin resistance ↓ Glucose utilisation and glycogen storage ↑ Gluconeogenesis ↓ Protein catabolism and reduced amino acid and protein synthesis in skeletal muscle ↑ Lipolysis and formation of ketone bodies ↓ Storage of fatty acids in the liver Osmotic diuresis with electrolyte loss and compromised circulating volume ↑ Risk of cerebrovascular accident, myocardial arrhythmias infarction electrolyte disorders ↑ Blood pressure and heart rate ↓ Peristalsis	Loss of lean body mass – impaired wound healing, ↓ resistance to infection Loss of adipose tissue Deficiency of essential amino acids, vitamins, minerals, and essential fatty acids Surgical complications Longer length of stay

[a] Norepinephrine is mostly augmented during surgery and epinephrine postoperatively. Stress stimulates glucagon secretion from the pancreatic alpha cells and together with growth hormone and cortisol, potentiates the effects of norepinephrine and epinephrine. Cortisol increases gluconeogenesis.

hepatic glucose output, lipolysis and insulin resistance. Unless these metabolic abnormalities are controlled, surgical stress increases the risk of DKA, Hyperosmolar states HHS, and lactic acidosis (see Chapter 7), infection, impaired wound healing, and cerebral ischaemia. The risk of HHS is high in procedures such as cardiac bypass surgery and has a high mortality rate (Dagogo-Jack & Alberti 2002).

In addition, anaesthesia and surgical stress, as well as medicines, induce gastrointestinal instability that can compound gastric autonomic neuropathy and lead to nausea, vomiting and predispose the individual to dehydration and exacerbate fluid loss via osmotic diuresis and blood loss during surgery. As a result, electrolyte changes, particularly in potassium and magnesium, increase the risk of cardiac arrhythmias, ischaemic events, and acute renal failure (Dagogo-Jack & Alberti 2002). The risk is particularly high in people with chronic hyperglycaemia (HbA$_{1c}$ > 8%), existing diabetes complications, older people, and those who are obese, all of which are associated with increased risk of interoperative and postoperative complications (Dickersen 2003).

Obesity is associated with functional risks in addition to the metabolic consequences of surgery that need to be considered when positioning the patient. The respiratory system is affected and functional residual capacity and expiratory reserve volume may be reduced possibly due to excess weight on the chest wall and/or displacement of the diaphragm. Severe obesity can lead to hypoventilation and obstructive sleep apnoea. These factors predispose the individual to aspiration pneumonia. Various cardiac changes increase the risk of heart failure and inadequate tissue oxygenation. In addition, the risk of pressure ulcers is increased due to the weight, and activity level is often compromised increasing the risk of venous stasis and emboli.

The need for nutritional support may be overlooked in obese individuals and protein deprivation can develop because protein and carbohydrate are used as the main energy sources during surgery rather than fat. In addition, energy expenditure is higher, which impacts on wound healing (Mirtallo 2008).

Different types of surgery present specific risks as do the person's age: the very young and older people are particularly at risk. The specific risks are summarised in Table 9.1. The blood glucose must be controlled to prevent DKA and HHS, promote healing and reduce the risk of infection postoperatively. The target blood glucose range in the perioperative period is 5–10 mmol/L (Australian Diabetes Society (ADS) 2012).

Hyperglycaemia inhibits white cell function and increases coagulability (Kirschner 1993). The magnitude of the metabolic/hormonal response depends on the severity and duration of the surgical procedure, metabolic control before, during, and after surgery, and the presence of complications such as sepsis, acidosis, hypotension, and hypovolaemia (Marks *et al.* 1998; ADS 2012). Significantly, metabolic disturbances can be present in euglycaemic states (De & Child 2001). Surgery is often performed as a day procedure, often without appropriate consideration of the effects of surgical and the related psychological stress on metabolic control. A multidisciplinary approach to planning is important.

Children with diabetes undergoing surgical procedures

Generally, children with Type 1 and Type 2 diabetes needing general anaesthesia should be admitted to hospital and must receive insulin to prevent ketosis even if they are fasting and should be managed with a glucose infusion if they need to fast for more than two hours to prevent hypoglycaemia (Betts *et al.* 2009). Blood glucose must be monitored hourly prior to and every 30 to 60 minutes during surgery to detect hypo- and hyperglycaemia. As in adults it is best to perform surgery when metabolic control is optimal and children should be first on the list if possible (Betts *et al.* 2009). An IV insulin-glucose infusion should be commenced two hours prior to surgery.

Older people with diabetes and surgical procedures

The Geriatric Surgery Expert Panel of the American College of Surgeons recently released a comprehensive guideline for assessing older people prior to surgery (Chow *et al.* 2012). The recommendations are not specific to people with diabetes but diabetes-related information could be incorporated into the guidelines. In addition to conducting a thorough history and physical assessment, the Expert Panel recommended assessing the individual's:

- Cognitive ability and capacity to understand the proposed surgery (give informed consent).
- Mental health: undertake a depression screen.
- Risk of developing delirium postoperatively.
- Alcohol, tobacco and other substance use.
- Functional status.
- Falls history.
- Frailty Index (score).
- Nutritional status.
- Medicine regimen to determine whether the regimen may need to be adjusted and to assess the level of polypharmacy. (Note information about insulin and other GLMs in this chapter) and adherence to their medicine regimen.
- Expectations of the surgery.
- Social and family support.
- Undertake appropriate investigations. These include renal function tests haemoglobin, and serum albumin and in some cases, white cell cont, platelet count, coagulation studies, electrolytes and blood glucose and a urinalysis to detect UTI.

Tests of physical and cognitive function are discussed in Chapter 12. Interestingly, the guidelines do not mention CAM use, but as indicated, people with diabetes use CAM and many herbal medicines interact with conventional medicines and increase the risk of adverse events.

Aims of management

(1) To identify underlying problems that could compromise surgery and recovery by undertaking comprehensive presurgical assessment (Dhatariya *et al.* 2012).
(2) To achieve normal metabolism by supplying sufficient insulin to counterbalance the increase in stress hormones during fasting, surgery, and postoperatively and avoid the need for prolonged fasting.
(3) To normalise metabolic control using regimens that minimise the possibility of errors and have the fewest adverse outcomes: target blood glucose range. 5–10 mmol/L and is best achieved with an insulin-glucose infusion (ADS 2012).
(4) To supply adequate carbohydrate to prevent catabolism, hypoglycaemia, and ketosis.
(5) To ensure that the patient undergoes surgery in the best possible physical condition.
(6) To prevent:
   - hypoglycaemia, children <5 years are prone to hypoglycaemia during anaesthesia and surgery (Kirschner 1993);
   - hyperglycaemia predisposing the patient to dehydration, electrolyte imbalance, ketoacidosis, and hyperosmolar states;

- complications of surgery;
- electrolyte imbalance;
- worsening of pre-existing diabetic complications;
- infection.

(7) To avoid undue psychological stress.

Preoperative nursing care

Good preoperative nursing care is important for both major and minor procedures. Preadmission clinics have an important role in identifying and managing preventable surgical risks. Sometimes people need to be admitted 2–3 days before major surgery to stabilise blood glucose levels and manage complications (see Table 9.2). Many procedures only require a day admission. In all cases careful explanation about what is required and *written* instructions that are at a suitable language level and are culturally relevant are vital.

The individual's blood glucose profile needs to be reviewed and their diabetes regimen may need to be adjusted prior to surgery to achieve good metabolic control. Erratic control could indicate the presence of infection that should be treated prior to surgery. Alternatively, it could indicate brittle diabetes that might require investigation because of the risk of hypoglycaemia and delayed gastric emptying depending on the underlying cause (Chapter 10). If possible, schedule for a morning procedure to avoid the need for prolonged fasting and counter-regulatory hormone release that leads to hyperglycaemia.

Nursing actions

(1) Confirm time and date of the operation and inform the patient.
(2) Explain the procedure and postoperative care to the patient and/or family members if appropriate, for example a child. Those patients on controlled GLMs may require insulin *during surgery and immediately post-operatively*. They should be aware of this possibility. Insulin during the operative period does not mean that diet- or tablet-controlled patients will remain on insulin when they recover from the procedure. People controlled by diet and exercise with good metabolic control (HbA$_{1c}$, 6.5%) may not require an IV insulin infusion for minor procedures but 1–2 hourly blood glucose monitoring is necessary (ADS 2012). Diet-controlled people who become hyperglycaemic may require supplemental insulin peri- and/or postoperatively. If control is suboptimal, and for procedures longer than one hour, an IV insulin/dextrose infusion is advisable (Dagogo-Jack & Alberti 2002; Kwon *et al.* 2003). In fact Kwon et al. (2003) suggested 'Perioperative glucose evaluation and insulin administration in patients with hyperglycaemia are important quality targets.' It should be noted that suboptimal control is common in diet-treated individuals.
(3) Ensure all documentation is completed:
   - consent form
   - medication chart
   - monitoring guidelines
   - chest X-ray and other X-rays
   - scans, MRI (magnetic resonance imaging)
   - ECG.
(4) GLMs: Sulphonylureas, Metformin, Repaglinide, Acarbose, TZDs and the incretins can be continued until the day of surgery to prevent preoperative hyperglycaemia (ADS 2012). Chlorpropamide should be given 36 hours preoperatively because it is

Table 9.2 Common complications of diabetes that can affect surgery and postoperative recovery. Many of these conditions may be documented in the person's medical record and they may undergo regular complication assessment but health status can change rapidly especially older people. Therefore, the current complication status should be assessed prior to surgery. Hyperglycaemia must be controlled.

Complication	Possible consequences	Preoperative evaluation
Cardiovascular	Hypertension Ischaemic heart disease Cardiomyopathy Myocardial infarction, which can be 'silent' and in the presence of autonomic neuropathy cause sudden tachycardia, bradycardia, and/or postural hypotension Cerebrovascular disease Increased resting heart rate is associated with increased risk of death in older people Daytime sleepiness is associated with 4.5-fold increased risk of stroke and other vascular events	Careful history and examination ECG Manage existing conditions such as heart failure Assess for silent cardiac disease autonomic neuropathy; indicators include: shortness of breath, palpitations, ankle oedema, tiredness, and atypical chest pain Assess resting heart rate Ask about daytime sleepiness or assess formally, for example, using the Epworth Sleepiness Scale (ESS)
Neuropathy Autonomic Peripheral	Cardiac as above Inability to maintain body temperature during anaesthesia Pressure areas on feet and ulceration Foot infection Falls postoperatively	Lying and standing blood pressure (abnormal if decrease >30 mmHg) Heart rate response on deep breathing (abnormal if increase >10 beats/min) Foot assessment, assess for active and occult infection and signs of neuropathy
Renal	Nephropathy, which may affect medication excretion Urinary tract infection (UTI), which may be silent and predispose to sepsis Acute renal failure and the need for dialysis UTI if catheterisation is needed	Urine culture to detect UTI, which should be treated with the relevant antibiotics Microalbuminuria and creatinine clearance, eGFR Blood electrolytes, correct potassium >5 mmol/L before surgery
Respiratory Airway	Obese people and smokers are prone to chest infections Obesity may be associated with reduced respiratory reserve and displacement of the diaphragm Reduced tissue oxygenation Soft tissue, ligament, and joint thickening that might involve the neck making it difficult to extend the neck and intubate and predispose the individual to neck injury and post operative pain	Counsel to stop smoking Chest physiotherapy Chest X-ray Blood gases Nebulised oxygen pre- and postoperatively if indicated See test for musculoskeletal disease (see page 341–342) Take extra care of the neck
Gastrointestinal	Autonomic neuropathy leading to gastric stasis delayed gastric emptying, gastric reflux, regurgitation and aspiration on anaesthesia induction Ileus May need to modify nutritional support if required postoperatively and given enterally	Assess history of heartburn or reflux and whether the person sleeps in an upright position A H_2 antagonist and metoclopramide might be indicated preoperatively Erratic food absorption can affect blood glucose levels
Eyes	Cataracts, glaucoma, and retinopathy can be exacerbated by sudden rise in blood pressure	Assess retinopathy stage
Neutrophil dysfunction	Increased risk of infection Inability to mount an appropriate response to infection	Check for possible foci of infection: including feet, teeth, and gums, UTI, Ensure optimal blood glucose control Optimise vascular function

Table 9.2 Continued.

Complication	Possible consequences	Preoperative evaluation
Polypharmacy	Risk of medicine interactions with anaesthetic agents and postoperative medicines Risk of lactic acidosis with Metformin Some medicines increase the risk of hyperglycaemia some hypoglycaemia	Medicine review Ask about complementary medicines Give the person clear, concise written instructions about how to manage their medicines preoperatively and postoperatively on discharge
Musculoskeletal	Difficulties with intubation and tube placement Falls risk	Assess, for example, prayer sign, Dupuytren's contracture, trigger finger Foot abnormality including Charcot's foot
Obesity	Increased systemic vascular resistance leading to reduced tissue oxygenation and increased risk of lactic acidosis in people on Metformin especially if renal function is compromised and those with surgical wound infections Sleep apnoea and associated daytime sleepiness with associated risk of cardiovascular events Difficulty intubating the person Assumption that the person is well nourished when in fact nutritional deficiencies especially protein are common High prevalence of hypertriglyceridaemia Cardiovascular and respiratory effects, which affect postoperative nutrition support if it is required Non-alcoholic fatty liver Risk of pressure ulcers	Assess nutritional status Assess cardiovascular and respiratory status. Ask about daytime sleepiness or assess formally, for example, using the ESS Skin condition

long acting; however, Chlorpropamide is rarely used nowadays and is no longer available in some countries e.g. Australia because of the significant hypoglycaemia risk. Metformin is traditionally ceased 24 hours preoperatively but there is little evidence that ceasing Metformin or continuing Metformin in the perioperatic period increases the risk of hyperglycaemia. Metformin is associated with a risk of lactic acidosis, although the risk is low; however, surgical procedures, hypotension secondary to blood loss, myocardial ischaemia, sepsis and anaestheic agents can contribute to the development of lactic acidosis, especially in people with renal impairment (Chapter 7). Thus a careful clinical assessment of the risks and benefits of ceasing/continuing Metformin in individual patients is essential Insulin therapy must be initiated before the procedure in people with Type 1 diabetes.

(5) Encourage patients who smoke to stop.

(6) Assess:
- Metabolic status: blood glucose control, ketones in blood and urine, hydration status, nutritional status, presence of anaemia, diabetic symptoms.
- Educational level and understanding of diabetes.
- Family support available postoperatively.
- Any known allergies or medicine reactions, which should include asking about complementary therapies, particularly herbal medicines, because some herbs predispose the person to haemorrhage and/or interact with anaesthetic agents and should be stopped at least 7 days prior to surgery (see Chapter 19).

- Presence of diabetic complications and other comorbidities, for example, renal, hepatic, cardiac disease (ECG for people >50 years to detect the risk of silent infarction is performed in some units), presence of neuropathy. Patients with autonomic neuropathy pose special problems during anesthesia: gastroparesis delays gastric emptying and the stomach can be full despite fasting and increases the possibility of regurgitation and inhalation of vomitus; or the vasoconstrictive response to reduced cardiac output may be absent and they may not recognise hypoglycaemia.
- Current medication regimen.
- Presence of infection, check feet and be aware of silent infection such as UTI.
- Self-care potential and available home support.

Note: Complications should be managed before the operation where possible (see Table 9.2).

Major procedures

Major surgery refers to procedures requiring anaesthesia and lasting longer than one hour (Dagogo-Jack & Alberti 2002).

Day of the operation

Premedication and routine preparation for the scheduled operative procedure should be performed according to the treatment sheet and standard protocols.

Where insulin is required, for example, Type 1 diabetes, major surgery, and poor control, an IV insulin infusion is the preferred method of delivering the insulin. The insulin dose should be balanced with adequate calories to prevent starvation ketosis, for example, saline/dextrose delivered at a rate that matches the insulin dose (Alberti & Gill 1997); see Chapter 5. Fluid replacement should be adequate to maintain intravascular volume; normal saline/dextrose in water is the preferred solution for this purpose. Preoperative hyperglycaemia especially if polyuria is present can cause significant fluid deficits and intracellular dehydration. Clinical signs of dehydration are:

- Thirst and a dry mouth: water loss <5% of body weight.
- Capillary refill >2 seconds (normal <2 seconds), reduced skin turgor, sunken eyes, reduced urine output, orthostatic hypotension, fainting on standing, low CVP/JVP: water loss 5–10% of body weight.
- Unconscious or shock: water loss >10% of body weight (French 2000).

Morning procedure

(1) Ensure oral medications were ceased on the operative day or earlier in specific circumstances.
(2) Fast from 12 midnight.
(3) Ascertain insulin regimen: commence insulin infusion.
(4) Monitor blood glucose 1–2-hourly. If the individual an insulin pump they should continue their usual basal rate (Joslin Diabetes Centre 2009).

Afternoon procedure

(1) Fast after an early light breakfast.
(2) Ensure oral medications are ceased.
(3) Ascertain insulin dose, usually 1/2 to 1/3 of usual dose (best given after IV dextrose has been commenced).

(4) It is preferable for IV therapy to be commenced in the ward to:
- prevent hyperglycaemia and dehydration;
- reduce the risk of hypoglycaemia. This will depend on the surgical and anaesthetic and usual hospital procedure. Some anaesthetists prefer to commence the infusion in theatre. It is preferable to insert the IV line in theatre in children unless blood glucose is <4 mmol/L (Werther 1994).

(5) Monitor blood glucose.

Practice points

- Sliding insulin scales are NOT appropriate to manage blood glucose postoperatively if they are used as the only method of managing uses blood glucose because it can lead to inadequate/inappropriate insulin administration and wide swing in the blood glucose levels.
- Supplemental insulin doses given in addition to the individual's medicine regimen is appropriate. Supplemental insulin is always short- or rapid-acting insulin and given before meals in addition to the insulin/GLM dose prescribed at that time.
- A daily review of the individual's blood glucose pattern and insulin requirements is essential to enable insulin doses to be calculated for the following day (ADS 2012).
- Persistent hyperglycaemia could indicate underlying infection or surgical or metabolic complications and severe pain.

The anaesthetist is usually responsible for the intraoperative blood glucose monitoring. Interoperative blood glucose monitoring is essential to detect hypo-and hyperglycaemia. The anaesthetic masks the usual signs of hypoglycaemia. Precautions are needed to avoid regurgitation and aspiration, cardiac arrhythmias, and postural hypotension in young children and patients with autonomic neuropathy. Hypoglycaemia increases the risk of seizures. In all cases careful explanation about what to expect and how to prepare for the procedure to the patient and their family/carers is essential.

The National Health Service in the UK released guidelines for managing people with diabetes in the perioperative period in 2012 (Dhatariya *et al.* 2012). The guidelines describe seven stages of the surgical journey including referrals from primary care, the surgical outpatient department, preoperative assessment, hospital admission, surgery, postoperative care and discharge. The guidelines highlight the value of insulin infusions and blood glucose monitoring during the operative process as well as the importance of patient education. The guidelines raise a number of areas of controversy such as whether high preoperative HbA_{1c} is associated with worse outcomes, using oral GLMS in the perioperative period and whether Metformin is associated with adverse events when radio contrast media are needed for investigative purposes.

The guidelines highlight two key points:

(1) Managing elective surgery in adults with diabetes should involve minimal fasting time e.g. only one missed meal and suggest that modifying the individual's usual medicine regimen is preferable to intravenous insulin infusions. However, this particular recommendation is not consistent with other experts who recommend insulin infusions during surgery.

(2) A poor glycaemic control leads to worse outcomes and more adverse events and should be addressed before surgery.

Postoperative nursing responsibilities

Immediate care

(1) Monitor and record vital signs.
(2) Monitor blood glucose and ketones initially 2-hourly.
(3) Observe dressings for signs of haemorrhage or excess discharge.
(4) Ensure drain tubes are patent and draining.
(5) Maintain an accurate fluid balance. Document all information relating to input and output, especially:

Input	Output
IV fluid	Drainage from wound
Oral	Vomitus
EN and TPN	Diarrhoea
	Urine

(6) Maintain care of IV insulin infusion.
(7) Ensure vomiting and pain are controlled.
(8) Ensure psychological needs are addressed, for example, change in body image.
(9) Ensure referral to appropriate allied health professional, for example, physiotherapist.
(10) Insulin therapy is continued for people on oral GLMs until they are eating a normal diet and blood glucose levels are stabilised. Plans for ceasing the insulin infusion and commencing GLM should be in place and usually commenced two hours before the infusion is stopped (Joslin Diabetes Centre 2009).
(11) Provide pressure care including high-risk neuropathic feet.

Ongoing care

(1) Document all data accurately on the appropriate charts.
(2) Prevent complications:
   • infection – aseptic dressing technique including IV sites;
   • venous thrombosis – anti-embolic stockings, physiotherapy, early ambulation, anticoagulants;
   • hypo/hyperglycaemia;
   • pressure ulcers.
(3) Diabetes education, instruct patient and their family/carers in wound care and medication management.
(4) Rehabilitation.

Antibiotics, heparin and other medicines should be administered according to individual patient requirements and medical orders.

Clinical observation

People sometimes complain of a sore throat for 24 hours after a general anaesthetic. They need to be reassured that this is normal and resolves spontaneously but advised to seek medical advice if it persists.

Minor procedures

Minor surgery may be performed on an outpatient basis. The metabolic risks are still a consideration if the person is expected to fast for the procedure. Ensure the procedure is fully explained to the patient at the time the appointment is made. Give *written* instructions about how to manage insulin, oral agents and other medications. Preoperative care is the same as for major surgery on the day of operation as regards:

- managing diabetes medicines;
- complication screening and managing complications when they are present;
- morning procedure is preferred.

Guidelines for informing patients about what they should do prior to surgical procedures

Examples of instructions for people undergoing outpatient procedures can be found in Example Instruction Sheets 2 (a) and (b) (see pages 298 and 299).

Note: These are examples only and protocols in the nurse's place of employment should be followed. Adjusting medications for investigations and day procedures is becoming more complex as the range of available insulin, oral agents, and other medicines increase, and multiple insulin injections, insulin pumps and combining insulin and oral agents is common practice.

It is important to consider the individual's blood glucose pattern, the medication regimen they are on and the type of procedure they are having when advising them about preoperative medication self-care.

Where people are on basal bolus regimes and scheduled for a morning procedure, the bedtime insulin dose may need to be reduced and the morning dose omitted. If the procedure is scheduled for the afternoon the morning dose may be given and the lunchtime dose omitted.

When people are on a combination of insulin and oral GLMs, the oral GLMs are usually withheld on the day of the procedure and the morning dose of insulin may be withheld for morning procedures. A reduced dose of insulin will usually be given if the procedure is scheduled for the afternoon.

> **Practice point**
>
> Advice about medications should also include information about medications and complementary therapies the person may be taking besides insulin and oral glucose-lowering medicines.

Morning procedure

(1) Insulin may or may not be withheld in the morning on the day of the procedure depending on the type of diabetes and blood glucose range.
(2) Test blood glucose and ketones if Type 1 before coming to hospital.
(3) Fast from 12 midnight.
(4) Some hospitals ask the individual to bring their insulin to hospital.
(5) Advise the patient to have someone available to drive him or her home after the procedure.

(6) Explain before discharge:
   (a) the risk of hypoglycaemia if not eating;
   (b) what to take for pain relief;
   (c) when to recommence OHAs/insulin;
   (d) what and when to eat;
   (e) any specific care, for example, wound dressings or care of a biopsy site.

Afternoon procedure

(7) Light breakfast (e.g. tea and toast).
(8) Fast after the breakfast. It may be necessary to explain what 'fasting' means.
(9) Test blood glucose and ketones in Type 1 before coming to hospital.
(10) Give insulin dose according to blood glucose test as ordered by the doctor.
(11) Explain before discharge:
   (a) the risk of hypoglycaemia if not eating;
   (b) what to take for pain relief;
   (c) when to recommence OHAs/insulin;
   (d) what and when to eat;
   (e) any specific care, for example, wound dressings or care of a biopsy site.

In both cases:

(i) Test blood glucose at the end of the procedure and before discharge and administer OHA or insulin dose.
(ii) Ensure the patient has appropriate follow-up appointments with doctors and other relevant health professionals, for example, diabetes educator and dietitian.
   (a) ensure the patient has someone to accompany them home;
   (b) allay concerns about the procedure;
   (c) provide appropriate care according to the medical orders;
   (d) inspect all wounds before discharge;
   (e) it is not advisable to drive, operate machinery or drink alcohol until the following day.

Clinical observations

It is important to ensure the patient and their family/carers understand what is meant by 'fasting' and 'light breakfast'. People have stated that they will 'come as fast as I can but I can only move slowly because of my hips'.

Insulin pump therapy in patients undergoing surgery

Insulin pumps or continuous subcutaneous insulin infusion (CSII) are becoming more common. The managing diabetes team in consultation with the patient, the anaesthetist and surgical team should determine the best way to manage the person's insulin needs during surgery. The patient must consent to continuing pump therapy in surgery.

If the person does continue pump therapy during surgery a clearly visible identification tag should state the person is wearing a pump.

The anaesthetist must have access to the pump during surgery and know how it operates and how to turn it off or disconnect it if necessary, for example in persistent hypoglycaemia. Once euglycaemia is restored the pump therapy can be recommenced at a lower basal rate, which may be temporary. Alternatively, the pump can be recommenced at the same basal rate and the rate of the glucose infusion increased, or the pump can be left off and an IV insulin infusion commenced (Queensland Health 2012).

If the decision is to continue to administer insulin using the pump then it is important to ensure the infusion site is secure and that the tubing cannot be inherently disconnected during transport to and from the operating room or surgery.

If the surgery is of short duration the usual basal insulin rate can be continued and an IV infusion of 5% glucose administered according to the individual's caloric requirement (Betts *et al.* 2009). The usual morning insulin bolus is not given except to correct hyperglycaemia.

Blood glucose must be monitored at least hourly pre- and postoperatively and every 30 minutes during surgery. If needed, correction insulin doses can be administered via the pump. However, if hyperglycaemia occurs it is important to ensure the pump is still functioning correctly, the infusion tubing is patent and the needle has not been dislodged from the infusion site. If the pump is not functioning an IV insulin-glucose infusion may be required to prevent ketosis and hyperglycaemia, which may compromise outcomes.

A bolus does of insulin is usually administered when the person is ready to eat postoperatively.

However, managing an insulin pump requires a great deal of knowledge and skill and should not be used if the surgical team does not have the necessary knowledge, skills and experience. Nassar *et al.* (2012) demonstrated inconsistent documentation of pump use and blood glucose monitoring throughout the perioperative period in 35 patients with insulin pumps who had surgical procedures in the US between 2006 and 2010. Likewise it was not clear whether the pump was functioning during most procedures. The authors recommended guidelines be developed. Their recommendation is interesting given least three such guidelines exist (Betts *et al.* 2009 (ISPAD); ADS 2012; Queensland Health 2012).

Emergency procedures

Approximately 5% of people with diabetes will need emergency surgery at some stage of their lives. These may be for general surgical emergencies such as appendicitis or diabetes-specific such as acute foot ulcer. Abdominal pain in the presence of DKA may not be an abdominal emergency. However, if the abdominal pain persists after the DKA is corrected an abdominal emergency should be considered. Likewise, functional problems associated with gastroparesis, gastroenteropathy and cyclical vomiting may be mistaken for a surgical emergency. Thus, even in an emergency situation it is important to undertake a thorough assessment and medical history.

The specific management will depend on the nature of the emergency. If possible, the metabolic status should be stabilised before surgery is commenced. Many patients requiring emergency surgery have suboptimal control. The minimum requirements are:

(1) Adequate hydration. IV access should be obtained and blood drawn for glucose, ketones, electrolytes, pH, and other tests as indicated by the presenting problem.
(2) If possible surgery should be delayed until the underlying acid–base derangement is corrected if ketoacidosis (DKA), hyperosmolar or lactic acidosis is present. Dehydration is often severe in hyperosmolar states and the fluid volume needs to be replaced quickly, taking care not to cause fluid overload or cerebral oedema. If the patient presents with an abdominal emergency ensure that it is not due to DKA before operating.

Specific treatment depends on the:

- Nature of the emergency.
- Time of the last food intake and the presence of autonomic neuropathy/gastric stasis.
- Time and type of the last insulin dose.
- Blood glucose level, which should be monitored hourly.
- Presence of complications such as cardiac arrhythmias and renal disease. Postoperative care will depend on the reason for the emergency and will encompass the care outlined earlier in the chapter.

Bariatric surgery

Bariatric surgery, a solution to obesity when other methods fail, is becoming safer and more acceptable. A recent study demonstrated that laparoscopic adjustable gastric banding (LAGB) and conventional diabetes management had five times the diabetes remission rate than other methods in 60 obese people with Type 2 diabetes (Dixon *et al.* 2008). Seventy three per cent achieved diabetes remission, there was an average weight loss of 20%, and average BMI fell from 36.6 to 29.5, and 80% achieved normoglycaemia. A recent report of a 15-year follow-up study involving 3000 Australians who had laparoscopic and adjustable banding surgery lost an average of 26 kg and maintained the weight loss for >10 years. (O'srien 2006). There were no deaths in the Australian cohort but one in 20 people had the band removed in the follow up period.

People who successfully lose weight after gastric banding are more likely to have improved insulin sensitivity, reduced fasting blood glucose and HbA_{1c}, especially those with Type 2 diabetes, and the lipid profile improves in people with Type 2 diabetes and those with impaired glucose tolerance (Geloneze *et al.* 2001). However, the risks and benefits need to be carefully considered on an individual basis.

Diabetes Australia recommends gastric banding should be a last resort for very obese adults when lifestyle changes are unsuccessful.

INVESTIGATIVE PROCEDURES

Key points

- Careful preparation and explanation to the patient and their family/carers.
- Never omit insulin in Type 1 diabetes.
- Radio-opaque contrast media may cause tubular necrosis in older people with diabetes so fluid balance must be monitored carefully.
- Complementary therapies especially herbs and topical essential oils may need to be stopped temporarily.

Rationale

Metabolic stress occurs to a lesser degree during investigative procedures than during surgical procedures but still occurs and needs to be managed appropriately to limit adverse outcomes.

Clear written instructions about managing medications and any specific preparation required can improve the individual's understanding and compliance with instructions.

Management protocols for patients undergoing medical tests/procedures such as X-rays, gastroscopy or laser therapy is not as intricate as those for ketoacidosis or major surgery. However, vigilant nursing care is equally important to prevent excursions in blood glucose levels and consequent metabolic effects, and psychological stress.

Note: Morning procedures are preferred.

The objectives of care

(1) It is important to prevent hyperglycaemia during surgical procedures to improve outcomes. Hyperglycaemia and insulin therapy can affect the uptake of the radio isotope fluorine-18-fludrodeoxyglucose in the area to be investigated using Positron Emission Tomography (PET) scans.
(2) To ensure correct preparation for the test.
(3) To ensure the procedure has been explained to the patient.
(4) To provide written instructions for the patient especially if the test is to be performed on an outpatient basis. These instructions should include what to do about their diabetes medications (insulin and oral agents) and any other medications they are taking and how to recognise and manage hypoglycaemia should it occur while they are fasting. They should also warn the person that it may not be safe for them to drive home depending on the procedure.

Usually, the doctor referring the person for a procedure should explain the procedure to the individual as part of the process for obtaining informed consent to undertake the procedure. Nurses have a duty of care to ensure instructions have been given and were followed.

General nursing management

(1) Be aware insulin pumps and continuous glucose monitoring devices should not be exposed to strong magnetic fields during X-rays, MRIs and CT scans, although they are designed to withstand common electromagnetic interference (ADS 2012).
(2) Insulin/oral hypoglycaemic agents:
  • insulin is *never omitted* in people with Type 1 diabetes;
  • if the patient needs to fast, insulin doses should be adjusted accordingly;
  • OHAs are usually withheld on the morning of the test;
  • ensure written medical instructions are available, including for after the procedure.
(3) Aim for a morning procedure if fasting is required and avoid prolonged fasting that results in a catabolic state and counter-regulatory hormone release (see Chapters 1 and 7).
(4) Monitor blood glucose before and after the test and during the night (3 a.m.) if fasting and in hospital.
(5) Observe for signs of dehydration. Maintain fluid balance chart if:
  • fasting is prolonged;
  • bowel preparations are required – some may lead to a fluid deficit especially in the setting of hyperglycaemia;
  • an IV infusion is commenced;

- dehydration in older people may predispose them to kidney damage if a radio-opaque contrast medium is used;
- An IV infusion may dilute some radio-opaque contrast media. The advice of the radiographer should be sought if IV therapy is necessary. Continue IV infusions and oral fluids after the procedure to wash out contrast medium.

(6) Control nausea and vomiting and pain, which can increase the blood glucose level.
(7) Ensure the patient can eat and drink normally after the procedure to avoid hypoglycaemia.
(8) Assess puncture sites (e.g. angiography) before discharge.
(9) Recommence medications as per the medical order.
(10) Counsel not to drive home if relevant.

Bowel procedures, for example, colonoscopy

(1) Iron, aspirin, and arthritis medications may need to be stopped one week before the procedure. Diabetes medications should be adjusted according to the procedures outlined for day procedures. Insulin doses may need to be reduced during the bowel preparation and people may only require long acting insulin. Oral medicines may not be absorbed because of the bowel preparation.
(2) The day before the colonoscopy only clear fluids are permitted and some form of bowel preparation is usually required to clean out the bowel and allow a better view of the mucosa. Bowel preparations should be diluted in water because cordial can contribute to diarrhoea. Older people are at risk of dehydration and should be carefully monitored. Modern preparations are not absorbed and do not usually lead to significant electrolyte disturbances.
(3) Fasting for at least 6 hours is usually necessary.
(4) If diabetes is unstable or the individual is hyperglycaemic and the procedure is urgent, admission to hospital and an IV insulin-glucose infusion during the procedure may be advisable (ADS 2012).
(5) Frequent blood glucose monitoring e.g. at least two hourly, is important especially for people who have unstable or brittle diabetes.

Eye procedures

People with diabetes are more prone to visual impairment and blindness than the general population. The eye manifestations of diabetes can affect all ocular structures. The time of appearance, rate of progression and severity of eye disease vary among individuals. However, most patients have some evidence of damage after 25 years of diabetes and vision is threatened in 10% of people with diabetes.

Retinopathy is symptomless and may remain undetected if an ophthalmologist or optician does not examine the eyes regularly. Retinal cameras are commonly used to assess the degree of retinopathy and do not require papillary dilation. Fluorescein angiography and retinal photography may aid in determining the severity of the disease. Management aims to conserve vision, and laser therapy is often effective in this respect.

Risk factors for eye disease include hypertension, pregnancy, nephropathy, hyperlipidaemia, and smoking (see Chapter 8).

Care of patient having fluorescein angiography

Fluorescein angiography is usually an outpatient procedure. The reasons for the test and the procedure should be carefully explained to the patient. They should be aware that:

- transient nausea may occur;
- the skin and urine may become yellow for 12–24 hours;
- drinking adequate amounts of fluid will help flush the dye out of the system;
- the dye is injected into a vein.

Care of the patient having laser therapy (photocoagulation)

'Laser' is an acronym for light amplification stimulated emission of radiation. There are many types of laser. The ones that are used to treat diabetic patients are the argon, krypton, and diode lasers. The lasers absorb light, which is converted into heat, which coagulates the tissue. Laser therapy is frequently used to treat diabetic retinopathy and glaucoma.

Goals of photocoagulation

To maintain vision:

- by allowing fluid exchange to occur and reducing fluid accumulation in the retina;
- by photocoagulating the retina, which is ischaemic, and thereby causing new vessels that are prone to haemorrhage, to regress.

Laser therapy is usually performed on an outpatient basis. Fasting is not required and medication adjustment is unnecessary.

Practice point

Laser therapy may not increase vision, but can prevent further loss of vision.

Nursing responsibilities

Ensure the purpose of laser therapy has been explained to the patient. Advise them to ask their doctor whether it is still safe to drive after the treatment – not just immediately after but generally. The majority can still drive safely but a driving assessment might be required.
(1) Before the procedure the patient should know that:
- the procedure is uncomfortable;
- the pupil of the eye will be dilated;
- anaesthetic drops may be used;
- the laser beam causes bright flashes of light;
- vision will be blurred for some time after the laser treatment;
- they should test their blood glucose before and after laser treatment;
- they should not drive home, and that they may have tunnel vision after the procedure, which can limit their visual field. The possible effects on driving should be explained (see Chapter 10).
(2) After the procedure the patient should know that:
- sunglasses will protect the eye and help reduce discomfort;
- spots may be seen for 24–48 hours;
- there can be some discomfort for 2–3 weeks;
- headache may develop after the procedure;
- paracetamol may be taken to relieve pain;

- activities that increase intraocular pressure, for example, lifting heavy objects, straining at stool, should be avoided for 24–36 hours;
- night vision may be temporarily decreased;
- lateral vision may be permanently diminished; this is known as 'tunnel vision'.

Practice point

Aspirin is best avoided because of its anticoagulant effect. If new vessels are present due to retinopathy they can bleed and threaten sight.

Other eye procedures include cataract operations.

Practice point

Blurred vision does not necessarily indicate serious eye disease. It can occur during both hypo- and hyperglycaemia. Vision often also becomes worse when diabetic control is improved, for example, after commencement of insulin therapy. Although this is distressing for the patient, vision usually improves in 6–8 weeks. Prescriptions for glasses obtained in these circumstances may be inappropriate. Glasses are best obtained when the eyes settle down.

The nursing care of people who are vision impaired is discussed in Chapter 14.

Care of the patient having radio-contrast media injected

Radio-contrast media are eliminated through the kidneys and can cause contrast-induced nephropathy that can result in lactic acidosis in people taking Metformin, especially if the radio-contrast media is injected IV (Klow *et al.* 2001). Metformin-induced lactic acidosis following injection of radio-contrast media almost always occurs in people with pre-existing renal impairment. Thus, the serum creatinine should be measured prior to the procedure. Most radiological services recommend withholding Metformin 24 hours prior and 48 hours after procedures requiring radio-contrast media.

Fasting is often required before the procedure and the patient can become dehydrated, especially if they are kept waiting for long periods, and kidney complications can occur. Patients most at risk:

- are over 50 years old;
- have established kidney disease;
- have had diabetes for more than 10 years;
- are hypertensive;
- have proteinuria;
- have an elevated serum creatinine, but note the limitations of serum creatinine discussed in Chapter 3.

Kidney problems caused by radio-contrast media may not produce symptoms. Reduced urine output following procedures requiring radio-contrast media may indicate kidney damage and should be investigated.

Management
(1) ensure appropriate preparation has been carried out;
(2) ensure the patient is well hydrated before the procedure (intravenous therapy may be needed);
(3) maintain an accurate fluid balance chart;
(4) avoid delays in performing the procedure;
(5) monitor urine output after the procedure;
(6) assess serum creatinine and/or other kidney function tests after the procedure;
(7) maintain good metabolic control;
(8) encourage the patient to drink water to help flush out the contrast media.

Complementary therapies and surgery and winvestigative procedures

A version of the following information was published in the *Australian Diabetes Educator* 2008; see also Chapter 19. Fifty per cent of patients undergoing surgical and investigative procedures use complementary medicines (CAM) and other CAM. Women aged 40–60 years are high users and often use CAM on the advice of friends (Tsen 2000; Norred 2000). Thus, CAM use is an important consideration for people with diabetes having surgical and/or investigative procedures.

Significantly, despite the high rates of CAM usage, most conventional practitioners do not ask about CAM use (Braun 2006). CAM use can improve health outcomes of patients undergoing surgery: for example, essential oil foot massage reduces stress and anxiety post CAGS (Stevenson 1994), essential oils lower MRI-associated claustrophobia and stress, acupuncture and peppermint or ginger tea reduce nausea, a range of strategies relieve pain and improve sleep and CQ10 prior to cardiac surgery improves post-operative cardiac outcomes (Rosenfeldt 2005).

However, there are also risks, which need to be considered in the context of the particular surgery or investigation required and overall management plan. Bleeding is the most significant risk. Other risks include hypotension, hypertension, sedation, and cardiac effects such as arrhythmias, renal damage, and electrolyte disturbances (Norred 2000, 2002). It is well documented that many conventional medicines need to be adjusted or ceased prior to surgery. Less information about managing CAM in surgical settings is available but a growing body of evidence suggests many CAM medicines may also need to be stopped or adjusted prior to surgery and some investigative procedures.

The following general information applies to people already using CAM medicines and those considering using them before or after surgery. Conventional practitioners may be able to provide general advice regarding CAM use but people with diabetes should be advised to consult a qualified CAM medicine practitioner because many therapies should be used under qualified supervision and for specific advice. Self-prescribing is not recommended in the surgical period because of the complex metabolic and neuroendocrine response to surgery.

Preoperative phase

People need written information about how to manage CAM medicines and conventional medicines in the operative period as well as any special preparation needed for the surgery or investigation. Conventional health professionals can provide such information if they are qualified to do so or refer the person to a qualified CAM practitioner. Such information should be provided in an appropriate format relevant to the individual's health literacy level; see Chapter 16.

Great care is needed for major and high risk such as heart, orthopaedic, or neurosurgery, if the person has renal or liver disease, or is very young or elderly. The conventional medication list is unlikely to include CAM medicines or supplements, although it should, thus health professionals should discuss CAM use with people during all structured medicine reviews and preoperative health assessments.

Some CAM medicines such as evening primrose oil, bilberry, cranberry, fish oils, ginger, Gingko, liquorice, guarana, willow bark, meadowsweet, and ginseng need to be stopped at least one week before surgery. St John's Wort and supplements such as vitamin E should be stopped two weeks before surgery, primarily because of the risk of bleeding. In addition, medicines such as St John's Wort, need to be stopped gradually (like conventional antidepressants). However, when CAM medicines are the main form of treatment, alternative management may be required to prevent the condition deteriorating and affecting the surgical outcome, for example, glucose-lowering herbal medicines.

In addition to the bleeding risk, some commonly used CAM medicines may/can interact with some anaesthetic agents and prolong their sedative effects, some affect blood pressure and heart rate, others cause changes in the major electrolytes, potassium, calcium, and sodium levels in the blood. Grapefruit juice interferes with the action of some antibiotics such as cyclosporine, which may be needed pre- or postoperatively. These problems do not occur in everybody who uses CAM in the same way that not everybody experiences adverse events associated with conventional treatments. It is sometimes difficult to predict who will or will not have problems. Some hospitals have policies and guidelines about using CAM and people who wish to continue using CAM in hospital should clarify such policies with the relevant hospital and surgeon before they are admitted. Most do not prescribe or supply CAM.

In addition to managing CAM and conventional medicines, achieving the best possible health status before surgery improves postoperative recovery. The preoperative assessment is an ideal time to revise the importance of eating a healthy balanced diet and exercise within the individual's capability, controlling blood glucose and lipids, which will support immune system functioning and enhance wound healing. Most people should continue their usual physical activity unless it is contraindicated to maintain strength and flexibility. Stress management strategies such as meditation, guided imagery, essential oils administered in a massage or via an inhalation, and music help reduce anxiety and fear about the surgery. Ginger capsules or tablets taken one hour before surgery reduces postoperative nausea (Gupta & Sharma 2001).

The preoperative assessment is also an ideal time to discuss postoperative recovery including managing pain and promoting sleep. CAM may be a useful alternative to some conventional medicines provided a quality use of medicines framework is adopted; see Chapter 5. For example, valerian, hops, and lavender in a vapourised essential oil blend, administered via massage or as herbal teas or medicines promote restful sleep and have a lower side effect profile than most conventional sedatives.

Postoperative phase

CAM users need information about whether and when it is safe to start using CAM again postoperatively considering any new conventional medicines that were prescribed, for example anticoagulants, which could influence the choice and/or dose of CAM medicines. Likewise, some non-medicine CAM therapies might need to be used with care such as needle acupuncture and deep tissue massage because they can cause bruising and/or bleeding.

A range of CAM strategies can be used to manage pain in the immediate postoperative phase as well as in the longer term is needed. Most are less likely to cause constipation and drowsiness than pethidine and morphine-based medicines. Alternatively, if these medicines are the best method of managing pain, high fibre CAM food/ medicines such as *Aloe vera* juice, probiotics, and psyllium can reduce constipation once oral feeding is permitted. Probiotics also increase bowel health and support natural bowel flora. Peppermint or ginger tea reduces mild-to-moderate nausea. Lymphatic drainage massage is very effective after some surgery to reduce swelling and relieve pain.

Some CAM products promote wound healing, for example, *Aloe vera*, Medihoney, and calendula and could be used depending on the wound. Arnica ointment reduces bruising but should not be used on open wounds. Comfrey poultices are very effective at reducing local oedema and local pain but should not be used on open wounds or taken internally.

Implications for nursing care

- CAM has both risks and benefits for people with diabetes undergoing surgery and investigative procedures.
- Not all the CAM therapies people use are medicines and not all CAM carry the same level of risk or confer equal benefits.
- Adopting an holistic quality use of medicines (QUM) approach can optimise the benefits and reduce the risks. A key aspect of QUM is asking about and documenting CAM use.
- People with diabetes who use CAM need written advice about how to manage their CAM during surgery and investigations.
- People with diabetes and cardiac or renal disease and those on anticoagulants, older people, and children are at particular risk if they use some CAM medicines.

References

Alberti, G. & Gill, G. (1997) The care of the diabetic patient during surgery, in International Textbook of Diabetes Mellitus (2nd edn.) (eds G. Alberti, R. DeFronzo & H. Keen). Wiley, Chichester, pp. 1243–1253.

Australian Diabetes Society (ADS) (2012) *Peri-operative Diabetes Management Guidelines*. ADS, Canberra.

Betts, P., Brink, S., Silink, M., *et al.* (2009) Management of children and adolescents with diabetes requiring surgery. *Paediatric Diabetes*, **10** (Suppl 12), 169–179.

Braun, L. (2006) Use of complementary medicines by surgical patients. Undetected and unsupervised, in Proceedings of the *Fourth Australasian Conference on Safety and Quality in Health Care*, Melbourne

Chow, W., Rosenthal, R., Merkow, R., Ko, C. & Esnaola, N. (2012) *Optimal Perioprative Assessment of the Geriatric Surgical Patient: A Best Practice Guideline From the American College of Surgeons National Surgical Quality Improvement Program and the American Geriatrics Society*. http://dx.doi.org/10.1016/jamcollsurg.2012.06.017 (accessed December 2012).

Dagogo-Jack, S. & Alberti, G. (2002) Management of diabetes mellitus in surgical patients. *Diabetes Spectrum*, **15**, 44–48.

De, P. & Child, D. (2001) Euglycaemic ketoacidosis – Is it on the rise? *Practical Diabetes International*, **18** (7), 239–240.

Dhatariya, L., Levy, N., Kilvert, A. *et al.* (2012) NHS Diabetes guideline for the perioperative management of the adult patient with diabetes. *Diabetic Medicine*, **29**, 420–433.

Dickerson L, Sack Y, Hueston W. (2003) Glycaemic control in medical inpatients with type 2 diabetes receiving sliding scale insulin regimens versus routine diabetic medicines: a multicentre randomized control trial. *Annals of Family Medicine* **1**, 29–35.

Dickerson, R. (2004) Specialised nutrition support in the hospitalized obese patient. *Nutrition in Clinical Practice*, **19**, 245–254.

Dixon J., O'srien P., Playfair J. *et al.* (2008) Adjustable gastric banding and conventional therapy for Type 2 diabetes: A randomized contolled trial. *Journal of the American Medical Association*, **299** (3), 316–323.

French, G. (2000) Clinical management of diabetes mellitus during anaesthesia and surgery. *Update in Anaesthesia*, **11** (13), 1–6.

Geloneze, B., Tambascia, M., Pareja, J., Repetto, E. & Magna, L. (2001) The insulin tolerance test in morbidly obese patients undergoing bariatric surgery. *Obesity Research*, **9**, 763–769.

Gill, G. (1997) Surgery and diabetes, in Textbook of Diabetes (eds. G. Williams & J. Pickup). Blackwell Science, Oxford, pp. 820–825.

Gupta, Y., & Sharma, M. (2001) Reversal of pyrogallol-induced gastric emptying in rats by ginger (*Zingber officinalis*). *Experimental Clinical Pharmacology*, **23** (9), 501–503.

Joslin Diabetes Centre (2009) Guideline for inpatient management of surgical and ICU patients with diabetes (pre, peri and postoperative care). The Joslin Centre Boston USA.

Kirschner, R. (1993) Diabetes in paediatric ambulatory surgical patients. *Journal of Post Anaesthesia Nursing*, **8** (5), 322–326.

Klow, N., Draganov, B., Os, I. (2001) Metformin and contrast media-increase risk of lactic acidosis? *Tidsskr Nor laegeforen* **121** (15), 1829.

Kwon, S., Thompson, R., Dellinger, P. *et al.* (2003) Importance of perioperative glycaemic control in general surgery: A report from the surgical care and outcomes assessment program. *Annals of Surgery*, **257** (1), 8–14.

Marks, J., Hirsch, J. & de Fronzo, R. (eds) (1998) Current Management of Diabetes Mellitus. C.V. Mosby, St Louis, pp. 247–254.

Mirtallo, J. (2008) Nutrition support for the obese surgical patient. *Medscape Pharmacist*, http://www.medscap.com/viewarticle/566036 (accessed February 2008).

Nassar, A., Boyle, M., Seifert, K., *et al.* (2012) Insulin pump therapy in patients with diabetes undergoing surgery. *Endocrinology Practice*, **18** (1) 49–55.

Norred, C. (2000) Use of complementary and alternative medicines by surgical patients. *Journal of the American Association of Nurse Anaesthetists*, **68** (1), 13–18.

Norred, C. (2002) Complementary and alternative medicine use by surgical patients. *AORN*, **76** (6), 1013–1021.

O'srien, P., Dixon, J. & Laurie, C. (2006). Treatment of mild to moderate obesity with laparoscopic adjustable gastric banding or an intensive medical program: A randomized trial. *Annals of Internal Medicine*, **144** (9):625-33.

Queensland Health (2012) Inpatient guidelines: Insulin infusion pump management. Queensland Health, Australia.

Rosenfeldt, F. 2005 Coenzyme CQ-10 therapy before cardiac surgery improves mitochondrial function and *in vitro* contractility of myocardial tissue. *Journal of Thoracic and Cardiovascular Surgery*, **129**, 25–32.

Stevenson, C. (1994) The psychophysiological effects of aromatherapy massage following cardiac surgery. *Complementary Therapies in Medicine*, **2** (1), 27–35.

Tsen, I. 2000) Alternative medicine use in presurgical patients. *Anaesthesiology*, **93** (1), 148–151.

Werther, G. (1994) Diabetes mellitus & surgery. Royal Children's Hospital Melbourne. http://www.rch.org.au/clinicalguide/cpg.cfm?doc_id=5190 (accessed February 2008).

Zhuang, U. *et al.* (2001) Do high glucose levels have differential effect on FDG uptake in inflammatory and malignant disorders? *Nuclear Medicine Communication*, **10**, 1123–1128.

Example Instruction Sheet 2(a): Instructions for people with diabetes on oral glucose-lowering medicines having procedures as outpatients under sedation of general anaesthesia

Person's Name: ....   UR...

Time & Date of Appointment: ....

Where to go:..

IT IS IMPORTANT THAT YOU INFORM NURSING AND MEDICAL STAFF THAT YOU HAVE DIABETES

Morning

If your diabetes is controlled by diet and/or diabetes tablets and you are going to the operating theatre in the morning:

- take nothing by mouth from midnight
- test your blood glucose and bring your blood glucose record to the hospital with you
- do not take your morning diabetes tablets.

Afternoon

If your diabetes is controlled by diet and/or diabetes tablets and you are going to the operating theatre in the afternoon:

- have a light breakfast only (coffee/tea, 2 slices of toast with spread), and nothing by mouth after that
- test your blood glucose and bring your blood glucose record to the hospital with you
- omit your morning diabetes tablets unless your doctor tells you to take them.

If you have any questions:

Contact: ....   Telephone: ....

Note: The inappropriate paragraph can be deleted or, better still, separate forms can be produced for morning and afternoon procedures.

Example Instruction Sheet 2(b): Instructions for people with diabetes on insulin having procedures as outpatients under sedation or general anaesthesia

Patient's Name: .... UR: ....

Time & Date of Appointment:...

where to go:..

IT IS IMPORTANT THAT YOU INFORM NURSING AND MEDICAL STAFF THAT YOU HAVE DIABETES

Morning

If your diabetes is controlled by insulin and you are going to the operating theatre in the morning:

- take nothing by mouth from midnight
- test your blood glucose and bring your blood glucose record to the hospital with you
- omit your morning insulin. OR Take units of insulin.

Afternoon

If your diabetes is controlled by insulin and you are going to the operating theatre in the afternoon:

- have a light breakfast only (coffee/tea, 2 slices of toast with spread), and nothing by mouth after that
- test your blood glucose and bring your blood glucose record to the hospital with you
- take .... units of insulin.

If you have any questions:

Contact:......................................   Telephone: ....

Note: The inappropriate paragraph can be deleted or, better still, separate forms can be produced for morning and afternoon procedures.

Chapter 10
Conditions Associated with Diabetes

Key points

- Some of the conditions described in this chapter are rare; others occur more often.
- Many are overlooked in the focus on achieving metabolic targets.
- Diabetes may be overlooked when managing conditions such as TB and HIV/ AIDs.
- Most conditions could be identified as part of routine diabetes assessment and preventative screening programmes.
- The concomitant presence of one or more of these conditions may influence diabetes management choices, health outcomes, diabetes self-care capability and mental health.

Introduction

This chapter outlines some conditions that are associated with diabetes. They are often managed in specialised services and some are very rare. A basic knowledge about these conditions can alert nurses to the possibility that they could be present, allow appropriate nursing care plans to be formulated and facilitate early referral for expert advice, which ultimately improves the health and well being of the individual.

The conditions covered in this chapter are:

- enteral and parenteral nutrition
- diabetes and cancer
- smoking and alcohol addiction
- brittle diabetes
- Illegal drug use
- oral health
- liver disease

Care of People with Diabetes: A Manual of Nursing Practice, Fourth Edition. Trisha Dunning.
© 2014 John Wiley & Sons, Ltd. Published 2014 by John Wiley & Sons, Ltd.

- breast mastopathy
- coeliac disease
- cystic fibrosis-related diabetes
- sleep disturbance
- tuberculosis
- HIV/aids
- hearing deficits
- musculoskeletal disorders
- corticosteroid and antipsychotic medications
- diabetes and driving
- fasting for religious observances.

ENTERAL AND PARENTERAL NUTRITION

Practice points

- The policies and procedures of relevant health service facilities and countries should be followed when caring for people with central lines, PEG tubes, and nasogastric tubes.
- Enteral and parenteral nutrition is used to supply nutritional requirements in special circumstances such as malnourished patients admitted with a debilitating disease and where there is a risk of increasing the malnourishment, for example, fasting states and palliative care. Malnourishment leads to increased mortality and morbidity thus increasing length of stay in hospital, especially in older people (Chapters 4 & 12) (Middleton *et al.* 2001). Malnourishment can also affect medicine choices. Often the patient is extremely ill or has undergone major gastrointestinal, head or neck surgery, or has gastroparesis diabeticorum, a diabetes complication that leads to delayed gastric emptying and can result in hypoglycaemia due to delayed food absorption, bloating, and abdominal pain. Alternatively, hyperglycaemia can occur. Gastroparesis is very distressing for the individual.

Aims of therapy

(1) Reduce anxiety associated with the condition requiring enteral therapy and the procedure by involving the individual in management decisions, explaining the process and why enteral feeing is necessary. In some cases family members/carers will need to be included in the education. Ample time should be allowed to enable people's concerns to be addressed.
(2) Prevent sepsis.
(3) Maintain an acceptable blood glucose range (4–8 mmol/L) except in frail older people when 6–8 mmol/L might be appropriate.
(4) Maintain normal urea, electrolytes, liver function tests, and blood gas levels.
(5) Supply adequate nutrition in terms of protein, fat, and carbohydrate to support normal body functions and promote growth and repair.
(6) Achieve positive nitrogen balance.
(7) Prevent complications of therapy.
(8) The long-term aim of enteral/parenteral feeding is the return of the patient to oral feeding. However, if life expectancy is reduced and/or in older people it may be

permanent (Chapters 4 and 12). In such cases decisions about when to discontinue the feeding should be made proactively, perhaps documented in an advanced care plan (Dunning *et al.* 2012). Blood glucose monitoring and reviewing the diabetes management regimen including medicines is essential when oral feeding resumes (Australian Diabetes Society (ADS) 2012).

It may also be necessary to consider the balance of bacteria in the gut and the role these organisms play in altering dietary and metabolic processes. Specific 'good bacteria' appear to play a role in reducing systemic inflammatory processes. They also appear to play a role in fasting hyperglycaemia, obesity, steatosis, insulin resistance and hyperinsulinaemia as well as in the secretion of gastrointestinal hormones such as the incretins see Chapter 1. Prebiotics and probiotics could be beneficial to gut and overall health but more research is required.

Complications of enteral nutrition

(1) Mechanical problems such as aspiration, poor gastric emptying and reflux can occur, especially if the person has altered mental status and/or a suppressed gag reflex.
(2) Metabolic consequences include hyperglycaemia and hypernatraemia depending on the feed used, the supplements added to the feed, and when a high feeding rate is used. Hyperglycaemia in people receiving enteral nutrition is associated with increased risk of cardiac complications, infection, sepsis and acute renal failure. Significantly people with mean blood glucose >9.1 mmol/L have a 10-fold greater risk of death than people with mean blood glucose 6.9 mmol/L, independent of age, gender and presence of diabetes complications (Australian Diabetes Society (ADS) 2912) Feeding into the small bowel rather than the stomach minimises metabolic disturbance. People who cannot indicate that they are thirsty and who have altered mental status, particularly older people, are at risk of these metabolic consequences. Hypoglycaemia can occur if food is not absorbed, the calorie load is reduced and if there are blockages in the feeding tubes. Medicine interactions can also contribute to hyper and hypoglycaemia, see Chapters 5 and 19.
(3) Gastrointestinal problems, the most common is diarrhoea, which is usually osmotic in nature. Gastroparesis may be present.

Routes of administration

Enteral feeds

The enteral route supplies nutrients and fluids when the oral route is inadequate or obstructed. Feeds are administered via a nasogastric, duodenal, jejunal or gastrostomy tube.

Enteral feeding is preferred over parenteral feeding when the gut is functioning normally and oral feeds do not meet the patient's nutritional requirements (McClave *et al.* 1999). Nasogastric tubes may be used in the short term. Nasogastric feeds have a significant risk of pulmonary aspiration. The tubes are easily removed by confused patients and cause irritation to the nasal mucosa and external nares that can be uncomfortable and is an infection risk in immunocompromised patients and people with hyperglycaemia.

Duodenal and jejunal tubes do not carry the same risk of pulmonary aspiration but the feeds can contribute to gastric intolerance and bloating, especially in the presence of gastroparesis; see Chapter 8.

Gastroscopy tubes are used in the long term when the stomach is not affected by the primary disease, which may preclude their use in people with established autonomic neuropathy that involves the gastrointestinal tract. The tubes can be inserted through a surgical incision and the creation of a stoma. More commonly, percutaneous endoscopic techniques (PEG) are used (Thomas 2001). Inserting a PEG tube involves making an artificial tract between the stomach and the abdominal wall through which a tube is inserted. The tube can be a balloon tube or a button type that is more discrete and lies flat to the skin. An extension tube is inserted into the gastroscopy tube during feeding.

Gastrostomy (PEG) feeds

Feeds can usually be undertaken 12–24 hours after the tube is inserted but can be given as early as 4–6 hours after tube insertion in special circumstances. The initial feed may be water and or dextrose saline depending on the patient's condition.

Mode of administration

(1) Bolus instillation: may result in distension and delayed gastric emptying. Aspiration can occur. Diarrhoea may be a complication. *This method is not suitable for people with diabetes who have autonomic neuropathy, especially gastroparesis.*
(2) Continuous infusion: via gravity infusion or pump. This can lead to hyperinsulinaemia in Type 2 diabetes because glucose-mediated insulin production occurs. The effect on blood glucose can be minimised by using formulas with a low glycaemic index. Administering insulin via the IV route enables the caloric input to be balanced with the insulin requirements, but is not suitable for long-term use or in some clinical settings.

The strength of the feeds should be increased gradually to prevent a sudden overwhelming glucose load in the bloodstream. An IV insulin infusion is an ideal method to control blood glucose levels. Blood glucose monitoring is essential to gauge the impact of the feed on blood glucose and appropriately titrate medication doses.

The feeds usually contain protein, fat, and carbohydrate. The carbohydrate is in the form of dextrose, either 25% or 40%, and extra insulin may be needed to account for the glucose load. A balance must be achieved between caloric requirements and blood glucose levels. Patients who are controlled by GLMs usually need insulin while on enteral feeding.

Parenteral feeds

Refers to administering nutrients and fluids by routes other than the alimentary canal, that is, intravenously via a peripheral or central line.

Mode of administration

Parenteral supplements are either partial or total.

(1) Peripheral: used after gastrointestinal surgery and in malabsorption states. Peripheral access is usually reserved for people in whom central access is difficult or sometimes as a supplement to oral/enteral feeds. It is not suitable if a high dextrose supplement is needed because dextrose irritates the veins, causing considerable discomfort. It can cause significant tissue damage if extravasation occurs.
(2) Central: supplies maximum nutrition in the form of protein, carbohydrate, fats, trace elements, vitamins, and electrolytes. For example, in patients with cancer or

burns, larger volumes can be given than via the peripheral route. In addition, it provides long-term access because silastic catheters can be left *in situ* indefinitely. If patients are at risk of sepsis, the site of the central line is rotated weekly using strict aseptic technique. Central lines enable the patient to remain mobile, which aids digestion and reduces the risk of pressure ulcers.

Choice of formula

The particular formula selected depends on the nutritional requirements and absorptive capacity of the patient. It is usual to begin with half strength formula and gradually increase to full strength as tolerated. The aim is to supply adequate:

- fluid
- protein
- carbohydrate
- vitamins and minerals
- essential fatty acids
- sodium spread evenly over the 24 hours
- preserve/enhance gut health.

Generally, feeds low in carbohydrate/dextrose and high in monosaturated fatty acids are preferred for people with diabetes (ADS 2012). Nutritional requirements can vary from week-to-week; thus, careful monitoring is essential to ensure the formula is adjusted proactively and appropriately.

Diabetes medication, insulin or oral agents, are adjusted according to the pattern that emerges in the blood glucose profile. The dose depends on the feeds used as well as other prescribed medicines, and the person's condition. Generally, the insulin/OHA doses are calculated according to the caloric intake.

There is very little good quality research into the effects of glucose lowering medicines on blood glucose in people receiving enteral/parental nutrition.

Nursing responsibilities

Care of nasogastric tubes

(1) Explain purpose of tube to patient.
(2) Check position of the tube regularly to ensure it is in the stomach to prevent pulmonary aspiration.
(3) Confirm the position of the tube with an X-ray.
(4) Change the position of the tube in the nose daily to avoid pressure areas.
(5) Flush regularly to ensure the tube remains patent.
(6) Check residual gastric volumes regularly to avoid gastric distension and reduce the possibility of aspiration, especially if gastroparesis is present.

Care of PEG tubes

The same care required for nasogastric tubes applies. Additional care:

(1) Monitor gastric aspirates at least daily.
(2) Elevate the head of the bed where there is a risk of pulmonary aspiration.
(3) Weigh the patient to ensure the desired weight outcome is achieved.

(4) Monitor nutritional status; see Chapter 4.
(5) Manage nausea and vomiting if they occur because they increase the risk of aspiration, represent fluid loss, and are uncomfortable for the patient. Record the amount and type of any vomitus. Antinausea medication may be required. Warm herbal teas such as chamomile, peppermint or ginger may be helpful non-medicine alternatives if oral intake is permitted.
(6) If the PEG tube blocks it can sometimes be cleared with a fizzy soft drink but local protocol should be followed because fizzy drinks can lead to electrolyte imbalances if they are used frequently.
(7) Ensure there is adequate fluid in the feeds to avoid dehydration and the consequent risk of hyperosmolar states; see Chapter 7 (Thomas 2001).

Care of IV and central lines

(1) Dress the insertion site regularly using strict aseptic technique according to usual protocols.
(2) Check position of the central line with a chest X-ray.
(3) Maintain strict aseptic technique.
(4) Maintain patency, usually by intermittently installing heparinised saline (weekly or when line is changed).
(5) Patients should be supine when the central catheter is disconnected and IV giving sets should be carefully primed to minimise the risk of air embolism.
(6) Check catheter for signs of occlusion (e.g. resistance to infusion or difficulty withdrawing a blood sample). Reposition the patient: if the occlusion is still present, consult the doctor.
(7) Observe exit site for any tenderness, redness or swelling. If bleeding occurs around the suture or exit site apply pressure and notify the doctor.
(8) Monitor the patient for signs of infection, for example, fever. Note that elevated white cell count may not be a sign of infection in people with diabetes if hyperglycaemia is present.

General nursing care

(1) Ensure the person is referred to a dietitian.
(2) Maintain an accurate fluid balance chart, including loss from stomas, drain tubes, vomitus, and diarrhoea.
(3) Monitor serum albumin, urea and electrolytes to determine nutritional requirements, nitrogen balance, and energy requirements.
(4) Weigh regularly (weekly) at the same time, using the same scales with the person wearing similar clothing to ensure energy balance and sufficient calories are supplied. Excess calories leads to weight gain and hyperglycaemia. Insufficient calories lead to weight loss and increase the risk of hypoglycaemia.
(5) Monitor blood glucose regularly, 4–6-hourly, initially. If elevated, be aware of possibility of a hyperosmolar event (see Chapter 7). If stable, less frequent monitoring might be appropriate.
(6) Record temperature, pulse and respiration and report if elevated (>38°C) or if any respiratory distress occurs.
(7) Check the label including the date and appearance of all infusions before they are administered.
(8) Medications are given separately from the formula; check with the pharmacist which medicines can be added to the formula. Follow pump instructions and local guidelines carefully. Be very careful with look-alike and sound-alike medicines.

Insulin therapy should include regular basal insulin (intermediate or long-acting) and prandial correctional doses if needed. If the blood glucose is unstable and intravenous insulin infusion might be indicated (ADS 2012). Sliding insulin scales are not recommended and increase the risk of hypoglycaemia (ADS 2102). However, prandial correction doses might be used; see Medicines, Chapter 5. Not all oral medicines can be crushed: it is essential to check before crushing medicines for oral administration via enteral tubes or orally.

(9)   Skin fold thickness and mid-arm muscle circumference measurement can also be useful to ascertain weight loss/gain.

(10) Skin care around tube insertion sites and stoma care for gastrostomy tubes to prevent infection.

Care when recommencing oral feeds

(1) Monitor blood glucose very carefully. Long-acting insulin is often commenced when oral feeds are resumed so there is a risk of hypoglycaemia. Only rapid or short-acting insulin can be given intravenously.

(2) Monitor and control nausea or vomiting, and describe vomitus.

(3) Maintain accurate fluid balance chart, usually 2-hourly subtotals.

DIABETES AND CANCER

Diabetes, especially Type 2, has been linked to various forms of cancer but the relationship is not straightforward. There appears to be an increased risk of cancer of the pancreas, liver, and endometrium, and endometrial cancer also appears to be associated with diabetes and obesity (Wideroff *et al.* 1997). Diabetes may be an early sign of pancreatic cancer (la Vecchia *et al.* 1994). A recent study demonstrated a significant increased risk for all cancers at moderately elevated HbA_{1c} levels (6–6.9%) with a small increased risk at high levels (>7%) (Travier *et al.* 2007). These findings support the hypothesis that abnormal glucose metabolism is associated with an increased risk of some cancers but may not explain the mechanism or causal relationship.

Other cancers such as lung cancer do not appear to be associated with an increased risk in people with diabetes, and the evidence for an association with kidney cancer and non-Hodgkin's lymphoma is inconclusive. Few researchers have explored the association between Type 1 diabetes and cancer (Giovannuci *et al.* 2010). Interestingly, diabetes appears to be associated with lower risk of prostate cancer and the risk of pancreatic cancer appears to be restricted to people with diabetes that precedes the diagnosis of pancreatic cancer by at least 5 years.

Researchers have also suggested that diabetes is an independent predictor of death from colon, pancreas, liver, and bladder cancer and breast cancer in men and women (Coughlin *et al.* 2004). Verlato *et al.* (2003) reported increased risk of death from breast cancer in women with Type 2 diabetes compared with non-diabetics and suggested that controlling weight reduced the mortality rate. Likewise, median survival time is shorter (Bloomgarden 2001).

Common risk factors for cancer and diabetes appear to be ageing, gender, obesity, physical inactivity, diet, excess alcohol consumption and smoking. Ethnicity and genetics also appear to play a role but the relationship is not straightforward. Likewise, the inter-related effect of hyperinsulinaemia, hyperglycaemia, inflammation and insulin-like growth factors (IGF) in carcinogenesis is unclear. There is limited evidence that specific glucose-lowering medicines cause cancer. Reported associations for an association between cancer and thiazolidinediones, sulphonylureas, incretins and insulin glargine may be confounded by factors such as the effects of other cancer risks and cancer not being a primary end point. More research is needed into these issues (Giovannuci *et al.* (2010). However, early evidence suggests, Metformin is associated with lower cancer risk, and research is continuing to clarify the association.

Management

People with diabetes should be encouraged to participate in appropriate cancer screening programmes the same as non-diabetics e.g. mammograms, bowel screens and prostate checks, event though prostate cancer may not be associated with diabetes, if it occurs glycaemic control is likely to be affected, and it is a common and devastating cancer. A healthy well-balanced diet low in fat and alcohol and regular exercise are important preventative strategies as well as part of diabetes and cancer management plans.

Cancer management is the same for people with diabetes as for people without diabetes; however, some extra considerations apply. Cancer cells trap amino acids for their own use, limiting the protein available for normal body functions, which sets the scene for weight loss, especially where the appetite is poor, and the senses of smell and taste are diminished. Malabsorption, nausea and vomiting, and radiation treatment further exacerbate weight loss. While weight loss may confer many health benefits, it is often excessive in cancer and causes malnutrition, which reduces immunity and affects normal cellular functioning and wound healing. Glucose enters cancer cells down a concentration gradient rather than through insulin-mediated entry and metabolism favours lactate production. Lactate is transported to the liver, increasing gluconeogenesis. Hypoalbuminaemia also occurs.

For the person with diabetes, lactate production can contribute to hyperglycaemia and reduce insulin production, with consequent effects on blood glucose control. Hyperglycaemia is associated with higher infection rates, and the risk is significantly increased in immunocompromised patients and those on corticosteroid medications. In addition hyperglycaemia-associated symptoms cause discomfort, (Dunning *et al.* 2011; Savage *et al.* 2012; Diabetes UK 2012).

Diabetes management should be considered in relation to the prognosis and the cancer therapy. Preventing the long-term complications of diabetes may be irrelevant if the prognosis is poor, but controlling hyperglycaemia has benefits for comfort, quality of life, and functioning during the dying process (Quinn *et al.* 2006; Dunning *et al.* 2012; Diabetes UK 2012). However, many people have existing diabetes complications such as renal and cardiac disease that need to be managed to promote comfort and quality of life (see Chapter 18). For example, the chemotherapeutic agent cisplatin causes renal insufficiency and can exacerbate existing renal disease; cisplatin, paclitaxel, and vincristine might exacerbate neuropathy. Side effects from chemotherapeutic agents are usually permanent. Where the prognosis is good, improving the complication status as much as possible and controlling blood glucose and lipids may help minimise the impact of chemotherapy.

Specific treatment depends on the type of cancer the patient has. Diagnosis of some types of cancer such as endocrine tumours can involve prolonged fasting and radiological imaging and/or other radiological procedures. The appropriate care should be given in these circumstances (see Chapter 9). Corticosteroid therapy is frequently used in cancer treatment and can precipitate diabetes in people without diabetes, especially if diabetes risk factors are present, and cause hyperglycaemia in people with diabetes. Corticosteroids may be required for a prolonged time or given in large doses for a short period. Therefore, blood glucose needs to be monitored regularly in patients on corticosteroid medications, which are discussed later in this chapter.

Objectives of care

Primary prevention

People with chronic diseases such as diabetes often do not receive usual preventative health strategies such as cancer screening (Psarakis 2006). For example, Lipscombe *et al.* (2005) found Canadian women with chronic diseases were 32% less likely to receive routine cancer screening even though their doctors regularly monitored them. The discrepancy in screening rates could not be explained by other variables. However, the current focus on individualised and person-centred care suggests general health advice and screening could, or even should, be encompassed in diabetes complication screening programs.

Proactive cancer screening and prevention programmes are important and should be promoted to people with diabetes, for example, mammograms, breast self-examination, and prostate checks. The findings also highlight another indication for normoglycaemia, controlling lipids, and weight management. Preventative health care also needs to encompass smoking cessation, reducing alcohol intake, and appropriate exercise and diet. In addition to the specific management of the cancer indicated by the cancer type and prognosis, diabetes management aims are to:

(1) Optimise cancer management considering the end of life stages: stable, unstable, deteriorating and terminal (Palliative Care Outcomes Collaboration (PCOC) 2008; Dunning *et al.* 2011) to meet the needs of the individual.
(2) Achieve as good a lifestyle as possible for as long as possible by optimising comfort, safety, quality of life, and enabling the person to make necessary life decisions by controlling symptoms and providing support and psychological care to the individual and their families.
(3) Achieve an acceptable blood glucose range in order to avoid the distressing symptoms associated with hyperglycaemia and hypoglycaemia and the consequent effect on comfort, cognitive function, mood and quality of life deepening on life expectancy (end of life phase), diabetes type and indications and contraindications for various glucose-lowering medicines (GLM) (Dunning *et al.* 2011; Savage *et al.* 2012; ADS 2012). Insulin may be required. The type of insulin and the dose and dose regimen depends on individual needs and the effects of other treatment such as medicines, feeding and pain on blood glucose levels. Insulin analogues such as levemir and glargine may provide adequate control in a simple regimen; see Chapters 5 and 18. The short-acting glitinides may be a useful GLM option if vomiting is not an issue. Pioglitazone has been associated with a small but absolute risk of bladder cancer (Lewis *et al.* 2011) and should be avoided in people with or at risk of bladder cancer. Metformin may be contraindicated depending on the cancer and the status of the gastrointestinal tract. As with all care planning, the individual and their relevant carers should be involved in care decisions
(4) Prevent/manage malnutrition, cachexia, dehydration, hyperglycaemia, which contributes to delayed healing and decreased resistance to infection and hypoglycaemia. Diet should be appropriate for the presenting cancer symptoms and in some cases is part of the treatment of some cancers. Sufficient protein and carbohydrate are needed for hormone synthesis and to maintain stores that are being depleted by the cancer. Small frequent feeds, enteral or parenteral (TPN) feeds may be needed. Enteral and TPN feeding can lead to hyperglycaemia and be exacerbated by corticosteroid medicines, stress, and infection. Short- or rapid-acting insulin may be needed, usually 1 unit of insulin to 10 g of carbohydrate initially but higher doses may be needed. As indicated previously, selecting formulas developed for people

with diabetes reduces the impact on blood glucose. High fibre diets can cause diarrhoea, vomiting, and bloating if the cancer involves the bowel.

(5) Adequately control pain. Hyperglycaemia exacerbates pain.

(6) Control nausea and vomiting, which are common side effects of chemotherapeutic agents as well as some cancers. Preventative measures to avoid ketoacidosis and hyperosmolar states that can require admission to hospital, must be factored into the care plan (Chapter 7). Other causes include bowel obstruction, gastroparesis, infection, liver disease, medicine interactions, and increased intracranial pressure such as cerebral oedema and radiation therapy. Nausea and vomiting can affect hydration status and physical comfort.

(7) Prevent trauma.

(8) Monitor renal and hepatic function before, during and after administering cytotoxic medicines and before using some GLMs such as Metformin.

(9) Encourage exercise within the individual's capacity.

(10) Provide education and psychological support. Prepare for end-of-life care such as advanced care plans (Chapter 18).

Nursing responsibilities

(1) Provide a safe environment.

(2) Consider the psychological aspects of having cancer and diabetes such as fear of death, body image changes, denial, and grief and loss.

(3) Involve the individual and their relevant carers in management decisions, proactively plan for end-of-life care including discussing documenting advanced care directives and plans, power of attorney and making a will.

(4) Ensure appropriate diabetic education if diabetes develops as a consequence of the altered metabolism of cancer or medicines.

(5) Proactively attend to pressure areas, including the feet and around nasogastric tubes.

(6) Provide oral care, manage stomatitis and mucositis, and ensure a dental consultation occurs.

(7) Control nausea, vomiting and pain, which contribute to fatigue and reduce quality of life.

(8) Manage radiotherapy. Fatigue often occurs as a consequence of radiotherapy; the rates vary between 14% and 90% of patients and can have a significant impact on quality of life and recovery (Faithful 1998). Radiotherapy is usually localised to a specific site and side effects are also usually localised but radiation-induced pneumonitis and fibrosis (late complication) can exacerbate fatigue and cause considerable discomfort, which compounds fatigue. The pattern of fatigue changes over the course of treatment and often declines on no-radiotherapy days. Ensuring the person understands and is given strategies to help them cope with fatigue is essential. Information should be oral and written. Stress management and relaxation techniques can be helpful as can providing an environment conducive to rest and sleep.

(9) Monitor blood glucose levels as frequently as necessary.

(10) Accurately chart fluid balance, blood glucose, TPR, weight.

(11) Ensure referral to the dietitian, psychologist, and diabetes nurse specialist/educator.

(12) Be aware of the possibility of hypoglycaemia if the patient is not eating, is vomiting or has a poor appetite. Where the appetite is poor and food intake is inadequate, hypoglycaemia is a significant risk. QID insulin regimens using rapid-acting insulin such as Novorapid or Humalog and/or long-acting insulin analogues may reduce the hypoglycaemia risk. GLMs with long duration of action may need to

be stopped because of the risk of hypoglycaemia. In addition, if hypoglycaemia does occur it can be more profound and the energy reserves in the liver and muscles may be insufficient to respond to the counter-regulatory response to hypoglycaemia (Chapters 1 and 6). Short-acting sulphonylureas or insulin may be indicated in Type 2 diabetes. Biguanides may be contraindicated if renal or hepatic failure is present because of the risk of lactic acidosis. TZDs take some time to have an optimal effect, are difficult to adjust in the short term, and contribute to oedema, and can reduce haemoglobin and contribute to fatigue. TZD are contraindicated in people with heart failure and those at high risk of fractures (Chapter 5). TZD may be useful if prolonged low-dose steroids are required (Oyer *et al.* 2006). Incretin mimetics reduce postprandial hyperglycaemia but research into their benefit in corticosteroid use is limited. In addition, they cause significant nausea, vomiting, and weight loss, which can exacerbate malnutrition and increase morbidity in people with cancer.

(13)   Be aware of the possibility of hyperglycaemia as a result of medications such as corticosteroids and antipsychotics, pain and stress.

(14)   Monitor biochemistry results and report abnormal results.

(15)   Provide appropriate care during investigative and surgical procedures; see Chapter 9.

(16)   Consider the possibility that people with cancer often try complementary therapies in an attempt to cure or manage their cancer. It is important to ask about the use of complementary therapies and provide or refer the person for appropriate information about the risks and benefits of such therapies (see Chapter 19).

(17)   Maintain skin integrity by appropriate skin care especially where corticosteroid medications are used. They cause the skin to become thin and fragile and it is easily damaged during shaving and routine nursing care, brittle hair, which can exacerbate the effects of chemotherapy, and bone loss. Corticosteroids are also associated with mood changes, which can cause distress to the patient and their relatives. Careful explanations and reassurance are required.

Clinical observations

(1) Narcotic pain medication can mask the signs of hypoglycaemia.

(2) Insulin/oral agents may need to be adjusted frequently to meet the changing metabolic needs and prevailing appetite and food intake. In the terminal stages of cancer these medicines can be withheld, as long as the individual is comfortable and not subject to excursions in blood glucose that can lead to uncomfortable symptoms, dehydration, and pain.

(3) People with diabetes in the end-of-life stages, and their family carers, want their blood glucose maintained in a range that avoids hypo- and hyperglycaemia to promote comfort and quality of life (Savage *et al.* 2012; Dunning *et al.* 2012).

Managing corticosteroids in people with cancer

People with cancer are often prescribed corticosteroids as a component of chemotherapy to prevent or manage nausea, reduce inflammation or following neurological procedures. These medicines cause postprandial hyperglycaemia by down-regulating GLUT-4 transporters in muscle, which impairs glucose entry into cells. They also promote gluconeogenesis. Not all glucocorticoids have the same effect on blood glucose.

The effect depends on the dose, duration of action, and duration of treatment. Morning prednisolone doses usually cause elevated blood glucose in the afternoon but the blood glucose usually drops overnight and is lower in the morning. Insulin is recommended to manage hyperglycaemia (ADS 2102), using morning basal insulin or a premixed insulin at the midday meal because the blood glucose tends to rise towards the afternoon. People already using insulin are likely to require higher doses while they are receiving corticosteroid medicines.

Complementary therapies and cancer

Many people with cancer use a variety of complementary therapies (CAM). Estimates vary from 7% to 83%: mean 31%. High usage occurs in children, older people, those with specific cancers such as prostate and breast cancer (Fernandez *et al.* 1998; Wyatt *et al.* 1999; Kao & Devine 2000). The type of CAM therapies used varies among countries and ethnic and cultural groups. Distinctive characteristics of CAM users with cancer include:

- women;
- younger age;
- higher education;
- higher socioeconomic group;
- prior CAM use;
- active coping and preventive health care behaviours, and a desire to do everything possible to maintain or improve health and quality of life, as well as take an active part in management decisions;
- participate in cancer support groups;
- have a close friend or relative with cancer who uses CAM;
- changed health beliefs as a consequence of developing cancer.

Many conventional practitioners are concerned that CAM holds out false hope of a cure, interferes with or delays conventional treatment, poses a risk of CAM medicine side effects and interactions, and because not all CAM is evidence-based. Many of these concerns are well-founded; see Chapter 19.

Where CAM is used, it needs to be integrated into the care plan to optimise the benefits of both CAM and conventional management strategies. Some benefits of CAM use are longer survival time and improved quality of life using mind body medicine (Eremin & Walker 2009); and reduction in chemotherapy-induced stomatitis (Oberbaum *et al.* 2001).

The Mayo Clinic (2012) suggests useful CAM strategies alone or in combination, include:

- Mind body therapies such as relaxation techniques, meditation, massage, and creative therapies such as music, art, and writing.
- Gentle exercises such as some forms of Tai Chi and Yoga, which combine meditative practices, and walking. The latter can include pet therapy e.g. walking the dog. In Australia women with breast cancer have participated in Dragon Boat racing.
- Essential oils can be used in psychological care as well as massage and education and some reduce stomatitis (Wilkinson 2008). The oils need to be chosen to suit the individual because some odours contribute to nausea or may provoke unpleasant memories. Alternatively they can recall happy memories. The Mayo Clinic website refers to fragrant oils, however, these are vastly different from essential oils chemically and

should not be applied to the skin, used in baths or taken orally but they can have useful emotional effects when inhaled.

- Nutritional medicine that focuses on a healthy well-balanced diet, whole foods, low in fat and sugar and using vitamin and mineral supplements, especially in immuno-compromised patients if they are not contraindicated. Probiotics can help sustain normal gut flora. Soy products and vitamin D supplementation improve bone mineral density.
- Acupressure and acupuncture to acupuncture point P6 reduces nausea, and is a useful addition to conventional methods of controlling nausea (Dibble *et al.* 2007).
- Herbal medicines such as milk thistle complement the action of chemotherapy agents and reduce the toxic effects on the liver in animal models (Lipman *et al.* 1997) and anti-inflammatory agents such as curcumin may have a role but more research is needed.

For information about advising people about the safe use of CAM see Chapter 19.

SMOKING, ALCOHOL, AND ILLEGAL DRUG USE

Substance use refers to intentionally using a pharmacological substance to achieve a desired effect: recreational or therapeutic. The term 'use' does not imply illegal use and is non-judgmental. However, the term 'substance abuse' is both negative and judgmental. Continued drug abuse can become an addiction. The American Psychiatric Association (2000) defined criteria for diagnosing psychiatric disease including drug abuse and drug addiction (see Table 10.1.)

Table 10.1 American Psychiatric Association criteria for drug abuse and drug addiction. Drug abuse is diagnosed when a person exhibits three of these criteria for 12 months.

Criteria for drug abuse	Criteria for drug dependence/addiction
Recurrent drug use and not fulfilling important/ usual life roles	Tolerance
	Withdrawal symptoms when not using
Using drugs in dangerous situations	Taking increasing amounts over time and for longer than intended (needing more drug to achieve an effect)
Encountering legal problems from using drugs	
Continuing to use drugs despite encountering problems	Wanting to or unsuccessfully trying to reduce use or quit
	Spending a considerable amount of time obtaining, using or recovering from drug use
	Usual activities are affected by drug use
	Continuing to use despite knowing it is harmful

Smoking

Giving up smoking is the easiest thing in the world. I know because I've done it thousands of times.

(Mark Twain)

The prevalence of smoking has decreased in many countries but smoking continues to be the most common morbidity and mortality risk factor (Australian Institute of Health and Welfare 2006). Smoking is hazardous to health regardless of whether the individual has diabetes or not. In addition, constantly being in a smoke-filled environment is a hazard for non-smokers causing ~50 000 deaths annually in the US (Surgeon General's Report 2004). Smoking during pregnancy has adverse effects on the foetus as well as the mother's health.

Smoking is a strong and independent risk factor for cardiovascular disease in a dose-dependent manner in the general population. Stopping smoking reduces the risk, but the degree of risk reduction depends on the duration of smoking (SIGN 2010). The evidence for an association between smoking and microvascular disease is unclear, although a Swedish study suggests people who smoke currently or up to five years before the study are at significant risk of chronic renal disease (Ejerblad *et al.* 2004) and may be at risk factor of retinopathy in Type 1 diabetes (Stratton *et al.* 2001).

Smoking is also associated with respiratory diseases such as emphysaema, chronic obstructive pulmonary disease (COPD), chronic bronchitis as well as oral, laryngeal, bladder and cervical cancers and tooth and gum disease (Orisatoki 2013). In addition, environmental tobacco smoke ('second hand smoking') can have the same or more adverse effects in non-smokers because there is three times the amount of tar and > six times the amount of nicotine in second-hand smoke (Orisatoki 2013). Second-hand smoke can affect the foetus and children. For example, infant death and preterm birth as well as low birth weight is associated with maternal smoking and there is a higher incidence of middle ear infections, coughing, wheezing and asthma (National Native Addiction Partnership Foundation 2006) and emotional and behavioural problems in children whose parents smoke (Weiser *et al.* 2010).

Nicotine is the primary alkaloid found in tobacco and is responsible for addiction to cigarettes. Tobacco also contains ~69 carcinogens in the tar, the particulate matter that remains when nicotine and water are removed, 11 of these substances are known carcinogens and a further 7 are probably carcinogens (Kroon 2007). Of these, polycyclic aromatic hydrocarbons (PAH) are the major lung carcinogens and are potent hepatic cytochrome P-450 inducers, particularly 1A1, 1A2 and possible 2E1. Thus, smoking and quitting can interact with commonly prescribed medicines and foods. Smoking status is an important aspect of routine medication reviews and when prescribing medicines.

Interactions that can occur between tobacco smoke and many commonly prescribed medicines include:

- Subcutaneous and inhaled insulin. Absorption of subcutaneous insulin may be reduced due to insulin resistance, which is associated with smoking. Inhaled insulin is rarely used, but when it is, smoking enhances absorption rates and peak action time is faster and insulin blood levels are higher than in non-smokers.
- Propanolol and other beta-blocking agents.
- Heparin: reduced half-life and increased clearance.
- Hormone contraceptives particularly combination formulations.
- Inhaled corticosteroids, which may have reduced efficacy in people with asthma.
- Tricyclic antidepressants.
- Other medicines such as olanzapine, clozapine, benzodiazepines, and opoids (Zevin & Benowitz 1999).

Other medicines and foods can also be affected leading to less than optional therapeutic effects and subtle malnutrition. Dose adjustments of many medicines may be required when people smoke and may need to be readjusted once they quit. The side effects of medicines may contribute to smoking withdrawal symptoms.

People most likely to smoke:

- Are members of some ethnic groups such as Indigenous Australians, African American, and Hispanics.
- Have a mental health problem, 70% of people with a mental health problem smoke. In addition, people often commence smoking when they develop a mental health problem.
- Use illegal drugs and/or alcohol.

Quitting smoking reduces the risk of cardiovascular disease, respiratory disease, cancer and a range of other diseases, and dying before age 50 by 50% in the following 15 years. The risk of developing many of these conditions is increased in the presence of obesity and uncontrolled diabetes. Smoking in middle and old age is significantly associated with a reduction in healthy life years (Ostbye & Taylor 2004; SIGN 2010). A recent meta-analysis of observational studies suggests smoking increases the risk of developing Type 2 diabetes in a dose-dependent manner (Willi *et al.* 2007). Willi *et al.* found smoking was independently associated with glucose intolerance, impaired fasting glucose and Type 2 diabetes.

Quitting smoking is difficult and requires significant behaviour change on the part of the individual and support form their family and friends. In order to change, the person must first recognise there is a problem and the scale of the problem. The desire to change may not be the same as wanting help to change. Almost 75% of smokers report they want to quit (Owen *et al.* 1992), but <7% remain smoke free after 12 months and the average smoker tries to quite 6–9 times in their lifetime (American Cancer Society 2007). Smoking at night appears to be a predictor of nicotine dependence and is a significant predictor of relapsing within 6 months of trying to quit (Bover *et al.* 2008). In addition, smoking at night is associated with poor treatment outcomes (Foulds *et al.* 2006). Bover *et al.* suggested health professionals should specifically ask about night smoking when assessing readiness to quit.

Research suggests timing smoking cessation interventions to coincide with the individual's readiness to change is important to success. In addition, sociologists highlight the importance of life course transitions in behaviour change and suggest the longer people live the more likely they are to make transitions in later life and the more likely such transitions are to be accompanied by changes in behaviour (George 1995). Thus targeting smoking cessation interventions to coincide with life transitions may be more likely to succeed.

For example, Lang *et al.* (2007) suggested individuals retiring from work are more likely to stop smoking than those who remain at work after controlling for retiring due to ill health. They recommended interventions be developed for those making the transition to retirement and employers should incorporate smoking cessation programmes into their retirement plans. Health events, particularly those that are disabling or affect work and lifestyle also affect smoking cessation rates (Falba 2005). These and other studies suggest several key transitions could be used target smoking cessation in addition to regular prevention messages.

However, population health models and strategies as part of every country's public health framework that focuses on all the inter-related personal and social factors involved is essential. Significantly, health professionals should be appropriate role models and not smoke.

Nicotine addiction

Nicotine receptors, a_4b_2 nicotinic acetylcholine receptors (nAChRs), are located throughout the central nervous system. Nicotine binds to these receptors, and acts as an agonist prolonging activation of these receptors and facilitating the release of neurotransmitters such as acetylcholine, dopamine, serotonin, and beta-endorphins, which engenders pleasurable feelings, arousal, reduced anxiety and relaxation. Nicotine action mode reinforces dependence in a cyclical manner: smoking stimulates dopamine, the dopamine level falls as the nicotine level falls producing withdrawal symptoms. Smoking again suppresses the cravings by restimulating the nAChRs receptors.

The area of the brain concerned with addiction appears to be the insula, a small structure within the cerebral cortex. People with damage to the insula from trauma or stroke often suddenly stop smoking and remain non-smoking (Naqvi *et al.* 2007). Five milligrams of nicotine per day is a large enough dose to cause addiction. Each cigarette contains between 0.13 and 2 mg of nicotine, thus even light smokers can be addicted. Nicotine is present in the blood stream within 15 seconds of smoking a cigarette, which provides immediate gratification (Watkins *et al.* 2000). Chronic nicotine use desensitises the receptors and increasing amounts of nicotine are required to achieve pleasurable effects.

Withdrawal symptoms usually occur within the first 24 hours and can be very stressful. Withdrawal symptoms include:

- craving tobacco;
- difficulty concentrating, which affects work and usual daily activities;
- headache;
- impaired motor performance;
- fatigue;
- irritability;
- anxiety and restlessness;
- sleep disturbances;
- nausea;
- hunger and weight gain; concern about putting on weight can be a barrier to quitting.

All of these symptoms can lead to neglect of diabetes self-care. Smoking cessation programmes need to help the individual manage these symptoms.

Assisting the person to stop smoking

Brief advice from general practitioners (GPs) and other health professionals has a limited effect: only 2–3% quit per year (Lancaster & Stead 2004) but the effect size can be increased if other strategies are also used. These include referral to Quitline and similar services, interested supportive follow up, setting achievable goals and pharmacotherapy. The 5As approach can be helpful. It consists of:

Ask about smoking habits and systematically document the information at each visit. Provide brief advice to quit in a clear supportive, non-judgmental manner regularly.

Assess interest in quitting so that advice can be appropriately targeted to the stage of change and to opportunistically support attempts to quit. Assess whether the individual has tried to quit in the past and the factors that prevented them from quitting and those that helped, as well as the level of nicotine dependence: ~70–80% of smokers are dependent on nicotine and will experience withdrawal symptoms when they try to quit. Nicotine addiction is a chronic relapsing condition (Wise *et al.* 2007). Repeated efforts to quit can be demoralising and set up learned helplessness. Helping the individual manage the symptoms can support their attempt. Sometimes mental health problems become apparent when a person stops smoking, thus mental health should be monitored.

Advise about the importance of quitting on a regular basis and provide new information as it arises. Advice can include information about smoking risks and quit programmes. Advice is more useful if it is tailored to the individual. In Australia some health insurance funds offer member discounts to quit programmes such as Allen Carr's Easy Way to Stop Smoking. This method consists of a combination of psychotherapy and hypnotherapy.

Assist those who indicate they want to quit by asking what assistance they feel would help them most, refer them for counselling, provide written information or recommend other therapies as indicated and follow up at the next visit. Relapsing after attempting to quit is common. Praise and support are essential as are exploring the reasons for relapsing and discussing strategies for continuing the quit process. Motivational interviewing can be a useful technique.

Arrange a follow-up visit preferably within the first week after the quit date (Torrijos & Glantz. 2006). Some pharmaceutical companies offer support programmes through newsletters and Internet sites. Fu *et al.* (2006) showed 75% of relapsed smokers were interested in repeating the quit intervention (behavioural and medicines strategies) within 30 days of quitting, which highlights the importance of support and constant reminders. Advising and supporting partners may also be important.

Non-pharmacological strategies can be combined with the 5As. These include opportunistic and structured counselling that encourages the individual to think about the relevance of quitting to their life, helps them identify their personal health risks, and helps them determine the barriers and facilitators they are likely to encounter develop strategies to strengthen the facilitators and overcome the barriers.

Improving nutrition is important to health generally. Diets rich in tyrosine, tryptophane, and vitamins B_6, B_3, C, and magnesium, zinc, and iron may stimulate the dopamine pathway and help reduce the effects of nicotine withdrawal by increasing serotonin levels (Osiecki 2006). Improving nutrition can also reduce oxidative damage, which is increased in smokers and help reduce weight gain.

CAM strategies may help manage withdrawal symptoms. These include acupuncture and acupressure to specific points to reduce the withdrawal symptoms (Mitchell 2008). Patients may be able to learn to self-stimulate specific acupressure points. Treatment consists of biweekly session for two weeks and then weekly for 2–6 weeks. Herbal preparations include green tea and lemon balm tea capsules, which improves focus and concentration and reduces anxiety without causing drowsiness; Ashwaganda capsules, an Ayurvedic medicine, which increases energy levels and wellbeing, *Silymarin* (milk thistle) before meals to control blood glucose and support the liver, flower remedies, melatonin and high-dose vitamin B. All of these interventions need to be combined with education, support, and counselling.

Self-help websites describe a time frame when symptoms resolve and people can expect to feel better, which gives them a goal to aim for. They also suggest some steps to stopping, which include:

- Making a firm decision to stop and ask for help without shame or guilt.
- Asking people who successfully quitted how they did it.
- Quitting with a friend to support each other.
- Wash your clothes and air out the house to get rid of the smell and if possible avoid smoke-filled environments.
- Writing down the reasons you want to quit and the things that can help you succeed.
- Obtaining information about all the quit options and decide which one/s is most likely to suit you.
- Setting small achievable goals.

These strategies can be used in combination and included in other strategies. In the past two years the Australian Government legislated for significant changes to labeling on tobacco packaging that included graphic pictures for example the effects of smoking on the mouth and gums, and advertising campaigns as well as regulating where people can smoke in public building and environments. The effects of these strategies are yet to be determined but an Australian Broadcasting Commission (ABC) news bulletin in January 2012 suggested smokers covered the tobacco package labels with masking tape.

Medicines to support smoking cessation

A number of medicines are available to assist smoking cessation but they are not a substitute for counselling and support, which need to continue if medications are indicated. Commonly used medicines to help people quit smoking are shown in Table 10.2. A combination of dose forms can be used, for example, patches and gums. In addition, nicotine replacement therapy can be prescribed for pregnant and lactating women but non-medicine options are preferred, people with cardiovascular disease, and young people aged 12–17 years (Tonstad *et al.* 2006).

Other medicines and an anti-nicotine vaccine are currently being developed to reduce the link between smoking and nicotine concentration in the brain to lower the related gratification. Transcranial magnetic stimulation (TMS) may be adapted in the future to specifically target the insula. Currently, TMS does not penetrate beyond peripheral tissues.

Many cultures smoke, chew or sniff a range of smokeless tobacco products such as Gul, Gutcha, Iq'mik, Pan Masal (betal quid), and different snuff preparations. These chemical products often contain chemicals such as bicarbonate and other ingredients such as spices. The Third International Conference on Smokeless Tobacco held in 2002 concluded there is evidence that smokeless tobacco causes cancer in humans especially in the oral cavity and increase the risk of head and neck cancer. In addition, they lead to other non-cancerous conditions and are as addictive, or more addictive, than nicotine (National Native Addictions Partnership Foundation 2006). The Third International Conference produced a number of fact sheets about these products that could be useful in cultures where smokeless tobacco products are used such as India and Native American Peoples.

Alcohol addiction

Alcohol is also an addictive substance associated with significant morbidity and mortality. Between 15% and 20% of GP consultations relate to alcohol (Lee 2008). Short-term consequences include injury and domestic violence; longer term effects include other risk-taking behaviours such as smoking, neglected self-care, driving while intoxicated, cognitive impairment, peripheral neuropathy, liver cirrhosis, and fetal damage in pregnant women. Hepatic encephalopathy (Gundling *et al.* 2013) and peripheral neuropathy are significant consequences of alcohol addiction.

Approximately 10% of Australians and 20% of Indigenous Australians drink more than the recommended level (National Health and Medical Research Council (NHMRC) 2007). Young people are also likely to consume higher than recommended amounts of alcohol. Recommendations for alcohol intake were discussed in Chapter 1 and are defined in the NHMRC and other guidelines such as the American Diabetes Association (2011) guidelines; generally one drink per day or less for women and two drinks per day or less for men.

Table 10.2 Medicines available to assist people to stop smoking. They should be combined with other counselling and support strategies and good nutrition and be considered as part of the medication record and their benefits and risks reviewed regularly while they are being used. The prescribing information should be consulted for specific information about each medicine.

Medicine	Dose	Duration of treatment	Side effects and precautions
Nicotine formulations: Gum (Nicorette)	2–4 mg: 1 piece of gum 1–2 hourly	Up to 12 weeks	Sore mouth, hiccups, dyspepsia Caution: unstable angina, 2 weeks post MI, serious cardiac arrhythmias Acidic drinks and caffeine affect absorption
Lozenge	2–4 mg: 1 lozenge 1–2 hourly for 6 weeks then 1 every 2–4 hours in weeks 7–9 and 1 every 4–8 hours in weeks 10–12 (9–20/day according to need)	Up to 12 weeks	Caution: uncontrolled hypertension, recent MI, arrhythmias, gastric ulcers, diabetes
Transdermal patch (NicoDerm CQ, habitrol)	Available in 7, 14, and 21 mg doses. Patch applied every 16–24 hours	8–10 weeks	Localised skin reactions, headaches, disturbed sleep Caution: unstable angina, 2 weeks after MI, cardiac arrhythmias
Inhaled	168 cartridges; 10 mg nicotine/cartridge but delivered dose is 4 mg; 1–2 doses/hour as required	Up to 8 weeks dose needs to be reduced in the last 4–6 weeks.	Nasal irritation Caution: unstable angina, 2 weeks after MI, cardiac arrhythmias Contraindicated if severe airways disease such as asthma and COPD is present
Nasal spray	100 mg nicotine/10 mL bottle, dose delivered per spray is 0.5 mg; one dose is 1 mg in each nostril (1 spray)	Up to 6 months	Nasal irritation May be contraindicated if severe airways disease such as asthma and COPD is present
Bupropion SR (Zyban)	Starting dose 150 mg/day for 3 days then 150 mg BD	Up to 24 weeks	Nausea, vomiting, constipation
Varenicline (Chantix)	Starting dose 0.5 mg/day for 3 days then 0.5 mg BD for 3 days followed by 1 mg BD	Up to 24 weeks	Nausea, vomiting, constipation Mercola (2011) suggested Chantix can cause extreme mind-altering behaviours and movement disorders by releasing dopamine in the brain and blocking the pleasure centres in the brain and can lead to severe depression. Chantix may also have adverse cardiovascular effects. Mercola listed the following psychological side effects: depression, anger, hostility, suicidal ideation, mania, paranoia, agitation, anxiety, confusion and sleep disorders

MI = myocardial infarction.

Excess alcohol >40 g/day increases the risk of liver disease, hypertension and violent death (SIGN 2010). Likewise drinking 2–3 units of alcohol/day may not result in hypoglycaemia but alcohol consumption reduces hypoglycaemia awareness. In addition, both alcohol and hypoglycaemia affect cognitive function in an additive manner (SIGN 2010). Alcohol is associated with both benefits and risks for cardiovascular disease and psychological well-being. Alcohol in small doses may prevent cardiovascular disease and death in people with Type 2 diabetes; however, the threshold for admission to hospital with an acute cardiac event occurs at a lower level of alcohol consumption: one glass of wine/day (SIGN 2010).

The criteria for alcohol dependence are the presence of three of the following seven features:

- alcohol tolerance;
- withdrawal symptoms;
- drinking more than the recommended level or for longer than planned;
- previous unsuccessful attempts to reduce consumption or stop drinking;
- spending a significant amount of time procuring or drinking alcohol;
- neglecting social interactions and work responsibilities because of alcohol;
- continuing to drink despite the actual and potential health risks.

The strategies outlined for helping people quit smoking can be adapted to help people reduce alcohol consumption to the recommended levels or stop drinking. Screening for alcohol dependence can be accomplished using the World Health Organization (WHO) Alcohol Use Disorders Identification Test (AUDIT) (Saunders *et al.* 1993). High AUDIT scores indicate the need for a comprehensive intervention and counselling. Support groups such as Alcoholics Anonymous have a well-recognised role in stopping drinking and preventing relapse. Anecdotally, Men's Sheds also play a supportive role in encouraging men to talk about their problems with peers, encouraging social interactions and hobbies and also have a positive impact on mental health and wellbeing.

Diabetes is difficult to manage because GLMs are often contraindicated because of the risk of lactic acidosis (Metformin) and hypoglycaemia. Insulin is often indicated but adherence is often suboptimal and is compounded by erratic intake and malnutrition, which put the individual at risk of hypoglycaemia. Withdrawal processes for heavy drinkers need to be supervised and people require a significant amount of support.

Medicines to assist alcohol withdrawal include Acamprosate and Naltrexon, which are generally well tolerated and can be continued if the person drinks alcohol. They are effective at preventing relapse, delaying return to drinking and reducing drinking days. Disulfiram (Antabuse) causes acute illness if the person drinks alcohol while taking the medication. Supervision is required if Antabuse is used because life-threatening reactions can occur. It is not the ideal first-line treatment and probably should only be prescribed by doctors with experience using it or use it under the guidance of such experts (Shand *et al.* 2003).

Illegal drug use

The effect of marijuana, cocaine, and other illegal drugs on diabetes is unclear. These substances are associated with poor health outcomes and risk-taking behaviours in non-diabetics and people with diabetes. In addition, illegal drugs and the associated risks may compound or contribute to short- and long-term diabetes complications. The fact that they are illegal makes illegal drug use harder to detect. Generally, illegal drugs fall into three main categories:

- Uppers, for example, ecstasy, ice, crystal meth, cocaine, snow, speed.
- Opiates, for example, morphine, heroin, smack.

Table 10.3 The effects of medicine or medicine combinations and duration of action.

Main class of illegal drug	Duration of action	Possible effect on blood glucose[a]	Some commonly reported effects
Uppers	Usually 4–6 but up to 24 hours	Hyperglycaemia from missing injections/OHA increasing the risk of ketoacidosis (DKA)/ hyperosmolar states (HONK) Hypoglycaemia due to inadequate intake, nausea, and vomiting	Increased energy Tachycardia Weakness and lethargy Heightened sensations Ecstasy can cause boundless energy and the user might not want to rest or eat Cocaine often reduces appetite Sleep disturbances and/or lethargy and prolonged sleep due to 'come down' as the effects of the drug wear off Dilated pupils Nausea and/or vomiting Weight loss Impaired memory and cognition These affect self-care and the ability to recognise hypoglycaemia
Opiates	4–24 hours	Hypo or hyperglycaemia due to inadequate self-care such as OHA/insulin mismanagement and increased risk of DKA/ HONK	Euphoria Hallucinations Relaxation Slurred speech Disinhibition Confusion and altered perception Diminished libido Constricted pupils Nausea/vomiting Pain relief (therapeutic use)
Hallucinogens	Often rapid onset, for example, Cannabis begins acting within 6–12 minutes and may be stored in fat deposits for weeks	Hyperglycaemia due to increased intake and/or forgetting to take OHA/ insulin Increased possibility of DKA/HONK Hypoglycaemia with some drugs such as large doses of marijuana	Euphoria and disorientation Hallucinations Disinhibition Marijuana increases appetite Difficulty with coordination, making judgement Tiredness Can lead to psychiatric disorders including depression and paranoia

[a]Note the effects on blood glucose may not be a direct effect of the drug but a consequence of cognitive impairment, effects on judgement, hypoglycaemia symptoms not recognised or confused with the effect of the drug, and inadequate self-care (Brink 2008 in Glick 2003). Frequent blood glucose testing is recommended if a person with diabetes uses illegal drugs but the cognitive effects of the drugs often means they do not test.

- Hallucinogens, for example, marijuana (cannabis, pot, weed), LSD, solvents such as petrol, glue, and paint. Table 10.3 outlines the effects of these substances and their impact on blood glucose.

In addition, many herbs have psychogenic properties. They may be stimulants, sedative, cognitive enhancing or analgesics as well as uppers, hallucinogens, or act in a similar way to opiates (Spinella 2005). Significantly, herbs may contain more than one chemical substance and are sometimes used to manufacture illegal drugs. Examples include but are not limited to:

- *Acorus calamus* (calamus). Ecstasy can be manufactured from calamus.
- *Salvia divinorum*
- Ephedra species
- *Amantia muscaria* (magic mushrooms)
- A herbal mixture called hoasia, yaje, or daime.

The effect of any drug depends on its pharmacokinetics and pharmacodynamics, bioavailability, and elimination. Thus, the effect depends on the administration route, how the individual metabolises drugs and is usually dose-dependent. Common routes of illegal drug administration are:

- Enteral;
  - oral
  - sublingual
  - rectal
- parenteral;
  - IV
- subcutaneous, for example, 'skin popping' heroin;
- inhalation smoking, pipe, cigarettes, hookah.

Effects on diabetes

Illegal drugs appear to have two inter-related consequences for people with diabetes: physical effects, although the pharmacological effects on blood glucose appear to be minor (Glick 2008), effect on cognitive processes, which disrupt problem-solving, decision-making, and self-care. Cognitive effects are significant and contribute to erratic blood glucose control. They are also associated with other general health risks such as sexually transmitted disease, malnutrition, and reduced immunity, which impact on diabetes related well being.

As well as contributing to the development of long-term diabetes complications through inadequate self-care and hyperglycaemia, addiction to some illegal drugs exacerbates existing diabetes complications. Illegal drugs exert significant haemodynamic and electrophysiological effects. The specific effects depend on the dose, the degree of addiction (see Table 10.3), and the drug formulation. Marijuana, the most commonly used illegal drug, is associated with cerebrovascular events and peripheral vascular events (Moussouttas 2004) and atrial fibrillation and increased cardiovascular morbidity (Korantzopoulos *et al.* 2008). Smoking exacerbates the vascular effects and nerve damage may be exacerbated by excessive alcohol use.

Cardiovascular effects include:

- slight increase in blood pressure especially in the supine position;
- rapid tachycardia, most likely due to enhanced automaticity of the sinus node, which increases cardiac output and reduces oxygen carrying capacity due to increased carboxyhaemoglobin when smoking marijuana;
- constriction of blood vessels increasing the risk of cardiovascular and cerebrovascular disease, for example, cocaine;

- reduced peripheral vascular resistance but the extent varies in different peripheral sites;
- angina and acute coronary syndromes especially in older people with postural or orthostatic hypotension.

Interactions with medicines

Information about interactions between illegal drugs and OHA and insulin is unclear but some drugs might affect OHA/insulin bioavailability. In addition, the different illegal drugs and the different dose forms (inhaled, smoked, intravenous, oral) are likely to have different pharmacodynamics and pharmacokinetics (Brown 1991). A significant problem is the fact that many such drugs are manufactured illegally and there are no quality control standard processes to ascertain purity, bioavailability, or the contents of the drug.

Management issues

Management is challenging and requires a great deal of tact and understanding. Referral to an appropriate 'drug and alcohol' service is advisable. Health professionals should be able to identify illegal drug use and refer early to reduce the likelihood of addiction developing (see Table 10.3). The effects of drug or drug combination and duration of action depends on a number of factors including the dose and frequency of use and individual factors. Long-term use can contribute to psychiatric disorders and conversely psychiatric disorders can trigger illegal drug use. Illegal drugs can interact with conventional and/or complementary medicines and sometimes alcohol. All can lead to addiction, which has social, professional and financial implications and increases the risk of inadequate diabetes care, coma, and death.

Strategies include:

- Providing an environment where patients feel safe and able to discuss difficult issues.
- Taking a thorough medical, work and social history, and monitoring changes.
- Assess whether there are any existing mental health problems and their relationship to illegal drug use.
- Assess diabetes status and self-care capacity and provide information about ways to enhance safety that are consistent with the advice of the specific drug service if they continue to use illegal drugs. Having appropriate information about how drugs work and their potential effects can help the individual develop strategies to reduce the risk of immediate and long-term adverse events if they continue to use drugs. Diabetes-specific advice might include:
  - importance of frequent blood glucose testing;
  - need to test for ketones if the blood glucose is high especially Type 1 diabetes;
  - need to continue OHA/insulin but the fact that the doses may need to be adjusted according to blood glucose tests; advice about how to make such adjustments may be needed;
  - importance of maintaining adequate fluid and food intake to avoid dehydration;
  - importance of being able to recognise and treat hypoglycaemia and strategies for distinguishing hypoglycaemia from the effects of the drug;
  - importance of seeking medical advice early if they are unwell, develop an infection, for example, at IV drug injection sites, have intractable nausea and/or vomiting, depression;

- ways to reduce personal risk such as:
  - making sure they obtain drugs from a reputable source;
  - using sterile techniques and not sharing needles (e.g. risk of HIV and hepatitis C) or pipes/hookahs (e.g. risk of TB, influenza);
  - not driving after using illegal drugs;
  - practicing safe sex;
  - using with a trusted person who can support their self-care and seek medical care if an adverse event occurs and using in a safe environment;
- safe sharps disposal.

Practice points

(1) Although the risk of psychiatric disorders is high, not all illegal drug users have psychiatric disorders and not all people with psychiatric conditions use illegal drugs.

(2) Co-occurring psychiatric disorders, substance addiction and diabetes are highly challenging to manage and there is very little evidence for the most effective strategies because such people are usually excluded from clinical trials (Wusthoff *et al.* 2012).

(3) Advice is easy to give but very difficult to follow because of the mental effects of most drugs on cognition, decision-making and judgement, which affect self-care capacity.

(4) Larger doses of drugs are often needed to achieve the desired effect as addiction worsens.

(5) Coffee, tea, and chocolate are also stimulants.

BRITTLE DIABETES

'Brittle diabetes' means different things to different people.

Introduction

There is no easy way to define brittle diabetes. Some experts consider it to be a psychological condition; others regard it as having a physical basis, it often has both physical and psychological components. Brittle diabetes usually refers to wide fluctuations in the blood glucose pattern despite optimal medical management. Vantyghem and Press (2006) suggested the term 'brittle diabetes' should be reserved for people in whom 'instability, whatever its cause, results in disruption of life and often recurrent and/or prolonged hospitalisation.' Whichever definition is used, brittle diabetes is difficult to manage, affects quality of life and emotional well being, and requires an holistic approach. Repeated admissions to hospital for bouts of DKA or severe hypoglycaemia often occur and could be an early indication of gastroparesis (Chapter 8).

Brittle diabetes affects 3/1000 people with Type 1 diabetes, mostly young women (Vantyghem and Press 2006). The causes of brittle diabetes are multifactorial. Three forms of brittle diabetes are described:

(1) recurrent diabetic ketoacidosis;
(2) predominant hypoglycaemic forms;
(3) mixed glucose instability.

Causes of brittle diabetes

Physical causes of brittle diabetes include:

- Impaired insulin response. This could be due to rare conditions such as degradation of insulin at the injection site. In these cases an insulin pump can improve insulin absorption. In other cases insulin absorption from specific injection sites can be reduced or delayed. Changing sites may help (Martin 1995).
- Communication problems such as dyslexia that can make education and therefore self-care difficult. People frequently hide their difficulty, and tactful questioning is needed to identify it.
- Drug addiction.
- Gastroparesis leading to erratic food absorption is discussed in Chapter 8. Other gastrointestinal problems can also be present, for example, coeliac disease and cystic fibrosis-related diabetes, which are discussed in this chapter, and should be excluded.
- Seizure disorders.
- Inappropriate management regimen.
- Presence of other endocrine disorders, for example, thyrotoxicosis. Two to three per cent of people with Type 1 diabetes have Hashimoto's thyroiditis.
- Eating disorders, either under- or overeating.
- Unrecognised hypoglycaemia and inappropriate insulin dose increases that lead to further hypoglycaemia, rebound hyperglycaemia and DKA.

Psychological causes include:

- Anger and non-acceptance of diabetes.
- Difficult relationships where diabetes is used to escape from the situation or to manipulate it, or gain attention.
- Sexual abuse.

Management

Management is protracted and requires a great deal of patience and support for the person with diabetes and their family. Taking a careful holistic history and a thorough physical assessment can identify physical causes. Processes used to quantify blood glucose variability include:

- mean amplitude of largest glycaemic excursions (MAGE);
- mean of daily differences (MODD);
- lability index (LI);
- low blood glucose index (LBGI);
- Clarke's score;
- hyposcore;
- continuous blood glucose monitoring;
- r range of psychometric measures to exclude/detect psychological causes; see Chapter 15.

A long-term management strategy is required that involves an agreed coordinated care plan that is communicated to all relevant health professionals and the patient and their family/carers. Managing the underlying organic problems where possible is important and optimising insulin therapy is essential. Continuous subcutaneous insulin therapy (insulin pump) might be indicated. In some cases an islet cell transplant can be considered provided the individual meets the criteria for transplantation: hypoglycaemic unawareness, BMI <25, normal renal function and no plans to become pregnant (Vantyghem and Press 2006).

Regular case conferencing with the relevant health professionals is important. Liaison with a psychiatrist is desirable if the underlying cause is psychological, and may help the individual come to terms with their diabetes by going back to the time of diagnosis and exploring the issues in operation at the time. The focus should be taken off 'diabetic control' and placed on quality of life, initially. If other issues are addressed metabolic control is easier to achieve. A basal bolus regimen using rapid-acting insulin can be commenced if it is not already being used.

Role of the nurse

Support and patience are required to manage people with brittle diabetes. Nurses need to be aware that it exists and that it can have a physiological basis as well as an underlying psychological component.

Nurses can play a key role in organising case conferences, supporting diabetes education and identifying barriers to learning, which might include inspecting injection sites and observing the person administering an injection and monitoring their blood glucose. Follow agreed management protocols and/or identify strategies to enhance management and ensure the person has follow-up appointments with appropriate health professionals on discharge. Regular blood glucose monitoring in hospital and continuous subcutaneous blood glucose monitoring can help identify excursions in blood glucose levels and identify unrecognised hypoglycaemia, which will assist with appropriate care planning.

ORAL HEALTH AND DIABETES

Introduction

People with diabetes are at increased risk of periodontal disease, a deep infection that affects bone caused by bacteria (plaque), which destroys the fibrosis attachment that anchors the teeth to the jaw (Southerland *et al.* 2006).In fact, periodontal disease has been called the 'sixth diabetes complication'. (Andersen *et al.* 2007) Increased glucose levels in saliva and reduced buffering power of saliva because of reduced saliva flow rates has been demonstrated (Connor *et al.* 1970). The pattern of dental decay and the decay rates vary between young and older people with diabetes but are largely unknown.

People with diabetes also have increased rates of oral candidiasis and a range of other oral cavity diseases, for example, lichen planus, painless swelling of the salivary glands (sialosis) that could be due to disordered fat metabolism, and changed taste sensation (Lamey *et al.* 1992).

Symptoms of oral cavity disease

- bleeding gums;
- swollen gums;
- Halitosis;
- inflamed receding gums;
- pus around the gums;
- loose teeth;
- oral candidia;
- dental plaque, caries loose, worn or chipped teeth or ill-fitting dentures;
- painful abscesses are a late symptom and indicate permanent damage (Dunning 2009).

Of people over 65, 67% have few or no natural teeth. This affects their overall food intake and the type of food selected. There is a propensity towards low fibre, low protein foods. This can represent a significant risk of hypoglycaemia and nutritional deficiencies, which in turn affect mental and physical functioning and quality of life; see Chapters 4, 15, and 12.

Ageing also leads to submucosal changes and increasing prevalence of gum disease due to hyperglycaemia and the resultant dry mouth as well as the effect on tissue and high sugar diets. Saliva production can be reduced (xerostomia) and is often exacerbated by medications that cause dry mouth (NHMRC 1999). The degree of metabolic control, duration, age, and dental hygiene influence the likelihood of gum disease occurring.

Younger people with diabetes are also at risk of tooth and gum disease primarily as a result of inappropriate diet and inadequate dental care.

Causal mechanisms

- uncontrolled diabetes;
- microangiopathy;
- increased collagen breakdown;
- defective neutrophil function such as reduced chemotaxis and phagocytosis during hyperglycaemia;
- depressed immune response during hyperglycaemia.

Insulin resistance and deteriorating metabolic control can occur as a result of oral infection and requires adjustment to the diabetic medication regime.

Management

- Consider the possibility of oral problems where signs of eating disorders, infection or deteriorating control are present.
- Include dental assessment in nursing history and assessment and annual complication screening programs.
- Provide opportunities for cleaning teeth during hospitalisation and in aged care facilities.
- Nurses have a responsibility to educate their patients about preventative oral hygiene. This includes:
  - the need to have regular dental checks and education about ways to maintain oral health;
  - choosing a good toothbrush and toothpaste;
  - good blood glucose control;
  - eating a healthy well-balanced diet;
  - seek dental advice early for any pain, bleeding, redness, and persistent bad breath so infection can be treated early;
  - correct method of brushing teeth, not gums, to reduce bleeding risk
- Refer for dental assessment if existing disease is identified.
- Check dentures regularly to ensure they fit.
- Educate dental practitioners about diabetes. Dental practitioners should also be aware of the possibility of hypoglycaemia occurring during dental procedures and how to manage it; see Chapters 6 and 9.

DIABETES AND LIVER DISEASE

Introduction

Research suggests liver disease is an important cause of death in people with Type 2 diabetes (Balkau *et al*. 1991; de Marco *et al*. 1999) and diabetes may be the most common cause of liver disease (US Organ Procurement and Transplantation Network 2004; Tolman *et al*. 2007). Some studies show cirrhosis accounts for 4.4% of diabetes-related deaths (Balkau *et al*. 1991). Hepatic steatosis, like insulin resistance might precede the onset of Type 2 diabetes (Zarrinpar & Loomba 2012). Bile acids have an important role in glucose homeostasis and their effects are mediated by the farneold X receptor (FXR) and the cell receptor TGR5 (Zarrinpar & Loomba 2012).

A range of liver diseases occur in Type 2 diabetes including:

- Abnormal liver enzymes. Elevated alanine transferase (ALT) is common in Type 2 diabetes and may be associated with liver disease. Some studies show elevated ALT is associated with liver disease in up to 98% of cases, commonly fatty liver (NAFLD) and chronic hepatitis. Alkaline phosphatase (AST) may also be elevated.
- Non-alcoholic fatty liver disease (NAFLD), the most common liver disease in Type 2 diabetes. NAFLD is defined as fatty liver disease with no alcohol intake or amounts <20 g/day (Caldwell *et al*. 1999; King 1996–2012). Insulin resistance is a significant contributing factor to NAFLD. It is estimated to occur in 34–74% of people with Type 2 diabetes, up to ~100% of obese Type 2 patients (Tolman *et al*. 2007). NAFLD is characterised by a range of liver diseases such as steatosis and non-alcoholic steatohepatitis (NASH). NASH is a similar condition that consists of steatosis, inflammation, necrosis, and fibrosis and can lead to cirrhosis. Fifty per cent of people with NAFLD have concomitant NASH and 19% have cirrhosis at diagnosis. These conditions rarely produce symptoms in the early stages. The exact cause is unknown. The associated lipid pattern, elevated triglycerides, low HDL, high LDL, and high cholesterol, also occur in Type 2 diabetes. Insulin resistance contributes to lipolysis and elevated free fatty acids (FFA), which overload the hepatic mitochrondrial b-oxygenation system, and FFAs accumulate in the liver and affect normal liver function. NAFLD has been described as the hepatic manifestation of insulin resistance (Marchesini *et al*. 2003). Adipokines may play a role in the development of NASH. NAFLD is associated with increased risk of early morbidity and mortality and may have worse overall survival than people with alcoholic liver disease (DDW 2012). In addition, moderate to severe sleep apnoea and hypoxia are common in people with NAFLD (Fuchs 2012).
- Cirrhosis, which is often due to alcohol addiction and is also associated with insulin resistance and reduced insulin secretion, which have implications for diabetes management. GLM therapy is limited by hepatic damage and the risk of hypoglycaemia (Gundling *et al*. (2013). Gundling *et al*. found the prevalence of diabetes in a cohort of people with cirrhosis (n=87) was 30.5% and 31% of these were prescribed medicines that could have serious adverse effect. Most continued to drink alcohol and 41.4% did not adhere to their medicine regimen. Only 28.7% of those with diabetes achieved HbA1c<6.5%; those who did achieve acceptable glycaemic control had lower risk of hepatic encephalopathy, hepatocellular carcinoma, arterial hypotension and hypercholesterolaemia. However, hepatic encephalopathy was significantly more common in people with diabetes then non-diabetics. The safety and risk of aiming for HbA_{1c} in people with cirrhosis needs to be considered because it affects liver glucose stores and the individual's ability to mount an effective counter-regulatory response (Chapters 1 and 6).

- Hepatocellular carcinoma, which appears to be associated with insulin resistance, increased lipolysis, accumulation of lipids in liver cells, oxidative stress leading to cell damage, fibrosis, and proliferation of procarcinogenic cells (El Serag & Everhart 2002).
- Acute liver failure. The exact mechanism is unclear. Contributing factors include some medications, and/or diabetes-related abnormalities.

Alcohol is also an addictive substance associated with significant morbidity and mortality. Between 15% and 20% of GP consultations relate to alcohol (Lee 2008). Short-term consequences include injury and domestic violence; longer term effects include other risk-taking behaviours such as smoking, neglected self-care, driving while intoxicated, cognitive impairment, peripheral neuropathy, liver cirrhosis, and fetal damage in pregnant women. Hepatic encephalopathy (Gundling *et al.* 2013) and peripheral neuropathy are significant consequences of alcohol addiction.

- There is an association between the hepatitis C medication a-interferon and Type 1 diabetes (Fabris *et al.* 2003).

Managing people with diabetes and liver disease

Managing people with diabetes and concomitant liver disease is complicated by changes in medicine metabolism, contraindication to medicines such as Metformin and increased risk of medicine interactions. Screening for liver disease consists of:

- liver function tests;
- abdominal ultrasound;
- computerised tomography;
- magnet resonance imaging;
- liver biopsy.

Management is essentially the same as for any patient with diabetes but the exact strategy depends on the severity of the liver disease and the blood glucose and lipid pattern. Identifying the presence of liver disease appears to be important. Counselling to help people realise the severity and consequences of the problem is essential. It is important to consider concomitant comorbidities such as sleep apnoea, obesity and cardiovascular disuse and manage these conditions.

Diet and exercise are important. Many people with liver disease are malnourished, which compromises their immune status and health outcomes. Nutrition and exercise are discussed in Chapter 4. Supplemental vitamins B_{12}, D, thiamine, and folic acid may be indicated. Alcohol and smoking should be avoided because of their toxic effects on the liver. Alcohol is a liver toxin and is high in calories. In addition, it contributes to vitamin deficiencies. Bile acid sequestrants such as colesevelum have been shown to improve glycaemic control. Likewise, enterohepatic bile acid recirculation can change after gastric bypass surgery and contribute to the improved glycaemic control noted after such surgery (Zarrinpar & Loomba 2012).

The usual contraindications to medicines should be considered. Liver failure, ascites, coagulopathy, and encephalopathy is associated with altered medicine metabolism. The risk of lactic acidosis with metformin needs to be considered. TZDs appear to improve ALT and liver histology (Harrison *et al.* 2005) but are associated with weight gain, see Chapter 5. ALT levels should be ascertained before commencing TZDs and monitored regularly. Insulin is frequently required. Lipid-lowering agents are usually also needed. The usual diabetes self-care and education is necessary; see Chapter 16 and consideration given to end of life care in end stage liver disease.

CAM medicines

CAM medicine use should be monitored. People often take CAM medicines 'to support liver function'. These include (*Silymarin marianum*) milk thistle, alpha-lipoic acid, vitamins E, C, and B, cysteine, and omega-3 fatty acids. Health professionals should monitor usage of CAM medicines because some can worsen liver problems and may interact with conventional medicines. The liver damage caused by CAM medicines is the same as other forms of liver damage due to conventional medicines (Chitturi & Farrell 2000).

People with the various forms of hepatitis and HIV infections frequently use CAM. There is some preliminary evidence that one medicine, Jianpi Wenshen Recipe, might help reduce the viral load of hepatitis B surface and e-antigen. Some studies show beneficial effects of Chinese herbal medicine formula used with interferon on viral clearance but the research methods are often flawed (Lipman 2007).

Prolonged ingestion or repeated exposure may play a role in the development of chronic damage with some medicines, for example, Jin Bu Huan. The type of herbs likely to be used depends on geographical location, but migration and travel means they are often widespread. Significantly, many CAM medicines contain a mixture of herbs and sometimes supplements so it can be difficult to identify the specific liver toxin, which might actually be due to contaminants rather than the herb itself if CAM medicines are not obtained from a reputable source. CAM medicines should be taken under the direction of a qualified practitioner. Some commonly used CAM medicines that are reported to cause liver damage are shown in the following list (see also Chapter 19):

- Chaparral.
- Dai-saiko to.
- *Chelidonium majus* (greater celandine).
- *Lycopodium serratum* (Jin Bu Huan).
- *Ephedra* species such as Ma-Huang.
- Oral ingestion of essential oils containing pulegone such as pennyroyal: pennyroyal is not usually used in aromatherapy.
- *Serenoa* species (saw palmetto) often used to manage prostate disease.
- *Valerian officinalis.*

Haemochromatosis

Haemochromatosis is an inherited disease and occurs secondary to thalassaemia, some types of anaemia, and excess alcohol consumption. It is characterised by increased iron absorption. The excess iron is deposited in the liver, pancreas, heart, and pituitary gland causing tissue damage that disrupts the normal function of these organs and glands. The liver is usually the first organ to be affected.

Sixty-five per cent of people with haemochromatosis have a family history of impaired glucose tolerance or a diagnosis of diabetes (Mendler *et al.* 1999). Men are ten times more likely than women to develop haemochromatosis. This could be due, in part, to iron loss with menstruation in women. Haemochromatosis is rarely seen before the age of 20 and the peak incidence occurs in people aged between 40 and 60 years.

Other diabetic complications such as nephropathy, neuropathy, and peripheral vascular disease are often also present. Arthropathy occurs in two-thirds of patients with acute crystal synovitis, which can make self-care tasks, for example, insulin administration, difficult (Sherlock 1981).

Iron overload

Iron overload is associated with various metabolic conditions besides diabetes. Steatohepatitis is an iron overload condition distinct from haemochromatosis. It is characterised by hyperferritinaemia and transferrin saturation. Liver damage includes steatosis and non-alcoholic fatty liver disease (NASH). Type 2 diabetes is often associated with NASH (Mendler *et al.* 1999). Obesity and hyperlipidaemia that can lead to fibrosis and cirrhosis of the liver are common. The excess iron can increase the risk of cancer, and most probably stroke. Diagnosis is by MRI, liver biopsy, and blood glucose and lipid levels.

Management

Management consists of:

- Venesection to remove excess iron. Hypoglycaemia can occur after venesection and the nurse needs to be aware of the possibility and know how to prevent and manage hypoglycaemia. The patient should be informed of the possibility of hypoglycaemia and how to manage their diet and medications on venesection days to reduce the hypoglycaemia risk.
- Blood glucose can be easy to control or the patient might require large doses of insulin because of insulin resistance. Oral hypoglycaemic agents often do not lead to acceptable blood glucose control and insulin is needed.
- Blood glucose monitoring to enable changes to medication and diet to be made early.
- Regular blood tests to monitor ferritin, iron levels, and metabolic control.
- Counselling and medication to manage depression, if indicated.
- Care during tests and procedures such as liver biopsy (see Chapter 9).

DIABETIC MASTOPATHY

Diabetic mastopathy is a rare disease that usually occurs in women with long-standing Type 1 diabetes around the time of the menopause. Most women with diabetic mastopathy also have microvascular disease and often other concomitant diseases such as autoimmune thyroid disease and cheiroarthropathy. There is relatively little information available about the causes of the disease but it is likely that it occurs as a result of an immune reaction to deposits in the breast as a result of hyperglycaemia.

The breast masses are usually firm-to-hard, poorly defined, freely movable and not fixed to the skin. It is important to exclude cancer to allay fear and anxiety and avoid unnecessary surgical intervention (Wilmshurst 2002).

Diagnosis

Investigations include:

- Mammogram or ultrasound.
- Fine-needle aspiration biopsy. This is often difficult to perform in people with diabetic mastopathy because the fibrous tissue is difficult to aspirate into the needle. Frequently, core or excision biopsy is required. The tissue is usually fibrous with lymphocyte infiltration but no glandular changes.

Management

(1) Counselling and reassurance is important.
(2) Regular annual follow-up is necessary with repeat mammogram and ultrasound on a regular basis.
(3) Single lesions can be removed. However, 63% of lesions are bilateral and often recur after excision.
(4) Supportive bras may help relieve breast discomfort.
(5) Regular breast self-examination and early help-seeking should be routine practice.

DIABETES AND COELIAC DISEASE

Coeliac disease, also known as gluten-sensitive enteropathy, is a chronic autoimmune disorder where the lining of the small intestine is damaged as a consequence of sensitivity to gluten (Marsh 2011). Coeliac disease leads to malabsorption and sometimes involves many body systems. The link among the various disorders and coeliac disease is clear for some but not all disorders (Duggan 2004; Juvenile Diabetes Research Foundation (JDRF) 2008). Coeliac disease can be present with few clinical signs and occurs in 0.5–1.0% of the population (Fasano *et al.* 2003).

The causal association between Type 1 diabetes and coeliac disease is currently under investigation and possibly involves similar HLA genes, which are associated with other autoimmune disorders such as Addison's disease and thyroid disease. The impact of environmental factors on the genetic predisposition is unclear. Current studies investigating these issues include the Disease Autoimmunity Research (CEDAR) study and the Diabetes Autoimmunity Study in the Young (DAISY). People with Type 2 diabetes may have gluten sensitivity but there is no known link between the two conditions because Type 2 is not an autoimmune disease.

Coeliac disease is caused by a complex immunological response to gliadin, the main protein in wheat. Rye, barley, and oats have smaller quantities of gliadin. T cells associated with HLA-DQ2 or HLA-DQ-8 antigen become sensitised to gliadin and produce cytokines, which causes tissue damage such as villous atrophy in the mucosa and activates plasma cells to produce antibodies to gliadin. Not everybody with the particular HLA antigens develop coeliac disease for unknown reasons. Interestingly, cigarette smoking reduces the risk of coeliac disease by 80% (Suman *et al.* 2003). Peak diagnostic times for coeliac disease occur at 3–5 years and during the 40s, and affects more women than men (Green & Jabri 2003).

Untreated coeliac disease can affect growth and development in children and cause long-term health problems in children and adults such as osteoporosis, infertility, miscarriage, tooth decay and increased risk of gastrointestinal cancers. It can also affect glycaemic control and represents a hypoglycaemia risk (Mohn *et al.* 2001). Consequently, glucose-lowering medicine doses may need to be reduced.

Commonly associated diseases include:

• Liver disorders such as fatty liver, transaminitis, or hepatitis.
• Dermatitis herpetiformis psoriasis.
• Type 1 diabetes. The prevalence of coeliac disease in Type 1 diabetes is between 1.3% and 6.4% (Farrell & Kelly 2002; Buysschaert & Tomasi 2005) and the prevalence of Type 1 diabetes in people with coeliac disease is 5% (Colin *et al.* 1994). There is limited information about whether a gluten-free diet relieves symptoms in people with Type 1 diabetes and coeliac disease (Duggan 2004). Cavallo (2004) suggests 1 in 20 people with Type 1 have coeliac disease and 1 in 10 test positive for transglutaminase IgA antibodies.

- Irritable bowel syndrome.
- Anaemia, which is often a result of malabsorption of iron and/or folate and which responds to iron supplements.
- Bone loss.
- Various cancers.
- IgA nephropathy.
- Epilepsy.
- Neuropathies.
- Myelopathies.
- Ataxias.
- Male and female infertility.

Signs and symptoms

Common signs and symptoms include:

- having a family history of coeliac disease;
- chronic tiredness, weakness and lethargy;
- poor appetite;
- weight loss, failure to thrive;
- delayed growth in children;
- abdominal symptoms such as bloating, discomfort, malabsorption syndromes, pot belly, diarrhoea if most of the intestine is involved;
- irritability and depression;
- discoloured tooth enamel;
- skin disorders such as psoriasis;
- unexplained hypo or hyperglycaemia;
- elevated transglutaminase and endomysial antibody titres;
- anaemia;
- histological changes on endoscopy and duodenal biopsy such as flattened villi;
- other less common signs and symptoms include easy bruising, mouth ulcers, muscle cramps if serum calcium levels are low, folate and vitamin B12, A, D, E and K (fat-soluble vitamins) deficiencies, memory and concentration deficits and bone/joint pain (Marsh 2011).

Diagnosis

Screening people with these symptoms and those with IgG antibodies and IgA deficiency may be useful because a gluten-free diet is likely to improve the symptoms and quality of life (Sjoberg *et al.* 1998; Green & Jabri 2003; Duggan 2004). Some experts suggest universal screening is not warranted and recommending a gluten-free diet when there are no symptoms may not be beneficial, may be socially restricting and may reduce quality of life. However, Buysschaert & Tomasi (2005) advocated screening all people with Type 1 diabetes and repeating the test every year for three years if the initial result is negative.

Likewise, the International Society for Paediatric and Adolescent Diabetes (ISPAD) recommends screening all children with Type 1 diabetes at diagnosis and that screening be continued annually for the first five years after diagnosis and then every two years (Kondonouri *et al.* 2007). In addition, screening should be undertaken if there are clinical signs and symptoms suggestive of coeliac disease, especially if the person has a first degree relative with coeliac disease.

Diagnosis usually consists of:

- Screening blood tests to measure antibodies: anti-tissue transglutaminase (tTG), deaminated gliadin peptide (DGP), IGA and IgG, which are sometimes used in place of anti-gliadin antibodies (AGA), and anti-endomyal antibodies (EMA). Note: these are screening tests rather than diagnostic tests because false positives can occur.
- Small bowel biopsies where tissue is biopsied from different sections of the small intestine. Atrophied villi confirm the diagnosis. However, if the person has been on a gluten-free diet, they must resume eating gluten-containing foods for at least six weeks before the biopsies are performed.
- Genetic testing by blood test or swab to detect HLA DQ2 or HA DQ8. However, genetic testing cannot be used alone because not everybody who carries these genes develops coeliac disease.

Management

Wheat, rye, barley, and oats need to be eliminated from the diet but the general principles of eating a healthy diet to manage blood glucose and lipids, applies. It is essential to ensure micronutrient intake is adequate to prevent anaemia and osteoporosis and other nutritional deficiencies such as vitamin B complex. Many gluten-free foods have a high GI and high fat content so referring the individual to a dietitian is essential. Grains such as buckwheat, chia and millet are acceptable alternative grains. The range of gluten-free foods available on the market is increasing, which makes it easier for people to adhere to the strict gluten free diet required to heal the intestine. Reading food labels to identify hidden gluten is essential.

Managing a gluten-free diet as well as balancing carbohydrate intake, insulin and activity can be challenging and stressful. However, the long-term consequences in people with diabetes include chronic hypoglycaemia (see Chapter 6) that can cause neurological deficits. The individual should carry gluten-free hypoglycaemia treatment at all times but should ingest gluten-containing food if that is all that is available because the risks associated with moderate to severe hypoglycaemia are significant. If hypoglycaemia unawareness is present the person might benefit from blood glucose awareness training. Managing intercurrent illness and optimal health to reduce the incidence and physiological impact of these illnesses is important. Regular screening for depression and quality of life might be indicated.

CYSTIC FIBROSIS-RELATED DIABETES

Cystic fibrosis (CF) is the 'most common lethal autsomal recessive disease in Caucasians, with a worldwide prevalence of 1/2500 live births.' (O'Riordan *et al*. 2009). Life expectancy for people with cystic fibrosis (CF) has improved over the past decade, thus complications, including cystic fibrosis-related diabetes (CFRD), the most common comorbidity of CF, are beginning to emerge. CFRD shares some characteristics in common with diabetes (Moran *et al*. 2010) but the pathophysiology of CFRD is not well understood. It is postulated that fatty infiltration in the pancreas leads to fibrosis and destruction of the beta cells that causes insulin deficiency, is the most likely cause. Identifying and treating people who develop CFRD early is important in order to maintain lung function and enhance survival. CFRD is more common in people with CF and liver disease. Recently, the Cystic Fibrosis Trust (CFT) (2004) in the UK recommended all people who develop CFRD be screened annually to detect diabetes and its complications. The SIGN (2010) guidelines recommend annual diabetes screening begins at age 10 and also recommends screening for associated conditions such as coeliac and thyroid disease. Both conditions can be present with few symptoms and can be missed during routine CF and CFRD care.

The prevalence of CFRD varies depending on the diagnostic criteria used. It can occur at any age but increases with age:

- 9% in 5–9 year olds;
- 26% in10–20 year olds;
- 50% by age 30 (O'Riordan *et al.* 2009).

However, SIGN (2010) suggested 20% of people with CF are likely to develop diabetes by age 20 and the incidence of CFRD increases thereafter to 80% by age 35.

CFRD mostly occurs in people with serious CF mutations that are associated with pancreatic insufficiency. Chloride channels are abnormal in people with CF, which results in thick viscous secretions obstructing the exocrine pancreas and fatty infiltration and progressive fibrosis that eventually affects the pancreatic alpha and beta cells. Thus the beta cell destruction in CFRD is not usually an autoimmune process.

Diagnosis

Few people with CF have normal blood glucose levels all the time for a number of reasons, thus diagnosing CFRD can be challenging and largely depends on detecting polyuria, polydipsia and weight loss, but such symptoms only occur in about 33% of individuals with CFRD (Dyce & Wallymahmed 2012) The CFT (2004) and Moran *et al.* (2010) recommend oral glucose tolerance testing (OGTT). However, the results can be misleading if the test is not conducted under ideal testing conditions and if the OGTT is performed when the individual is unwell or when they are on high doses of corticosteroids, which also increase the risk of Type 2 diabetes.

Variable intermittent post-prandial hyperglycaemia is the earliest sign followed by impaired glucose tolerance, then diabetes without fasting hyperglycaemia and diabetes with fasting hyperglycaemia (O'Riordan et al. 2009). Significantly, a diagnosis of normal glucose tolerance on and OGTT does not exclude abnormal post-prandial blood glucose levels at home when the person is consuming their usual amount of carbohydrate as distinct from the 75 grams used in an OGTT.

Some experts recommend the individual undertake regular blood glucose monitoring for a period of time to help diagnose the condition (CFT 2004). Blood glucose monitoring should be undertaken when corticosteroids are not being used for diagnostic purposes to make the blood glucose pattern easier to interpret. However, diabetes often presents when insulin resistance is increased such as acute pulmonary infections and lung disease, which can cause hyperglycaemia especially when corticosteroid medicines are used to control the inflammatory response. Other insulin resistance-inducing factors include oral, intravenous, nasogastric, gastrostomy high carbohydrate supplements and feeds, and immunosuppressive therapy e.g. after a transplant.

CF-specific factors that cause fluctuating blood glucose levels include:

- respiratory infections and inflammation;
- increased energy expenditure;

- gastrointestinal abnormalities that affect food absorption, change intestinal motility and liver disease;
- glucagon deficiency.

HbA_{1c} is currently being considered as a diagnostic test for diabetes but false negative results can occur in people with cystic fibrosis because of the increased red blood cell turnover. Fructosamine might be a useful alternative to monitoring diabetes control once the diagnosis is made.

Signs and symptoms

CFRD usually develops insidiously. Some signs and symptoms that should prompt investigation for CFRD include:

- unexplained polyuria and/or polydipsia;
- inability to maintain or gain weight despite optimal nutrition;
- poor growth;
- delayed puberty;
- unexplained decline in lung function.

Management

Managing blood glucose is important but challenging. People might require insulin during exacerbations of CF that require corticosteroid treatment (see information in this chapter). A high calorie high fat diet is recommended in CF (O'Riordan *et al.* 2009), thus an appropriate insulin regimen is usually required. Insulin is the only glucose-lowering medicine recommended for CFRD (Moran *et al.*1999) but the insulin regimen should be tailored to suit the individual.

The person needs to learn or have access to health professional support to increase insulin doses during acute illnesses, when the corticosteroid dose increases and when they are receiving parenteral supplements or feeds and in hospital. In these circumstances the insulin dose may increase up to four times the usual insulin dose (Moran *et al.* 1999). The insulin dose must be reduced when these circumstances are managed to avoid hypoglycaemia.

Diabetes education and involving the individual in care decisions is essential as is individualising the management plan to suit the individual. The plan should include plans for managing CFRD during period of wellness and plans for managing diabetes during exacerbations of CF including adjusting glucose lowering medicines to manage blood glucose excursions; diabetes and driving if they are insulin treated.

SLEEP DISTURBANCE AND DIABETES

Chronic sleep deprivation increases the risk of obesity, insulin resistance and diabetes (Shaw *et al.* 2008). Obstructive sleep apnoea is the most common type; central sleep apnoea occurs when the brain signals to the muscle that control breathing are affected. Often both types occur together. In addition, obese people and people with diabetes are more likely to develop obstructive sleep apnoea (OSA). Disturbed sleep results in daytime drowsiness. Shift workers are at increased risk of obesity and Type 2 diabetes, possibly due to changes in insulin sensitivity and appetite regulation when meals are consumed in normal sleep time (at night).

Possible pathways linking OSA and diabetes include:

- Activation of the sympathetic nervous system resulting in hypoxia and repeated arousal from sleep.
- Hypoxia effects on insulin sensitivity.
- Systemic inflammatory effects. OSA engenders increased inflammatory markers such as CRB and IL6 independently of other causes of inflammation.
- Disruption of the Hypothalamic-Pituitary Adrenal Axis, which leads to elevated cortisol levels, which affect insulin secretion and glucose disposal.
- Suppressed slow wave sleep. Slow wave sleep is thought to be important to metabolic and emotional restoration. Lack of slow wave sleep leads to insulin resistance independently of hypoxia and total sleep time.
- Fatigue form OSA and chronic sleep disturbance leads to less physical activity, which contributes to obesity and Type 2 diabetes risk.
- Autonomic nerve dysfunction due to chronic hyperglycaemia, which affects sleep regulation and can contribute to OSA and/or reduce the person's response to hypoxia generated by existing OSA.
- OSA is independently associated with hypertension and exacerbated cardiovascular risk.

Sleep apnoea can develop at any age and occurs in both men and women, but it is more common in men, especially men over age 30 and high BMI. Quality slow wave sleep is important to the way people process and store information they collect consciously and subconsciously during the day. Thus, sleep apnoea can affect memory.

Diagnosis

Common signs and symptoms include:

- unrefreshing sleep especially if the person snores;
- insomnia;
- snoring, startling and choking episodes during sleep;
- nocturia;
- night sweats;
- sexual dysfunction;
- cognitive impairment, difficulty concentrating, forgetfulness;
- depression;
- sleep-related driving incidents;
- systemic pulmonary hypertension;
- cardiac arrhythmias and angina at night (Young *et al.* 2002).

Physical examination should include neck circumference, which is often enlarged. In addition, microagnathia and enlarged tonsils might also be present. An oxygen desaturation index (ODI) >3–4% below baseline per hour of sleep represent severe OAS. Normal ODI is <5, and ODI >29 indicate severe OSA. The gold standard diagnostic test for OSA is polysomnography (ISG), which measures oral-nasal airflow, respiratory effort and oxyhaemoglobin desaturation, which is undertaken in sleep laboratories.

However, OSA can be measured at home using oximeters and noting symptoms of day-time drowsiness. In addition, valuable information can be obtained using the Insomnia

Severity Index, the Epworth Sleepiness Scale or the Berlin Questionnaire (Department of Veterans Affairs US 2013). Depression and OSA often coexist and may share some common aetiologies (Allen 2012). Thus, screening for and managing depression is also important.

Management

Management consists of weight loss and optimising blood glucose and lipid levels are essential because hyperglycaemia contributes to lethargy and sleepiness, exacerbates OSA and increases the risk of death. It is important to avoid stimulant foods such as caffeine and spices at night and to limit alcohol. Likewise, avoiding sedatives is important.

Mouth appliance that opens the airways and continuous positive airway pressure (CPAP) improve sleep duration and quality (McDermott 2012).

Screening people with OSA for metabolic derangements and asking about symptoms including snoring and daytime sleepiness is important. People who live with the individual can contribute important information.

Counselling about the risks associated with driving is essential. Significantly, partners should be involved unless the individual objects because they can often contribute important information to help health professionals support the couple and because sexual counseling might be beneficial.

Modern CPAP machines are not as noisy as the older models but they do emit an electric humming noise that can disturb partner's sleep.

DIABETES AND TUBERCULOSIS

There is strong evidence for a link between diabetes and tuberculosis (TB): people with diabetes and TB have higher rates of TB treatment failure and death, even when TB treatment is appropriate (Dooley *et al.* 2009; Sullivan & Ben Amor 2012). People with diabetes have a 2–3 times higher risk of developing TB than people without diabetes; approximately 10% of TB cases are linked to diabetes. The link between diabetes and TB will become increasingly important because of the expected increase in obesity and diabetes in countries that have a high TB prevalence, for example Africa.

TB is often not diagnosed or diagnosed late in a large number of people with concomitant diabetes and TB (WHO 2011). Thus, everybody with TB should be regularly screened for diabetes and screening for diabetes in people with TB should be considered in high risk populations. It should be noted that such populations might exist in countries where TB has been eradicated such as Australia and the UK, due to migration and refugees from TB-prevalent countries coming to these countries. In addition, many migrants and refugees are often also at high risk of diabetes. Although health checks are conducted before migrants and refugees enter Australia and other countries, diabetes and TB can be latent and become active at a later date.

Management

Studies are currently in progress to determine whether diagnosing and treating diabetes early in people with TB can improve TB outcomes (Dooley *et al.* 2009). Early detection and management may improve outcomes. Blood glucose and lipids, blood pressure control and complication screening should be individualised (Chapter 1). Active TB should be treated and TB status monitored. Relevant family and community members should be educated about diabetes and infection control processes. Systematically documenting and sharing outcomes could contribute to the evidence base for managing these two conditions when they occur together.

DIABETES AND HIV/AIDS

HIV/AIDs results in changes in glucose homeostasis possible through increased non-oxidative glucose disposal and increased glucose production in the liver (Spollett 2006). HIV is characterised by deficient immune status and is treated using combination therapy such as nucleoside reverse transcriptase inhibitors (NRTIs) and HIV-1 protease inhibitors (PI). The latter has been linked to hyperglycaemia, which resolves when the PI is discontinued or replaced with another class of medicine (Martinez *et al.* 1999). Other medicines such as Megestrol acetate, which is used as an appetite stimulant in people with AIDs-related cachexia has glucocorticoid effects that predispose people with diabetes risk factors to hyperglycaemia and weight gain (Rathgaber *et al.* 1992). The benefits of these medicines for treating HIV most probably outweigh the risk of diabetes.

Management

There appears to be three groups of people with HIV and diabetes:

- people with HIV and undiagnosed diabetes;
- people who develop diabetes during treatment for HIV;
- people who have diabetes and develop HIV.

The optimal method of screening for diabetes in people with AIDs is still under debate and may differ among ethnic groups. Screening is recommended for people who have the classic risk factors for diabetes, especially women, because of the dual risk to the baby of HIV and diabetes-related foetal abnormalities including Type 2 diabetes (Chapter 1) (Howard *et al.* 2005). However, there is some controversy over the best screening method to use. OGTT might detect diabetes more effectively than other methods in people with HIV (Spollett 2006). Some experts recommend performing fasting plasma glucose and a diabetes risk screen before commencing HIV treatment, especially with PIs are used because of the known hyperglycaemia risk associated with these medicines.

Choosing HIV medicines carefully and limiting the use of PIs where possible, especially in people at risk of diabetes or those who already have diabetes is a key strategy. However, the risk of developing/exacerbating diabetes needs to be considered in light of the benefits to be gained by reducing the HIV viral load and improving immune status.

Eating a healthy diet and exercising are key management strategies but need to be tailored to the individual's HIV status and capability. Nutrition supplements may be needed in HIV-related cachexia. GLMs might be indicated especially when PIs are used. Liver function should be tested before Thiazolidinediones (TZD) are prescribed and during treatment with TZDs (Chapter 5). Before Metformin is used the individual should screened for lactic acidosis and abnormal serum creatinine levels (Aberg *et al.* 2004).

People receiving NRTI therapy, especially if the treatment lasts longer than six months, may be at higher risk of lactic acidosis. Stavudine, Zidavudine and Didanosine are more likely to precipitate lactic acidosis than other antiviral medicines. Although Metformin is not contraindicated in people using antiviral medicines, clinicians must be aware of the possibility of lactic acidosis and educate the person accordingly. Insulin may be indicated for some people and the type of insulin and dose regimen needs to be individualised.

Diabetes complications need to be detected early and managed to improve outcomes. For example people with HIV and diabetes, especially those with a high viral load, prescribed the antiretroviral medicines Ziagen and the combination medicines Kivexa and Trizvier, have a high prevalence of albuminuria: two-fold greater than for either disease alone (Kim. 2011).

There is limited research on interactions between glucose-lowering medicines and antiretroviral medicines, but such interactions are possible because both groups of medicines use similar metabolic pathways. Blood glucose monitoring is important to detect hypo- or hyperglycaemia, which could indicate an interaction. Significantly safe disposal of sharps is paramount in people with diabetes and HIV.

Managing hyperglycaemia and its consequences is important to the individual's comfort and most likely outcomes. However, the added responsibility of managing diabetes as well as HIV may be overwhelming and compound/lead to depression. People with HIV and diabetes need tailored diabetes education that considers their HIV self-care, medication regimen and other relevant personal information. People who are prescribed Metformin need advice about recognising lactic acidosis (Chapter 7) and liver-related symptoms such as abdominal tenderness, ascites and peripheral oedema (Aberg *et al.* 2004).

Although survival is improving for people with HIV and diabetes, end of life care should also be considered proactively and include diabetes management and management directions the individual chooses to document (Chapter 18).

DIABETES AND HEARING LOSS

A recent meta-analysis suggests there is a higher prevalence of hearing impairment in people with diabetes compared with people without diabetes (Horikawa *et al.* 2012) and the association appears to be stronger in younger than older people (Bainbridge 2013). The prevalence of hearing loss appears to be approximately 30% higher in people with diabetes than in non-diabetics.

The pathophysiology of diabetes-related hearing loss is not clear but might be due to neuropathic changes in the vascular and/or neural systems in the inner ear. Autopsy evidence shows sclerosis of the internal auditory artery, thicker vessel walls in the stria vascularis and basilar membrane, demyelinisation of the cochlear nerve, atrophy of the spiral ganglion and loss of outer ear hair cells. However, age-related hearing changes need to be considered.

Causes of hearing loss

The causes of hearing loss are multifactorial and include:

- Older age, the most common cause of hearing loss. One in three people aged 65–74 have some degree of hearing loss and after 75 the ratio increases to one in two people (Wilson *et al.*1999). Genes and exposure to noise may play a role in aged-related hearing loss.
- Loud and continuous noise e.g. in some workplaces, musicians, the military and people who constantly listen to loud music on I-phones or in nightclubs. Wearing earplugs and limiting exposure to noise is important.

- Some medicines including antibiotics, chemotherapy medicines, aspirin, loop diuretics and medicines used to treat malaria and erectile dysfunction; some 200 medicines are reported to trigger hearing loss.
- Some illnesses such as cardiovascular disease, hypertension and diabetes, which affect the blood supply to the inner ear and infections.
- Trauma that involves the eardrum, or skull. (WebMD 2013).

Sudden hearing loss >30 decibels is uncommon and not particularly related to diabetes. It can occur over hours or days and often only affects one ear. The cause is often hard to identify. The degree of hearing loss is classified as mild, moderate, severe or profound. As the hearing loss progresses, the ability to accurately understand conversational speech declines, and people become isolated and maybe depressed. Progressive hearing loss associated with ageing often affects the high frequency sounds first. Therefore, in the early stages high-pitched sounds such as women's voices and speech sound such as 'S' and 'F' become inaudible, while other lower pitched sounds may still be heard at relatively normal levels.

Other signs of hearing loss include:

- difficulty understanding telephone conversations;
- trouble hearing when there is background noise;
- difficulty following conversations that involve several people speaking at once;
- feeling people are mumbling;
- misunderstanding what people say, which can lead to miscommunication and adverse events especially in health care settings;
- needing to ask people to repeat themselves;
- ringing, hissing or other sounds in the ear;
- other people complain about TVs, radios being too loud.

Diagnosis is through audiology testing.

Management

The earlier detection and management of hearing loss produces better outcomes. The earlier it is detected the easier it is to treat. Unmanaged hearing loss has a negative impact on quality of life; appropriately managed hearing loss improves quality of life. However, hearing loss often occurs gradually and may go unnoticed by the individual concerned, although people around him/her may be aware of the changes. Diabetes-related hearing loss is typically high frequency sensorioneural hearing loss that can be managed using hearing aids. Ear infections that lead to temporary hearing loss can be treated with antibiotics, however the specific treatment depends on the underlying cause and frequent middle ear infections could permanently compromise hearing.

Clinicians need to be aware of the subtle changes in hearing and speak directly to the person while looking them in the face, be sure you have the person's attention before you speak. Supplementing oral information with written information is helpful, provided it is at an appropriate literacy level and is culturally relevant. Given the prevalence of hearing loss and the effects on outcomes clinicians need to encourage people to have their hearing assessed and refer them to an audiologist or an ear specialist for assessment and appropriate management.

Group education programmes may be challenging for people with hearing loss but there is a range of options that can improve hearing and enable people with mild-to-moderate hearing loss to participate in groups. People with severe hearing loss would benefit more from individual education unless sessions are conducted with AUSLAN (Australian sign language) interpreters. Learning AUSLAN takes time and it is recognised as a minority language. Learning sign language is rarely an option for older people with diabetes-related hearing loss..

In hospital settings background noise may be distracting and consultations and beds should be placed in the quietest possible location with as few noise distractions as possible. A recent study also suggests much higher prevalence of hearing loss among hospital patients.

DIABETES AND MUSCULOSKELETAL DISEASES

Musculoskeletal disorders associated with diabetes are often overlooked in usual clinical diabetes care. Diabetes is associated with several specific musculoskeletal disorders and others occur concomitantly. Diabetes-related musculoskeletal disease reflects the multisystem effects of defects in glucose homeostasis. Potential causal mechanisms include:

- non-enzymatic glycosylation of protein resulting in advanced glycated end products (age) and stiffened connective tissue;
- increased deposition of connective tissue as a result of myofibroblast proliferation;
- neuropathy;
- autoimmune diseases associated with Type 1 diabetes;
- obesity-related changes and strain on joints;
- hyperinsulinaemia and associated hormonal abnormalities such as elevated growth hormone (Brown *et al*. 2001; Smith *et al*. 2002).

Activities of daily living (ADL), quality of life, and driving safety are often associated with stress and lowered mood. Some cause chronic pain. Thus they affect diabetes health outcomes. The prevalence of these conditions tends to increase with long duration of diabetes especially associated with chronic hyperglycaemia. These conditions include:

- shoulder adhesive capsulitis, which is painful and limits movement;
- shoulder–hand syndrome, which consists of painful shoulder capsulitis and swollen, tender hands;
- cherioarthropathy (limited joint mobility) is specific to diabetes and causes stiffening of the small joints in the hands;
- Dupuytren's contracture, which is associated with vision-threatening retinopathy, increased risk of foot ulceration, and other musculoskeletal disorders in Type 1 and Type 2 diabetes;
- carpal tunnel syndrome, which is also associated with hypothyroidism; the causal process is usually not due to inflammation;
- hyperostosis and Forestier's disease, which commonly occurs in obese middle-aged men with Type 2 diabetes; the thoracic spine most commonly affected;
- gout, pseudogout and osteoarthritis;
- osteopenia, usually in Type 1 diabetes may be associated with retinopathy; bone density is usually normal or increased;
- prayer sign;
- flexor tenosynovitis (trigger finger);
- diabetic foot diseases such as Charcot's foot; see Chapter 8.

Management

Specific management depends on the cause. Usually the diagnosis is made on clinical grounds but X-ray, MRI, and ultrasound may be required. Muscle biopsy, EMG testing may be useful. Improving metabolic control using an appropriate diet and exercise is essential. Strength and flexibility training programmes such as progressive weight training and some forms of gentle Tai Chi, physiotherapy massage and appropriate pain management using non-medicine options where possible are helpful.

Some conditions such as carpel tunnel syndrome may require surgical management. The impact on quality of life, ADLs, and safety such as driving and falls risk need to be regularly assessed for example during annual complication screening programmes or driving license renewal assessment.

CORTICOSTEROID AND ANTIPSYCHOTIC MEDICATIONS AND DIABETES

Key points

- Corticosteroid medications predispose the person to insulin resistance, dose-related hyperglycaemia, and hyperinsulinaemia.
- They are used to control disease processes or are given as hormone replacement therapy for some endocrine diseases, for example, pituitary tumours. In the latter case corticosteroid doses are usually small or physiological levels and are less likely to cause hyperglycaemia.
- Non-diabetics on high doses, long-term or intermittent corticosteroids should be monitored and should test their blood glucose. People with diabetes should test their diabetes and their medicines should be adjusted proactively.
- Corticosteroids and atypical antipsychotic medicines can precipitate hyperosmolar states.

Introduction

Steroids are naturally occurring hormones produced by the adrenal glands under the control of the pituitary hormone ACTH. There are three major classes of steroid hormones:

(1) glucocorticoids
(2) mineralocorticoids
(3) androgens and oestrogen.

Glucocorticoid effects on blood glucose

Corticosteroid medicines are an essential part of the management of inflammatory disease processes, haematologic malignancies, allergic reactions, and shock. The long-term use, especially in high doses, predisposes the individual to steroid-induced diabetes or to hyperglycaemia in people with established diabetes. Corticosteroids have the propensity to cause insulin resistance, increased hepatic glucose output, reduced glucose transport, and to inhibit insulin secretion resulting in hyperglycaemia.

Effect on blood glucose

The effect on blood glucose depends to some extent on the biological action of the particular preparation used and the length of time it is required. Hyperglycaemia usually occurs with doses of Prednisolone (or equivalent) >7.5 mg/day.

Specific short courses of corticosteroids usually only affect the blood glucose temporarily or not at all, but hyperglycaemia occurs if the dose is increased or the medication is needed intermittently or in the long term (Williams & Pickup 1992). If given for <1 week even large doses do not usually present problems, although impaired glucose tolerance can be present and can occur within 48 hours. IV steroids usually have a shorter duration of action than steroids given by other routes and do not increase the blood glucose if only 1–2 doses are given (Jackson & Bowman 1995).

Predisposing factors

People with existing risk factors for diabetes run the greatest risk of developing steroid-induced diabetes. These risks are described in Chapter 1. They include the following conditions:

- old age;
- existing impaired glucose tolerance;
- current or previous GDM;
- cardiac disease;
- psychosis.

The presence of one or more of these risk factors may influence the decision to use steroids, the duration of the treatment, and the dose. In many cases steroids are the medicines of choice and management strategies should be implemented to minimise the impact on the blood glucose.

Management

- Screen for the risk factors for diabetes before commencing corticosteroids.
- Where diabetes is present, GLM and/or insulin need to be reviewed and may require adjustment according to the blood glucose profile. In most cases the postprandial blood glucose increases during the day but drops overnight and the fasting glucose may not be significantly elevated (Oyer *et al.* 2006).

Over 50% of people with Type 2 diabetes treated with GLMs require insulin if they require corticosteroids, sometimes permanently (Williams & Pickup 1992). Shapiro (2007) suggested TZDs might be useful to overcome steroid-induced insulin resistance but recommended considering the individual characteristics before prescribing a TZD. However, TZD have a slow onset of action so they would not be beneficial when steroids are needed in the short term. When steroids are used in the long term they exacerbate cardiovascular risk factors and lead to weight gain. In such cases TZD may increase because they also cause oedema and exacerbate heart failure.

Other GLM may be effective depending on the individual cautions and contraindication. The GLP-1 agents might be effective in some patients but more research is needed (van Raalte 2009). The risk of lactic acidosis associated with Metformin may preclude its use in many people with diabetes. Sulpuonylureas have a limited role in managing corticsteroid-induced hyperglycaemia (ADS 2012).

Therefore, insulin is often required. Dose flexibility is greater with insulin and the rapid onset of action and ease of dose titration are advantages. The insulin dose and dose regimen need to be individualised. Insulin regimens to manage steroid-induced hyperglycaemia include:

- Morning Isophane insulin or morning premixed insulin.
- Long-acting insulin in the morning, with or without rapid-acting insulin at meal times, which prevents new onset diabetes following immunosuppressive therapy following renal transplants.

Insulin can be given by injection or insulin pump. In a small study (n = 10) people with Type 1 diabetes on 80 mgs Prednisolone per day managed on insulin pumps required dose increases between 30–100% (ADS 2012).

Management

- Select the optimal route of corticosteroid administration for the particular problem: oral, IV, inhaled, topical cream.
- Use the lowest effective corticosteroid dose for the shortest possible time.
- Monitor blood glucose 4-hourly if the person has diabetes and at least weekly if they do not.
- Monitor for ketones, especially in Type 1 diabetes because steroids predispose them to DKA.
- Explain to the patient the reasons for the blood glucose monitoring, especially if they do not have diabetes. Reassure them that steroids are the medicine of choice for their condition and that hyperglycaemia can be controlled.
- Steroids required on a temporary basis must be withdrawn gradually to allow the pituitary–adrenal axis to return to normal activity (Jackson & Bowman 1995).
- If GLM/insulin doses were commenced or increased they will need to be reduced as the steroid dose is reduced to avoid hypoglycaemia.
- Prolonged steroid use depresses the immune system. Aseptic technique is important if any invasive procedures are required and the immune system should be supported with a healthy diet and regular activity within the individual's tolerance level.

Steroids can mask some of the signs and symptoms of infection, as can diabetes. Common infection sites should be closely monitored, for example, injection sites, feet, mouth and gums, and the urinary tract.

- The skin can become thin and fragile and easily damaged if corticosteroids are required in the long term, predisposing the individual to bruising, skin tears, ulcers, and other trauma, especially older people. A protective skin care regimen is important.
- Protecting older people from falls that predispose them to trauma is essential where long-term corticosteroids are required because of the effects on bone and the increased risk of fractures if they fall.
- Alternate-day steroid regimens show greater effects on the blood glucose on the day steroid medications are taken. OHA/insulin regimes for steroid and non-steroid days may be needed.
- Insulin is often required for people on GLMs if long-term steroids are required or if hyperglycaemia persists despite compliance with their GLMs, and an appropriate diet.
- Where permanent steroid therapy is required, for example, after surgery for a pituitary tumour, the steroid dose usually needs to be increased during illness or surgery. Careful, *written* instructions detailing how to manage steroid dose reductions in

these circumstances and close liaison with their endocrinologist is essential. OHAs/insulin will also need to be adjusted in these circumstances.

- Achieving acceptable growth and development in children on permanent steroids is important and should be closely monitored. Growth hormone may be required.
- Body changes can occur such as weight gain, moon face, thinning hair, and acne which can affect body image.
- Steroids can cause mental changes ranging from mild changes to psychosis, which can affect the person's self-care. If psychosis occurs it will need to be managed appropriately. The help of a psychiatrist may be necessary.

Corticosteroids and osteoporosis

Corticosteroids can also reduce bone formation and the viability of osteoblasts and osteocytes, reduce calcium absorption from the intestine and increase renal calcium excretion predisposing the individual to osteoporosis and fractures (Romas 2008). These negative effects can be managed with supplemental oral calcium and vitamin D or calcitriol. In some cases, gonadal hormone production can be affected, which exacerbates the other bone effects. Changes are noted even at low doses of corticosteroids and fractures can occur soon after commencing these medicines, especially in high-risk individuals.

Risk factors include:

- age;
- female gender;
- post menopausal women who are at the highest risk;
- low bone mineral density.

Bone mineral densitometry and dual energy X-ray absorptiometry of the lumbar spine and neck of the femur are warranted for all patients on corticosteroid therapy >3 months. Using a non-steroid medicine if possible and using these medicines in the lowest possible dose for the shortest time helps reduce the risk of adverse effects. Oral bisphosphonates with vitamin D are important primary prevention medicines for people in the high fracture risk category.

Recent research suggests there is a significant inverse association between serum 25-dehydroxyvitamin D levels and the risk of developing Type 2 diabetes (Chiu et al. 2004).

See Chapter 18 for information about corticosteroids and end-of-life care.

Antipsychotic medicines

Antipsychotic medicines more than double the risk of gestational diabetes in pregnant women using these medicines (Boden *et al.* 2012). The effect may be due to weight gain, insulin resistance and hyperlipidaemia. Significantly, infants of mothers taking Olanzapine and Clozapine are at double to risk of being born with larger than normal heads after adjusting for maternal risk factors. Thus, women using antipsychotic medicines should be closely monitored.

Some antipsychotic agents are also associated with prolonged QT intervals, which predisposes the individual to cardiac arrhythmias (O'Brien & Oyebode 2003). A number of different pharmacological mechanisms are proposed and vary among the different antipsychotic medicine groups. Prexisting cardiac disease and factors that predispose the individual to cardiac arrhythmias in crease the risk.

There is considerable overlap between other cardiovascular risk factors including excess alcohol consumption, smoking, lack of physical activity. In addition antidepressants independently exacerbate dyslipidaemia, hyperglycaemia and the metabolic syndrome.

Close monitoring of risk factors, especially in individuals at risk, is essential. Education about self-care and seeking medical advice is also important. It is important to choose the antipsychotic medicine with the least effect on blood glucose and cardiovascular functioning and use it at the lowest effective dose. However, managing the person's psychiatric diagnosis and enabling them to function as normally as possible is essential.

DIABETES AND DRIVING

The association among diabetes, diabetes complications, medications, coexisting comorbidities, intercurrent illness, alcohol intake, environmental conditions and driving accidents is complex and multifactorial. Individual driving risk needs to be assessed and monitored regularly, for example, when a complication is diagnosed, when the medication regimen is modified, as the person grows older, and following a crash. In addition, the ability to operate other vehicles such as motorised 'wheelchairs' and farm vehicles also needs to be considered.

Diabetes can have a significant impact on driving safety, yet many current diabetes management guidelines and diabetes complication screening programmes do not make provision for proactive structured assessment of driving ability, which usually only occurs when the driving license needs to be renewed or following a serious hypoglycaemic event or traffic accident. Often license renewal may not be required for several years and the health status can change significantly between renewal periods. Statistically young men and older people are most at risk of road crash but people need to be assessed on an individual basis. Diabetes-specific effects on driving are shown in Table 10.4.

Guidelines for assessing fitness to drive exist in most countries, for example, the Australian AUSTROADS (2012) standards, which is currently under review. Although the Australian standards are comprehensive, outline how health issues can impact on driving safety, and include standards for private and commercial licenses, they do not stress the cumulative impact of comorbidities on driving safety, even where the standards are cross-referenced. Such guidelines recommend counselling people with diabetes about their rights and responsibilities with respect to driving and increasingly recognise that hyperglycaemia, as well as hypoglycaemia affects cognitive function.

Prevalence of and risk factors for driving crashes

Evidence about driving crash rates in people with diabetes is confusing. Some old research suggests the traffic crash rate is similar between diabetics and non-diabetics (MacLeod 1999). Others report a lower mileage-adjusted crash rate per million miles driven in people with diabetes than in the general population (Eadington & Frier 1989;). Older drivers generally appear to have a higher crash rate than any other age group except people <25 years (Guerrier *et al.* 1999; McGwin *et al.* 2000; Braver & Trempel 2004). Older women with heart disease, stroke, or arthritis are at high risk (McGwin *et al.* 2000). If they are in an accident, older people are more likely to suffer serious injury or die. The presence of diabetes was not reported in these studies.

Table 10.4 Possible pharmacological mechanisms of various antipsychotic medicines responsible for cardiovascular effects.

Antipsychotic medicine	Pharmacological mechanism likely to contribute to cardiovascular disease
Tricyclic antidepressants	Affect a broad range of receptor pathways that are implicated in therapeutic as well as adverse outcomes. For example, they inhibit central cholinergic neurotransmission, which affects autonomic functions such as tachycardia, which is accompanied by neuronal uptake of norepinepherine, which can exacerbate tachycardia. They can block alpha-adrenergic receptors, which can reduce systemic vascular resistance and cause hypotension or orthostatic hypotension. High doses increase sympathetic and reduce parasympathetic influences on heart rate variability. They inhibit sodium channel conduction, which delays phase 0 cardiac depolarisation, which can result in slower conduction within the His-Purkinje fibres and the ventricles, which prolongs the QRS complex.
Selective serotonin reuptake inhibitors	Cause cardiovascular effects mostly because of the release of excess serotonin within the central nervous system, which can cause mild systemic hypotension. Citalopram and Escitalopram can cause generalised seizures. The two medicines can lead to dose-dependent prolongation of the QT interval.
Monoamine oxidase inhibitors	Enhance the concentration of a broad range of central neurotransmitters including norepinephrine. Tachycardia and hypertension might occur as a consequence, particularly at high doses. The onset of cardiovascular effects might not occur for 12–24 hours after the medicine is taken because it takes time for the concentration of central neurotransmitters to accumulate. Consuming foods or medicines high in tyramine can precipitate severe hypertension; the so called 'cheese effect.' Cardiovascular effects may also be due to serotonin accumulation and include tachycardia and hypotension especially when Monoamine oxidase inhibitors are combined with serotonin reuptake inhibitors.
Serotonin and norepinephrine reuptake inhibitors	Venlafaxine, Reboxetine and Duloxetine appear to stimulate cardiac sympathetic nerve activity, which cause mild tachycardia and systemic hypertension. If sympathetic activity is excessive, more serious tachyarrhythmias are possible especially if cardiomyopathy is present. Venlafaxine can block cardiac sodium conduction.
Lithium	Might be associated with several cardiac conduction defects such as complete heart block and impaired atrioventricular conduction and prolonged QTcB intervals. The onset of cardiotoxicty might be delayed after commencing lithium due to the delay in reaching equilibrium in cardiac tissue concentrations.

However, many older drivers voluntarily restrict their driving, for example, not driving at night or in peak hour traffic (Penckofer *et al.* 2007).

Other modern risk factors for driving and other accidents include using mobile phones and other distractions while driving, especially if concentration is impaired by hypo- or hyperglycaemia, depression, alcohol or other drugs or medicines such as sedatives. The prevalence of accidents relating to these issues is unknown.

Falls in older people, especially a fall in the previous year, increases crash risk (Margolis *et al.* 2002). Falls are more likely to occur when the following factors are present. Almost all of these apply to diabetes:

- unstable balance;
- neurological problems;
- musculoskeletal problems;
- cardiovascular disease;
- vision deficits;
- cognitive impairment;
- insulin treatment;
- significant postural hypotension;
- female gender (Gregg *et al.* 2000).

Although insulin treatment is assumed to carry a higher crash risk, people managed by diet and exercise are also at significant risk (Sagberg 2006). Sagberg found a significant risk of road crashes and the presence of medical conditions, symptoms, and some medicines in drivers of all ages. In particular, Sagberg found significant associations among crash risk and diabetes, previous MI, wearing glasses while driving, myopia, difficulty getting to sleep, frequent tiredness, depression, and taking antidepressant medicines. Koepsell *et al.* (1994) also found increased crash risk when diabetes and heart disease were both present, people on insulin or OHA, and duration of diabetes >5 years. Experts suggest diabetes-related crashes involving insulin-treated people are often due to hypoglycaemia (Clark *et al.* 1980; Frier *et al.* 1980; Steel *et al.* 1981; Koepsell *et al.* 1994). However, McGwin *et al.* (1999) found no significant difference in crash rates according to diabetes treatment mode or in people with diabetes overall.

In some countries people on insulin are not permitted to drive articulated vehicles or other heavy vehicles such as passenger buses. However, there are no restrictions on driving other heavy vehicles such as tractors and farm vehicles in rural areas. Crashes involving these vehicles cause significant injury. Laberge-Nadeau *et al.* (2000) reported a higher crash rate associated with people with diabetes driving non-articulated but not articulated trucks. In contrast, Laberge-Nadeau *et al.* (2000) found no significant differences in crash rates between people with diabetes and non-diabetics driving either type of truck. Interestingly, non-insulin users and those with no diabetes complications were more likely to be involved in a crash while driving trucks.

Cox *et al.* (2000) used driving simulators to determine the effect of hypoglycaemia on driving ability in young people with diabetes. No effect was detected at blood glucose 3.6 mmol/L but significantly more swerving, driving over the line or off the road, and compensatory slow driving occurred at 2.6 mmol/L. Fifty per cent indicated they would not drive if their blood glucose were low. In a second simulator study, Cox *et al.* (2000) progressively lowered blood glucose to <2.8 mmol/L. Most participants recognised they were hypoglycaemic but only a minority treated the hypoglycaemia or stopped driving despite impaired driving performance.

Lee *et al.* (2003) used a PC-simulator to assess older people's driving ability. Driving skill declined significantly with increasing age. Sommerfield *et al.* (2003) reported significant impairment in working memory, ability to make decisions under pressure, and less confidence driving at speed in a group of older people. It is not clear whether any of the participants in these studies had diabetes but the findings mostly likely also apply to older people with diabetes.

However, driving simulators, particularly in research settings, may not be an appropriate way to assess actual driving behaviour because of distractions such as intravenous lines, wearing an EEG cap and being asked questions while driving, as occurred in Cox *et al.*'s study. In addition, a different set off skills is needed to drive in simulators from driving on the road. Simulators can cause stress and anxiety as well as being distracting, all of which affect driving skill and compound the effects of medical conditions. Some people may enjoy 'playing the game'.

Driving can also be affected by weather and road conditions, level of vehicle maintenance, and the age and type of vehicle (Evans 2004). Some of these factors are significantly different from conditions operating when some older studies were undertaken. Likewise, many of the newer glucose-lowering agents (OHA) and insulin analogues, and the trend towards using shorter acting OHA and insulin analogues have reduced the risk of hypoglycaemia.

Diabetes-related effects on driving

Diabetes-related factors that affect driving ability include:

- The duration of diabetes. Risk increases with increasing duration of diabetes largely because of the increasing risk of diabetes complications.
- Usual metabolic control. Hypoglycaemia is a recognised crash risk but hyperglycaemia also has short-term effects on driving ability and long-term consequences as a result of complications (see Table 10.5).
- Functional impairment and disability, for example, arthritis, and common diabetes complications; hypertension, stroke, and transient ischaemic attacks (TIA) are associated with functional decline (Stuck *et al.*1999). Diabetes-related musculoskeletal disease can make it difficult to grip the steering wheel or feel the pedals and affect the degree of control over the vehicle and/or make turning to view traffic and road signs difficult and may compound the effects of arthritis and vision deficits.
- Impaired cognitive functioning due to age-related changes, hypo- or hyperglycaemia or other factors. Hyperglycaemia is linked to impaired cognitive functioning (Meneilly *et al.*, 1993), slows recovery from injury following an accident (Scalea *et al.* 2007) and leads to tiredness and sleep disturbance, which affect concentration in the daytime.
- Long-term complications that cause functional and cognitive deficits such as cardiovascular disease, musculoskeletal problems, renal disease, retinopathy, and other vision deficits. Diabetic retinopathy is associated with a high rate of driving-related fear, Coyne *et al.* (2004). Autonomic neuropathy causing hypoglycaemic unawareness represents significant crash risk in insulin-treated people.
- Medicines likely to affect physical and/or mental functioning such as insulin and OHA, antihypertensive agents, sedatives, antidepressive agents, some herbal medicines and illegal drugs. Polypharmacy is common in diabetes and medicine interactions and adverse events can occur that affect driving safety. Many people with diabetes use complementary medicines (CAM) and some CAM medicines can interact with conventional medicines, for example, glucose-lowering herbal medicines.
- Self-care knowledge and behaviours, which encompasses diabetes-related and general self-care and safety considerations such as:
  - testing blood glucose before driving and not driving if it is low or goes low while driving;

Table 10.5 Diabetes-related complications that can affect driving ability and safety. Frequently more than one factor is present, therefore, the cumulative effect on driving ability needs to be considered. MI = myocardial infarction; 'Hypo' = hypoglycaemia.

Complication	Effects	Possible consequences while driving
1. Short term		
Hypoglycaemia	Cognitive impairment Impaired decision making Vision changes Symptoms may be distracting Hypoglycaemic unawareness. If nocturnal, daytime lethargy Risk of falls Risk of coma	Can be distracting, for example, reaching for glucose to treat the 'hypo' May not be convenient to stop to treat the 'hypo' so mild hypoglycaemia progresses Impaired decision-making, not recognising the need to stop or treat the hypo Symptoms not recognised and episode not treated Inability to control the vehicle due to cognitive and functional changes Slow reaction time and erratic driving Difficulty reading road signs Loss of consciousness
Hyperglycaemia	Increased rate of intercurrent infection and if severe risk of ketoacidosis and hyperosmolar states Tiredness and lethargy Changed cognitive functioning Polyuria and polydipsia Vision changes Lowered mood Compromised self-care Risk of falls	Distractions, for example, need to pass urine Slowed reaction time Inability to control the vehicle Difficulty reading road signs Impaired decision-making Fall asleep while driving
2. Long term		

Microvascular disease:
(a) Retinopathy
	Vision impairment
	Visual field defects
	Self-care deficits
	Risk of falls
		Distractions.
		Slow reaction time as a consequence of the difficulty:
		    gauging distance
		    seeing oncoming vehicles
		    reading road signs
		    loss of peripheral vision
		Impact on night driving
		Wearing appropriate glasses for driving and ID necessary
		Effect of investigations such as retinal screening, angiograms and laser therapy

(b) Nephropathy	Changed medicine pharmacokinetics and pharmacodynamics Hypotension especially if on dialysis Increased hypo risk especially on dialysis days Discomfort Muscle weakness Lethargy Depression Risk of falls	Distractions Slow reaction time Inability to control the vehicle Difficulty reading road signs Impaired decision-making

Table 10.5 Continued.

Complication	Effects	Possible consequences while driving
Macrovascular disease:		
(a) Cardiac	Cardiac dysrhythmias	Distractions
	Silent MI	MI during driving
	Disorientation and confusion	Sudden death while driving
	Tiredness	Impaired decision-making
	Lightheadedness	Daytime sleepiness
	Depression	
	Risk of falls	
(b) Cerebral	TIAs, stroke	Slow reaction time
	Not recognising 'hypos'	Impaired decision-making
	Cognitive changes	Reduces strength in affected limbs
	Risk of falls	Difficulty operating pedals
(c) Peripheral	Intermittent claudication	More likely to use a car because of difficulty walking
Neuropathy:		
(a) Peripheral	Reduced sensation in feet and unstable gait	Difficulty operating pedals
	Pain	Distraction
	Risk of falls	
(b) Autonomic	Postural hypotension	Distractions
	Hypoglycaemic unawareness	Slow reaction time
	Gastroparesis	Inability to control the vehicle
	Incontinence	Erratic driving
	Unstable blood glucose pattern	'Hypo' not recognised and not treated
	Depression	May not be convenient to stop to treat a 'hypo'
	Silent MI	
	Silent UTI	Difficulty reading road signs
	Communication difficulties	Impaired decision-making
	Lethargy	Sudden death
	Inadequate self-care	
	Depression	
	Suicide	
Musculoskeletal e.g.	Reduced fine motor skill affecting dexterity	Distractions
Carpal tunnel	Weakness	Slow reaction time
syndrome	Pain	Difficulty controlling the vehicle
Dupuytren's	Falls risk	Difficulty turning the head
contracture		
Joint stiffness		
Sleep apnoea usually	Pain	Distraction
occurs as a	Day time lethargy	Fall asleep while driving
consequence of		Difficulty fitting seat belts
obesity.		

Reproduced with permission from Chapter 8 Dunning (2009) in Odell (ed) 2009.

- carrying hypoglycaemia treatment;
- not consuming alcohol or taking illegal drugs before driving;
- maintaining the vehicle in a roadworthy condition;
- considering environmental factors such as the weather when planning a trip;
- stopping regularly on long drives;
- wearing seat belts;
- obeying road rules;
- knowing what to do if an accident occurs.

Hypoglycaemia effects on driving

Hypoglycaemia is the most significant side effect of insulin and most OHAs; see Chapter 5. Cox *et al.* (2000) undertook a simulator study and showed driving performance and decision-making were impaired during mild hypoglycaemia. Unless mild hypoglycaemia is treated, the blood glucose usually continues to fall. However, Marrero & Edelman (2000) suggested the blood glucose range at which driving is impaired and the specific driving actions that are impaired vary among individuals. Generally, judgement is impaired during moderate-to-severe hypoglycaemia.

Low blood glucose triggers a counter-regulatory response: at about 3.5–3.7 mmol/L adrenergic symptoms such as sweating and trembling appear. Fine motor skills, coordination, mental processing, concentration, and some memory functions are impaired <3.0 mmol/L (Heller & Macdonald 1996; Sommerfield *et al.* 2003) and affect driving safety. Sommerfield *et al.* (2003) suggested decision-making ability is affected when blood glucose <3.0 mmol/L. However, McAulay *et al.* (2001) found no significant effect on problem-solving ability but significant effects on attentional ability.

The Edinburgh Hypoglycaemia Scale is often used to grade hypoglycaemia severity in research projects and could help define driving risk National Health Service (NHS) 2010):

- Grade 1, mild: the person is aware of hypoglycaemia and responds and self-treats appropriately.
- Grade 2, moderate: the person cannot respond to hypoglycaemia and needs help. Oral treatment corrects the blood glucose level.
- Grade 3, severe: the person is semi- or unconscious and unable to self-treat. Glucagon or IV glucose may be required to correct the blood glucose.

Interpreting driving risk according to these grades suggests the person is at risk of an accident and should stop and treat hypoglycaemia immediately they recognise the symptoms. They are unlikely to manage alone and will be at greater risk if hypoglycaemia is moderate or severe. However, other factors that can affect judgement need to be considered. These include hypoglycaemic awareness, and alcohol and illegal drug use, which cloud judgement and may mask hypoglycaemic symptoms. If present, these factors significantly increase the risk of crash. Testing blood glucose before driving, not driving if the blood glucose is low and not drinking alcohol or using illegal drugs and driving reduce crash risk.

Most people recover from severe hypoglycaemia (Cryer 2007) without permanent effects on driving. The possibility of hypoglycaemia is increased with the trend towards stringent blood glucose targets but the effects on driving crashes is unknown and the overall rate of severe hypoglycaemia is difficult to establish. Severe hypoglycaemia occurred in 0.4–2.3% of insulin-treated Type 2 people per year compared with 0.4% on diet or sulphonylureas, in the UKPDS1998).

In a later UKPDS substudy, Wright *et al.* (2006) reported hypoglycaemia grades 1 and 2 occurred in 0.8% in the diet group and 1.7% in the Metformin group per year; and grades 2–4 in 0.1% and 0.3% respectively, compared to 7.9%, and 1.2% in the sulphonylurea group. Hypoglycaemia increased significantly in the basal insulin group; 21.2% and 3.65; and 32%, and in those on basal bolus insulin, 5.5%. Hypoglycaemia frequency and severity in Type 2 diabetes is lower than Type 1 (Yki-Jarvinen *et al.* 1999).

The rate of OHA-induced hypoglycaemia may be lower than insulin-induced hypoglycaemia but when it does occur it is often prolonged and can recur within 24 hours despite treatment, and carries a mortality rate of 4–10% (Shorr *et al.* 1997; Stahl & Berger 1999). In addition 5% of survivors have permanent neurological damage (Salas & Caro 2002; Veitch & Clifton-Bligh 2004).

People on insulin have a higher crash risk than the general population but serious hypoglycaemia during driving is rare. Harsch *et al.* (2002) reported more hypoglycaemia in Type 1 diabetes; the accident rate was 0.19–8.26 or 0.02–0.63 per 100 000 kilometers per year per driver depending on the intensity of the insulin regimen. Harsch *et al.* also found fewer events in those on basal bolus therapy and insulin pumps: 0.09–0.49 events per 100 000 kilometers or 0.007–0.01 per driver per year. Likewise, Ziemer *et al.* (2007) found lower hypoglycaemia risk in people on basal bolus insulin regimens and no increase in driving risk.

Lower accident risk with basal bolus regimens might be due to the fact that rapid-/short-acting insulins have a shorter duration of action and smaller frequent doses significantly reduces the insulin depot. Long-acting insulin analogues also have a lower hypoglycaemic profile (see Chapter 5). Temporary driving restrictions usually apply if a person has severe hypoglycaemia. The license may not be renewed until blood glucose is stabilised and is in a safe range. Loss of their driving license can cause considerable hardship for the individual involved and sometimes their families and is a threat to independence and access to essential services including health professionals especially in outer suburban and rural areas.

If hypoglycaemic unawareness is a contributing factor, Blood Glucose Awareness Training (BGATT) may help the individual learn to recognise impending hypoglycaemia and improve their safety and confidence. Cox *et al.* (2000) reported 6.8 crashes in a group of people participating in a BGATT programme per million miles driven versus 29.8 in the control group in a four-year observational study. BGATT did not improve the decision not to drive when blood glucose levels were low. In contrast, Broers *et al.* (2005) found a significant improvement in deciding not to drive during hypoglycaemia in BGATT participants. They also had a lower crash rate compared to controls: 0.6 versus 0.2 per patient per year. These findings of the BGATT programmes may be a useful addition to driver rehabilitation/safety programmes for people with severe hypoglycaemia.

Strategies to enhance driving safety

Health professionals could adopt a more proactive, holistic education and risk management approach to diabetes and driving safety. Such an approach includes:

* Conducting regular structured driving assessments as part of care planning, and annual complication screening as well as during significant health and treatment changes, would enable declining functional and cognitive ability and the potential effects on driving safety to be identified and remedial strategies implemented. If relevant, geriatric, mental health and/or driving assessments should be sought. Such an approach would enable a gradual, planned transition to stopping driving to occur and reduce the physical and mental impact on the individual.
* Undertaking opportunistic driving assessments instead of only at license renewal time or when a severe hypoglycaemic event or a driving accident occurs. For example, during an emergency department/hospital presentation, when medicines are changed, and during the annual complication assessment, changes in mental and physical capabilities.
* Assessing the individual's level of risk and counselling them appropriately about how to reduce their risk. Circumstances and the level of risk sometimes change rapidly, thus forward planning for such contingencies is helpful especially for older people. This could include developing a proactive driving/transport plan and recognising when to suggest the individual implements their plan. The driving plan could include making plans to cope during temporary incapacity, for example, during acute illness, investigative procedures, or surgery as well as a long-term plan to eventually stop driving.

- Being aware of the general and diabetes-related risk factors that contribute to unsafe driving and ensure they are considered when undertaking education, health assessments, and formulating management plans.
- Knowing the relevant driving legislation and where/how to access information for themselves and patients. When providing information it needs to be relevant to the individual and in a format they are likely to use, for example, older people like and refer to written information, whereas Cox *et al.*'s (2000) simulator studies suggest computer programs that involve 'playing a game' may be appropriate to younger people.
- Knowing the commonly used classes of medicines that can impair driving skills such as:
  - anticonvulsants
  - antihistamines
  - antipsychotics
  - benzodiazepines
  - OHA and insulin
  - muscle relaxants
  - opioid analgesics
  - serotonin reuptake inhibitors
  - tricyclic and tetracyclic antidepressants
  - sympathomimetics (Drummer 2008).
- Considering driving safety when managing medicines including when undertaking medicines reviews including home medicine reviews (HMRs) as a key aspect of the Quality Use of Medicines (QUM). Ask about complementary therapy use, particularly herbal medicines and supplements.
- Ensuring diabetes and other relevant education programmes encompass driving responsibilities and safety.

Information for people with diabetes to help them drive safely

The following information can be included in patient education programmes and supportive information such as handouts. It could also be used as a framework for assessing driving knowledge:

- Be aware of your responsibilities as a driver. Make sure you comply with legislation such as informing traffic authorities that you have diabetes especially if you use insulin or glucose-lowering tablets.
- Regularly think about your driving ability, to help you decide your level of risk and whether a formal driving assessment or attending a driving safety class would be useful. Advanced driving classes can be very helpful at improving driving safety for non-diabetics as well as people with diabetes and adapted for younger and older drivers in some countries. They can reduce the likelihood of an accident or improve the way you manage in high-risk driving situations. Formal driving assessment might be needed, for example, if you have a driving accident, a period of illness or your vision declines.
- Consider your own safety, that of your passengers, and other road users when you drive, for example, test your blood glucose before you drive if you are on insulin or diabetes tablets and do not drive if your blood glucose is low. Always carry glucose with you and wear a medical alert 'bracelet' containing relevant health information.
- Decide whether somebody should accompany you and/or whether you should inform relatives or friends where you are going.
- Discuss the factors likely to affect your driving safety with health professionals and your family on a regular basis, for example, when you have your annual diabetes

complication check or winter influenza vaccinations. Make sure you have written advice about what to do when you are sick, have a hypo, need surgery, or an investigation such as an eye test. It may be advisable not to drive in these situations. Knowing beforehand will enable you to make other arrangements.

- Develop a formal driving/transportation plan to ensure you have strategies in place when you can no longer drive safely and ease the transition to not driving.
- Consider factors likely to affect driving safety before you drive. These include your health at the time and other factors such as the weather, distance to cover, road works, and the time of the day or night. Having a mobile phone enables you to call for help but should not be used while the vehicle is moving.
- Follow regulations such as wearing a seat belt, not speaking on a mobile phone while driving and not consuming alcohol or illegal drugs before or while driving. Make sure children and pets cannot move around in the car and place other objects such as groceries in the boot or secure them so they cannot move around and injure passengers if you have to stop suddenly.
- Stop regularly when driving long distances especially if you feel tired or have trouble concentrating. Test your blood glucose, walk around, have a powernap and a drink and some food.
- If you feel unwell, stop and pull over immediately. Check your blood glucose and treat a hypo if your blood glucose is low. If you have chest discomfort, feel dizzy or lightheaded call an ambulance.
- Make sure you know what to do if you have an accident.
- Be aware that motorised wheelchairs/vehicles, and farm machinery such as tractors can also cause 'traffic' accidents and result in significant injury. Safe driving advice also applies to these vehicles, particularly farm machinery.

Diabetes and fasting for religious observances

Religious observances such as fasting are important to many people. Muslim and Buddhist rituals include fasting: Ramadan and Buddhist Lent (Vassa) respectively. Some Christians also fast. Fasting can have an impact on blood glucose and put the individual at risk of an adverse event. Exception from fasting for people with diabetes is permitted in many countries, but many people want to observe their religious conventions.

Ramadan is known as partial feasting because people are not permitted food or fluids from sunrise to sunset for a month each year. Alcohol is not permitted during Ramadan (Al Maatouq 2012). Vassa is observed for three months in the rainy season. Fasting occurs from noon to midnight followed by a 12-hour period when the fast is broken (Latt & Kaira 2012). Glycaemia may improve, worsen or stay the same during religious fasting periods.

Potential effects of fasting:

- Hypoglycaemia (Chapter 6). Severe hypoglycaemia in people with Type 2 diabetes requiring hospital treatment increases during Ramadan (Salti *et al.* 2004) and occurs in~20% of people on sulphonylureas (Al Maatouq 2012). Hypoglycaemia symptoms may go unnoticed e.g. when meditating during Vassa or praying. Likewise hypoglycaemia can impair the meditation.
- Hyperglycaemia. Symptomatic hyperglycaemia can occur if people stop taking their GLM or reduce the dose inappropriately during fasting. Salti *et al.*(2004) reported a five-fold increase in hyperglycaemia during Ramadan. Excessive food intake during the non-fasting hours contributes to hyperglycaemia. Hyperglycaemia can cause polyuria, polydipdia and lethargy, which contribute to dehydration.

- Dehydration and volume depletion. Dehydration and volume depletion may be exacerbated in hot climates due to insensible fluid loss. Dehydration can lead to hyperosmolar states, orthostatic hypotension that can lead to syncope, falls and injuries. The risk of postural hypotension is higher in people who have autonomic neuropathy. Older people may also be at increased risk because they may not experience thirst. (Chapter 7)
  - Cognitive changes due to hyper- and hypoglycaemia that affect decision-making.
  - Overeating after the fasting period.

Education and counselling

Advice needs to be tailored to the individual and the way the manage Ramadan/Vassa and could include:

- The risks associated with fasting.
- How to determine the individual's risk level from hypo-and hyperglycaemia (Chapters 6, 7 and 12).
- How to adjust the medicine regimen for periods of fasting and non-fasting.
- The importance of monitoring blood glucose to determine the blood glucose pattern sand using the information to manage the food and medicine regimen.
- When to test ketones, especially people with Type 1 diabetes.
- Hypoglycaemia and hyperglycaemia management may need to be reviewed and include specific information about when to break the fast for safety reasons. Al Maatouq (2012) recommends breaking the fast if the blood glucose is < 3.9 mmol/L early in the fast because the blood glucose is likely to continue to fall., or if it is <3.3 mmol/L during the fast. These levels may be too low for some people at particular risk of hypoglycaemia such as older people and children. No specific levels were recommended for hyperglycaemia.
- When to seek advice.
- Avoiding calorie-rich foods during non-fasting periods.

> ### Practice points
>
> - Reflect on how having diabetes and two other commitment diseases would affect your mental health, work and social functioning and other aspects of your everyday life.
> - What education, care and advice would you expect your health care providers to provide?
> - How would you manage all the self-care tasks involved including medicines management if various health professionals gave you different information/advice?

References

Enteral and parenteral nutrition

Australian Diabetes Society (2012) *Guidelines for Routine Glucose Control in Hospital Australian Diabetes Society*, ADS, Canberra.

McClave, S., Snider, H. & Spain, D. (1999) Use of residual volume as a marker for enteral feeding intolerance: prospective blinded comparison with physical examination and radiographic findings. *Journal of Parenteral and Enteral Nutrition*, **16**, 64s–70s.

Middleton, M., Nazarenko, G., Nivison-Smith, I. & Smerdley, P. (2001) Prevalence of malnutrition and 12-month incidence of mortality in two Sydney teaching hospitals. *Medical Journal of Australia*, **31**, 455–461.

Thomas, B. (2001) *A Manual of Dietetic Practice*. Blackwell Science, Oxford.

Diabetes and cancer

Bloomgarden, Z. (2001) Diabetes and cancer. *Diabetes Care*, **24**, 780–781.

Coughlin, S., Calle, E., Teras, L., Petrelli, J. & Thun, M. (2004) Diabetes mellitus as a predictor of cancer mortality in a large cohort of US adults. *American Journal of Epidemiology*, **159**, 1160–1167.

Dunning, T., Savage, S., Duggan, N. & Martin, P. (2011) *Guidelines for Managing Diabetes at the End of Life*. Centre for Nursing and Allied Health Research, Deakin University and Barwon Health http:// clearinghouse.adma.org.au/browse-resources/guideline/guidelines-for-managing-diabetes-at-the-end-of-life/details.html

Dunning, T., Savage, S., Duggan, N. & Martin, P. (2102) Diabetes and end of life: Ethical and methodological issues in gathering evidence to guide care. *Scandinavian Journal of Caring Sciences, DOI: 10.111/j.1471-6712.2012.01016x.*

Dibble, S., Luce J. & Cooper, B. (2007) Acupressure for chemotherapy-induced nausea and vomiting: A randomized clinical trial. *Oncology Nursing Forum*, **34**, 813–820.

Eremin, O. & Walker, M. (2009) Immuno-modulatory effects of relaxation training and guided imagery in women with locally advanced breast cancer undergoing multimodality therapy: a randomised controlled trial. *Breast*, **18** (1), 17–25.

Faithful, S. (1998) Fatigue in patients receiving radiotherapy. *Professional Nurse*, **13** (7), 458–459.

Fernandez, C., Stutzer, C., MacWilliam, I. & Fryer, C. (1998) Alternative and complementary use in pediatric oncology patients in British Columbia: Prevalence, reasons for use and nonuse. *Journal of Clinical Oncology*, **16** (4), 1279–1286.

Giovannuci, E., Harlan, D., Archer, M. *et al.* (2010) Diabetes and cancer: a consensus report. *Diabetes Care*, **33** (7), 1674–1685.

Jung, R.T. & Sikora, K. (1984) *Endocrine Problems in Cancer*. Heinemann Medical Books, London.

Kao, G. & Devine, P. (2000) Use of complementary health practices by prostate carcinoma patients undergoing radiotherapy. *Cancer*, **88** (3), 615–619.

Lewis, J., Ferrara, A., Peng, T. *et al.* (2011) Risk of bladder cancer among diabeteic patients treated with pioglitazone. *Diabetes Care*, **34**, 916–922.

Lipman, T. (2007) The role of herbs and probiotics in GI wellness for older adults. *Geriatrics and Aging*, **10** (3), 182–191.

Lipscombe, L., Hux, J. & Booth, G. (2005) Reduced screening mammography among women with chronic medical diseases. *Archives of Internal Medicine*, **165**, 2090–2095.

Mayo Clinic (2012) http://www.mayoclinic.com/health/cancer-treatment/CM00002/NSECTIONGROUP= 2 (accessed January 2012).

Oberbaum, M., Yaniv, I. & Beg, G. (2001) Treating chemotherapy-induced stomatitis with Traumeel. *Cancer*, **92** (3), 684-690.

Oyer, D., Shah, A. & Bettenhausen, S. (2006) How to manage steroid diabetes in the patient with cancer. *Supportive Oncology*, **4** (9), 479–483.

Palliative Care Outcomes Collaboration (PCOC)—CareSearch (2008) www.caresearch.com.au/ caresearch/tabid/99/Default.aspx (accessed February 2013).

Psarakis, H. (2006) Clinical challenges in caring for patients with diabetes and cancer. *Diabetes Spectrum*, **19**, 157–162.

Quinn, K., Hudson, P. & Dunning, T. (2006) Diabetes management in patients receiving palliative care. *Journal of Pain and Symptom Management*, **32** (3), 275–286.

Savage, S., Dunning, T., Duggan, N. & Martin, P. (2012) The experiences and care preferences of people with diabetes at the end of life. *Journal of Hospice and Palliative Nursing*, **14**, 293–323.

SIGN (Scottish Intercollegiate Guidelines Network) (2010) *A National Clinical Guideline*. SIGN, Edinburgh.

Travier, N., Jeffreys, M., Brewer, N. *et al.* (2007) Association between glycosylated hemoglobin and cancer risk: A New Zealand linkage study. *Annals of Oncology*, **18** (8), 1414–1419.

la Vecchia, C., Negri, E., D'Avanzo, B. & Boyle, P. (1994) A case-control study of diabetes mellitus and cancer risk. *British Journal of Cancer*, **70** (5), 950–953.

Verlato, G., Zoppini, G., Bonora, E. & Muggeo, M. (2003) Mortality from site specific malignancies in Type 2 diabetes patients from Verona. *Diabetes Care*, **26**, 1047–1051.

Wideroff, L., Gridley, G., Mellemkjaer, L. *et al.* (1997) Cancer incidence in a population-based cohort of patients hospitalised with diabetes mellitus in Denmark. *Journal of the National Cancer Institute*, **89** (18), 1360–1365.

Wilkinson, J. (2008) "Good gargling": Evaluation of the use of an essential oil mouthwash in the management of radiation-induced mucositis of the oropharyngeal area. *Proceedings of the 3rd International Congress on Complementary Medicine*, Sydney, March 2008, p. 26.

Wyatt, G., Friedman, L., Given, C. & Beckrow, K. (1999) Complementary therapy use among older cancer therapy patients. *Cancer Practice*, **7** (3), 136–144.

Smoking, alcohol, and illegal drug use

American Cancer Society (2007) *Cancer Facts and Figures*. American Cancer Society, Atlanta, GA.

American Psychiatric Association (APA) (2000) *Diagnostic and Statistical Manual of Mental Disorders* (4th edn) Text Revision (DSM-1V-TR), APA, Washington DC.

Australian Institute of Health and Welfare (AIHW) (2006) *Australia's Health*. Catalogue number AUS 73. AIHW, Canberra.

Bover, M., Foulds, J., Steinberg, M., Richardson, D. & Marcella, S. (2008) Waking at night to smoke as a marker for tobacco dependence: Patient characteristics and relationship to treatment outcome. *International Journal of Clinical Practice*, **62** (2), 182–190.

Brink, S. (2008) in Glick D. (2003) Legal and illegal drugs: what every person with diabetes should know before they party. *Diabetes and Health*, http://www.diabeteshealth.com/read/2003/11/0i/3163.html (accessed August 2008).

Brown, L. (1991) Clinical aspects of drug abuse in diabetes. *Diabetes Spectrum*, **4** (1), 45–47.

Department of Health and Human Services (DHHS) (2006) *The Health Consequences of Involuntary Exposure to Tobacco Smoke: A Report of the Surgeon General – Executive Summary*. Department of Health and Human Services (DHSS, Public Health Service, Center for Disease Control, Center for Chronic Disease Prevention and Health Promotion, Office of Smoking and Health, USA.

Ejerblad, E., Fored, C., Lindblad, P. *et al.* (2004) Association between smoking and chronic renal failure in a nationwide population-based case-control study. *Journal of the American Society of Nephrology* **15** (18), 2178–2185.

Falba, T. (2005) Health events and the smoking cessation of middle aged Americans. *Journal of Behavioural Medicine*, **28**, 21–33.

Foulds, J., Gandhi, K. & Steinberg, M. (2006) Factors associated with quitting smoking at a tobacco dependence treatment clinic. *American Journal of Health Behaviour*, **30**, 400–412.

Fu, S., Partin, M. & Snyder, A. (2006) Promoting repeat tobacco dependence treatment: Are relapsed smokers interested? *American Journal of Managed Care*, **12**, 235–243.

Kroon, L. (2007) Drug interactions with smoking. *American Journal of Health-Systems Pharmacy*, **64** (18), 1917–1921.

George, L. (1993) Sociological-perspectives on life transitions. *Annual Review of Sociology*, **19**, 353–373.

Glick, D. (2003) Legal and illegal drugs: What every person with diabetes should know before they party. *Diabetes and Health*, http://www.diabeteshealth.com/read/2003/11/0i/3163.html (accessed August 2008).

Korantzopoulos, P., Liu, T., Papaioannides, D., Li, G. & Goudevenos, J. (2008) Atrial fibrillation and marijuana smoking. *International Journal Clinical Practice*, **62** (2), 308–313.

Lancaster, T. & Stead, L. (2004) Physician advice for smoking cessation. *Cochrane Database of Systematic Reviews*, Issue 4, Art. No. CD000165.

Lang, I., Rice, N., Wallace, R., Guralnik, J. & Melzer, D. (2007) Smoking cessation and transition into retirement: analysis from the English longitudinal study. *Age and Aging*, **36** (6), 638–643.

Lee, N. (2008) Alcohol intervention: What works? *Australian Family Physician*, **37** (1/2), 16–19.

Mercola.com (2011) *Drug used to help people stop smoking may cause suicide*. http://articles.mercola.com/sites/articles/archive2011/06/13/drug-used-to-help-people (accessed December 2012).

Mitchell, D. (2008) Pushing the pin on smoking. *Journal of Complementary Medicine*, **7** (2), 55 and 63.

Moussouttas, M. (2004) Cannabis use and cerebrovascular disease. *Neurologist*, **10**, 47–53.

Naqvi, N., Rudrauf, D., Damasio, H. & Bechara, A. (2007) Damage to the insula disrupts addiction to cigarette smoking. *Science*, **315** (5811), 531–534.

National Health and Medical Research Council (NHMRC) (2007) *Draft Australian Drinking Guidelines for Low Risk Drinking*. www.nhmrc.gov.au/consult (accessed November 2007).

National Native Addictions Partnership Foundation (2006) keeping the sacred in tobacco: a toolkit for tobacco cessation http://www.nnapf.org/tobacco-sacred (accessed November 2012).

Orisatoki R. (2013) The public health implications of the use and misuse of tobacco among Aboriginals in Canada. *Clinical Journal of Health Science*, 5 (1); 28–34.

Osiecki H. (2006). *The Physician's Handbook of Clinical Nutrition*. Bio Concepts Publishing, Eagle Farm, Australia.

Ostbye, T. & Taylor, D. (2004) The effect of smoking on years of healthy life (YHL) lost among middle-aged and older Americans. *Health Services Research*, 39, 531–532.

Owen, N., Wakefield, M., Roberts, L. & Esterman, A. (1992) Stages of readiness to quit smoking; Population prevalence and correlates. *Health Psychology*, 11, 413–417.

Saunders, J., Aasland, O. & Babor, T. (1993) Development of Alcohol Use Disorders Identification Test (AUDIT). WHO collaborative project on early detection of persons with harmful alcohol consumption. Part 2. *Addiction*, 88, 791–804.

Shand, F., Gates, J., Fawcett, J. & Mattick, R. (2003) *Guidelines for the Treatment of Alcohol Problems*. National Drug and Alcohol Research Center, Sydney.

Spinella, M. (2005) *Concise Handbook of Psychoactive Herbs*. Haworth Herbal Press, Oxford.

Stratton, I., Kohner, E., Aldington, S. *et al.* UKPDS 50 (2001) Risk factors for incidence and progression of retinopathy in type 2 diabetes over 6 years from diagnosis *Diabetologia*, 44 (2), 156–163.

Surgeon General's Report (2004) *The Health Consequences of Smoking: Surgeon General's Report 2004*. Department of Health and Human Services (DHSS, Public Health Service, Centre for Disease Control, Center for Chronic Disease Prevention and Health Promotion, Office of Smoking and Health. DHSS publication number CDC 099-7830.

Third International Conference on Smokeless Tobacco, (2002) Smokeless tobacco fact sheets. Stockholm September 22 – 25.

Torrijos, R. & Glantz, S. (2006) The US Public Health Service Treating tobacco use and dependence clinical practice guidelines as a legal standard of care. *BMC Journal of Tobacco Control*, 15 (6), PMC2563672.

Tonstad, S., Tonnesesn, P. & Hajek, P. (2006) Effect of maintenance therapy with varenicine. *Journal of the American Medical Association*, 296, 64–71.

Watkins, S., Koob, G. & Markou, A. (2000) Neural mechanisms underlying nicotine addiction: acute positive reinforcement and withdrawal. *Nicotine Tobacco Research*, 2 (1):, 19–37.

Weiser, M., Zarka, S., Webeloff, N., Kravitz, E. & Lubin, G. (2010) Cognitive test scores in male adolescent cigarette smokers compared to non-smokers: A population-based study. *Addiction*, 10 (2), 358–363.

Willi, C., Bodenmann, P., Ghali, W. A. , Faris, P. D. & Cornuz, J. (2007) Active smoking and the risk of type 2 diabetes: A systematic review and meta-analysis. *Journal of the American Medical Association*, 298, 2654–2664.

Wise, R., Sims, T. &Taylor, R. (2007) Smoking cessation–A practical guide for the primary care physician. *Primary Care Reports*, 13 (4), 49–60.

Zwar, N. (2008) Smoking cessation: What works? *Australian Family Physician*, 37 (1/2), 10–14.

Brittle diabetes

Martin, F. (1995) Brittle diabetes. *Diabetes Communication*, July, 7–8.

Vantyghem, M. & Press, M. (2006) Management strategies for brittle diabetes. *Annals of Endocrinology* 67 (4), 287–296.

Oral health and diabetes

Andersen C, Flyvbjerg K, Holmstrup P. (2007) periodontitis is associated with aggravation of prediabetes in Zuker rats. *Journal of Periodontology*, 78 (3), 559–565.

Connor, S., Iranpour, B. & Mills, J. (1970) Alteration in the parotid salivary flow in diabetes mellitus. *Oral Surgery*, 30, 15.

Dunning, T. (2009) periodontal disease 0 the overlooked diabetes complication *Nephrology Nursing Journal*, 36: 171–181.

Holmes, S. & Alexander, W. (1997) Diabetes in dentistry. *Practical Diabetes International*, 14 (4), 107–110.

Lamey, P., Darwazeh, A. & Frier, B. (1992) Oral disorders associated with diabetes mellitus. *Diabetic Medicine*, 9 (5), 410–416.

National Health Medical Research Council (NHMRC) (1999) *Dietary Guidelines for Older Australians*. Commonwealth of Australia, Canberra.

Southerland J, Taylor G, Moss K, Beck J, Offenbacher S. (2006) Commonality in chronic inflammatory diseases: Periodontitis, diabetes, and coronary artery disease. *Periodontology* **40**, 130–43.

Proceedings of the World Workshop in clinical **periodontics** 1996) Position Paper (Diabetes and periodontal disease. *Journal of Peridontology*, 67, 166–176. https://www.thieme.de/medias/ sys.../9783131698032_extras_1.pdf?...(accessed December 2012).

Diabetes and liver disease

Balkau, B., Eschwege, E., Ducimetiere, P., Richard, J. & Warnet, J. (1991) The high risk of death by alcohol-related diseases in subjects diagnosed as diabetic and impaired glucose tolerant: The Paris Prospective Study after 15 years follow-up. *Journal of Clinical Epidemiology*, **44**, 465–474.

Caldwell, S., Oelsner, D., Iezzoni, J. *et al.* (1999) Cryptogenic cirrhosis: Clinical characterisation and risk factors for underlying disease. *Hepatology*, **29**, 664–669.

Cantley, L. (2002) The phosphoinositide 3-kinase pathway. *Science*, **296**, 1655–1657.

Chitturi, S. & Farrell, G. (2000) Herbal hepatotoxicity: An expanding but poorly defined problem. *Journal of Gastroenterology and Hepatology*, **15**, 1093–1099.

De Marco, R., Locatelli, F., Zoppini, G. *et al.* (1999) Cause-specific mortality in type 2 diabetes: The Verona Diabetes Study. *Diabetes Care*, **22**, 756–761.

El-Serag, H. & Everhart, J. (2002) Diabetes increases the risky of acute liver failure. *Gastroenterology*, **122**, 1822–1828.

Fabris, P., Floreani, A., Tositti, G., *et al.* (2003) Type 1 diabetes mellitus in patients with chronic hepatitis C before and after interferon therapy. *Alimentary Pharmacology Therapy*, **18**: 549–558.

Fuchs, M. (2012) Non-Alcoholic Fatty Liver Disease: The Bile Acid-Activated Farnesoid X Receptor as an Emerging Treatment Target. *Journal of Lipids*, DOI:10.1155/2012/934396.

Gundling, F. Seidl, H., Haler, B. *et al.* (2013) Clinical manifestations and treatment options in patients with cirrhosis and diabetes mellitus. *Digestion* **87** (2):75–84.,

Harris, M., Flegal, K., Cowie, C. *et al.* (1998) Prevalence of diabetes, impaired fasting glucose, and impaired glucose tolerance in US adults: The Third National Health and Nutrition Examination Survey 1988–1994. *Diabetes Care*, **21**, 518–524.

Harrison, S., Belfort, R., Brown, K. *et al.* (2005) A double-blind, placebo controlled trial of pioglitazone in the treatment of non-alcoholic steatohepatitis (NASH). *Gastroenterology*, **128** (Suppl. 2), A681.

King, M. (1996–2012) themedicalchemistrypage.org.LLC/info@themedicalchemistrypage.org (accessed November 2012).

Lipman, T. (2007) The role of herbs and probiotics in GI wellness for older adults. *Geriatrics and Aging*, **10** (3), 182–191.

Marchesini, G., Bugianesi, E., Forlani, G. *et al.* (2003) Nonalcoholic fatty liver, steatohepatitis and the metabolic syndrome. *Hepatology*, **37**, 917–923.

Mendler, M.H., Turlin, B., Moirrand, R. *et al.* (1999) Insulin resistance-associated iron overload. *Gastroenterology*, **117**, 1155–1163.

Sherlock, S. (1981) *Diseases of the Liver and Biliary System*. Blackwell Science, Oxford.

Tolman, K., Fonseca, V., Dalpiaz, A. & Tan, M. (2007) Spectrum of liver disease in type 2 diabetes and management of patients with diabetes and liver diseases. *Diabetes Care*, **30**, 734–743.

US Organ Procurement and Transplantation Network and Scientific Registry of Transplant Recipients (2004) Annual Report. http://www.optn.org/AR2005/904a_rec-dgn_li.htm (accessed January 2007).

Zarrinpar, A. & Loomba, R. (2012) Review article: The emerging interplay among the gastrointestinal tract, bile acids and incretins in the pathogenesis of diabetes and non-alcoholic fatty liver disease. *Alimentary Pharmacology Therapeutics*, **36**, 909–921.

Diabetic mastopathy

Wilmshurst, E. (2002) Facts about diabetic breast disease all women should know. *Diabetes Conquest*, Autumn, 13.

Diabetes and coeliac disease

Buysschaert, M. & Tomasi, J. (2005) Prospective screening for biopsy proven celiac disease, autoimmunity and malabsorption markers in Belgian subjects with type 1 diabetes. *Diabetic Medicine*, **22**, 889–892.

Cavallo, J. (2004) Celiac disease: Sometimes silent, often misleading, always serious. *JDRF* (Juvenile Diabetes Research Foundation) *Countdown*, Summer.

Colin, P., Reunala, T. & Pukkala, E. (1994) Coeliac disease – Associated disorders and survival. *Gut*, **35**, 1215–1218.

Duggan, J. (2004) Coeliac disease: The great imitator. *eMedical Journal of Australia* http://www.mja.com.au/public/issues/180_10_170504/dug10818_fm.html (accessed November 2007).

Fasano, A., Berti, I. & Gerarduzzi, T. (2003) Prevalence of celiac disease in at-risk and not-at-risk groups in the United States. *Archives of Internal Medicine*, **163**, 286–292.

Green, P. & Jabri, B. (2003) Coeliac disease. *Lancet*, **362**, 383–391.

Juvenile Diabetes research foundation (JDRF) (2008). Type 1 diabetes and celiac disease. http://www.jdrf.org.au/living_w_diabetes/newsitem.asp?newsid=166 (accessed January 2008).

Kondonouri, O., Maguire, A. & Knip, M. (2006) ISPAD Clinical Practice Consensus Guidelines 2006–2007. Other complications and associated conditions. *Paediatric Diabetes*, **8** (3),171–176.

Marsh, K. (2011) Coeliac disease and type I diabetes. *The Australian Diabetes Educator*, **14** (3),18–21.

Mohn, A., Cerruto, M., Lafusco, D. *et al.* (2001) Coeliac disease in children and adolescents with type I diabetes: Importance of hyperglycaemia. *Journal of Paediatric Gastroenterology and Nutrition*, **32**, 37–40.

Sjoberg, K., Eriksson, K. & Bredberg, A. (1998) Screening for celiac disease in adult insulin-dependent diabetes mellitus. *Journal of Internal Medicine*, **243**, 133–140.

Suman, S., Williams, E. & Thomas, P. (2003) Is the risk of adult celiac disease causally related to cigarette exposure? *European Journal of Gastroenterology Hepatology*, **15**, 995–1000.

Diabetes and cystic fibrosis-related diabetes

Cystic Fibrosis Trust (2004) *Guidelines for the Management of Cystic Fibrosis-Related Diabetes*. Cystic Fibrosis Trust, Bromley, Kent, UK.

Dyce, P. & Wallymahmed, M (2012) Evaluating screening for long-term complications of cystic fibrosis-related diabetes. *Journal of Diabetes Nursing* **16** (6), 240–246.

Moran, A., Hardin, D., Rodman, D. *et al.* (1999) Diagnosis, screening and management of cystic fibrosis related diabetes mellitus: A consensus conference report. *Diabetes Research and Clinical Practice* **45**, 61–73.

Moran, A., Becker, D. & Castella, S. (2010) Epidemiology, pathophysiology and prognostic implications of cystic fibrosis-related diabetes. *Diabetes Care* **3**, 2677–2685.

O'Riordan, S., Robinson, P., Donaghue, K. & Moran, A. (2009) Management of cystic fibrosis-related diabetes in children and adolescents. ISPAD Clinic Practice Compendium. *Paediatric Diabetes* **10** (Suppl 12), 43–30.

Sleep apnoea

Allen, R. (2012) Home sleep studies. *Australian Prescriber* **25**, 62–64.

McDermott R. (2012) Sleep disturbance as an independent risk factor for diabetes *Diabetes Managment Journal* **39**:4–5.

Department of Veteran's Affairs USA. https://www.myhealth.va.gov/mhv-porta-web/anonymous.portal (accessed December 2012).

Shaw J, M. Punjabi N, Wilding J, Alberti G, Zimmet P. (2008) Sleep-disordered breathing and type 2 diabetes A report from the International Diabetes Federation Taskforce on Epidemiology and Prevention. *Diabetes Research and Clinical Practice*, **81**, 2–12.

Diabetes and tuberculosis

Dooley, K., Tang, T., Golub, J, Dorman, S. & Cronin, W. (2009) Impact of diabetes mellitus on treatment outcomes of patients with active tuberculosis *American Journal of Tropical Medicine and Hygiene*, **80**, 634–639.

Dooley, K. & Chaisson, R, (2009) Tuberculosis and diabetes mellitus: convergence of two epidemics. *The Lancet Infectious Diseases*, **9**, 737–746.

Sullivan, T. & Ben Amor, V. (2012) The co-management of tuberculosis and diabetes: Challenges and opportunities in the developing world. *PloS Med*, **9** (7) e10011269.doi.10.1371/journal.pmed.1001260.

World Health Organization (WHO) (2011) *Tuberculosis and Diabetes: Collaborative Framework for Care and Control of Tuberculosis and Diabetes*. WHO www.who.int/tb (accessed November 2012).

HIV/AIDS and diabetes

Aberg, J., Gallant, J., Anderson, J. *et al.* (2004) Primary care guidelines for the management of persons infected with human immunodeficiency virus: Recommendations of the HIV Medicine Association of the Infectious Diseases Society of America. *Clinics of Infectious Diseases*, **39**, 609–629.

Howard, A., Floris-Moore, A., Amsten, J. *et al.* (2005) disorders of glucose metabolism in HIV infected women. *Clinics of Infectious Diseases* **40**, 1492–1499.

Kim, P. (2011) Increased prevalence of albuminuria in HIV-infected adults with diabetes. *PloS One*, **6** (9), e24610,doi.10.1037/journal.pone.0024610,2011.

Martinez, E., Conget, I., Lozano, L., Casamitjana, R. & Gatell, J. (1999) Reversion of metabolic abnormalities after switching from HIV-1 protease inhibitors to nevirapine. *AIDS* **13**, 805–810,

Rathgaber, H, Sullivan, C. & McCabe K. (1992) Diabetes mellitus induced by megestrol acetate in patients with AIDS and cachexia. *Annals of Internal Medicine*, **116**, 53–54.

Spollett, G. (2006) Hyperglycaemia in HIV/AIDS. http://spectrum.diabetesjournals.org/content /18/3/163 (accessed October 2012).

Diabetes and hearing loss

Bainbridge, K. (2013) *Diabetes and Hearing Impairment: An Epidemiological Perspective.* American-Speech-Language-Hearing Association, http://www.asha.org/aud/articles/diabetes-hearing-impairment/ (accessed December 2012).

Horikawa, C., Kodama, S., Tanaka, S. *et al.* (2012) Diabetes and Risk of Hearing Impairment in Adults: A Meta-Analysis *Journal of Clinical Endocrinology and Metabolism* 2012-2119v1 98/1/51.

WebMD (2013) *Hearing Loss.* http://www.wedmed.com/a-to-z-guides/hearing-loss-causes-symptoms-treatment (accessed January 2013).

Wilson D., Walsh P., Sanchez L. *et al.* (1999). The epidemiology of hearing impairment in an Australian adult population. *International Journal of Epidemiology*, **28** (2), 247–252.

Diabetes and musculoskeletal diseases

Brown, D., McRae, F. & Shaw, K. (2001) Musculoskeletal disease in diabetes. *Practical Diabetes International*, **18** (2), 62–64.

Chiu K. Chu A, Go V et al. (2004) Hypovitaminosis D is associated with insulin resistance and β cell dysfunction. *The American Journal of Clinical Nutrition*, **79** (5), 820–825.

Gregg E, Pereira M, Caspersen C. (2000) Physical activity, falls, and fractures among older adults: a review of the epidemiologic evidence. *Journal of the American Geriatrics Society*, **48**, 883–893.

Smith, L., Burnet, S. & McNeil, J. (2002) *Musculoskeletal Manifestations of Diabetes Mellitus.* www.bjsm.bmj (accessed March 2008).

Corticosteroid medications and diabetes

Australian Diabetes Society (ADS) (2012) *Guidelines for Routine Glucose Control in Hospital.* Australian Diabetes Society, Canberra. 13–14.

Diabetes UK (2012) Hyperglycaemia symptoms. www.nhs.uk/Conditions/Hyperglycaemia/Pages/Symptoms.aspx (accessed February 2013).

Dunning, T. (1996) Corticosteroids medications and diabetes mellitus. *Practical Diabetes International*, **13**, 186–188.

Jackson, R. & Bowman, R. (1995) Corticosteroids. *Medical Journal of Australia*, **162**, 663–665.

O'Brien P, Oyebode F. (2003) Psychotropic medication and the heart. *Advances in Psychiatric Treatment* 9: 414-423 DOI: 10.1192/apt.9.6.414

Romas, E. (2008) Corticosteroid-induced osteoporosis and fractures. *Australian Prescriber*, **21** (2), 45–49.

Williams, G. & Pickup, J. (1992) *Handbook of Diabetes.* Blackwell Science, Oxford.

Shapiro K (2007) . What Is the Role of Rosiglitazone in Steroid-Induced Diabetes? *Medscape.* Mar 06, www.medscape.com/viewarticle/552606 (accessed October 2012).

van Raalte D, Ouwens D, Diamant M. (2009) Novel insights into glucocorticoid-mediateddiabetogenic effects: Towards expansionof therapeutic options? *European Journal of Clinical Investigation*, **39**, 81–93.

Diabetes and driving

AUSTROADS (2012) *Assessing Fitness to Drive.* National Transport Commission, Sydney.

Braver, E. & Trempel, R. (2004) Are older drivers actually at higher risk of involvement in collisions resulting in deaths or non-fatal injuries among their passengers and other road users? *Injury Prevention*, **10**, 27–32.

Broers, S., van Vliet, K., le Cessie, S. *et al.* (2005) Blood glucose awareness training in Dutch type 1 diabetes patients: One year follow up. *Netherlands Journal of Medicine*, **63**, 164–169.

Clark, B., Ward, J. & Enoch, B. (1980) Hypoglycaemia in insulin dependent diabetic drivers. *British Medical Journal*, **281**, 586.

Clark, D., Stump, T. & Wolinsky, F. (1998) Predictors of onset of and recovery from mobility difficulty among adults aged 51–61 years. *American Journal of Epidemiology*, **148** (1), 63–71.

Cox, D., Gonder-Frederick, L., Julian, D. *et al.* (1991) Intensive versus standard blood glucose awareness training (BGAT) with insulin-dependent diabetes: Mechanisms and ancillary effects. *Psychosomatic Medicine*, **53**, 453–462.

Cox, D., Gonder-Frederick, L., Kovatchev, B., Julian, D. & Clarke, W. (2000) Progressive hypoglycaemia's impact on driving simulation performance: Occurrence, awareness and correction. *Diabetes Care*, **23**, 163–170.

Coyne, K., Margolis, M., Kennedy-Martin, T. *et al.* (2004) The impact of diabetic retinopathy: Perspectives from patient focus groups. *Family Practice*, **21**, 447–453.

Cryer P. (2007) Hypoglycaemia, functional brain failure and brain death. *Journal of Clinical Investigation* **117**:868–870.

Diabetes Control and Complication Trial Research Group (DCCT) (1991) Epidemiology of severe hypoglycaemia in the Diabetes Control and Complications Trial. *American Journal of Medicine*, **90**, 450–459.

Diabetes Control and Complication Trial Research Group (DCCT) (1997) Hypoglycaemia in the diabetes control and complications trial. *Diabetes*, **46**, 271–286.

Drummer, O. (2008) The role of drugs in road safety. *Australian Prescriber*, **31** (2), 33–35.

Eadington, D. & Frier, B. (1989) Type 1 diabetes driving experience: An eight year cohort study. *Diabetic Medicine*, **6**, 137–141.

Deary, I., Hepburn, D., MacLeod, K. *et al.* (1993) Partitioning the symptoms of hypoglcaemia using multi-sample confirmatory factor analysis, *Diabetologia*, **36**, 771–777

National Health Service (NHS) (2010) The Hospital Management of Hypoglycaemia in Adults in Hospital www.diabetes.nhs.uk/document.php?o=217 –(accessed January 2013).

Edinburgh Hypoglycaemia Scale. http://www.datadictionaryadmin.scot.nhs.uk/isddd/15647.html (accessed December 2012).

Evans, L. (2004) Overview of traffic fatalities, in *Traffic Safety*. Evans L. (ed) Bloomfield Hills, MI, Science Serving Society, pp. 57–58.

Frier, B., Mathews, D., Steel, J. & Duncan, L. (1980) Driving and insulin-dependent diabetes. *Lancet*, **8180**, 1232–1234.

Guerrier, H., Manivannan, P. & Nair, N. (1999) The role ofworking memory, field dependence, visual search, and reactiontime in left turn performance of older female drivers. *Applied Ergonomic*, **30**, 109–119.

Harsch, I., Stocker, S., Radespiel-Troger, M. *et al.* (2002) Traffic hypoglycaemias and accidents in patients with diabetes mellitus treated with different antidiabetic regimens. *Journal of Internal Medicine*, **252**, 352–360.

Heller, S. & Macdonald, I. (1996) The measurement of cognitive function during acute hypoglycaemia: Experimental limitations and their effect on study of hypoglycaemic unawareness. *Diabetic Medicine*, **13**, 607–615.

Henderson, J., Allen, K., Deary, I. & Frier, H. (2003) Hypoglycaemia in insulin-treated type 2 diabetes: Frequency, symptoms and impaired awareness. *Diabetic Medicine*, **20** (12), 1016–1021.

Koepsell, T., Wolf, E. & McCloskey, L. (1994) et al. Medical conditions and motor vehicle collision injuries in older adults. *Journal American Geriatric Society*, **42** (7), 695–700.

Laberge-Nadeau, C., Dionne, G. & Ekoe, M. (2000) Impact of diabetes on crash risks of truck-permit holders and commercial drivers. *Diabetes Care*, **23** (5), 612–7.

Lee, H., Lee, A., Cameron, D. & Li-Tsang, C. (2003) Using a driving simulator to identify older drivers at inflated risk of motor vehicle crashes. *Journal of Safety Research*, **34** (4), 453–459.

MacLeod, K. (1999) Diabetes and driving: Toward equitable evidence-based decision-making. *Diabetes Medicine*, **16**, 282–290.

Margolis, K., Kerani, R., McGovern, T. *et al.* (2002) Study of osteoporotic fractures research, risk factors for motor vehicle crashes in older women. *Journal of Gerontology. Series A, Biological Sciences and Medical Sciences*, **57**, M186–M191.

Marrero, D. & Edelman, S. (2000) Hypoglycaemia and driving performance: A flashing yellow light? *Diabetes Care*, **23** (2), 146–147.

McGwin, G., Sims, R., Pulley, L. & Roseman, J. (1999) Diabetes and automobile crashes in the elderly: A population-based case control study. *Diabetes Care*, **22**, 220–227.

McGwin, G., Sims, R., Pulley, L., Roseman, M. (2000) Relations among chronic medical conditions, medications, and automobile crashes in the elderly. *American Journal of Epidemiology*, **152** (5), 424–431.

Meneilly, S., Cheung, E., Tessier, D., Yakura, C. & Tuokko H. (1993) The effect of improved glycemic control on cognitive functions in the elderly patient with diabetes. *Journal of Gerontology*, **48** (4), M117–M121.

Penckofer, S., Ferrans, C., Velsor-Fredrich, B. & Savoy, S. (2007) The psychological impact of living with diabetes: Women's day-to-day experiences. *The Diabetes Educator*, **33** (4), 680–690.

Sagberg, F. (2006) Driver health and crash involvement: A case control study. *Accident Analysis and Prevention*, **38** (1), 28–34.

Salas, M. & Caro, J. (2002) Are hypoglycaemia and other adverse effects similar among sulphonylureas? *Adverse Drug Reactions Toxicology Review*, **21**, 205–217.

Scalea, T., Bochicchio, G. & Bochicchio, K. (2007) Tight glycaemic control in critically injured trauma patients. *Annals of Surgery*, **246**, 605–610.

Shorr, R., Ray, W., Daugherty, J. & Griffin, M. (1997) Incidence and risk factors for serious hypoglycaemia in older persons using insulin or sulphonylureas. *Archives of Internal Medicine*, **157**, 1681–1685.

Sommerfield, A., Deary, I., McAuley, V. & Frier, B. (2003) Short-term delayed, and working memory are impaired during hypoglycaemia in individuals with type 1 diabetes. *Diabetes Care*, **26**, 390–396.

Stahl, M. & Berger, W. (1999) High incidence of severe hypoglycaemia leading to hospital admission in type 2 diabetic patients treated with long-acting sulphonylureas versus short-acting sulphonylureas. *Diabetic Medicine*, **16**, 586–590.

Steel, J., Frier, B., Young, R. & Duncan, L. (1981) Driving and insulin dependent diabetics. *Lancet*, **2** (8242), 354–356.

Stuck, A., Walthert, J., Nikolaus, T. *et al.* (1999) Risk factors for functional status decline in community-living elderly people: A systematic review. *Social Science Medicine*, **48**, 445–469.

UKPDS (United Kingdom Prospective Diabetes Study) (1998) Intensive blood glucose control with sulphonylureas or insulin compared with conventional treatment and risk of complications in patients with Type 2 diabetes (UKPDS 33). *Lancet*, **352**, 837–853.

US Department of Transportation Federal Highway Safety Information http://safety.fhwa.dot.gov. older_users (accessed March 2013).

Wright A, Cull C, Macleod K, et al. (2006) for the UKPDS Group Hypoglycemia in Type 2 diabetic patients randomized to and maintained on monotherapy with diet, sulfonylurea, metformin, or insulin for 6 years from diagnosis: UKPDS73. *Journal of Diabetes Complications*, **20**, 395–401.

Wusthoff, T., Smee, C., Merchant, N., *et al.*, (2012). Prediction of neurodevelopmental outcome after hypoxic-ischemic encephalopathy treated with hypothermia by diffusion tensor imaging analyzed using tract-based spatial statistics. *Pediatric Research*, **72**, 63–69.

Veitch, P. & Clifton-Bligh, R. (2004) Octreotide treatment for sulfonylurea- induced hypoglycaemia. *Medical Journal of Australia*, **180** (10), 540-541.

Yki-Jarvinen, H., Ryysy, L., Nikkila, K. *et al.* (1999) Comparison of bedtime insulin regimens in patients with type 2 diabetes mellitus. A randomised, controlled trial. *Archives of Internal Medicine*, **130**, 399–396.

Ziemer B, Barnes C Tsui C. (2007) hypoglycaemia is not associated with intensification of diabetes therapy. American Diabetes association Scientific sessions, June 24th 2007, Chicago Illinois.

Fasting for religious observances

Al Maatouq M. (2012) Pharmacological approaches to the management of type 2 diabetes in fasting adults during Ramadan. *Diabetes Metabolic Syndrome and Obesity: Targets and Therapy*, **20** (25), 109–119.

Latt, T. & Kaira, S. (2012) Managing diabetes during fasting – Afocus on Buddhist Lent. *Diabetes Voice*, **57** (4), 42–45.

Salti I, Benard E, Detournay B. (2004) EPIDIAR study. A population-based study of diabetes and its characteristics during the fasting month of Ramadan in 13 countries: Results of the epidemiology of diabetes and Ramadan 1422/2001 study. *Diabetes Care*, **27**, 2306–2311.

Chapter 11
Diabetes and Sexual and Reproductive Health

Key points

- Sexual problems are common in the general population but people with diabetes are at increased risk.
- The presence of a sexual problem and diabetes does not mean one led to the other: other causative factors need to be discussed.
- Physical, psychological, environmental, and social factors that affect sexual health should be considered.
- The needs and perceptions of both partners are important.
- Addressing sexual health and sex education should be part of preventative, holistic diabetes care.
- The sexual health needs of older people are often overlooked and not addressed.
- There is a fine line between taking a sexual history and voyeurism.
- The focus should be on what is normal and achievable for the individual/couple rather than dysfunction or 'performance.'
- Health professionals need to be comfortable with their own sexuality to advise other effectively.

Rationale

Nurses are often the person's first point of contact. People with diabetes expect nurses to be knowledgeable about the impact of diabetes on their sexual health. Sexuality is an integral component of health and sexual problems affect all aspects of health and well being. Sexual dysfunction in men with diabetes is well documented but sexual dysfunction among women with diabetes is still not well understood. The sexual response is an interaction between two (usually) people. Sexual dysfunction is also likely to involve both partners in the relationship (Masters & Johnson 1970). Nurses are ideally placed

Care of People with Diabetes: A Manual of Nursing Practice, Fourth Edition. Trisha Dunning.
© 2014 John Wiley & Sons, Ltd. Published 2014 by John Wiley & Sons, Ltd.

to be able to emphasise the need for primary prevention and early identification of sexual difficulties and to dispel common sex myths.

Sexual health

Sexual health is a core aspect of an individual's general health and wellbeing and is the result of an integration of many components into a unified complex system—endocrine hormonal regulators, and the vascular, nervous, and psychological systems. Diabetes can profoundly affect the individual's sexual identity and the physical ability to engage in sexual activity. Maximising sexual health should be an integral part of an holistic management plan for people with diabetes. Management should include education about screening for where relevant and managing diabetes-related complications and issues such as safe sex, contraception, sexually transmitted diseases, and the importance of planning pregnancies. Thus, a life continuum approach to sexual health is recommended.

Contraception

Female contraception is described in Chapter 14. Contraception options for men include:

- Condoms;
- Withdrawing before ejaculating, which is not recommended and has a high failure rate for pregnancies and sexual satisfaction;
- Billing's method, which requires cooperation from female partners;
- Vasectomy;
- Male contraceptive agents are currently under study (see Chapter 14).

Sexual issues are highly sensitive and must be approached with tact and consideration of the person's culture, sexual beliefs, and their privacy and confidentiality. Thus, although partners can often provide important information about their partner's sexual functioning, they should not be included in the consultation unless the individual agrees. The World Health Organization (WHO) (2010) stressed the importance of sexuality as an integral component of health and defined sexual health as:

> A state of physical, emotional, mental and social wellbeing in relation to sexuality; it is not merely the absence of disease, dysfunction or infirmity. Sexual health requires a positive, respectful approach to sexuality and sexual relationships and the possibility of having pleasurable and safe sexual experiences, free of coercion, discrimination and violence. For sexual health to be attained and maintained, the sexual rights of all persons must be respected, protected and fulfilled.
>
> (WHO 2010)

By the WHO definition, the majority of the general populations, including people with diabetes, do not achieve sexual health!

Masters and Johnson first described the human sexual response in 1970. They described four phases: arousal, plateau, orgasm, and resolution (Masters & Johnson 1970). These phases blend into each other and sexual difficulties can occur in one or all of them. Kaplan (1979) described a biphasic response that involved parasympathetic nerve activity—vasocongestion, vaginal lubrication and erection; and sympathetic nerve activity—reflex muscle contraction, orgasm, and ejaculation. Kaplan's description makes it easier to understand how diabetes can affect physical sex given that autonomic neuropathy causes nerve damage, which is a component of erectile dysfunction; see Chapter 8.

Sex counsellors continue to utilise many of the sexual counselling techniques Masters and Johnson developed. Sexual difficulties do not occur in isolation from other aspects of an individual's life and relationships and a thorough assessment and history is necessary to identify the underlying inter-related causal factors. Masters and Johnson found that age and chronic disease processes do not affect female sexual responsiveness as severely as they affect male sexuality and stated the sexual response is more varied in women than in men. However, other studies suggest diabetes has a pervasively negative effect on women with type 2 diabetes' sexual health and well being, which begins after the diagnosis of diabetes (Albright 2012).

Sexual development

Sexual development occurs across the lifespan:

- Chromosomal sex is determined at fertilisation.
- 3–5 years – diffuse sexual pleasure, fantasies and sex play. Often form a close relationship with a parent of the opposite sex.
- 5–8 years – interest in sexual differences, sex play is common.
- 8–9 years – begin to evaluate attractiveness and are curious about sex.
- 10–12 years – preoccupation with changing body and puberty. Adolescents are often sexually active by this age, thus sex education should start early and information provided in accordance to the child's capacity to understand and using appropriate language.
- 13–20 years – puberty, development of self-image and sexual identity.
- Late 30s–early 40s – peak sexual responsiveness.
- Menopause – variable onset and highly individual effect on sexuality.
- Old age – physical difficulties and limited opportunity.

Effective sex and diabetes education should be part of the diabetes management plan so that problems can be identified early and optimal sexual functioning maintained. Health professionals and people with diabetes often have limited information about the impact diabetes can have on their sexual health. Sex education, good metabolic control, early identification, and management of sexual problems are important, but often neglected, aspects of the diabetes care plan and should be included in annual complication screening programmes. When a sexual problem is identified the focus is often on dysfunction and performance rather than on what is normal or achievable, which can have a negative psychological impact on sexuality. Changing the focus to what can be achieved and focusing on feelings, intimacy, love, and warmth have a big impact on general and sexual well being.

Sexual problems

Sexual satisfaction is a combination of physical and emotional factors. Sexual problems can be:

- Primary – usually defined as never having an orgasm.
- Secondary – difficulties occur after a period of normal sexual functioning. Most sexual difficulties fit into this category.
- Situational – where the situation itself inhibits sexual activity, other sexual problems may also be involved.

Possible causes of sexual difficulties and dysfunction

Sexual difficulties usually involve two people. The problem may be shared or each person may have individual issues that need to be considered. Interpersonal factors, the relationship and environmental and disease factors need to be explored with the individuals and couple involved.

(1) Individual factors
   - Ignorance and misinformation, which are common, despite today's sexually permissive society and the surfeit of explicit sex in movies, books and television programmes and advertisements (sell it with sex). A great deal of readily available literature in magazines and on television over emphasise performance set up unreal expectations.
   - Guilt, shame, and fear, which may be fear of getting pregnant, contracting a sexually transmitted disease, not pleasing their partner or being rejected by them.
   - Gender insecurity/uncertainty and sexual preference.
   - Non-sexual concerns, for example, worry about finances, children, and job.
   - Past sexual abuse.
   - Physical condition, for example, presence of diabetes especially diabetes complications such as autonomic neuropathy and vascular disease.
   - Age related changes and the menopause in women.
(2) Interpersonal factors
   - Sexual relationships are one of the most complex undertakings people ever make; yet most people prepare for sexual relationships and their sexual health casually and in an uninformed way.
   - Communication problems – the most common sexual difficulty.
   - Lack of trust.
   - Different sexual preferences and desires, for example, frequency of intercourse.
   - Relationship difficulties that can include difficulties associated with incompatibility, alcohol and violence or be related to disease process, including diabetes.
   - Changes in lifestyle, for example, having children, retrenchment, retirement, and illness including diabetes.
(3) Chronic disease sequelae
   (a) Psychological.
      - Depression, anger, guilt, anxiety, fear, feelings of helplessness, changed body image and self-identification as a victim, lowered self-image and self-esteem may or may not accompany the disease. Loss of libido is one of the classic signs of depression.
   (b) Physical changes, for example, arthritis and diabetic neuropathy.
      - Pain, debilitation associated with changed mobility, for example, arthritis, bad odour associated with infections and candidia, cardiac and respiratory problems and sleep apnoea, and snoring. Some people worry about resuming sexual activity after an MI or having a heart attack during sexual activity. Education can help allay such fears.
      - Disease processes and hormonal imbalance, including diabetes, as well as other endocrine and reproductive conditions.
      - Medications, for example, antihypertensive and antidepressive agents.
   (c) Diabetes-related.
      - Hypoglycaemia during intercourse can be frightening and off-putting, especially for the partner, and inhibit spontaneity and enjoyment in future encounters.
      - Tiredness and decreased mood and decreased arousal and libido are associated with hyperglycaemia.

- Mood disorders such as depression and other psychological problems may be present but mood can change with hypo- and hyperglycaemia and can cause temporary sexual problems.
- Autonomic neuropathy leading to erectile dysfunction in men and possibly decreased vaginal lubrication in older women. Vaginal dryness is also associated with normal ageing, not being aroused and painful intercourse and has not been definitively linked to diabetes as a cause.
- Men with diabetes are likely to have low testosterone levels especially if they have poor glycaemic control. Low testosterone is associated with increased risk of death. Testosterone supplementation improves glycaemic control (HbA$_{1c}$), lipids and well being (Heulelder 2012).

(e) Infections, for example, vaginal/penile thrush.

(f) Musculoskeletal diseases that limit mobility, dexterity and may cause pain; see Chapter 10.

(4) Environmental factors.
- Lack of privacy.
- Limited opportunity, for example, older people generally and especially those who live in aged care facilities.
- Uncomfortable, noisy surroundings.
- Drugs and alcohol.
- Health professional and population agist attitudes concerning older people's sexual needs

Sexuality and older people

Older people are capable of having fulfilling sexual relationships but often lack the opportunity or are constrained by environmental factors, ageist attitudes, sexual stereotypes and disease processes (see Chapter 12). Sensory impairment can change the individual's response to sexual stimulation and the multiplicity of medications required by many older people can inhibit sexual functioning. Touch is important throughout life and caring touch as distinct from providing nursing care is often lacking. Touch can provide a great deal of sexual pleasure when intercourse is not possible. Many older people are deprived of touch when a partner dies and in aged care facilities.

Women

The biological effect of diabetes on male sexual functioning has been well documented. The effects of diabetes on sexual function in women are poorly understood and the evidence for any effect is less conclusive than the evidence for the effects on male sexual functioning (Leedom *et al.* 1991). Physicians regularly ask men about their sexual functioning but not women (Albright 2012 Copeland *et al.* 2012).

Women with diabetes are twice as likely to report low sexual satisfaction then women without diabetes (Copeland *et al.* 2012). In a study (n=2000) women on insulin were more likely to report difficulty with vaginal lubrication and 80% reported difficulty achieving orgasm. Not surprisingly, women with diabetes complications such as peripheral neuropathy, renal dysfunction and cardiovascular disease were more likely to report less sexual activity and les satisfaction than controls. However, a number of factors besides diabetes contribute to sexual dissatisfaction as indicated in the previous section.

Women who have difficulty accepting that they have diabetes report higher levels of sexual dysfunction than those who accept their diabetes. Type 2 diabetes has a pervasively negative effect on women's sexuality (Schriener-Engel *et al.* 1991). There appears to be little or no effect in women with Type 1 diabetes but they often have concerns about pregnancy, childbirth, and hypoglycaemia during sex in the younger years (Dunning 1994). There is a positive association between the degree of sexual dysfunction and the severity of depression that illustrates the connection between physical and psychological factors and the need for an holistic approach.

Fluctuating blood glucose levels can have a negative transient effect on desire and sexual responsiveness and women often report slow arousal, decreased libido and inadequate lubrication during hyperglycaemia. Desire can fluctuate with stages of the menstrual cycle but this also occurs in women without diabetes. Polycystic Ovarian Disease and its effects could have adverse psychological effects, which in turn affect sexual health (see Chapter 14). Obesity can contribute to physical difficulties during sexual intercourse.

The developmental stage of the individual should also be considered when assessing sexual health and planning sex education and counselling.

- Children and adolescents—diabetes can affect normal growth and development if it is not well controlled and menarche and puberty can be delayed. This could impact negatively on body image and the development of sexual identity and self-esteem. Eating disorders and insulin manipulation can compound the problem.
- Young adulthood—attracting a partner, successful pregnancy and birth can be areas of fear and concern that affect sexual health (Dunning 1994). Hyperglycaemia can occur during menstruation resulting in tiredness, decreased arousal and libido. Vaginal thrush is common and causes itch and discomfort during sexual intercourse. It may be associated with taking oral contraceptives or antibiotics for intercurrent illness. Thrush and balanitis can inhibit male sexual activity. Brittle diabetes (chapter 14) may also inhibit sexual functioning and health.
- Older age group— hormonal changes due to menopause and associated fatigue and depression inhibit sexual enjoyment. Often a long-term partner's life courses are different and can affect their sexual relationship. There are fewer partners and opportunities for sexual activity for older women especially those in care facilities.

Specific problems should be investigated depending on their presentation. Diabetes management should be revised to achieve good glycaemic control and a medicines review may be indicated. Preventative sexual health care such as breast self-examination, mammograms, and cervical (pap) smears should be part of the care plan. Contraception is discussed in Chapter 14.

Men

Diabetes has physical effects that cause erectile dysfunction (ED). Other ED causes include:

- Andropause, which leads to a normal, gradual reduction in male hormones such as testosterone and sex hormone binding globulin (SHBG) akin to the menopause in women. Andropause can result in depression, low libido, erectile dysfunction and irritability. Men with diabetes tend to experience andropause earlier and the symptoms are more pronounced then men without diabetes.
- Vascular damage, both systemic atherosclerosis and microvascular disease.
- Neurological diseases such as spinal cord damage, multiple sclerosis, and diabetic neuropathy.
- Psychological causes such as performance anxiety, depression and mood changes may be associated with hypo- or hyperglycaemia.

- Endocrine diseases that result in lowered sex hormones: testosterone, SHBG, prolactin, FSH, and LH. Hypogonadism can occur in chronic disease.
- Obesity can contribute to physical difficulties during sexual intercourse.
- Surgery and trauma to genitalia or its nerve and vascular supply.
- Anatomical abnormalities, for example, Peyronie's contracture, which is often associated with Dupuyten's contracture and other glycosylation diseases including diabetes; see Chapter 10.
- Medicines such as thiazide diuretics, beta blockers, lipid lowering agents, antidepressants, SSRI, smoking, alcohol, and illicit drug use.
- Normal ageing.

ED is defined as the inability to achieve or maintain an erection sufficient for satisfactory sexual performance – penetration and ejaculation. It is common in men with diabetes especially if other diabetic complications are present. It occurs in 50% of men 10 years after the diagnosis of diabetes especially those who smoke. ED is gradual, insidious and progressive (Krane 1991). ED may be a predictor of cardiovascular risk and there is a higher incidence of undiagnosed coronary disease in men with ED. Elevated blood fats and hypertension and antihypertensive agents also play a part in the development of ED. Lowered sperm counts are associated with obesity, smoking and poor diet.

ED significantly reduces the man's quality of life especially in the emotional domain and has a negative effect on self-esteem. However, ED also has a significant effect on the man's partner. Partners play a key supportive role in the man's treatment and treatment success (Dean *et al.* 2008). When sexual functioning improves, improvement in mental and social status follows. Other sexual issues for men are fatigue, fear of performance failure, and concern about not satisfying their partners, but most men do not involve their partners when they seek advice about ED (Dean *et al.* 2008).

Aboriginal and Torres Strait Islander men have higher incidence of ED; ~ 10% in men younger than 35 years and 28% in men 55–74 years. Those with a chronic disease or living in remote areas are more likely to have moderate to severe ED and a similar low level of help-seeking as non-Indigenous men. Barriers to help-seeking in Indigenous men are shame, cultural inappropriate services and lack of awareness (Adams *et al.* 2013). In is not clear whether similar issues apply to other Indigenous peoples. Sexual health assessment, education and management programmes need to be culturally sensitive and should be developed by/with relevant Indigenous people.

Investigation and management

A thorough history and physical examination are required. Some of the questions that need to be asked are very personal, which may be difficult and stressful, thus time, privacy, and tact are essential. The assessment includes diabetic complication status and blood glucose and lipid control, identifying the cause and determining the extent of the dysfunction, for example, using rigiscan and snap gauge to determine whether nocturnal erections occur, and sleep apnoea studies. There is an association between poor sleep, sleep apnoea and ED. Doppler studies are carried out to determine local blood flow. Testosterone, FSH, LH, SHBG, and prolactin levels are measured.

Management consists of:

- Good metabolic control to prevent ED and improve andropause symptoms. If the testosterone is low, supplementation might improve symptoms. Testosterone can be given by injection, patch, topical gel and implants. Complementary medicines include L-arginine and *Gingko biloba* (Andropause Report 2013).

- Early intervention if ED occurs.
- Assessing fitness for sex and modifying risk factors, for example, losing weight, managing pain, smoking cessation, and reducing alcohol intake.
- Appropriate diet and exercise programme. Tai Chi and strength training can improve flexibility and strength and general well being in older men.
- Sex education that includes setting realistic expectations and planning for regular sexual health checks, for example, prostate disease.
- Diabetes education.
- Counselling, which should include partners and inform them about treatment options to help the couple find fulfilling sexual alternatives if the man cannot achieve erections.

Men are often reluctant to seek help, especially for sexual difficulties. Programmes such as Men's Sheds in Australia have had a positive effect on mental health and well being as well as helping men develop life skills in a peer education environment. It is not clear whether men discuss sexual health in Men's Sheds but diabetes educators have been invited to discuss diabetes in these sheds.

Medication management for ED

Oral medicines

Medication management includes oral phosphodiesterase type 5 (PDE-5) inhibitors Sildenafil (Viagra), Vardenafil (Levitra), and Cialis, which are vasodilators that enhance the natural sexual response. They can cause visual disturbances ('blue vision'), transient hypotension and can unmask cardiac ischaemia. PDE-5 medicines are contraindicated if nitrate medications are used and when cardiovascular disease is present. Cimetidine and Ketoconozale can increase Viagra levels and Rifampicin decreases them. Other oral medicines currently under study include sublingual apomorphine (UPRIMA), which acts centrally and enhances the response to stimulation and oral phentolamine (VASOMAX), which improves penile blood flow (Endocare 2004).

Urethral and injected medicines

Urethrally introduced medicines such as MUSE have a success rate between 30% and 50% of men. Side effects include urethral pain and burning in 7–10% of men who use this medicine. Intracavernosal therapy or penile injections such the vasoconstrictor agents papaverine, alprostadil (Caverject), VIP, and the vasodilator phentalamine. Men and/or their partners need to learn the technique of penile injections, which should be done under supervision. A rare but serious side effect is priapism, which requires urgent treatment to reverse the effects of the vasoconstricton. Other side effects include the formation of scar tissue, bruising, and rarely infection at injection sites. Caverject sometimes causes pain in high doses.

Non-pharmacological therapy

Non-pharmacological therapy includes external vacuum pumps. Vacuum devices are a simple effective method of achieving an erection. A man suffering from ED invented a device called ErecAid® in the 1960s. It consists of a clear plastic cylinder, which has either a manual pump or batteries and a special tension ring. The penis is placed into the cylinder and the man or his partner holds the device firmly against the body to form an airtight seal and then pumps the air out of the cylinder, which creates a vacuum and causes the penis to become erect. The special tension ring is inserted over the device around the base of the penis to maintain the erection, and the device is removed. The whole process takes about two minutes and the erection is maintained for about 30 minutes (longer than natural erections). The ring *must* be removed after intercourse.

Vacuum pumps have very few side effects. Sometimes, small red dots called petechiae and bruising can occur on the penis but these are not harmful. They are more likely to occur if the individual is on anticoagulant medicines. The temperature in the penis drops 1–2 degrees, which is caused by the tension ring. The device can be difficult to use, so learning how to use it, is important. It can reduce sexual spontaneity so it is very important that the man discusses sexual issues and their management options with his partner.

Hormone replacement therapy

Hormone replacement therapy (testosterone) might be indicated in 3–4% of men, but is contraindicated in men with liver disease, cardiovascular disease, renal disease, and prostate cancer. These contraindications probably apply to many men with diabetes. See subheading Men.

Complementary medicines for sexual problems (CAM)

Men with sexual health problems commonly use CAM especially if they receive conflicting advice and worry a lot about the problem (Trutnovsky *et al.* 2001). CAM can be used to improve general health and well being and mange stress that can have benefits for sexual health, see Chapter 19. Likewise, recommendations about the importance of eating a healthy diet and exercise and adequate rest and sleep to sexual health are important CAM as well as conventional strategies. Often CAM practitioners recommend supplements such as flaxseed oil, vitamins E, and C and zinc. However, rigorous evidence for a beneficial effect for most herbal medicines is lacking and some are harmful. CAM therapies appear to target three main sexual health issues: improving sexual 'stamina', aphrodisiacs, and overcoming erection problems.

Commonly used CAM medicines to improve libido and erections include the following. They are often used in combination:

- Horney goat weed
- Passion treatment
- Damiana
- Yohimbe
- Asian Ginseng
- Goji berries, which are sometimes referred to as 'natural viagra' and also come chocolate coated.

Many so-called aphrodisiacs carry significant health risks (often for animals as well as men) and are not recommended. These include powdered rhino horn, crushed pearls, Spanish fly, and animal testicles.

The risks and benefits of these medicines are not known and they may interact with conventional medicines including those used to manage sexual problems. Therefore, it is important to ask men and women with sexual health problems about CAM use. The US FDA warned people about two unapproved dietary supplements sold online to treat

ED: 'Blue Steel' and 'Hero', which contain active ingredients with similar actions to sildenafil. These products could interact with conventional nitrate medicines and cause hypotension. People might unwittingly seek such alternatives if conventional ED medicines are contraindicated or if they do not feel comfortable discussing sexual health with their health professionals.

Involving partners in ED management

Partners may be able to contribute important information about the man's general health and sexual history but should only be involved if they are willing and the man agrees. The man, and ideally his partner, needs to be involved in selecting the best management option. Partner's attitudes affect the man's uptake of and adherence to ED treatment and long-term management is more successful if the partner is involved (Fisher *et al.* 2005). The Index of Sexual Life (ISL) (Chevret *et al.* 2004) is a validated tool developed to assess women's sexual desire and satisfaction when their partner has ED.

Chevret *et al.* (2004) and Fisher *et al.* (2005) found partners of men with ED had significantly reduced sexual drive, orgasm, satisfaction, and frequency of sex compared with partners of men who did not have ED, and prior to the onset of ED. In addition, partners of men with ED are more likely to have sexual dysfunction or avoid sexual activity. A number of studies demonstrate significant improvements in sexual function, satisfaction, and quality of life for both partners following treatment, especially with PDE-5 medicines (Fisher *et al.* 2005) but discontinuation rates with these medicines appear to range between 10 and 45% (Madduri 2001).

Clinical observations

- Improving sexual functioning can lead to positive changes in the relationship; it can also result in conflict and disharmony, especially if both partners are not involved in management decisions.
- Women have reported acute cystitis when their partners begin using Viagra due to the increased sexual activity, so-called 'honeymoon cystitis'.
- Sex education is part of the management for both men and women, and needs to include:
- Focus an what is achievable and not on improving 'performance.'
- Revision of diabetes knowledge and self-care and the importance of blood glucose and lipid control.
- Knowledge about sex and sexuality and 'normal' sexual functioning.

Sexual counselling

Good communication and trust is essential to sexual relationships. It is also essential to sexual counselling. Health professionals need knowledge of the human sexual response, normal ageing, and the potential effects of diabetes on sexual health, to counsel effectively. Questions about sexual health can be included when taking a nursing history. Including sexual questions in the nursing history can be simple and identify sexual problems that require specific questions to obtain a more detailed history or referral to a sex specialist. Respect and regard for the person and empathetic understanding and privacy are essential (Ross & Channon-Little 1991). The main areas to be covered when taking a sexual history are:

(1) Social aspects
   - Childhood experiences;
   - Marital status;
   - Family relationships;
   - Number and sex of any children;
   - Interests, activities;
   - Job demands/unemployment;
   - Religious and cultural beliefs.
(2) Sexual aspects
   - Sexual knowledge, education, fears, fantasies.
   - Previous sexual experiences.
   - Contraception method.
   - If there is a current problem:
     - Whose problem does the person believe it to be?
     - Description of the problem in the person's own words.
     - Is the partner aware of the problem?
     - Does the problem follow a period of poor diabetic control or illness?
     - Have there been any previous sexual problems?
     - What were those problems?
     - How were they resolved?
(3) Psychological aspects
   - Acceptance of diabetes by self and partner.
   - Body-image concepts.
   - Presence of depression or other psychological problem.
(4) Diabetes knowledge
   - Self-care skills and knowledge of effects of poor diabetic control.

In addition questions to assess the level of communication among partners could include:

- Have you discussed your problem with your partner? Be specific about the problem after the individual explains what the problem is, and address each problem separately if there is more than one problem.
- Do you know what your partner thinks about the problem?
- Is your partner supportive of you seeking treatment to improve the problem?
- Does your partner have any question or concern about the treatment?
- Do you think your partner would come with you to discuss ways to improve your sex life?
- Does your partner have any concerns about his/her sexual function or general health?
- Is there anything else you would like to tell me to help me understand the problem?

The ISI questionnaire could also be useful to understand the woman's perspective.

Measuring sexual health

General measures of well being and psychological are useful indicators of mood and the effects of diabetes on these parameters see Chapter 15. Following are examples of some of the many tools available. Some are old, but most are valid and reliable:

- Derogatis Sexual Function Inventory (DSFI);
- Sexual Concerns Checklist (SCC);

- Sexual Interest Questionnaire (SIQ);
- Harvard Sex Questionnaire;
- Sexual Anxiety Scale (SAS);
- Body Attitude Scale (BAS).

Interpersonal relationships can also be measured if indicated using tools such as:

- Marital Satisfaction Inventory;
- Index of Marital Satisfaction;
- Caring Relationship Inventory;
- Sexual Communication Inventory.

Specific training in sexual counseling might be required to use these tools and interpret the findings and to use the information to help the individual. Some of the tools could be administered in stage one or two of the PLISSIT Model (next section) and forwarded to a sexual health counselor with a referral for specific sexual counselling.

The WHO produced a manual: *Measuring sexual health: conceptual and practical considerations and related indicators* (2010) that contains 17 global indicators governments can use to legislating for sexual health, equality and safety. There are a number of tools clinicians can use as part of sexual counseling, with the PLISST model and as part of diabetes complication screening programmes.

The PLISSIT model

PLISSIT is an acronym for Permission–Limited Information–Specific Suggestions–Intensive Therapy. The model uses four phases to address sexual problems and moves from simple to complex issues. It can be used in a variety of settings and adapted to the individual's needs (Anon 1975). It is an old model but it is still effective and follows education theory, thus the framework can be used to investigate other health issues.

(1) Permission-giving
- Being open and non-judgemental allows the person to discuss their problem by:
  - offering reassurance.
  - accepting the person's concerns;
  - Being open and non-judgemental;
  - establishing acceptable terminology;
  - being truly present in the consultation (Dunning 2013).

Questions about the person's sexuality can be asked or the nurse can respond to sexual questions the person asks. These actions establish that it is appropriate and acceptable to discuss sexual issues.

(2) Provide limited information
- This involves giving limited information and general suggestions that might include practising safe sex, contraceptive advice, diabetes, and sex education and giving:
- accurate, limited information.
- some reference information for home reading.

(3) Specific suggestions
- These are usually made by a qualified sex therapist and often include sensate focus exercises and the squeeze technique for premature ejaculation.
- involve the partner.
- provide sex education.

(4) Intensive therapy

Therapy at this stage requires referral to a sex psychologist/psychiatrist. Techniques include a range of counselling techniques, behavioural therapy and a range of other therapies.

Practice points

(1) The nurse must have adequate knowledge to undertake steps 3 and 4 in the PLISSIT model and know when and how to refer the person appropriately.
(2) Examples of information to give in stage 1 includes information about the differences between men and women, for example, women take longer to become aroused than men and need sufficient quality foreplay to be able to achieve orgasm; the effects of medications, smoking, alcohol, and diabetes on sexual responsiveness.

Role of the nurse

The nurse has an important role in the early identification of sexual problems and helping the individual or couple develop a health plan that includes sexual health. Some sexually transmitted diseases must be notified to government health authorities in some countries. Some specific nursing actions include:

- Being aware of the possibility that a sex problem may exist and allowing people to discuss their concerns.
- Debunking sexual myths, for example, old people who have sex are 'dirty old men/women'.
- Identifying sexual problems and addressing them or referring appropriately.
- Providing relevant care and information during investigative procedures and surgery.
- Medication advice and management.
- Advice about safe sex and contraception. People can be referred to family planning clinics, sexual health clinics, clinics that manage sexually transmitted disease if relevant. There is a great deal of useful information on the Internet but people need to be careful about the sites they access and the information provided. One useful booklet that can be downloaded free is *A Couple's Guide for the Treatment of Erectile Dysfunction* (Endocare 2004) available at www.osbonerecaid.com.
- Advice about monitoring quality sexual health.
- Advice about self-care and when it is safe to resume sex after hospitalisation, for example, after a myocardial infarct or cardiac surgery.
- In care homes for older people and rehabilitation settings, providing an appropriate environment and opportunities for couples to enjoy a sexual relationship might be possible.

References

Adams, M., Collins, V., Dunne, M., deKrester, D.& Holden, C. (2013) Male reproductive health disorders among Aboriginal and Torres Strait Islander men: A hidden problem? *Medical Journal of Australia*, **198** (1), 33–38.

Albright, A. (2012) *Women, Sex and Diabetes*. Diabetes Health Centre http://diabetes.webmed.com/features/women-sex-and-diabetes (accessed December 2012).

Andropause Report (2013) *All About Diabetes, Testosterone Replacement and Andropause*. http//andropausereport.com/all-about-diabetes-testosterone-replacement-and-andropause (accessed January 2012).

Anon (1975) *The Behavioural Treatment of Sexual Problems*. Enabling Systems, Honolulu.

Chevret, M., Jaudinot, E. & Sullivan, K. (2004) Impact of erectile dysfunction (ED) on sexual life of female partners: Assessment with the Index of Sexual Life (ISL) questionnaire. *Journal of Sex and Marital Therapy*, **30**, 157–172.

Copeland, K., Brown, J., Creasman, J. et al. (2012) Diabetes Mellitus and Sexual Function in Middle-Aged and Older Women *Obstetrics & Gynecology* **120** (2), 331–340.

Dean, J., Rubio-Aurioles, E., McCabe, M. et al. (2008) Integrating partners into erectile dysfunction treatment: Improving the sexual experience for the couple. *International Journal of Clinical Practice*, **62** (1), 127–133.

Dunning, P. (1994) Having diabetes: Young adult's perspectives. *The Diabetes Educator*, **21** (1), 58–65.

Dunning, T. (2013) The teacher: Moving from good to exceptional, in *Diabetes Education: Art, Science and Evidence*, Dunning, T. (ed.), Wiley Blackwell, Chichester UK pp. 62–77.

Endocare (2004) *A Couple's Guide for the Treatment of Erectile Dysfunction* (available at www.osbonerecaid.com).

Fisher, W., Rosen, R. & Mollen, M. (2005) Improving the sexual quality of life of couples affected by erectile dysfunction: A double blind, randomized, placebo controlled trial of vardenafil. *Journal of Sex Medicine*, **2**, 699–708.

Kaplan, H. (1979) *Making Sense of Sex*. Simon & Schuster, New York.

Krane, R. (1991) Commentary on erectile dysfunction. *Diabetes Spectrum*, **4** (1), 29–30.

Leedom, L., Feldman, M., Procci, W. & Zeidler, A. (1991) Severity of sexual dysfunction and depression in diabetic women. *Journal of Diabetic Complications*, **5** (1), 38–41.

Madduri, S. (2001) After 2 years, did Viagra live up to its expectations? *Mo Medicine*, **98**, 243–245.

Masters, W. & Johnson, V. (1970) *Human Sexual Inadequacy*. Little Brown Company, Boston.

Ross, M. & Channon-Little, L. (1991) *Discussing Sexuality. A Guide for Health Practitioners*. MacLennan & Pretty, Sydney.

Schriener-Engel, P., Schiavi, P., Vietorisz, D. & Smith, H. (1991) The differential impact of diabetes type on female sexuality. *Diabetes Spectrum*, **4** (1), 16–20.

Trutnovsky, G., Law, C., Simpson, J. & Mindel, A. (2001) Use of complementary therapies in a sexual health clinic setting. *International Journal of STD and AIDS*, **12** (5), 307–309.

WHO (2010) Measuring sexual health: Conceptual and practical considerations and related indicators. WHO, Geneva.

Further reading

Dunning, P. (1993) Sexuality and women with diabetes. *Patient Education and Counselling*, **21**, 5–14.

ED-Alliance Group (2000) Erectile Dysfunction Alliance Guidelines. *Practical Diabetes International*, **17** (5), 139–140.

Heulfelder, A. (2012) *Testosterone deficient diabetic men benefit form testosterone replacement*. Presented at the Endocrine Society 89th annual meeting, June 5th in Toronto. (Abstract number OR55.5).

House, W. & Pendelton, L. (1986) Sexual dysfunction in diabetics. *Postgraduate Medicine*, **79**, 227–235.

Chapter 12
Diabetes in Older People

Key points

- An holistic proactive and integrated approach is needed to achieve effective diabetes management, manage age- and diabetes-related health risks and ensure management strategies are appropriate for the individual.
- Increasing age is associated with insulin resistance that predisposes older people to diabetes.
- Diabetes is common in people over 65. Most have Type 2 diabetes but Type 1 and LADA also occur in older people.
- Older people rarely present with the textbook symptoms of hyperglycaemia, the onset of diabetes is often insidious and the non-specific symptoms are often mistaken for advancing age or other conditions.
- Long-term complications are often present at diagnosis and often coexist with other functional defects and comorbidities.
- The individual should be encouraged to maintain independent self-care within their capabilities for as long as possible, but carer assistance is often needed, especially during illnesses.
- There is limited evidence for metabolic targets in older people. Targets must be appropriate to the individual and limit the risk of adverse events such as hypoglycaemia, hyperglycaemia, and falls.
- Pharmacovigilance is essential because age-related changes affect medicine absorption, distribution, metabolism and elimination leading to serious adverse events. Being hospitalised can lead to a decline in physical and cognitive functioning in older people.
- Where relevant, carers' well-being needs to be considered.

Care of People with Diabetes: A Manual of Nursing Practice, Fourth Edition. Trisha Dunning.
© 2014 John Wiley & Sons, Ltd. Published 2014 by John Wiley & Sons, Ltd.

Rationale

People over age 65 are usually regarded as old. Older people with diabetes are not a heterogeneous group. Some are healthy and active; others are frail and have multiple health problems. Thus, care needs can differ among older individuals of the same age. Clinically relevant categories of older people that can help determine diabetes management needs are:

- Healthy older people who are independent and self-caring.
- Older people who manage most activities of daily living independently but require some assistance.
- Frail older people whose care needs to be considered on an individual basis depending on their functional (physical and mental) status.
- Older people at the end of life.

Managing diabetes in older people is a complex and increasingly important aspect of nursing care as the population ages and because the incidence and prevalence of diabetes increases with increasing age. Diabetes manifests differently in older people and their healthcare needs are different from younger people. Likewise, diabetes and its complications are likely to adversely affect many activities of daily living including, socialising and driving as well as physical and mental functioning, all of which affect self-care ability, independence and psychological well-being.

Evidence suggests older people with diabetes use more primary care services than older people without diabetes and frequently require hospital care and/or care in aged care facilities (Sinclair 2011). Optimal management could reduce the high cost of care and help older people with diabetes live more fulfilling lives.

Introduction

The ageing process refers to a progressive deterioration of bodily functions over the lifespan (US National Institute of Health (NIH) undated) whose characteristics are destructive, progressive, intrinsically determined and universal. Ageing occurs at different rates among individuals and among individual organs and tissues in the body. There are many theories, but no consensus, about what causes ageing. The two major schools of thought are: (1) ageing is programmed and (2) ageing is random, each accompanied by specific theories (see Table 12.1). These theories give rise to the question: Can ageing be cured (anti-ageing research) or should it be managed better to maintain wellness for longer with a short decline to death because aging is a natural process? Strategies to maintain wellness include:

- Counselling and supporting the individual to reduce risk factors that accelerate aging such as smoking, obesity, hypertension, and diabetes.
- Improving micronutrient deficiencies and using antioxidant supplements based on the Ames hypothesis that an adaptive triage process occurs in the body when micronutrients are scarce that favours short-term survival over long-term and health-energy pathways are favoured over DNA repair (Ames 2006).
- Anti-ageing strategies such as:
  - optimal nutrition that includes adequate calories essential amino acids, fats and micronutrients

Table 12.1 Theories of ageing. Currently there is no general agreement about the causes of ageing but most experts favour cellular damage theories. These seem to apply to uncontrolled diabetes where similar theories have been proposed for the development of diabetes complications. See Chapter 8.

Programmed theories *Ageing is a designed process (built in obsolescence)*	Damage theories *Ageing is due to accumulated molecular damage especially to DNA and proteins that causes cell, organ, and system dysfunction*
Disposable soma Organisms exist to reproduce and then die	Systematic damage theories: Immune system failure Failure of neuroendocrine regulation Failure to adapt
Antagonistic pleiotropy Genes that are essential and advantageous in young people cause damage in older people Developmental programming Ageing is regulated by genes and damage only begins to occur after development is complete Neuroendocrine programming Biological clock regulated by the hypothalamus. Hormone production eventually diminishes and causes changes associated with ageing Rate of living (live fast die young) Every person has a fixed metabolic potential that can be affected by lifestyle, also known as metabolic burnout Genetic programming Ageing is preprogrammed in genes that might affect germ cell function, cell division, and cell death	Cellular damage theories caused by free radical damage by reactive oxygen species (ROS), hyperglycaemia causing advanced glycated end products (AGE) and binding of AGE receptors (RAGE) to AGE resulting in oxidative and inflammatory effects (accelerated in diabetes), and/or chronic inflammation caused by inflammatory cytokines and eicosanoids, which with infection can induce oxidant-generating enzymes such as NADPH oxidase and nitric oxide synthase that produce ROS and reactive nitrogen species (RNS) that react with each other to form more potent reactive species that damage DNA and contribute to diseases such as cancer by activating oncogenes and/or suppressing tumour suppressor proteins Damage to cell membranes Somatic mutations Failure of repair processes

- anti-ageing nutrient supplements to reduce inflammation and oxidative stress such as SOD, CQ-$_{10}$, Gingko, Ginseng, Brahmi
- hormones such as melatonin
- medicines to improve insulin sensitivity, vasodilators, and mind stimulants
- keeping physically active
- keeping mentally active e.g. brain training.
- Under research: gene therapy, therapeutic cloning, cell therapy, nanotechnology (Grossman 2005).

Advancing age is associated with glucose intolerance, changes in renal function which alter medicine pharmacodynamics and pharmacokinetics, reduced sense of smell, hearing, sight, mobility, reduced muscle mass, and changed cognitive functioning, all of which increase the individual's vulnerability to ill health. Significantly, chronological age is not the most important factor to consider when deciding management options. The functional status and biological age are more important determinants of care (National Health and Medical Research Council (NHMRC) 2009). Some of the particular problems encountered in older people are shown in Table 12.2. It is important to realise that older people in hospital or living in residential aged care facilities do not represent the majority of older individuals living in the community (Australian Institute of Health and Welfare (AIHW) 2002).

Table 12.2 Particular problems encountered in older people with diabetes and the resultant risks associated with the problem. Individuals are likely to have more than one of these conditions and or other geriatric syndromes. Most of these conditions affect activities of daily living and extended activities of daily living. They represent a cumulative health burden and almost all represent a falls risk and many contribute to or complicate delirium and depression and increase the risk of driving accidents.

Problem	Associated risk
Hyperglycaemia leading to:	Constipation Postural hypotension Dehydration and electrolyte imbalance Polyuria and nocturia, which may present as urinary incontinence Hyperosmolar coma and ketoacidosis Impaired cognition Thrombosis Infection, for example, UTI Impaired wound healing Postural hypotension Decreased pain threshold Exacerbated neuropathic pain Lowered mood, lethargy, compromised self-care Driving deficits Falls
Chewing problems and swallowing difficulties	Hypoglycaemia Nutritional deficiencies: • Impaired immune response • Infection risk • Decreased plasma protein Impaired wound healing: • Higher fat intake • Dehydration • Muscle wasting and reduced strength in the lower limbs, which affect ADLs • Increased risk of systemic diseases such as cancer and cardiovascular diseases • Driving deficits • Difficulty swallowing medicines Inappropriate fluid and nutrition replacement at end of life that actually increases risks Energy deficits Increased morbidity and mortality Falls
Cerebral insufficiency	Stroke Non-recognition of hypoglycaemia Trauma Impaired cognition TIAs being confused with hypoglycaemia Increased prevalence of vascular dementia and Alzheimer's disease and other dementias Falls Driving deficits
Cardiac insufficiency	Myocardial infarction Confusion Poor wound healing Poor peripheral circulation Foot ulcers Driving deficits Falls

Table 12.2 Continued.

Problem	Associated risk
Autonomic neuropathy	Postural hypotension
	Gustatory sweating
	Urinary tract infections and incontinence
	Unrecognised hypoglycaemia
	Silent myocardial infarction
	Decreased/delayed food and medicine absorption and glycaemic variability if the gastrointestinal tract is affected
	Poor nutrition
	Infections, pain
	Decreased motor skills
	Erectile dysfunction
	Driving deficits
	Falls
Peripheral insufficiency	Trauma
	Foot/leg ulcers
	Claudication
	Falls
Peripheral neuropathy	Unstable gait
	Foot ulcers
	Depression
	Driving deficits
	Falls
Other neuropathies such as Bell's palsy	Reduced self-care
	Loss of independence
	Body image changes
Visual impairment	Self-care deficits
Changed colour perception (red, blue, green, violet)	Depression
	Loss of independence
	Social isolation
	Education difficulties with types of materials used and, differentiating medications
	Driving deficits
Skin atrophy	Pressure ulcers, skin tears
	Infection
	Progression of acute wounds to chronic wounds
	Stress and depression
	Oedema
Communication problems	Misunderstanding
	Confusion
	Inaccurate self-care
	Stress
	Social isolation
Stress and depression	Inadequate self-care
	Hypertension
	Hyperglycaemia

(Continued)

Table 12.2 Continued.

Problem	Associated risk
	Hypoglycaemia
	Impacts on wound healing
	Driving deficits
	Suicide risk
	Falls
Renal disease associated with diabetes and normal age-related renal changes	Decreased medicine clearance and prolonged activity
	End-stage renal disease requiring dialysis
	Difficulty interpreting investigative blood tests
	Malnutrition
	Reduced choice of GLM
	Dehydration
	Hyperosmolar coma
	Lactic acidosis
	Driving deficits
	Falls
Failure to recognise thirst (normal ageing process)	Dehydration
	Hyperglycaemia
	Confusion
	Driving deficits
	Falls
Cognitive impairment	Self-care deficits
	Education difficulties
	Reduced quality of life
	Falls
	Driving deficits
Musculoskeletal disorders such as Dupytren's contracture, cherioarthropathy, flexor tenosynovitis, carpal tunnel syndrome	Difficulty performing activities of daily living
	Pain and discomfort
	Driving deficits
	Falls

The Department of Health Victoria (2013) identified several specific issues that need to be addressed to maintain functional status:

(1) optimising nutrition;
(2) increasing functional mobility;
(3) preserving skin integrity;
(4) reducing incontinence;
(5) avoiding and reducing the incidence of falls;
(6) detecting and managing delirium and dementia;
(7) reducing medicine-related risks and maximising the benefits;
(8) supporting and maintaining self-care;
(9) detecting and managing depression.

DHS (2003) also noted the need to ensure relevant services are available and that they function optimally and to consider the health and well-being of carers. An early NHMRC series on clinical care of older people (number 3, 1994) that focused on reducing hospital admissions and preventing complications in hospital encompassed most of these issues and highlighted the need for multidisciplinary health professional care. In particular, The NHMRC emphasised the atypical presentation of many illnesses in older people, including diabetes. More recent guidelines such as ADA (2013) and ADS (2012) and position statements (Sinclair *et al.* 2012) make similar recommendations about individualising management targets.

Many illnesses present with atypical symptoms, which can delay appropriate diagnosis and management and result in death or significant morbidities and geriatric syndromes including:

- failure to thrive;
- immobility;
- postural instability;
- incontinence;
- confusion and delirium;
- depression;
- fatigue and lethargy;
- weight loss;
- undetected hyperglycaemia (IGT) can be present in non-diabetic older people and diabetes triggered by an intercurrent illness, a diabetes complication or emotional stress, and present as:
  - constipation
  - dehydration
  - postural hypotension
  - confusion
  - polyuria or urinary incontinence
  - infections such as UTI and URTI.

Older people with diabetes usually have multiple health problems, some of which are the result of diabetes-related complications and are present at diagnosis in >20% of people (NHMRC 1992). Thus, actively screening older people for diabetes and its complications in hospital and care facilities is warranted. Bayliss *et al.* (2007) found an average of 8.7 chronic diseases present per person in a cross-sectional survey of people aged >65 years. Compared with newly diagnosed non-diabetics, older people have a 9% mortality rate, 40% more lower leg complications (claudication, cellulitis), double the risk of cardiovascular disease including heart failure, double the risk of end-stage renal disease, and are 60% more likely to have vision problems (Kirkman *et al.* 2012). They are also at great risk of falling, especially in hospital.

Managing diabetes, its complications, and other comorbid diseases requires multiple medicines, and often several doses per medicine per day. Many commonly used laboratory tests have lower specificity and sensitivity in older people, which can further complicate the clinical picture clinical decision-making. For example, serum creatinine may not detect renal impairment especially in normal weight or underweight individuals (Giannelli *et al.* (2007) and contraindicated medicines may not be stopped.

Fasting blood glucose may not be an appropriate screening test for older people, even though blood glucose levels increase with age. Loss of the first phase insulin response means older people with normal fasting glucose can have high post prandial blood glucose levels that require treatment (Abdo & Flack 2012). Likewise, HbA_{1c} <7% increases the risk of hypoglycaemia and its consequences. HbA_{1c} >10% has significant physiological effects as well as effects on neutrophil function and wound healing (Shekelle & Vijan 2007). Thus, the risks and benefits for the individual need to be considered when interpreting clinical assessment and laboratory data.

Evidence for ideal HbA_{1c} targets in older people is limited, apart from the UKPDS (1998), which focused on preventing long-term complications rather than safety and maximising functioning. The Australian Diabetes Educators Association (ADEA) (2003) proposed targets based on a systematic review; however, the ADEA targets were not intended for older people in aged care facilities. Brown *et al.* (2003) suggested $HbA_{1c} < 7\%$ for most older people; and <8% in frail older people because preventing the short-term consequences of hypo- and hyperglycaemia and their associated symptoms and risks to safety and quality of life, might be more important than preventing long-term complications. Most diabetes-related guidelines published in the last four years recommend HbA_{1c} 7–7.5% (53–58 mmol/mol) in general but stress the need to individualise glycaemic targets, and recommend $HbA_{1c} \sim 8\%$ in frail older people (Sinclair et al. 2012, Australian Diabetes Society (ADS) 2012; American Diabetes Association 2013). However, management also depends on the individual's functional status, risk profile and quality of life.

Interestingly, despite the association among obesity and morbidity and mortality (Hu *et al.* 2004; Chen *et al.* 2008; Masters *et al.* 2013) being overweight is associated with longer life expectancy in men and women >80 years and underweight with shorter life expectancy, even when other comorbidities are present (Takata *et al.* 2007). Weight loss is associated with total mortality in older people, independently of low body weight (Keller *et al.* 2004). These findings suggest recommending older overweight people lose weight may actually put them at risk.

Determining functional status

Functional ability refers to an individual's ability to perform activities of daily living (ADL). There are two main types of ADL: physical (PADL) that encompasses essential daily activities such as bathing and dressing; and instrumental (IADL), which enable the individual to live independently in society and are more complex (Kock & Garratt 2001). IADL assessment must be based on activities relevant to the individual and take account of their physical surroundings, culture, and interests. For example, assessing an older person when they are in hospital and their blood glucose levels are in the optimal range may not accurately reflect their ADL and adverse event risk level at home (Dunning & Alford 1993). Significantly, older people with diabetes have more functional impairment than age- and gender-matched controls in the same community (Sinclair et al. 2008) as well as cognitive impairment that affects self-care capacity.

Older people in hospital and care facilities are a vulnerable group and the latter often receive suboptimal care (Kirkland 2000). Sinclair *et al.* (1997) found 40% of residents in aged care facilities were on long-acting sulphonylureas: fewer than 1 in 10 had any regular diabetes follow-up, they had more hospital admissions than people without diabetes, stayed in hospital longer and had more complications. In addition, staff and resident knowledge about diabetes was deficient. Likewise, functional decline occurs in 30–50% of older people during hospitalisation and ~30% >70 years return home with ADL deficits (Royal Melbourne Hospital 2002). Functional decline is associated with long duration of hospitalisation and manifests gradually as malnutrition, reduced mobility, compromised skin integrity, incontinence, falls, delirium, depression, geriatric syndromes and inadequate self-care.

The degree of disability is likely to change over time, sometimes rapidly, and during illness, and affect the amount of assistance the individual needs, either on a temporary basis or in the longer term. Changing circumstances often have financial implications for the individual and the health system. Table 12.3 suggests some key questions that can help decide the level of assistance needed and appropriate management. In addition, geomaps and ecomaps can provide a great deal of information about the individual's

Table 12.3 Key issues that need to be considered when assessing disability in older people with diabetes. Repeat measures may be needed especially during acute illnesses when the physical and mental condition can change rapidly. These issues should be considered as part of the standard diabetes complication screening process. (Dunning T [2005]).

Questions	Implications
(1) What activities are limited and to what degree?	A precise description of the disability is important in order to plan appropriate medical and nursing care and evaluate outcomes.
(2) Which disease processes are causing the disability?	Attributing disability to 'old age' is not an appropriate diagnosis. Common causes of disability include arthritis, cardiovascular disease, respiratory disease, stroke and visual impairment. One or more of these comorbidities often coexist with diabetes. Polypharmacy is likely. In some cases the medicine of choice for some comorbidities increases blood glucose levels.
(3) What is the person's mental state? Various assessment tools are used to assess mental status, for example the Mini-Mental, however their limitations need to be considered.	Evidence of memory loss, disorientation, confused behaviour and personality change may indicate diseases of the brain, dementia states or metabolic changes such as high or low blood glucose levels that impair mental processing. Consideration should also be given to the presence of anxiety, depression and the individual's general mental approach to life (positive or pessimistic) and hearing deficits.
(4) What is the person's social situation? See Figure 2.1	Disability implies dependence on others. It is important to identify the services and people likely to be able to support the individual if they do require help. In addition, it is important to ensure the person who takes on the care is supported and their personal health and well-being considered preventing stress, sleep disturbance and ill health in the carer, especially if they are also old.

social network and relationships; see Chapter 2. Annual diabetes complication screening should encompass screening for hypo- and hyperglycaemia risk, depression, comorbidities, falls risk, incontinence, pain and memory deficits, degree of frailty, functional status including driving ability, and a structured medicines review. The current Australian complication review (annual cycle of care in general practice) does not encompass these issues and needs to be used in conjunction with other screening tools when assessing older people.

Determining the frailty level (frailty index FI) might help identify older people likely to suffer adverse health effects (Kulminski *et al.* 2007). Frailty is a consequence of declining physical reserve and altered functioning in multiple physiological systems, which make the individual vulnerable to physical and mental stressors (Bortz 2002; Fried *et al.* 2004). Several definitions of frailty exist including the following:

> *The frailty state can be described using a cumulative index of health and well being deficiencies that is assessable for each individual ... the fraction of deficits in a list of items that measure health and well being* [constitutes the frailty index (FI)]
> (Kulminski *et al.* 2007)

A number of methods of estimating the FI have been proposed. The most useful enable clinicians to use health information already being collected to predict older people at risk of adverse health outcomes and proactively plan preventative care. Frailty could be calculated for older people with diabetes as part of the annual complication screening process and be monitored proactively and prospectively.

Geriatric syndromes

The term 'geriatric syndromes' refers to commonly occurring comorbidities in older people that makes managing diabetes, and the associated syndromes, very complex and challenging. The American Geriatrics Society (2012) described six commonly occurring geriatric syndromes:

- polypharmacy; see Chapter 5;
- depression (Chapter 15 and this chapter);
- cognitive impairment;
- urinary incontinence;
- injurious falls;
- pain.

Other authors include delirium, renal disease, cardiovascular disease, infections and frailty. As indicated, all of the coexisting comorbidities need to be identified and adequately treated as part of individuaised care.

Cognitive functioning

Non-pathological age-related cognitive changes are a normal part of aging, however pronounced, severe cognitive changes may reflect pathological changes such as Alzheimer's disease. However, normal age-related cognitive changes can impair usual functioning such as managing finances, diabetes self-management including medicine self-management, remembering information and medical appointments (Vance 2012). Some researchers suggest cognitive reserve acts as a neurological reservoir that can sustain cognitive functioning during illness, substance abuse, depression and underlying metabolic abnormalities associated with diabetes (Carmichael *et al.* 2010).

Cognitive reserve refers to the neuronal connections that organise, store and transmit information. The strength of the neuronal connections affects the brain's ability to cope with damage before cognitive function is disrupted (Vance *et al.* 2012). Neuronal connections need to be used to remain efficient. Some experts recommend various 'brain training' activities to maintain/enhance neuronal reserve; however, cognitive reserve is difficult to measure and different factors affect cognitive reserve. Table 12.4 depicts some of the positive and negative factors that affect cognitive reserve.

Cognitive decline in older people with diabetes is multifactorial due to advancing age and vascular dementia but not other forms of dementia (Allen *et al.* 2004), hyperglycaemia (Morley & Flood 1990), and hypoglycaemia, and increasing duration of diabetes. Large community studies suggest older people with diabetes have worse cognitive functioning than non-diabetics (Croxon *et al.* 2000; Gregg *et al.* 2000; Logroscino *et al.* 2004), and the decline is more rapid in those with diabetes (Biessels *et al.* 200 6). The Framingham Study suggests hypertension and diabetes are independent risk factors for poor performance on memory and visual organisation tests (Elias *et al.* 2005). In contrast, Asiakopoulou *et al.* (2002) demonstrated minimal effects on verbal and logical memory when blood glucose control is optimal.

Older people with dementia have more hospital admissions, comorbidities and mortality than those without dementia (Zuliani 2012). People with dementia in Zuliani's study (50 000 admissions and data collected over 6 years) had high rates of cardiovascular disease, pneumonia and hip fractures. Dementia was associated with secondary diagnoses such as delirium, immobility, dehydration and pressure ulcers. These findings might be expected, but they could also suggest some admissions could be prevented by optimal assessment and proactive, preventative care planning.

Table 12.4 Positive and negative factors that affect cognitive reserve. Good cognitive reserve protects against age-related cognitive changes. The theory supports the need for and importance of proactive, lifelong optimal health-related self-care and regular comprehensive physical, spiritual and mental assessments.

Factors that contribute to positive neuroplasticity and enhance cognitive reserve	Factors that contribute to negative neuroplasticity and reduce cognitive reserve
Mental stimulation and cognitive-enhancing activates (use it or lose it)	Low education and health literacy level. Low health literacy predicts mortality (Bostock & Steptoe 2012) and compromise participation in activities that enhance cognition
Positive thinking, spirituality and resilience	Mood disorders including depression, which are associated with negative thinking and compromised resilience
Healthy diet	Inadequate nutrition (similarly muscle reserve protects older people from sarcopenia)
Optimal health status.	Health status e.g. cardiovascular risk factors are associated with faster cognitive decline in older people (Dregan et al. 2012) and there is an association between higher Framingham risk score and worse cognitive functioning (Kaffashian *et al.* 2011).
Regular physical activity	Inactivity
Using few medicines and avoiding medicines and addictive substances that affect cognition	Some prescribed medicines as well as alcohol and drug abuse and smoking
Social engagement and stimulation	Social isolation

During acute illnesses it is important to differentiate cognitive decline from hypoglycaemia, hyperglycaemia, and hyperosmolar states, delirium, MI, and other causes. Delirium is often not diagnosed and is associated with:

- prolonged hospitalisation, poor outcomes and admission to aged care facilities;
- functional declin;
- increased use of chemical and other restraints that increase the falls risk and may increase delirium;
- presence of infection, which can precipitate hyperosmolar states;
- multiple comorbidities (geriatric syndromes);
- severe illness;
- dehydration, which can precipitate hyperosmolar states and may lead to a diagnosis of diabetes in undiagnosed at risk individuals; see Chapter 7;
- alcohol abuse;
- falls and fractures;
- prescribed psychotropic medications.

Delirium, but not the severity, can be distinguished from non-reversible cognitive impairment using the Confusion Assessment Method (CAM) (Waszynski 2004); also see Table 12.5. The CAM has concurrent validity with the MMSE but has not been tested in clinical settings and is associated with a 10% false-positive rate. The key aspects of the CAM are shown in the following list. A diagnosis of delirium is made if 1 and 2 and either 3 or 4 are present:

(1) acute onset and fluctuating course during the day;
(2) inattention such as being easily distracted and finding it difficult to recall what was said last;
(3) disorganised thinking and unpredictable switching from topic-to-topic;
(4) altered consciousness (Inouye *et al.* 1990; Waszynski 2004).

Table 12.5 Some of the presenting feature of dementia, delirium and depression.

Parameter	Dementia	Delirium	Depression
Onset	Usually slow and progressive occurring over years	Usually occurs over hours or days	May be sudden and often occurs during significant life transitions such as death of a loved one and admission into an aged care home. Changes persist for at least two weeks.
Course	Symptoms are irreversible and gradually progress over time	The course is usually short and cognitive changes may fluctuate over the day and may be worse at night. Once the underlying cause/s is/are identified and treated, symptoms usually abate to the individual's predelirium state	Usually worse in the morning but could be seasonal (Chapter 15) Usually improves with treatment (non-medicine options and medicines as a last resort)
Duration	Depends on the type of dementia present and varies from months to several years	Usually less than four weeks	Variable from weeks to years
Cognition (1) Alertness (2) Attention span (3) Thinking	Generally alert Usually normal in the early stages Often have difficulty finding words and remembering and recalling people, and events. Difficulty learning new information. May wander, become agitated, especially in the afternoon (Sundowner's syndrome) or withdrawn and may have coexisting depression Multiple cognitive deficits may be present	Varies from lethargic to hyperactive. Depends on the degree of delirium. Have difficulty organising thoughts Several types of delirium are described: • Hyperactive (agitation, restlessness, hallucinations) • Hypoactive (sleepy, difficult to rouse) • Mixed (combination of hyper- and hypoactive symptoms).	Normal but may be apathetic. Depends on interest and severity of the depression. Thinking is usually intact but can be disordered. Disinterest in activities and usual activities Withdrawn Appetite often changes
Mood	May be associated with depression	Mood changes: may be angry, afraid, tearful	

Table 12.5 Continued

Parameter	Dementia	Delirium	Depression
Commonly used screening and diagnostic tools *	• Mini-Mental Status Exam (Folstein) • Clock Drawing Test. • Mini-Co Dementia Screen. • Cohen-Mansfield Agitation Inventory (CMAI) if behavioural issues are present.	• Confusion Assessment Method (CAM) • IWATCH DEATH (Infections, **W**ithdrawal, **A**cute metabolic, **T**oxins, drugs **C**NS pathology, **H**ypoxia, **D**eficiencies, **E**ndocrine, **A**cute vascular, **T**rauma, **H**eavy metals	• Geriatric Depression Scale (GDS) and the GDS Short Form • Cornell Scale for Depression • Patient Health Questionnaire (PHQ) and PHQ-2. • Whooley Depression Screen. • SIG ECAPS (DSM-1 V Criteria
Laboratory investigations	TSH, electrolytes, Ca Blood glucose and ketones	Na, K+, Na, Ca, Urea and electrolytes, creatinine, liver function tests, Hb, white cell count (which can be elevated in hyperglycaemia without indicating infection) Blood glucose and ketones Oxygen saturation, blood gasses, urinalysis and culture Alcohol/drug screen Chest X-ray	TSH, Vitamin B12, folate, Ferritin, Iron, K+, Hb, ESR, Albumin, Full blood count

*See Chapter 15 for commonly used diabetes-specific tools to identify diabetes-related distress.

Recognising cognitive decline

The following strategies can slow cognitive decline and enhance mental health:

- Determine and monitor cognitive status as part of diabetes complication screening programmes. For example, incorporate ADL assessment such as Barthel Index and the 'Get up and Go' test; and cognitive assessment such as Mini-Mental State Examination (MMSE), the Clock test and screen for depression using tools such as the Geriatric Depression Score (Sinclair 2011).
- Regularly screen for diabetes-related complications that can impair cognitive function such as cardiovascular disease (American Diabetes Association 2013).
- Establish individuals' risk of low cognitive reserve, delirium and depression and the presence of geriatric syndromes.
- Make an accurate diagnosis, which might require referral to a geriatrician and/or psychiatrist. Making an accurate diagnosis includes differentiating between the '3Ds' dementia, delirium and depression. Be aware that hypoglycaemic symptoms in older people are predominantly neurological and can be mistaken for delirium.
- Develop an appropriate care plan to manage the condition, which might include behavioural or psychosocial interventions and 'brain training'. Involve older people in group diabetes education programmes and diabetes self-care activities to the level of their ability, which can improve glycaemic control (Beverly *et al.* 2012). In aged care homes consider how the environment could affect mental health and well-being positively or negatively, including disrupting sleep.
- Managing diabetes by individualising management targets and medicine use and avoiding polypharmacy when possible.
- Undertake a comprehensive medicine review and, where possible, stop medicines that affect cognitive functioning. These include medicines prescribed to manage 'behaiours of concern' and sliding scales of insulin. For example, refer to the Beers criteria (American Geriatrics Society 2012). Consider medicine contraindications and interactions and ask about herbal medicine use.
- Manage pain.

Poor blood glucose control is associated with reduced cognitive functioning and problem-solving and planning skills. Cognition sometimes improves when the blood glucose pattern improves (Gradman *et al.* 1993). Screening for cognitive impairment can be incorporated into the diabetes management plan using screening tools such as the Mini Mental State Examination (MMSE) and the results used to plan diabetes education strategies (Sinclair 1995).

Dehydration

Fluid balance disturbances are common in older people largely as a result of changes in body water composition, declining renal function, and reduced thirst perception. Dehydration is common in community dwelling older people (Warren *et al.* 1994) occurring in ~6.7% of those >65 years in hospital and is the principal diagnosis in 1.4% (Warren *et al.* 1994). Dehydration is present in 50% of residents in aged care facilities with a febrile illness who are often referred to hospital due to dehydration (Bourdel-Marchasson *et al.* 2004). Dehydration should be preventable in hospital and aged care facilities. Management guidelines should encompass strategies to do so considering the following information.

Dehydration is associated with hyperglycaemia and DKA and HHS (see Chapter 7), thromboembolism, infections, renal calculi, falls and constipation, and causes up to

50% mortality if it is not adequately managed (Wilson & Morley 2003), and poor mental functioning (Wilson & Morley. 2003; Faes *et al.* 2007). Early diagnosis is difficult because of the atypical presentation in older people and because there is no absolute definition of dehydration (Weinberg *et al.* 1995). A commonly used definition is:

> … a clinically relevant decrease of an individual's optimal Total Body Water (TBW) amount and may occur with or without loss of electrolytes.

> (Faes *et al.* 2007)

Thus, the degree of dehydration depends on the relative rather than the actual total intracellular and extracellular water loss. People with low body weight show signs of dehydration after losing small amounts of water. Significantly, ~25% of older people drink <1 litre of fluid per day, especially those over 85 (Volkert *et al.* 2005). Risk factors for dehydration include:

- age over 85 years;
- female;
- having ≥ chronic diseases;
- using ≥5 medicines;
- medicine-related factors such as high protein oral or enteral feeds, laxatives, antidepressants, and diuretics;
- fasting for surgery or investigative procedures;
- fluid loss such as diarrhoea, vomiting, hyperglycaemia;
- being confined to bed/chair;
- poor mobility including manual dexterity;
- poor eye-hand coordination;
- communication difficulties;
- inability to feed themselves;
- social isolation;
- hot weather;
- having Alzheimer's disease and other cognitive disturbances (Lavizzo-Mourey *et al.* 1988).

The diagnosis is made on clinical signs such as recent weight loss >3% body weight, presence of an intercurrent illness, dry mucous membranes, coated tongue, sunken eyes, confusion, hypotension, muscle weakness in the upper body, and falls. Laboratory investigations such as serum osmolality, creatinine, blood urea nitrogen (BUN), BUN/ creatinine ratio, and electrolytes as well as urine pH and output are useful. Three forms of dehydration occur:

- hypertonic: sodium >150 mmol/L or serum osmolality >300 mosmol/L;
- isotonic dehydration occurs when water and electrolyte loss are balanced, for example, diarrhoea and vomiting;
- hypotonic dehydration results when electrolyte loss is greater than water loss, for example, overuse of diuretics.

The prevalence of the isotonic and hypotonic dehydration has not been studied systematically and may be under-recognised. Having a high level of suspicion and care strategies to ensure optimal fluid intake such as prompting older people to drink are important preventative measures. Specific treatment depends on the clinical assessment and may include IV fluid replacement, preventing venous stasis, pressure ulcers and falls, as well as managing the underlying cause, and uncontrolled hyperglycaemia. Care must be taken not to over-hydrate the individual and cause cerebral oedema or water intoxication.

Depression and older people with diabetes

Given the increasing prevalence of diabetes in older people, the fact that depression is a risk factor for diabetes, and the 2-fold increased risk of depression in people with diabetes (Bogner *et al.* 2007), it is likely that many older people have undetected diabetes as well as undetected depression, which is a concern given that depression in older people is treatable in 65–75% of people (Ragan & Kane 2010). Undiagnosed depression contributes to physical and mental functional impairment and is a known risk factor for suicide (Cahoon 2012). Older people with depression require higher levels of informal care, even after adjusting for other comorbidities, and place a significant burden on family caregivers (Langa 2004). Managing depression reduces depression-related caregiver burden (Martire 2010)

Depression frequently precedes and may be the factor that leads to admission to an aged care facility. Depression may be due to grief over loss of functional and self-care ability and independence (Fleming 2002) and is significantly correlated with quality of life (Goldney *et al.* 2004). Depression is often associated with diabetes-related complications such as cardiovascular disease (Fenton & Stover 2006; Cahoon 2012), diabetes (Verma 2010), chronic pain, and unhealthy diet. Depression is more likely to be recurrent in older people (Cluning 2001) and leads to inadequate self-care, unstable blood glucose patterns, and affects cognitive functioning. Comorbidities need to comprehensively evaluated because when one comorbidity worsens, others also worsen, and if all comorbidities are not detected then treatment could be ineffective (Cahoon 2012). Treating depression in older people reduces mortality by 50% (Bogner *et al.* 2007).

Commonly used depression screening tools are shown in Table 12.5. Some clinical indicators of depression in older people are:

- constantly talking about physical symptoms and believing they have a serious illness (Cluning, 2001);
- grief over loss and lost opportunities, abilities, and self-determination;
- withdrawing from communal activities;
- experiencing chronic pain;
- having had a stroke or cardiovascular event;
- not receiving any visitors at least once a week in hospital and aged care facilities;
- difficulty establishing relationships with staff and other aged care residents in the first four weeks after admission.

Depression management is discussed in Chapter 15. When possible, non-pharmacological options should be used first.

Dementia

The prevalence of dementia increases with age and ranges from 63% to 81% (Zimmerman *et al.* 2007). Approximately one in four Australians over age 85 have dementia (Gray *et al.* 2002). There are two main forms of dementia: Alzheimer's disease (AD) accounting for 70% of known dementias and Vascular Dementia (VD) accounting for the remaining 20%. Both AD and VD are present in ~20% of people especially those with diabetes (Stewart & Liolitsa, 1999). The association between diabetes and dementia may be due to:

- cardiovascular disease: TIAs and stroke that can cause multifocal brain damage;
- hypoglycaemia, especially if it is frequent and recurrent, which may cause permanent neuronal destruction;
- persistent hyperglycaemia increases protein glycosylation and contributes to the development of advanced contributes to AGE (see Chapter 8) found in AD plaques (Phillips & Popplewell, 2002).

Nay and Garratt (1999) outlined three main stages of AD. The first is characterised by absent-mindedness, emotional instability and poor concentration. These symptoms can include spatial disorientation, disturbed perception, changes in personal appearance and hygiene, a tendency to blame others for a range of occurrences, and an inability to successfully perform ADLs. Depression is often present in the early stages because the person is aware that something is 'not quite right' and they realise 'things are slipping away' from them (Katona, 1994).

Stage two lasts up to 12 years. The person may withdraw and behaviour is often variable including anger, transient crying, poor sleep patterns, disorientation, and profound short-term memory loss. Gait often changes, people have difficulty recognising their own face in a mirror, and continence issues emerge as well as other behaviours such as exhibitionism. The person cannot live safely by themselves in the community.

Stage three is often the shortest, lasting up to 2 years. Profound physical and cognitive decline occurs, finally resulting in stupor and coma. Depression, delirium and dementia can occur concommitanly and have cumulative and compounding effects on physical and mental functioning. It can be difficult to differentiate among the three states: Table 12.5 compares some of the features to help differentiate among them to ensure treatment is timely and appropriate; refer to Table 12.5, which outlines some differences among dementia, delirium and depression.

Managing diabetes in older people

Age, life expectancy, other health problems and the person's social situation should be considered when planning care. Achieving near-normal blood glucose levels and preventing long-term complications may not be priority management aims. It is important to control uncomfortable symptoms (polyuria, polydipsia, lethargy), maintain quality of life (QoL) and wellbeing and minimise the risk of hypoglycaemia and the attendant risk of falling.

Suboptimal metabolic control is associated with urinary incontinence, leg/foot ulcers, infections, nutritional deficiencies, exacerbates neuropathic pain, affects communication and cause confusion and aggression (Kirkland 2000). Strategies and care priorities need to be implemented using a stepwise approach and non-pharmacological measures where possible. Planning should include planning for end of life care (Chapter 18).

Management aims

Managing older people is complicated and diabetes adds to the complexity. Various models of care exist biased on the chronic disease model and the governments of some countries are introducing policies and service models to cope with the aging population and the increasing prevalence of diabetes. For example, the Australian Government introduced a suite of reforms for the aged care sector in 2012 that are currently being implemented; some of which aim to support people to remain living at home for longer.

Other strategies include Geriatric Evaluation Units (GEM) in hospitals, which provide comprehensive assessment and plan care with the individual and their families/carers to support community-dwelling older people remain independent and self-caring for as long as possible. Older people managed in GEM units spend less time in hospital, are discharged taking fewer medicines and have better outcomes (Verschoor 2012).

The Eden Alternative, an innovative to residential aged care, has a philosophical approach that changes the focus in aged care facilities from medical to creating environments that address common problems people living in aged care facilities face: loneliness, boredom and helplessness. The Eden Alternative encourages contact with children, companion pets, hobbies and indoor and outdoor gardens. Benefits include fewer infection and lower medicine use.

The main aims of care are to:

- Optimise nutrition.
- Prevent hypo- and hyperglycaemia.
- Undertake a structured medication management programme using a quality use of medicine framework, considering the Beers Criteria (American Geriatrics Society (2012) and deprescribing where possible to limit polypharmacy.
- Proactively screen for and prevent and/or manage diabetic complications, comorbidities, depression, and maintain independent self-care as long as possible.
- Undertake general preventative health measure such as vaccinations and health checks, for example, mammograms, prostate checks. Flu vaccine prevents respiratory illnesses, pneumonia, hospital admissions and death in older people (Gross et al. 1995). However, in years without influenza, booster vaccinations may not confer added benefits if routing trivalent vaccination does not produce seroprotection (Gaughran et al. 2007). Research suggests people with chronic diseases are less likely to receive preventative care despite attending health professionals frequently (Beckman et al. 2001; Lipscombe et al. 2005).
- Manage coexisting illnesses to improve physical and mental functional ability and improve quality of life.
- Maintain or enhance a positive attitude (cognitive reserve).
- Maintain a safe environment to limit adverse events such as falls.
- Regularly assess driving safety and help the individual develop and maintain a transportation plan to make the transition to stop driving. Be aware that operating motorised wheelchairs, Go-Fors, and farm machinery may also constitute a driving risk.
- Develop and end of life care plan to ensure a comfortable and peaceful death when the time comes.
- Undertake regular diabetes complication screening that includes geriatric syndromes, medicines and mental health. Such screens may need to be undertaken at any change in physical and mental health status, not juts annually.

Factors that affect management decisions

- Age, but age alone may not give an accurate picture of an individual's ability to cope with self-care tasks and activities of daily living. Functional level should be assessed using appropriate tools in an appropriate familiar setting.
- Current diabetes control and complication status including the presence of liver and kidney disease.

- Presence and severity of comorbidities.
- Life expectancy.
- Mental and physical capacity to self-care.
- Nutritional status. Inadequate nutrition predisposes the person to hypoglycaemia, falls, decreased immunity, delayed wound healing and infections, and other diseases.
- Learning capacity, which is influenced by the individual's learning style, sight, hearing and cognitive ability, interest in the topic, and the way the individual presents the information, see Chapter 16.
- Social support from family and the community.
- Financial status and access to services.
- Advanced Care Plan (Chapter 18).

Nutritional management

Older people are often malnourished. Malnourishment is associated with adverse outcomes and weight change in older people is associated with longer length of stay in hospital, and increased mortality (Middleton *et al.* 2001) and is particularly concerning in frail older people (Devitt 2011). The causes of poor nutrition are shown in Table 12.6. Sometimes it is difficult to distinguish between the effects of malnutrition and disease processes, which are closely related (World Health Organization 1999). Significantly under nutrition is often under-recognised and under diagnosed.

It is important to take a broad approach to nutritional assessment and management in older people with diabetes rather than the usual focus on reducing dietary fat and sugar. Energy requirements usually reduce in older people but they require nutrient-rich

Table 12.6 Risk factors for inadequate nutrition and malnutrition in older people are mulitfactorial and encompass the factors shown in the table.

Risk factor	Potential outcome
Living in an institution	Forced food choices and meal times, loss of control over environment, depression Not being able to reach food and/or feed themselves Not being exposed to sunlight leading to vitamin D deficiency
Diminished hunger sensation, anorexia, dysphagia, mouth pathology	Reduced intake Weight loss
Malabsorption	Bacterial infections, coeliac disease, medicines, disease processes and diabetes complications such as gastric autonomic neuropathy
Neurological deficits	Stroke, dementia, neuropathy
Medicines	Digitalis, alcohol, sedatives and metformin is known to affect the absorption of vitamin B12
Sensory deficits	Impaired sight and/or hearing, taste and smell
Dentition and swallowing difficulties	Ill-fitting dentures, caries, missing teeth, gum disease, malnutrition
Social circumstances	Isolation, poverty, inability to shop or prepare food, depression, malnutrition
Medical problems	Chronic disease, pneumonia, heart failure, chronic infection, thyroid disease, malnutrition, low immunity

foods to ensure essential nutrients are included in the diet. Generally caloric requirements reduce by 20–30%. Caloric requirements should be individualised according to age, gender, body size and composition, activity and medicine regimen.

Older people need to be encouraged to:

- Incorporate omega-3 foods into the diet.
- Eat a variety of nutritious foods in at least three meals every day.
- Eat plenty of cereals, wholegrain bread and pasta especially those with a low Glycaemic Index; 50–60% of total intake.
- Have adequate protein intake, consisting of at least 15% of the total intake and not <0.8 gms/kg/day Protein requirements increase during wound healing and stress conditions such as infections and might decrease in end stage renal disease.
- Eat plenty of fruit and vegetables to reduce the risk of cardiovascular and degenerative diseases and supply essential vitamins and minerals, such as calcium.
- Have an adequate fluid intake, including water (about 1500 millilitres per day) to reduce the likelihood of dehydration, especially in hot weather, unless fluid restriction is indicated.
- Drink alcohol in moderation. Because of the reduced muscle mass, the volume in which alcohol is distributed is reduced; therefore, the concentration of circulating alcohol is higher, putting the person at risk of cognitive impairment, hypoglycaemia, and falls. However, moderate consumption of alcohol might have health benefits.
- Use low salt food and only add small amounts of salt to food to help prevent hypertension (National Health and Medical Research Council 1999).

Practice points

(1) Many older people are malnourished even though they appear overweight. Malnutrition is common: 15% of homebound community dwelling, 35–65% of hospitalised people and 50% of residential aged care residents (Szony 2004). Malnutrition is associated with longer length of stay in hospital and is a strong predictor of readmission and is associated with pressure ulcers, delirium, and depression.
(2) There is limited data about the nutritional needs of very old people.
(3) People over the age of 70 have special nutritional needs (Drewnowski & Warren-Mears 2001) especially if they have diabetes.
(4) Enteral feeding and supplements are often required but can affect blood glucose levels unless the formula is carefully selected and the risks and benefits of enteral feeding are carefully considered..

Malnourishment can occur while older people are in hospital (McWhirter & Pennington 1994). In care facilities rates between 36% and 43% are reported (Friedman & Kalant 1998). Concomitant diseases that increase the risk of malnutrition in older people with diabetes include:

(1) Psychiatric disorders including depression, see Chapter 15.
(2) Parkinson's Disease.
(3) Chronic obstructive pulmonary disease.
(4) Polypharmacy, which is common in diabetes.
(5) Renal failure.
(6) Neurological dysfunction.

(7) Dental problems and chewing and swallowing difficulties. The latter also increases the likelihood that nasogastric or enteral feeding will be needed as well as the risk of coughing and choking during feeding and increases the risk of chest infections. Swallowing difficulties affect ~10% of hospitalised older people (Hudson *et al.* 2000).
(8) Disabled house-bound individuals.
(9) People with cancer or HIV/AIDS.
(10) At the end stages of life.

Specific nutritional deficits include vitamin D and calcium, which increases the risk of osteoporosis and fractures. Low intake of vitamin K-rich vegetables affects the stability of the INR in people on anticoagulant therapy (Franco *et al.* 2004). Factors that help maintain optimal nutrition for people over 80 living in the community are supportive family and friends, having a microwave oven, transportation, and proximity to a grocery store (Callan & Wells 2003). The Australian Nutrition Screening Initiative was developed to highlight the importance of identifying older people at risk of malnutrition. The tool can help nurses decide when a comprehensive nutritional assessment is required and refer the individual to a dietitian.

The Hydration Assessment checklist detects hydration problems in older people (Zembrzuski 1997) and the Mini Nutritional assessment (MNA) detects actual and potential malnourishment in people over 65 (Reilly 1996) and may predict mortality in older people (Persson 2002). Other nutrition assessment tools are listed in Chapter 4.

Biochemical assessments include plasma proteins, recognising the concentration can be influenced by non-nutritional factors such as liver disease, some cancers, sepsis, and inflammatory bowel disease. Protein intake can be calculated using the blood urea nitrogen (BUN) with the serum creatinine. If the creatinine is low, protein intake is low. If both the creatinine and BUN are low, a state of tissue catabolism such as that associated with hyperglycaemia, exists. Low serum albumin indicates chronic protein deficiency. However, albumin has a long half-life (~20 days), thus, it is not an accurate indicator of temporary protein lack (Baines & Roberts 2001). Specific tests for deficiencies such as zinc and vitamins may be indicated. Indicators of malnutrition include:

- Significant weight change: 10% of body weight in six months. Weight loss in older people often means loss of muscle mass, which affects strength and functional ability.
- Body Mass Index <22 or >27.
- Mid arm circumference < 10th percentile. Mid are circumference is often easier to measure in older people, especially frail older people and those in aged care homes.
- Triceps skin fold <10th or >90th percentile.
- Serum:
  - prealbumin <16 mg/dl
  - transferring <200 mg/dl
  - albumin <3.5 g/dl
  - cholesterol <160 mg/dl (Mooradian *et al.*1999)

Nutritional supplements are a simple way of increasing the energy and nutrient content of the diet of older people. Even when the daily intake of vitamins and minerals is adequate these nutrients may not be bioavailable and supplements may be needed (Truswell 2003). For example, omega-3 supplementation may be beneficial to lower triglycerides of people with heart disease if the RDI cannot be consumed by eating oily fish. The American Heart Foundation (AHA) (Orford *et al.* 2002) recommended doctors supervise omega-3 supplementation in older people. Omega-3 supplements may cause gastrointestinal disturbances and hyperglycaemia and may interact with warfarin and cause bleeding.

Enteral therapy

An increasing number of older people, particularly those living in aged care facilities, require enteral feeding. Usually, glucose lowering medicines (GLMs)/insulin should be administered and blood glucose tests performed before administering the enteral feed but other medications may need to be administered separately from feeds to ensure they are absorbed. Nasogastric tubes are usually used when temporary enteral feeds are needed. Gastroscopy, jejunostomy or PEG tubes are usually preferred when enteral feeding is required long term. Enteral therapy enables fluid and macronutrients to be provided to meet the individual's metabolic and nutritional requirements (see also Chapter 10).

Feeds are administered slowly initially to prevent Refeeding Syndrome and to limit the metabolic and haemodynamic effects. For example, electrolyte shifts can precipitate congestive cardiac failure, cardiac arrhythmias, and neuromuscular and respiratory dysfunction (Crook *et al.* 2001). The formula used depends on the indication, for example, the need to reduce CO_2 production in respiratory disease when CO_2 excretion is compromised. There are no specific guidelines for people with diabetes at risk of malnutrition who require nutritional support. General dietary recommendations for people with diabetes may not be appropriate for older malnourished people with diabetes (Elias *et al.* 2005). Formulas with less impact on blood glucose are available for people with diabetes. Types of formulas include:

- Standard, which are often used when commencing enteral feeding. These are high in carbohydrate and low in fat and fibre and can cause hyperglycaemia because of their rapid transit time and nutrient absorption and lead to post prandial hyperglycaemia due to impaired muscle and splanchic glucose uptake (Basu *et al.* 2001).
- Hypercaloric, used if fluid intake needs to be restricted, for example, end-stage renal disease.
- Fibre to reduce constipation.
- A range of specialty formulas exists for renal, hepatic, respiratory disease, wound management, and cancer. Specialty formulas for people with diabetes include Nutrison low energy for diabetes, Nutrison diabetes, Resource diabetes, and Glucerna, which are all generally low GI. These formulas used as enteral feeds or supplements have less effect on blood glucose than standard feeds (Elia *et al.* 2005). Glucerna has less effect on blood glucose than Enrich, Ensure HN and Compleat Modified (Peters & Davidson 1992). Diabetes-specific formulas contain fructose, fibre mono-unsaturated fatty acids, protein and antioxidants. High GI feeds can precipitate osmotic diarrhoea, dehydration, and hyperosmolar states. If high GI foods are indicated they should be commenced slowly and increased slowly and oral hypoglycaemic agents/insulin adjusted according to the blood glucose pattern. Blood glucose should be monitored regularly.
- Elemental and sub-elemental formulas are easily digested and may be suitable for people with autonomic gastroparesis.
- Modular formulas, which contain a single nutrient, enable feeds to be tailored to the individual.

The effects on the individual need to be considered when commencing enteral feeding: these include isolation, depression, and reduced QoL. In addition, enteral feeds may not prevent malnutrition, even when they are carefully tailored. They may delay wound healing if they lead to hyperglycaemia, pressure sores and infection can develop around the tube insertion site and the nasogastric tubes can become dislodged and cause aspiration pneumonia and are associated with increased risk of mortality. They can be a burden on carers, and incorrect administration of medicines through enteral feeding methods occurs in home, aged care and hospital settings, for example crushing enteric-coated long-acting medicines.

Guidelines for administering diabetes medicines with enteral feeds

The policies and guidelines of the relevant facility should be followed. In addition, advice is available Department of Health and Aging *Guidelines for Medicine Management in Residential Aged care facilities* (DOHA 2012). Generally:

(1) Liquid dose forms are the preferred formulations. If there are no contraindications to crushing tablets or opening capsules they should be crushed to a fine powder and mixed with 10–15 mL of water.
(2) The feed should be stopped 30 minutes before the scheduled medication administration time and flushed with 30 mL water before administering the medicines when medicines need to be administered on an empty stomach and recommenced 30 minutes after all the medicine is administered.
(3) If medicine/enteral formula incompatibilities are possible; alternative medicines or formulas should be prescribed if possible. It is not possible, the feed should be stopped 2 hours before medicine administered as a single daily dose and recommenced 2 hours after the medicine is administered. If more frequent doses are prescribed one hour should be allowed before and after the medicine/s are administered. However, this method does *not* guarantee complete bioavailability of the medicines but no incompatibility between commonly used diabetes medicines and enteral feeds were identified.
(4) Medicines should be remixed before they are administered using a syringe clearly labelled for oral dosing to avoid the possibility of a wrong route medication error. Allowed the medicines to flow in by gravity. If the mixture does not flow easily the plunger can be depressed very gently. Medicines should not be pushed through enteral tubes because they can obstruct the tube.

Different medicines should never be mixed together in a syringe

The syringe should be flushed with 5 mL of water between medicines when several medicines need to be administered at the same time. The tube should be flushed with 30 mL of water and clamped after all the medicines are administered. The feeding can then be recommenced. A feeding record should be maintained and the amount of water used to flush the tubing should be documented, especially when the person has oedema or renal disease. Medicines should be documented on the medication record.

It is advisable to consult a pharmacist before crushing medicines or opening capsules and administering them through enteral feeding tubes. Some medicines are more toxic if they are crushed, others have reduced efficacy, and the possibility of medicine interactions increases. If possible, liquid formulations should be used for enteral administration. Other dose formulations such as topical applications, intranasal sprays, patches, suppositories or injections should be used if applicable. Many lipid lowering agents and antihypertensive medicines should not be crushed.

The Product Information sheets and quality medicine handbooks detail specific information about administering medicines in relation to food, solubility, and information about administering via enteral routes. For example, some medicines are absorbed from specific areas of the gastrointestinal tract and need to be enteric coated to reach the area before being absorbed.

Practice points

(1) During acute illness, surgical procedures and trauma blood glucose levels can be controlled more effectively with insulin.
(2) Insulin may be preferable and reduce the risk of adverse medicine events if enteral feeding is required temporarily and in the long term.
(3) GLM may be contradicted in some disease states, see Chapter 5.
(4) Diabetes medication management must relate to enteral therapy routines and not usual medication/meal administration times. For example, if the individual is scheduled for an enteral feed five times a day, for example, at 6 a.m., 10 a.m., 2 p.m., 6 p.m., and 10 p.m., the diabetes medicines must be administered and blood glucose tested considering these feed times. Thus, many diabetes medications need to be administered at 6 a.m. with the first feed and not at 8 a.m. when breakfast is served. Capillary blood glucose testing should be performed before an enteral feed and/or 2 hours after the feed to determine postprandial glucose clearance.

There is no specific information about compatibility between various enteral feeds and many medicines. Therefore, patients should be monitored according to the indication for the medicine and the enteral feed to ensure management aims are met. Enteral feeding may not be a contraindication to medicines, but administering some medicines via enteral tubes can alter their bioavailability. For example, crushing may increase the absorption and affect the action profile of some medicines and increase the possibility of adverse events (Gilbar, 1999; Engle & Hannawa 1999; Young 2004).

Nutrition in dementia

Inadequate nutritional intake is common in people with dementia who accept or refuse meals erratically and may be anorexic. When a person refuses meals they can be encouraged to consume fluids and light foods such as hot chocolate, milkshakes, ice cream, fruit, yoghurt, and custard. Repeating favourite foods can sometimes help. For example, if the person likes breakfast foods, breakfast can be repeated at dinnertime. Nutritional supplements may also be useful, for example, 60 mL Two-Cal® administered with normal prescribed medications four times a day will increase protein intake.

Education approaches

Diabetes education is discussed in detail in Chapter 16. Factors that affect learning in older people include the environment, the time the education is delivered, the duration of the session, the type of education materials used and the person's physical and mental state (Table 12.6). Where appropriate, people should have their glasses (spectacles) and hearing aid with them during diabetes education sessions (Jennings 1997; Rosenstock 2001).

Spouses and/or carers should be included in diabetes education sessions when appropriate especially when cognition is impaired for whatever reason. Support groups have long-term benefits for knowledge retention, psychosocial functioning and improved metabolic control and improve socialisation (Gilden *et al.* 1992). In the absence of dementia, the factor most likely to affect an older person's ability to learn, retain, and recall new information and skills and problem-solve depends on whether they are actively involved in their community. For example, an older person who participates in social activities is more likely to want to learn about their diabetes management than socially isolated older people.

Many diabetes education programmers are not age-specific and often occur in groups, which makes it difficult for hearing and vision impaired people to participate. Computer-generated learning packages are also difficult to see, access and use for some older people. In addition, many older people have low literacy skills. Small font sizes and/or text printed on shiny or coloured paper with insufficient contrast between the text and the background also compromises comprehension. Despite these limitations older people like to receive written information, are likely to refer to it and use it in their diabetes care.

Participating in education programmes can provide mental stimulus and help preserve mental functioning as well as reduce hospital admissions and improve QoL. Memory, learning, information retrieval and cognitive deficits have been demonstrated in people with Type 2 diabetes particularly when metabolic control is poor (Gilden *et al.* 1992). Several factors affect memory and learning besides cognitive function and vision changes. These include:

- Degree of wellness.
- Physical, psychological, and biological capacity.
- Social situation and available support.
- Degree of adjustment to being older and age-related changes, for example, wearing glasses.
- Sensory loss, tiredness, and incontinence can be barriers to effective education.
- Interest in the topic.
- Educator's style and skill. Diabetes education strategies must include methods of increasing concentration and enhancing attention especially when vision and hearing are impaired. Incorporating relaxation techniques and other complementary therapies into the education session can relieve stress and enhance learning, see Chapter 19.
- The environment in which the education occurs.

When recommending self-care equipment to older people consider factors such as whether they can hold it easily, numbers on meters and insulin devices are large and clear enough to see. Memory prompts and cues can be helpful for some people.

Self-care

Self-care is important and independent self-care should be maintained as long as possible. Older people may need help with some self-care tasks but not others. Health professionals need to realise that diabetes self-care is relentless and demanding. Self-care can be an added burden to carers who may be old and have illnesses themselves. Self-care capacity should be assessed regularly as part of the annual complication assessment, following a hospital admission, and when medicine or medicine doses change. Barriers to self-care include declining physical and mental functioning, depression, intercurrent illness, comorbidities, and the effects of medications. Specific factors associated with inadequate self-care include:

- geriatric syndromes and frailty;
- lower levels of physical functioning;
- inadequate knowledge about the medical condition/s;
- limited participation in social activities;
- depression;
- financial constraints;
- male gender;
- low perceptions of health status;
- high number of concomitant conditions (Bayliss *et al.* 2007).

Potential barriers include high levels of morbidity, cumulative effects of comorbidities, inadequate health professional/patient communication, and health professional clinical inertia. In addition, self-perception, the desire to remain independent, health beliefs and attitudes play a role. For example, in general older people are reluctant to use walking aids. However, sudden changes in walking ability and positive cultural views about ageing make a difference to their willingness to accept a walking aid (Gooberman-Hill & Ebrahim 2007).

The person's home blood glucose testing record might provide important clues to self-care. For example, if it is smeared with blood it might indicate visual, eye-hand coordination, or manual dexterity deficits. Food- and blood-stained record books and blood glucose meters might indicate testing from contaminated fingers. If these deficits are suspected the issue needs to be approached with tact and in a non-judgmental manner. Record books can be used proactively and constructively to help people understand the effects of food, activity, medicines and stress on their blood glucose, help them find solutions to problems and involve them in planning their care. Wetzels *et al.* (2007) undertook a systematic review of the relevant literature that showed using a pre-visit record book in combination with an education session or consultation led to more questions and more self-reported health care.

Some older people find the print too small in commercial blood glucose record books and prefer to use 'exercise books'. Paper-based patient-held records are still popular with many people despite modern meters that automatically record blood glucose results and have the capacity to download the results directly onto computers (Davis 2003).

Factors that can affect metabolic control

'Barriers to good control are often in the minds of physicians rather than the capacity of the elderly person with diabetes' (Halter 2001). A current term is 'clinical inertia'. For example, many GPs are reluctant to commence insulin in older people when metabolic control deteriorates, even when the patient and their family/carers are willing. It is important to consider the health professional's influence on an individual's healthcare, especially when the individual is old. Health professionals often judge older people in general by the older people they manage in aged care facilities who may not accurately represent the majority of self-caring elderly people living in the community. Some of the factors that can affect diabetes control in the elderly are shown in Table 12.7.

Table 12.7 Factors that can affect diabetes control and management in older people.

Health professionals	Attitudes and beliefs Inadequate knowledge about diabetes and/or about teaching and learning Inappropriate advice, education materials Ageist approaches to services and diabetes management choices Clinical inertia Constraints on time and services
Altered senses	Communication difficulties Diminished vision, hearing and smell, altered taste, decreased proprioception Not understanding instructions
Cognitive status	Diminished cognition affects learning, memory and recall May be temporarily affected by hypo- or hyperglycaemia
Food difficulties	Purchasing, preparing and consuming food, understanding nutritional requirements, poor appetite, early satiety, gastrointestinal problems Disease processes Dental and oral problems
Disease processes/effects	Tremor, arthritis, poor dentition, gastrointestinal abnormalities, altered thirst sensation, altered renal and hepatic function, infection (acute and chronic)
Mobility	Limited ability to exercise Self-imposed driving restrictions or withdrawal of driving license
Medicines	Alcohol, medications such as glucocorticoids, interactions, self-prescribed medications
Complementary therapies	Hypo- or hyperglycaemia, medicine/herb interactions, herb/herb interactions
Malabsorption	Owing to diabetes medications, disease processes, medicine interactions, diabetes complications
Psychological issues	Bereavement, depression, cognitive deficits
Social factors	Social isolation, living alone or in care facilities, family expectations
Financial status	Purchasing recommended foods, monitoring equipment, diabetes complication screening, podiatry services

Access and equity to diabetes services

Older people are often unable to attend mainstream diabetes services especially where they are fragmented and essential services are offered on different days. Appointments scheduled to allow a 'one stop' approach to diabetes management enhance attendance rates. People are often required to attend different sites to have their eyes, kidneys, and feet checked for diabetic complications. Therefore, integrated care and careful transition care, discharge planning, and involving the GPs is essential. In Australia, the GP incentive schemes and integrated care planning and assessment strategies and the National Service Framework in the UK have significantly improved diabetes care in general practice.

Infection

The presence of infection can significantly affect the health status of older people. Any sudden increase in blood glucose that cannot be accounted for by dietary changes, inactivity, medicines, or stress should be investigated. The temperature should be recorded.

Foot inspection is important to exclude occult infection. Reduced mobility and sitting with feet in the dependent position can cause lower leg oedema, which puts pressure on fragile, less flexible older skin causing small ruptures, weeping and increase the risk of infection and chronic ulcers. Mental stress associated with non-healing wounds delays wound healing.

Urinary tract infections are common in older people. A urine dipstick test for white cells and nitrate should be performed. There is growing evidence that consuming cranberry formulations on a daily basis can prevent UTI in older people with diabetes. Cranberry formulations can interact with warfarin so caution is needed in people on these medicines. As indicated, annual influenza vaccination should be part of the individual's routine health management plan.

An holistic approach to healing is needed that includes proactive screening for occult infections, optimal nutrition, education, and strategies that encompass physical, spiritual, and mental health. A single point of care coordination is desirable but the expertise of several health professional groups may be needed. For example, podiatrist, orthotist, endocrinologist, diabetes educator, dietitian, vascular surgeon, orthopedic specialist, infectious diseases physician and a wound consultant might all be required to manage an infected foot.

Quality of life

Quality of life refers to an individual's enjoyment of life and might or might not include prolonging life see Chapter 15. QoL issues specific to the individual are more likely to accurately gauge life enjoyment than objective QoL tools even those well validated and frequently used tools. Such tools are essential if the objective is to compare individuals. However, they may be less relevant if the objective is to sequentially monitor individual QoL. For example, pets enhance QoL and are treasured companions for many older people, yet pets are not mentioned on any QoL tools. Older people identify QoL as being more important than length of life (Medical Research Council, 1994).

Many factors affect QoL in addition to personal QoL factors, these include:

- General health and medical issues such as diabetes type, treatment regimen, level of metabolic control and presence of complications. The greater the severity and effects of diabetes-related complications the greater the effect on QoL. Sexual health is often overlooked in older people. It is an important aspect of QoL often compromised by medical conditions, medications, the effects of age, and health professional and societal attitudes.
- Management strategies. The level of glycaemic control rarely relates to the level of well being (Testa *et al.* 1998) but diabetes symptoms of hypo or hyperglycaemia are more directly related to QoL.. Maaravi *et al.* (2000) identified nutritional status as a major determinant of QoL in a community dwelling people over 70 years. There are conflicting about the effects of the different types of diabetes treatment on the QoL of older people. QoL is lower in people treated with insulin (Petterson *et al.* 1998; Rutherford *et al.* 2006; Speight *et al.* 2011). In contrast, Reza *et al.* (2002) reported better mental health, social functioning, and vitality and less carer strain associated with insulin.
- Cognitive functioning is affected by acute and chronic blood glucose fluctuations. The associated neuropsychological changes can reduce QoL of both the person with diabetes and their family.

- Health, diabetes, cultural, and general attitudes and beliefs, which influence factors such as self-efficacy and locus of control. Strategies that focus on understanding the individual's beliefs and attitudes, and encompass empowerment theories improve an individual's sense of well being and involvement in their care.
- Demographic factors such as gender, education level ethnicity, age, and social support. Men report better QoL than women and young people better than older people. Higher education is associated with a higher QoL. Individuals with good support generally have a better QoL and reduced risk of depression.

Various tools to measure QoL and other related factors are shown in Chapter 15.

Safety

In many respects diabetes management in older people encompasses managing risks regardless of whether the individual lives in the community, in a care facility, or is being cared for in acute, ambulatory, or primary care settings. Safety is multifactorial and risks are often cumulative as can be seen from Table 12.2. Many safety programmes focus on falls, but driving and other safety issues also need to be addressed.

Falls are the sixth leading cause of death in older people with and without diabetes, but having diabetes significantly increases the risk. People who fall, do so repeatedly, and falls are a common cause of placement in an aged care home. Falls are a result of a combination of accumulated effects of disease processes, impairment, and medications (Quayle 2001). It can be seen from Table 12.2 that a significant number of diabetes-related problems significantly increase the likelihood that an older person with diabetes will fall.

General factors that increase the risk of falling include:

- fell in the last year;
- have difficulty with mobility and/or sensory deficits;
- are on four or more medications particularly oral GLMs, insulin, and antihypotensive and antidepressive agents;
- have an acute illness;
- were recently discharged from hospital;
- have reduced strength and require a walking stick or frame;
- wear inappropriate footwear;
- live where there are environmental hazards;
- have balance problems;
- have diabetes complications such as autonomic neuropathy and vision loss;
- are sedated, especially in an unfamiliar environment such as hospital or aged care facilities where the person can become disorientated and fall going to the toilet at night.

Diabetes is associated with a two-fold increased risk of older people falling (Sinclair 2006) and older women are at increased risk of sustaining a fracture if they fall (Gregg *et al.* 2002). Ninety per cent of those who fall are likely to fracture a hip, shoulder, or foot (Schwartz *et al.* 2001). Women with diabetes aged 70–79 are more likely to fall if their HbA_{1c} is ≤6.8% and they are on insulin (Schwartz *et al.* 2003), which suggests hypoglycaemia may be implicated in many falls in older women with diabetes. Significantly, the presence of diabetes predicts failure to recover from mobility deficits, which increases the likelihood the individual will require supported care

(Clark *et al*. 1998). Some diabetes-specific factors related to falls are shown in Table 12.2. Others include:

- Insulin treatment leading to hypoglycaemia. Sulphonylureas, particularly long-acting agents also cause hypoglycaemia but less frequently than insulin. The association between hypoglycaemia and OHA might be partly due to reduced renal clearance of active OHA metabolites of long-acting agents. Falls are associated with high levels of cystatin-c, an indicator of kidney function (Schwartz *et al*. 2008).
- Postural and postprandial hypotension. Hypertension is also associated with haemodialysis on dialysis days. See Chapter 10 and cardiovascular disease Chapter 8.
- Postural instability, and gait, and balance problems due to a wide range of health problems including erratic blood glucose pattern, muscle wasting and reduced lower limb strength, musculoskeletal problems, low vision and environmental factors.
- Weight loss and nutritional deficiencies.
- Neurological problems that may slow recognition of and response to falls risk situations.
- Cardiovascular disease: ~77% of presentations to emergency department due to unexplained falls have their basis in cardiovascular disease (van der Velde *et al*. 2007). Poon & Braun (2005) suggested orthostatic hypotension might be contributory factor in up to 32% of falls associated with cardiovascular disease. Postprandial hypotension is also a falls risk. Postprandial hypotension is described as a blood pressure fall of 20 mmHg, an hour after eating. In aged care facilities postprandial hypotension is associated with an increased incidence of falls, syncope, stroke, and new coronary events (Aronow & Ahn 1997).
- Withdrawing medicines that contribute to orthostatic hypotension reduces the falls rate. Tilt table tests might be useful to detect hypotension (van der Velde *et al*. 2007). However, this equipment is unlikely to be readily available in most clinical situations.
- Cognitive impairment, which might be due to hyper- or hypoglycaemia, hypotension, neurological problems, vascular disease, depression, dementia or a number of other causes.

Interestingly, Oates *et al*. (2007) showed older people, >80 years (n=4071 from 10 US veteran's affairs sites) had lower 5-year survival rates if they had low blood pressure than those with higher blood pressure, which suggests current blood pressure targets might be harmful in very old people, particularly given the associated falls risk. Research in other populations also demonstrated better outcomes in older people with higher than recommended target blood pressure levels (Vidan *et al*. 2010). However, blood pressure targets need to be considered in light of hypertension-associated risks such as stroke and cardiovascular events. All of these factors support the need for individualised, structured medicines reviews that are undertaken in the context of cumulative risk and QoL.

However, there is some evidence to support:

- Exercise and/physical therapy with vitamin D supplementation in community-dwelling older people (Moyer 2012).
- Tai chi, which improves balance and stability (Li 2012).
- LIFE programme (Lifestyle integrated Functional Exercise, which improve functional capcity (Clemson *et al*. 2012).
- Yoga, (Patel et al 2012) but studies are small with different methodologies and yoga styles.
- In hospital:

○ bedside handover;
○ hourly rounding;
○ ensuring the individual can reach walking aids and call bells and the environment is free from obstacles;
○ nursing rosters to ensure adequate staffing is maintained (Digby 2012).

Multifactorial strategies are usually needed to prevent and manage falls. Interestingly, a meta-analysis of the literature about hospital falls prevention programmes demonstrated falls reduction between 30% and 49% but few studies used sound methodologies or represent strong evidence for their benefit (Coussement *et al.* 2008). After adjusting for falls risk, Coussement *et al.* 2008 suggested current falls prevention programmes may only be useful in long stay care units. They suggested more research into primary falls prevention in hospitals is needed in which the number of fallers, the effect of the setting in which the fall occurred, and individual falls risk are examined to determine the effect of the separate components of falls reduction programmes. A recent literature undertaken by the author and one of her PhD students suggests Coussement *et al.*'s suggestions have not been implemented. That is it is difficult to combine data because of methodological differences and deficits.

Pharmacovigilance

Medications are discussed in detail in Chapter 5. Medication-related problems are 'common and costly and often preventable in older people:' adverse medicine events occur in 42% older people living in aged care facilities, most during prescribing and monitoring (American Geriatrics Society 2012). Age-related medicine pharmacokinetic and pharmacodynamic changes, nutritional status, cardiovascular status, and risk of polypharmacy and its consequences must be considered when deciding whether to use a medicine, which medicine, dose and dose interval, to use (Australian Medicines Handbook 2010).

Inappropriate high risk medicines should be avoided and non-medicine options used where possible (Quality Use of Medicines). The American Geriatrics Society (2012) Beers Criteria was developed for use to guide medicine use for people > 65 years in all care settings in the US, but is used in many countries. The Beers Criteria were designed to enhance clinical judgement and highlight the need to seek safer alternative medicines and 'less-is-more.' The criteria encompasses most classes of medicines, describes the rationale for the recommendation, the recommendation and quote the quality of the evidence. The criteria strongly recommends avoiding sliding scales of insulin and long acting sulphonylureas in older people with diabetes.

The Australian National prescribing Service (NPS 2004) developed a range of education programmes and multi media campaigns to enhance medicine self-management in older people such as Medimate and other programmes such as home medicine reviews.

As indicated in Chapter 5, declining renal function is a normal consequence of ageing, consequently long-acting medicines may be contraindicated if they have a prolonged half-life. Liver damage and inadequate or erratic food intake or food low in carbohydrate increases the risk of hypoglycaemia in insulin-treated individuals and with some CLMs. When swallowing difficulties are present medication dose forms may need to be reviewed. Suggested strategies to improved medicine safety when swallowing difficulties are present include:

• identifying medications that cannot be crushed and discuss these with the individual's doctor (hospital or GP) and pharmacist to determine whether the medicines are still required. if so, decide whether a non-medicine option could be used or whether there is an alternative dose form;

- placing a medication alert and a swallowing alert in the person's medical record;
- communicate the alerts to the relevant carers and health professional carers especially when transferring among services;
- providing education for people with diabetes, their carers and health professionals;
- regularly reviewing medications.

Practice point

The medicine dose forms that cannot be crushed are enteric coated, extended release, sublingual, medicines that irritate the oral mucous membranes, have a bitter taste, contain incipients and dyes that could stain the teeth, when specific protection is required when handling the medicine (Mitchell 2011).

Antipsychotic medicines should be used with caution in older people with dementia because they are associated with increased risk stroke and a moderately increased risk of MI when corrected for age, gender and cardiovascular risk (Parlente 2012).

Some medicines affect nutritional status by altering appetite, taste or sense of smell and affect food appreciation. Medicines such as antidepressants, sulphonylureas, and glucocorticoids contribute to weight gain. Others, such as anticholinergic medicines lead to dry mouth and difficulty in swallowing. Some medicines impair absorption, of vitamins and minerals, for example, antacids reduce iron and iron tablet absorption whereas vitamin C enhances iron absorption. There is increasing evidence that people with diabetic renal disease are at earlier risk of renal-associated anaemia but the exact mechanism and role of nutrition in this process is not known.

Phenytoin is sometimes used to manage painful diabetic peripheral neuropathy as well as seizures. It can inhibit absorption of vitamin D and folic acid. Some foods modify the absorption of some medicines, which explains why the timing medication doses in relation to food is important, especially in enteral feeding regimens.

Exercise/activity

Regular exercise has physical and mental benefits for people with and without diabetes of all ages. Exercise helps reduce the risk of developing diabetes and cardiovascular disease as well as improving mental wellbeing. Any movement of the body or limbs helps reduce cardiovascular fatalities by up to 50% and the chance of a second myocardial infarct by 25% as well as reducing hypertension and stroke risk (Department of Health Victoria 2004).

However, exercise is difficult for many older people because of the decline in muscle mass and general mobility, strength, and energy. These factors increase the risk of falls, injury, and fractures. Thus, exercise needs to be planned and individualised considering safety. At least 30 minutes of aerobic exercise per day and strength training exercises help maintain muscle mass and energy. In addition, adequate nutrition, especially protein, is important to preserving muscle mass and mobility, reduce falls, and improve well being (Viatkevicius *et al*. 2002: Stressman *et al* 2002;) It is not appropriate to merely recommend an older person to begin an exercise programme without assessing his/her physical status first. Assessment can be incorporated in usual care and includes assessing:

- Vascular status and detecting cardiac. Well older people in the community may require a graded exercise test. Blood pressure, lipid profile and assessment for autonomic neuropathy, which could lead to silent MI is advisable (Flood & Constance 2002).
- The feet to detect peripheral neuropathy and any other foot pathology that could increase the risk of foot injury during exercise.
- The eyes to detect the presence and status of retinopathy.
- Gait and balance.
- Blood glucose pattern and do not encourage activity if the blood glucose is <6 mmol/L or >10 mmol/L.
- Self-care knowledge. Be aware of the signs of hypoglycaemia, such as sweating, faintness, weakness, and dizziness, can be missed or attributed to the effect of the exercise, especially if hypoglycaemic unawareness is present, or could have other causes such as angina, or silent MI. Important information includes:
  - Knowing some physical activity can lower blood glucose for up to 48 hours therefore, an adequate high GI intake is required when aerobic activities are planned and activity levels increased gradually.
  - The importance of wearing appropriate clothing and footwear that does not restrict blood flow and breathing or put the feet at risk.
  - The need to warm up and cool before and after exercise.
  - How to incorporate exercise/activity into the usual daily routine.
  - The need to consider their personal safety and be aware of risks such as being attacked when out walking, risk of falling on poorly maintained footpaths.

The Society of Geriatric Cardiology recommend older people participate in physical activity programmes that include aerobic and strength training activities for example, Tai chi, which reduces blood pressure, blood glucose, and lipids, improves balance and well-being (Lan *et al.* 1998; Tsai *et al.* 2003). Resistance training reduces bone loss, improves strength, and makes routine activities such as carrying groceries and gardening easier (Meuleman *et al.* 2000; Simkin 2004). Walking 30 minutes/day or for 10 minutes three times per day is ideal. Swimming has the benefit of being non-weight bearing and might be easier for overweight people to manage. A great deal of incidental activity occurs during usual activities such as playing with grandchildren, housework, and gardening.

Hypoglycaemia

Hypoglycaemia is the most important side effect of insulin and GLMs, see Chapters 5 and 6. Hypoglycaemia occurring in older people managed using GLMs can be difficult to recognise. Usually the counter-regulatory response is triggered when the blood glucose drops below ~3.5–3.7 mmol/L, which triggers adrenergic symptoms such as sweating and trembling. Fine motor coordination, the speed of mental processing, concentration, and some memory functions are when blood glucose is <3 mmol/L (Sommerfield *et al.* 2003) The effects on decision-making are unclear. Some researchers suggest attentional ability is compromised but problem-solving ability remains intact (McAulay *et al.* 2001). Prolonged hypoglycaemia can result in neurological damage or death but these are rare (Cryer 2007).

The usual hypoglycaemia signs and symptoms can be masked or absent in older people and hypoglycaemia can present as chronic confusion, and not be recognised. The presentation of hypoglycaemia may resemble a cerebrovascular accident or mental confusion leading to an incorrect diagnosis of impaired mental function and delayed treatment or failure to treat the hypoglycaemia. The need to consider hypoglycaemia in older people with diabetes presenting to emergency departments has improved with education and since the introduction of capillary blood glucose testing on all unconscious patients presenting to emergency departments.

Hypoglycaemia caused by GLMs, especially long acting agents, is often profound and prolonged and can become chronic or fatal. If it is prolonged it can cause brain damage or provoke a MI (Tiengo 1999). If a person on insulin and a sulphonylurea or Glitinide starts to feel unwell, test their blood glucose to exclude/confirm hypoglycaemia as a cause. The risk of hypoglycaemia in the elderly is increased by:

- Treatment with oral hypoglycaemic agents, especially long-acting agents such as Glibenclamide (now rarely used in Australia and the UK) and Amaryl, see Chapter 5.
- Renal and/or hepatic disease that leads to impaired metabolism and excretion of medications and accumulation of medicines with long half-lives, and increased risk of medicine interactions (Jennings 1997; Howes 2001).
- Patients on multiple medicines where the risk of interactions is high.
- Impaired cognitive function where the individual fails to recognise hypoglycaemia and the signs can be confusing for family, carers, and health professionals.
- Patients who are sedated.
- Inadequate nutrition and malnutrition where glucose stores are inadequate to respond to the counter-regulatory hormone response to hypoglycaemia.
- Autonomic neuropathy, which can mask the symptoms of hypoglycaemia so the patient is unaware their blood glucose is low. These asymptomatic hypoglycaemic episodes are not recognised and therefore not treated early enough to avoid a severe episode. Alternatively, autonomic neuropathy can cause upper body sweating that can be mistaken for hypoglycaemia, see Chapter 6.
- Patients who are fasting for medical procedures or investigations.
- Excessive consumption of alcohol.
- Inadequate communication between health professionals caring for the patient and between health professionals and the patient, leading to confusion and management mistakes.

It is important to monitor the blood glucose of older peoples and residents presenting with these risk factors and to be aware that usually more than one risk factor is operating. The more risk factors present the greater the likelihood of hypoglycaemia occurring.

Managing hypoglycaemia
The method of treating hypoglycaemia must reflect the functional level of the individual:

- People on a normal oral diet:
  - Treat with a high glycaemic index food such as 10 g of glucose powder dissolved in water *or* 1 glass Glucozade *or* 5 glucose jelly beans
- People having thickened fluids/vitamised diets:
  - 15 g tube glucose gel
- People fed through a PEG tube:
  - 15 g tube glucose gel in the mouth
- 10 g of glucose powder dissolved in water and inserted into the PEG tube.

Practice points

- Hypoglycaemia leading to unconsciousness is rare in older people. However, such an event is very stressful and can precipitate an MI. An ECG should be performed.
- In cold weather prolonged hypoglycaemia can lead to hypothermia, which has a poor outcome.

Regular vaccinations against influenza and pneumonia are recommended for older people. A recent report recommended vaccinating infants as young as six months if they are in contact with frail elderly grandparents/relatives to reduce the spread of infection (Jackson & Janoff 2008). Interestingly, researchers found that, although people's immune response depends on the vaccination they received, the side of their brain that is most active also had an effect on the degree of the response (Davidson *et al.* 2003).

Davidson *et al.* (2003), found people aged 57–60 with left-sided brain activity in the prefrontal cortex developed stronger immunity. The prefrontal cortex is associated with a positive outlook on life. While the study is small, it demonstrates the effect of psychological parameters on physical status. Another earlier study (Graham *et al* 2006), demonstrated that chronic stress reduces immune function in older people and impaired antibody responses to influenza vaccinations. These findings also apply to older carers. These studies suggest that chronically stress older people including carers may be vulnerable to infection and because they are not able to mount an adequate immune response. Therefore, infection control procedures and appropriate preventative measure must be in place.

Nursing care

- Careful assessment of the individual from an holistic approach that incorporates physical, psychological, social, spiritual and relationship functioning. The latter includes relationships with health professionals.
- Strategies need to be in place to assess and minimise the risk of falling. These include providing a safe environment, orientating the person to the ward, considering protective measures to avoid pressure ulcers such as hip protectors, careful discharge planning, and early referral to the social worker, domiciliary or aged care team for home assessment.
- Timing meals, PEG, and enteral feeds and medication rounds to reduce the risk of hypoglycaemia.
- Adequate preparation of the patient for surgical and investigative procedures, see Chapter 9.
- Reminding the person to drink, especially in hot weather.
- Monitoring blood glucose and taking steps to correct persistent levels outside the target range.
- Providing clear, careful explanations when relevant and checking the person understands what is required of them. Written information enhances verbal information.
- Identifying stress and depression and ensuring appropriate assessment and management ocurs.
- Identifying the barriers to self-care and recognising and changing those things that can be changed and those that cannot.

- Bed rest may be required initially, but it should not be prolonged because of the loss of muscle mass especially in the lower limbs, venous stasis, skin tears, pressure ulcers and falls risk. Thus, it is important to ensure timely assessment when an older person presents to the emergency department and to consult an aged care expert early in the admission to ensure appropriate management and reduce the likelihood of repeated presentations.

WHO (1983) emphasised the importance of helping older people live safe, dignified lives in society with their families and friends if possible. Similarly, the Victorian Department of Human Services (2003) recognised the important role carers play in supporting older people in the community. Carers should be included in assessment and health planning and outcome monitoring processes where appropriate. Carers are concerned when they are not consulted when their older relative is hospitalised from an aged care facility (Hong *et al.* 2004). Written action plans can support carers to manage older people at home but need to be relevant to the carer and the older person and revised regularly bearing in mind the burden of care.

Having such strategies in place for respite and end of life care can relieve the burden of care and improve outcomes for carers and older people (Berthold *et al.* 1991). Carers presenting with health problems:

- Have long standing health problems.
- Experienced health problems in the previous year.
- Are concerned about their health.
- Experience a high level of frustration.
- Perform personal tasks such as bathing and dressing the older person, which can be distressing for both parties. Many older people do not want 'physical help' from their family and friends (Connell 1991), even when they need it. Providing support when it is not wanted, even if it is needed, can result in negative outcomes and be perceived as interference. Carers often tread the fine line between support and 'interference' on a daily basis
- Have difficulty communicating with the older person (Toraski 2004).
- Do not have adequate respite care/support services in place.
- Feel depressed and 'burnt out' (Toraski 2004).

An education programme for caregivers that includes information about how to manage their relative's behaviour can foster closer relationships between the carer and their older relative, and fewer incidents of acute confusion and faecal incontinence during hospital admissions and fewer depressive symptoms (Hong *et al.* 2004).

References

Abdo, S. & Flack, J. (2012) Diabetes as the years progress: How does management differ? *Endocrinology Today* **2**, 6–14.

Allen, K. V., Frier, B. M. & Strachan, M. W. (2004) The relationship between type 2 diabetes and cognitive dysfunction: longitudinal studies and their methodological limitations. *European Journal of Pharmacology*, **490**, 169–75.

American Diabetes Association (2013) *Clinical Guidelines – Diabetes in Older People*. http://www.ndei.org/ADA-2013-Guideline-Diabetes-Older-Adults.aspx (accessed January 2013).

American Geriatrics Society (2012) Updated Beers Criteria for potentially inappropriate use in older adults. *Journal of the American Geriatrics Society*, DOI: 10.111/j.1532-5415.2012.03923.x.

Ames B. (2006) Low micronutrient intake may accelerate degenerative diseases of aging through allocation of scarce micronutrients by triage. *Proceedings of National Academy of Science USA*, **103** (47), 17589–17594.

Aronow, W. & Ahn, C. (1997) Association of post prandial hypotension with incidence of falls, syncope, coronary events, stroke, and total mortality at 29 months follow-up in 499 older nursing home residents. *Journal of the American Geriatrics Society*, **45**, 1051–1053.

Australian Diabetes Society (ADS) (2012) Guidelines for Routine Glucose Control in Hospital, ADS, Canberra.

Australian Institute of Health and Welfare (AIHW) (2002) *Aged Care*. www.aihw.gov.au/agedcare/ (accessed October 2012).

Australian Medicines Handbook (AMH) (2010) Aged Care Companion (3rd edn) AMH, Melbourne.

Australian Quality Council (1998) Accreditation Standards for Aged Care. Australian Quality Council, Canberra.

Australian Diabetes Educators Association (ADEA) (2003) Guidelines for the Management and Care of Diabetes in the Elderly. ADEA, Canberra.

Asimakopoulou, S. & Hampson, E. (2002) Cognitive Functioning and Self-Management in Older People With Diabetes. *Diabetes Spectrum*, **15** (2), 116–121.

Baines, S. & Roberts, D. (2001) Undernutrition in the community. *Australian Prescriber*, **24** (5),113–115.

Basu, A., Basu, R., Sha, P. *et al*. (2001) Type 2 diabetes impairs splanchnic uptake of glucose but does not alter intestinal glucose absorption during enteral glucose feeding. *Diabetes*, **50**, 1351–1362.

Bayliss, E., Ellis, J. & Steiner, J. (2007) Barriers to self-management and quality of life outcomes in seniors with multimorbidities. *Annals of Family Medicine*, **5** (5), 395–402.

Berthold, H., Landahl, S. & Svanborg, A. (1991) Intermittent care and caregivers at home. *Ageing*, **3** (1), 51–56.

Beverly, E., Fitzgerald, S., Sitnikov, L. *et al*. (2012) *Do older adults aged 60 to 70 years benefit from diabetes behavioural interventions?* http://creativecommons.org/licenses/hy-ne-nd/3.0 (accessed December 2012).

Biessels, G., Staekenborg, S., Brunner, E. *et al*. (2006) Risk of dementia in diabetes mellitus: A systematic review. *The Lancet Neurology*, **5** (1), 64–74.

Bogner, H., Morales, K., Post, E. & Bruce, M. (2007) Diabetes, depression, and death: A randomized controlled trial of a depression treatment program for older adults based in primary care (PROSPECT). *Diabetes Care*, **30**, 3005–3010.

Bortz, W. (2002) A conceptual framework of frailty: A review. *Journal of Gerontology*, **75** (5), 283–288.

Bourdel-Marchasson, I., Proux, S. & Dehail, P. *et al*. (2004) One-year incidence of hyperosmolar states and prognosis in a geriatric acute care unit. *Gerontology*, **50** (3), 171–176.

Bostock, S. & Steptoe, A. (2012) Association between low functional health literacy and mortality in older adults: Longitudinal cohort study. *British Medical Journal*, **3**, 344 DOI: http://dx.doi.org/10.1136/bmj.e1602.

British Diabetic Association (1999) Guidelines for Residents with Diabetes in Care Homes. British Diabetic Association, London.

Brown, A., Mangione, C., Saliba, D. & Sarkisian, A. (2003) California Healthcare Foundation/American Geriatrics Society Panel on Improving Care for Elders with Diabetes. Guidelines for improving the care of the older person with diabetes mellitus. *Journal of the American Geriatric Society*, **55** Suppl Guidelines, S265–S280.

Cahoon, C. (2012) Depression in older adults *American Journal of Nursing*, **112** (11), 22–30.

Carmichael, O., Schwarz, C. & Drucker, D. (2010) Alzheimer's Disease Neuroimaging Initiative. Longititudinal changes in white matter disease and cognition in the first year of the Alzheimer's disease neuroimaging initiative. *Archives of Neurology*, **67** (11), 1370–1378.

Callan B, Wells T. (2003) Views of community-dwelling old-old people on barriers and aids to nutritional health *Journal of Nursing Scholarship*, **35** (3), 257–262.

Chen, X., Beydoun, M. A. & Wang, Y. (2008) Is sleep duration associated with childhood obesity? A systematic review and meta-analysis. *Obesity*, **16** (2), 265–274.

Connell, F., Shaw, C. & Will, J. (1991) Lower extremity amputations among people with diabetes: Washington State. Olympia Washington State Department of Health Diabetes Control Program *MMWR* **40**, 737–739.

Clemson, L., Fiatarone Singh, M., Bundy, A. *et al*. (2012) Integration of balance and strength training into daily life activity to reduce rate of falls in older people (the LIFE study): Randomized panel trial. *British Medical Journal*, **340** (c2244), 1042–1043.

Cluning, T. (2001) Aging at Home: Practical Approaches to Community Care. Ausmed Publications, Melbourne.

Coussement, J., De Paepe, L., Schwendimann, R. *et al.* (2008) Interventions for Preventing Falls in Acute- and Chronic-Care Hospitals: A Systematic Review and Meta-Analysis *Journal American Geriatric Society*, **56**, 29–36.

Crook Hally, V. & Panteli, J. (2001) The importance of the refeeding syndrome. *Nutrition*, **17**, 632–637.

Croxon, S. (2000) Diabetes in United Kingdom care homes *Practical Diabetes International*, **17** (3), 1868–1869.

Cryer, P. (2007) Hypoglycaemia, functional brain failure, and brain death. *Journal of Clinical Investigation*, **117**, 868–870.

Davidson, R., Kabat-Zinn, J., Schumacher, J., *et al.* (2003) Alterations in brain and immune function produced by mindfulness meditation. *Psychosomatic Medicine*, **65** (4), 564–570.

Davis, T. (2003) Patient-managed records: Their use in diabetes care. *Diabetes Management Journal*, **5** (18), 4–7.

Department of Health (2001) Care Homes for Older People: National Minimal Standards. Care Standards Act 2000. HMSO, London.

Department of Health and Aging (DOHA) (2012) Guidelines for Medicine Management in Residential Aged care facilities. DOHA, Canberra.

Department of Health Victoria (2004) VicFit Active Life programs www.health.vic.gov.au/archive/archive2005/.../programs.htm (accessed January 2013).

Department of Health Victoria (2013) Improving Care for Older People. www.health.vic.gov.au/older/policy.htm (accessed February 2013).

Devitt, H. (2011) Exploring nutrition for older people with diabetes. *Australian Diabetes Educator*, **14** (2), 16–19.

Digby, R. (2012) Focus on falls prevention. *Australian Nursing Journal*, **10** (17), 35.

Dregan, A., Stewart, R. & Gulliford, M. (2012) *Age and Aging*. DOI: 10.1093/aging/afs/66 (accessed December 2012).

Drewnowski, A. & Warren-Mears, V. (2001) Does aging change nutrition requirements? *Journal of Nutrition, Health and Aging*, **5** (2), 70–74.

Dunning, P. & Alford, F. (1993) Dilemmas in the management of the elderly diabetic. A community or medical problem? *Medical Journal of Australia*, **3**, 158–164.

Egede, L., Xiaobou, Y., Zheng, D. & Silverstein, M. (2002) The prevalence and pattern of complementary and alternative medicine use in individuals with diabetes. *Diabetes Care*, **25**, 324–329.

Elias, M., Ceriello, A., Laube, H. *et al.* (2005) Enteral nutrition support and use of diabetes-specific formulas for patients with diabetes. *Diabetes Care*, **28**, 2267–2279.

Engle, K. & Hannawa, T. (1999) Techniques for administering oral medications to critical care patients receiving continuous enteral nutrition. *American Journal of Health Systems Pharmacy*, **56** (14), 1441–1444.

Faes, M., Spigt, M. & Olde Rikkert, M. (2007) Dehydration in geriatrics. *Geriatrics and Aging*, **10** (9), 590–596.

Fenton, W. & Stover, E. (2006) Mood disorders: Cardiovascular and diabetes comorbidity. *Current Opinion in Psychiatry*, **19**, 421–427,

Fleming, R. (2002) Report of Federal Department of Health survey into depression in the elderly. *Australian Doctor*, March 14, 10–11.

Flood, L. & Constance, A. (2002) Diabetes and exercise safety. *American Journal of Nursing*, **102** (6), 47–55.

Franco, V., Polanczyk, C., Clausell, N., *et al.* (2004). Role of dietary vitamin K intake in chronic oral anticoagulation: Prospective evidence from observational and randomized protocols. *American Journal of Medicine*, **116**, 651–656.

Fried, L., Ferrucci, L., Darer, J. *et al* (2004) Untangling the concepts of disability, frailty, and comorbidity: implications for improved targeting and care. *Journal of Gerontology American Biological Science Medical Science*. 59 M255–M263.

Friedman, R. & Kalant, N. (1998) Comparison of long term care in an acute institution and a long term care institution. *Canadian Medical Association Journal*, **159** (9), 1107–1113.

Gaughran, F., Walwyn, R., Lambkin-Williams, R. *et al.* (2007) Flu: Effect of vaccine in elderly care home residents: A randomized trial. *Journal of the American Geriatric Society*, **55** (12), 1912–1920.

Giannelli, A., Patel, K. & Windham, G. (2007) Magnitude of underascertainment of impaired kidney function in older adults with normal serum creatinine. *American Geriatric Society*, **55** (6), 816–823.

Gilbar, P. (1999) A guide to enteral drug administration in palliative care. *Journal of Pain and Symptom Management*, **17** (3), 197–207.

Gilden, J., Hendryx, M., Clar, S., Casia, C. & Singh, S. (1992) Diabetes support groups improve health care of older diabetic patients. *Journal of the American Geriatric Society*, **40**, 145–150.

Gradman, T., Laes, A., Thompson, L. & Reaven, G. (1993) Verbal learning and/or memory improves with glycaemic control in older subjects with non insulin-dependent diabetes mellitus. *Journal of the American Geriatrics Society*, **41**, 1305–1312.

Graham, J., Christian, L. & Kiecolt-Glaser, J. (2006) Stress, Age, and Immune Function: Toward a Lifespan Approach. *Journal of Behavioral Medicine*, **29** (4), 9057–9064.

Gray, L., Woodward, M., Scholes, R., *et al.* (2002) Geriatric Medicine, 2nd edn, Ausmed Publications, Melbourne.

Gregg, E., Yaffe, K., Cauley, J., *et al.* (2000) Is diabetes associated with cognitive impairment and cognitive decline among older women? *Archives of Internal Medicine*, **160**, 174–180.

Gregg, E., Mangione, C., Cauley, J., *et al.* (2002) Diabetes and incidence of functional disability in older women. *Diabetes Care*, **25**, 61–67.

Gross, P. A., Hermogenes, A., Sacks, H., Lau, J. & Levandowski, R. (1995) The efficacy of influenza vaccine in elderly persons. A meta-analysis and review of the literature. *Annals of Internal Medicine*, **123** (7), 518–527.

Grossman, T. (2005) Latest advances in anitaging medicine. *Keio Journal of Medicine*, **54** (2), 85–94.

Goldney, R., Phillips, P. & Fisher L. (2004) Diabetes, depression and quality of life. *Diabetes Care*, **27**, 1066–1070.

Gooberman-Hill, R. & Ebrahim, S. (2007) Making decisions about simple interventions: Older people use of walking aids. *Age and Aging*, **36** (5), 569–573.

Halter, J. (2001) Report of the American Diabetes Association Meeting. *Practical Diabetes International*, **18** (7), 251–258.

Howes, L. (2001) Dosage alteration in the elderly – Importance of mild renal impairment. *Current Therapeutics*, **42** (7), 33–35.

Hong, K., Ngyuen, Y. & Ogden, J. (2004) Understanding HIV and AIDS-Related Stigma in Vietnam. International Center for Research on Women Research Report. ICRW, Washington.

Hu, G., Eriksson, J., Barengo, N.C., *et al.* (2004). Occupational commuting and leisure-time physical activity in relation to total and cardiovascular mortality among Finnish subjects with type 2 diabetes. *Circulation*, **110**, 666–673.

Hudson, H., Daubert, C. & Mills, R. (2000) The interdependency of protein-energy malnutrition, aging, and dysphagia. *Dysphagia*, **15** (1), 31–38.

Inouye, S., van Dyck, C., Alessi, C. *et al.* (1990). Clarifying confusion: The confusion assessment method. *Annals of Internal Medicine*, **113** (12), 941–948.

Jackson, L. & Janoff, E. (2008) Pneumococcal vaccination of elderly adults: new paradigms for protection. *Clinical Infectious Diseases*, **47**, 1328–1338.

Jennings, P. (1997) Oral antihypoglycaemics: Considerations in older patient with non insulin-dependent diabetes mellitus. *Drugs and Aging*, **10** (5), 323–331.

Kaffashian, S., Dugravot, A. & Nabi, H. (2011) Predictive utility of the Framingham general cardiovascular risk profile for cognitive function: Evidence from the Whitehall 11 Study. *European Heart Journal* **32**, 2326–2332.

Katona, C. (1994) Depression in Old Age. John Wiley and Sons, New York.

Keller, H. *et al.* (2004) Nutritional risk predicts quality of life in elderly community-living Canadians. *Journal of Gerontological Association Biological Science Medical Science*, **59** (1), 68–74.

Kirkman, S., Briscoe, V., Clark, N., *et al.* (2012) Diabetes in Older Adults: A Consensus Report. *Journal of the American Geriatric Society*, DOI: 10.1111/jgs.12035

Kock, S. & Garratt, S. (2001) Assessing Older People: A Guide for Health Care Workers. McLennan and Petty, Eastgardens NSW, Australia.

Kulminski, A., Ukrantseva, S., Akushevic, I., Arbeev, K. & Yashin, A. (2007) Cumulative index of health deficiencies as a characteristic of long life. *Journal of the American Geriatric Society*, **55** (6), 935–940.

Lan, C., Lai, J., Chen, S. & Wong, M. (1998) 12-month Tai Chi training in the elderly: its effect on health fitness. *Medicine Science Sports Exercise*, **30** (3), 345–351.

Langa, R. (2004) Extent and cost of informal caregiving for older Americans with symptoms of depression. *American Journal of Psychiatry*, **161** (5), 857–863.

Lavizzo-Mourey, R., Johnson, J. & Stolley, P. (1998) Risk factors for dehydration among elderly nursing home residents. *Journal of the American Geriatric Society*, **36**, 213–218.

Li, F. (2012) Tai Chi and postural stability in patients with Parkinson's disease. *New England Journal of Medicine*, **366** (5), 511–519.

Lipscombe, L., Hux, J. & Booth, G. (2005) Reduced screening mammography among women with diabetes. *Archives of Internal Medicine*, **165**, 2090–2095.

Logroscino, G., Kang, J. & Grodstein, F. (2004) Prospective study of type 2 diabetes and cognitive decline in women aged 70–81 years. *British Medical Journal*, **328**, 548–551.

Maaravi, Y., Berry, E., Ginsberg, G. *et al.* (2000) Nutrition and quality of life in the aged: the Jerusalem 70-year olds longitudinal study. *Aging*, **12** (3), 173–179.

Martire, L. (2010) Treatment of late-life depression alleviates caregiver burden. *Journal of the American Geriatrics Society*, **58** (1), 23–29.

Masters, R., Powers, D. & Link, B. (2013) Obesity and US mortality risk over the adult life course *American Journal of Epidemiology*, DOI: 10.1093/aje/kws325.

Mathiesen, B. & Borch-Johnsen, K. (1997) Diabetes and accident insurance: A three year follow up of 7,599 insured diabetic individuals. *Diabetes Care*, **20** (11), 1781–1784.

McAulay, V., Deary, I. & Frier, B. (2001) Symptoms of hypoglycaemia in people with diabetes. *Diabetic Medicine*, **18**, 690–705.

McWhirter, J. & Pennington, C. (1994) Incidence and recognition of malnutrition in hospitals. *British Medical Journal*, **306**, 945–948.

Meuleman, J, Brechue, W. & Kubilis, P., (2000) Exercise training in the debilitated aged: strength and functional outcomes. *Archives of Physical Medicine and Rehabilitation*, **81**, 312–318.

Medical Research Council (1994) The Health of the UK's Elderly People. Medical Research Council London.

Middleton, M., Nazarenko, G., Nivison-Smith, I. & Smerdely, P. (2001) Prevalance of malnutrition and 12-month incidence of mortality in two Sydney teaching hospitals. *International Medicine Journal*, **31**, 455–461.

Miller, C. (1999) Nursing Care of Older Adults, 3rd edition. Lippincott Williams and Wilkins, Philadelphia.

Mitchell, J. (2011). *Oral dosage forms that should not be crushed.* http://www.ismp.org/tools/donot-crush.pdf (Accessed March 2013).

Morley, J. & Flood, J. (1990) Psychological aspects of diabetes mellitus in older persons. *Journal of the American Geriatrics Society*, **38**, 605–606.

Mooradian R, McLaughlin S, Boyer C (1999) Diabetes care for older adults *Diabetes Spectrum*, **12**, 70–77. .

Moyer, A. (2012) Prevention of falls in community-dwelling older adults: US Preventative Services Taskforce recommendations. *Annals of Internal Medicine*, May 29, www.annals.org (accessed November 2012).

Nay, R. & Garrat, S. (1999). Sexuality in aged care, in Nursing Older People: Issues and Innovations, (eds R. Nay, & S. Garrat). MacLennan & Petty Pty Ltd, Sydney.

NHMRC (National Health and Medical Research Council) (1994) *Health Care and The Elderly: Series on Clinical Management Problems in the Elderly*, www.nhmrc.gov.au/_files_nhmrc/publications/attachments/ac3.pdf (accessed December 2012)

NHMRC (National Health and Medical Research Council) (2009) NHMRC Guidelines to reduce risks from alcohol www.nhmrc.gov.au/_files_nhmrc/publications/.../ds10-alcohol.pdf (accessed November 2012).

NPS (National Prescribing Service) (2004) *NPS Service Newsletter*. www.nps.org.au (accessed October 2012).

Oates, D., Berlowitz, D.& Glickman, M., *et al.* (2007) Blood pressure and survival in the oldest old. *Journal American Geriatric Society*, **55**, 383–388.

Orford, J., Sesso, H., Stedman, M. *et al.* (2002) A comparison of the Framingham and European Society of Cardiology coronary heart disease risk prediction models in the normative aging study. *American Heart Journal*, **144** (1), 95–100.

Paolisso, G., Gambardella, A., Verza, M. *et al.* (1992) ACE-inhibition improves insulin-sensitivity in age insulin-resistant hypertensive patients. *Journal of Human Hypertension*, **6**, 175–179.

Parlente, A. (2012) Antipsychotic use and Myocardial infarction in older patients with treated dementia. *Archives of Internal Medicine*, **172** (8), 648–653.

Patel, N., Newstead, A. & Ferrer, R. (2012) The effects of yoga on physical functioning and health related quality of life in older adults: A systematic review and meta-analysis *Journal of Alternative and Complementary Medicine*, **18** (10), 902–917.

Persson, M., Brismar, K., Katzarski, K. *et al.* (2002) Nutritional status using mini nutritional assessments and subjective global assessments predicts mortality in geriatric patients. *Journal of the American Geriatrics Society*, **50** (12), 1992–200.

Peters, A. & Davidson, M. (1992) Effects of various enteral feeding products on postprandial blood glucose response in patients with type 1 diabetes. *Journal of Parenteral and Enteral Nutrition*, **16** (1), 69–74.

Petterson, T., Young, B., Lee, P., *et al.* (1998) wellbeing and treatment satisfaction in older people with diabetes. *Diabetes Care*, **21** (6), 930–935.

Phillips, P. & Popplewell, P. (2002) Diabetes and Dementia. *Medicine Today*, **3** (11), 30–40.

Poon, I. & Braun, U. (2006) High prevalence of orthostatic hypotension and its correlation with potentially causative medications among elderly veterans. *Journal of Clinical Pharmacy Therapy*, **30** (2), 173–178.

Quayle, S. (2001) Gains of minimising falls: Managing the older patient. *Australian Doctor*, **July**, 43–44.

Ragan, M. & Kane, C. (2010) Meaningful lives: Elders in treatment for depression. *Archives of Psychiatric Nursing*, **24** (6), 408–417.

Reilly, H. (1996) Screening for nutritional risk. *Proceedings of the Nutrition Society*, **55**, 841–853.

Reza, M., Taylor, C. & Towse, *et al.* (2002) Insulin improves wellbeing for selected elderly type 2 diabetic subjects. *Diabetes Research and Clinical Practice*, **55** (3), 201–207.

Rosenstock, J. (2001) Management of Type 2 diabetes in the elderly: Special considerations. *Pulsebeat*, **Oct–Nov**, 5.

Royal Melbourne Hospital (2002) Project report: The prevention of **functional decline** in elderly patients, www.rmh.mh.org.au/project-reports/w1/i1017258/ (accessed December 2012).

Rutherford, A., Wright, E. D, Hussain, Z & Colagiuri, R. on behalf of the Australasian DAWN Advisory Group. (2004) DAWN: Diabetes Attitudes, Wishes and Needs – The Australian Experience. Novo Nordisk Australia, Sydney.

Schwartz, M., Woods, S., Porte, D., Seeley, R. & Baskin, D. (2000) Central nervous system control of food intake. *Nature*, **404**, 661–671.

Schwartz, A., Sellmeyer, D., Ensrud, K., *et al.* (2001) Older women with diabetes have an increased risk of fracture: a prospective study. *Journal of Clinical Endocrinology Metabolism*, **86**, 32–38.

Schwartz, A., Vittinghoff, E., Sellmeye, D, *et al.* (2003) Health, Aging, and Body Composition Study Diabetes-related complications, glycemic control, and falls in older adults. *Diabetes Care*, **3**, 391–396.

Schwartz, A., Vittinghoff, E., Sellmeyer D, *et al.* (2008) Diabetes-related complications, glycaemic control and falls in older adults *Diabetes Care*, **31** (3), 391–396.

Shekelle, P. & Vijan, S. (2007) ACOVE: Quality indicators for the care of diabetes mellitus in vulnerable elders. *Journal American Geriatric Society*, **55** Suppl S, S312–S317.

Simkin, B. (2004) Even frail elderly patients can benefit from exercise. *Geriatric Times*, **3** (4) 331–334.

Simpson, C. (2005) Crushed medications: An emerging guideline. *Australian Nursing Journal*, **13** (1) Clinical Update, 1–4.

Sinclair, A. (1995) Initial management of NIDDM in the elderly, in Diabetes in Old Age (eds P. Funacane & A. Sinclair). John Wiley & Sons, Chichester, pp. 181–201.

Sinclair, A. (2006) Special considerations in older adults with diabetes: meeting the challenge. *Diabetes Spectrum*, **19**, 218–219.

Sinclair, A., Allard, I. & Bayes, A. (1997) Observation of diabetes care in long-term institutional settings with measures of cognitive function and dependency. *Diabetes Care*, **20** (5), 778–786.

Sinlcair, A., Conroy, S. & Bayer, A. (2008) Impact of diabetes on physical function in older people. *Diabetes Care*, **31** (2), 233–235.

Sinclair, A. (2011) Diabetes care for older people: A practical view on management. *Diabetes and Primary Care* **13** (1), 29–37.

Sinclair, A., Morley, J., Rodriguez, L., *et al.* (2012) Diabetes mellitus in older people: Position statement on behalf of the International Association of Gerontology and Geriatrics (IAGG), the European Diabetes Working Party for Older People (EDWPOP), and the International Taskforce of Experts in Diabetes. *Journal of Applied Research and Clinical Issues*, **13** (6), 497–502.

Speight, J., Brown, J.L., Holmes-Truscott, E., Hendrieckx, C. & Pouwer, F. (2011) Diabetes MILES – Australia 2011 Survey Report. Diabetes Australia, Canberra.

Sommerfield, A., Deary, I., McAuley, V., *et al.* (2003) Short term delayed and working memory are impaired during hyperglycaemia in individuals with type 1 diabetes. *Diabetes Care*, **26**, 390–396.

Stewart, R. & Liolitsa, D. (1999) Type 2 diabetes mellitus, cognitive impairment and dementia. *Diabetic Medicine*, **16**, 93–112.

Stressman, J., Hammerman-Rozenberg, R., Maaravi, Y. *et al.* (2002) Effects of exercise on ease in performing activities of daily living and instrumental activities of daily living from age 70 to 77: The Jersalem longitudinal study. *Journal of the American Geriatrics Society*, **50** (12), 1934–1938.

Szony, G. (2004) Investigating weight loss in the elderly. *Medicine Today*, 5 (9), 53–57.

Takata Y., T. Ansai I. Soh S. Akifusa, *et al.* (2007). Association between body mass index and mortality in an 80-year-old population. *Journal of the American Geriatrics Society*, 55 (6), 913–917.

Testa, M., Simonson, D., Turner, R. (1998) Valuing quality of life and improvements in glycaemic control in people with type 2 diabetes. *Diabetes Care*, **21** (suppl. 3), c44–c52.

Tiengo, A. (1999) Burden of treatment in the elderly patient: Reducing the burden of diabetes. *Diabetes Care*, **11**, 6–8.

Toraski C (2004) Care giving demands increase with depression symptoms in the elderly. *American Journal of Psychiatry*, **16**, 1857–1863.

Truswell, A. (2003) Nutrient Supplements. *Australian Doctor*, **21**, March:i–iv.

Tsai, J., Wang, W., Chan, P. *et al.* (2003) The beneficial effects of Tai Chi Chuan on blood pressure and lipid profile and anxiety status in a randomized controlled trial. *Journal Alternative and Complementary Medicine*, **9** (5), 747–754.

UK Prospective Diabetes Study (UKPDS) Group (1998). Intensive blood-glucose control with sulphony-lureas or insulin compared with conventional treatment and risk of complications in patients with type 2 diabetes (UKPDS 33). *Lancet*, **352**, 837–853.

US National Institutes of Health (NIH) (undated) *Aging Under the Microscope: A Biological Quest.* http://www.nia.nih.gov/HealthInformationPublications/AgingUndertheMicroscope/   (accessed February 2008).

VaikeResa , P., Ebersold, C., Shah, M., *et al.* (2002) Effects of aerobic exercise training in community-based subjects aged 80 and older: A pilot study. *Journal of the American Geriatrics Society*, **50** (12), 2009–2013.

Vance, D. (2012) Potential factors that may promote successful cognitive aging. *Nursing Research and Reviews*, **2**, 27–32.

van der Velde, N., van den Meiracker A., Pols, H. *et al.* (2007) Withdrawal of Fall-Risk-Increasing Drugs in Older Persons: Effect on Tilt-Table Test Outcomes. *Journal of the American Geriatric Society*, **55** (5), 734–739.

Verschoor, R. (2012) GEM unit a plus for older patients. *Australian Nursing Journal*, **10** (17), 36.

Verma, S., Luo, N., Subramaniam, M. et al (2010) Impact of depression on health related quality of life in patients with diabetes. *Annals of Academic Medicine Singapore*, **39** (12), 913–917.

Victoria Department of Health (2003) Recognising and supporting care relationships for older Victorians. www.health.vic.gov.au/agedcare/.../agedcare_action_plan_0806.pdf (accessed January 2013).

Vidan, M., Bueno, H., Wang, Y., *et al.* (2010) The relationship between systolic blood pressure on admission and mortality in older patients with heart failure *European Journal of Heart Failure*, **12** (2),148–155.

Volkert, D., Kreuel, K. & Stehle, P. (2005) Fluid intake of community-living, independent elderly in Germany – a nationwide representative study. *Journal of Nutrition Health Aging*, **9** (5), 305–309.

Warren, L., Bacon, W., Harris, T., *et al.* (1994) The burden and outcomes associated with dehydration among US elderly. *American Journal of Public Health*, **84**, 1265–1269.

Waszynski, C. (2004) *The Confusion Assessment Method (CAM) Best Practice in Nursing Care of Older Adults* (13), Revised 2012. New York University, New York.

Weinberg, A. D., Minaker, K. L., Council on Scientific Affairs AMA. (1995) Dehydration: Evaluation and management in older adults. *Journal of the American Medical Association*, **274** (19), 1552.

Wetzels, R., Harmsen, M., van Weel, C., Grol, R. & Wensing, M. (2007) Interventions for improving older patients' involvement in primary care episodes. *Cochrane Database of Systematic Reviews*, Issue 1, Art. No.: CD004273. DOI 10. 1002/14651858. CD004273.pub2.

Wilson, M. & Morley, J. (2003) Impaired cognitive function and mental performance in mild dehydration. *European Journal of Clinical Nutrition*, **57** (Suppl 2), S24–S29.

World Health Organisation (1983) Healthy Aging Profiles www.euro.who.int/document/e91887.pdf (accessed December 2012).

World Health Organization (1999) Guidelines for Older Australians. Commonwealth of Australia, Canberra.

Young, C. (2004) Pharmacy Drug Information Paper Prepared in Response to a Personal Enquiry About Administering Commonly Used Diabetes Medications Via Enteral Tubes. St Vincent's Hospital, Melbourne.

Zembrzuski, C. (1997) A three dimensional approach to hydration of elders: Administration, clinical staff, and in service education. *Geriatric Nursing*, **18** (1), 20–26.

Zhao, W., Chen, H., Xu, H. *et al.* (1999) Brain insulin receptors and spatial memory. *Journal of Biological Chemistry*, **274**, 34893–34901.

Zimmerman, S., Sloane, P. D., Williams, C. S. *et al.* (2007) *Journal of the American Geriatric Society*, **55** (9), 1349–1355. (Residential care/assisted living staff may detect undiagnosed dementia using the minimum data set cognition scale.)

Zuliani G. (2012) Discharge diagnosis and comorbidity profile in hosptalised older patients with dementia. *International Journal of Geriatric Psychiatry* **27** (3), 313–320.

Chapter 13
Diabetes in Children and Adolescents

Key points

- A supportive family is an important aspect of diabetes management.
- Family stress and marital disharmony affect the child's metabolic control.
- Clinicians caring for with children and adolescents with diabetes must diplomatically assess the family structure and social situation and help the family to support their child.
- Management and education strategies must be applicable to the age and developmental stage of the individual.
- Most children have Type 1 diabetes and insulin should never be withheld in these children.
- There is increasing prevalence of Type 2 diabetes in children and adolescents and complications are often evident at diagnosis or occur soon after diagnosis, thus a complication assessment should be part of the initial assessment.
- Management strategies are different for children with Type 1 and Type 2 diabetes but both require an appropriate nutritious diet and regular exercise to sustain normal growth and development.

Rationale

Diabetes management in children and adolescents changes during the various transitions that occur as the child grows and develops. Diabetes and its management impacts on the family dynamics and can affect quality of life and mental well being. Family support is essential if the child is to achieve euglycaemia and psychological well being. Thus, the family needs to be included in education and management decisions. Management plans need to make provision for normal growth and development and a gradual transition to independent self-care and often transition from paediatric to an adult care

Care of People with Diabetes: A Manual of Nursing Practice, Fourth Edition. Trisha Dunning.
© 2014 John Wiley & Sons, Ltd. Published 2014 by John Wiley & Sons, Ltd.

service, which is often also stressful and often occurs when other major life changes are occurring such as entering university or starting work.

Introduction

The number of children diagnosed with Type 1 diabetes is increasing globally and Type 2 diabetes in children is an emerging global problem. The incidence varies but ~70/000 children <14 years are diagnosed annually and an estimated 440/000 children have diabetes worldwide (EURODIAB 2000; Soltesz 2007; Alberti *et al.* 2004). Lee (2008) reported a 38% increase in the number of hospital admissions with diabetes in children aged 0–29 years between 1993 and 2004. The hospitalisation rate was higher in girls, 42% versus 29% for males.

In most countries girls and boys are equally affected by diabetes but the rate is not the same among age groups. Diabetes tends to increase with age, peaking around puberty, usually slightly earlier in girls, which is consistent with the earlier onset of puberty. The global incidence is estimated to increase by ~50% in the next 15 years (Soltesz 2007). In Australia ~1 in 500 children <15 years have Type 1 diabetes.

A number of forms of diabetes occur in childhood. Type 1 was formerly the most common especially in children <10 years, but the incidence of Type 2 in children and adolescents is increasing, as indicated.

- Type 1, which accounts for ~98% of diabetes diagnosed in children and results from beta cell destruction leading to absolute insulin deficiency, immune-mediated or idiopathic (Craig *et al.* 2009).
- Type 2, which has an increasing prevalence.
- Other specific types:
  ○ Type 2 diabetes, which mostly occurs in overweight children and adolescents.
  ○ Monogenic defects of beta cell function, for example, familial diabetes, neonatal diabetes. Neonatal diabetes presents in the first 6 months of life (Srinivasan & Donaghue 2007; Craig *et al.* 2009). About 50% have transient neonatal diabetes and insulin treatment is usually not required with ~3 months, but may recur in the second or third decade.
  ○ Diabetes as a consequence of diseases of the exocrine pancreas, for example, cystic fibrosis-related diabetes (Chapter 10).
  ○ Diabetes associated with endocrine diseases such as Cushing's syndrome and hyperthyroidism.
  ○ Medicine-or chemical-induced diabetes, for example, chemotherapy, glucocorticoids.
  ○ Diabetes associated with genetic syndromes such as Trisomy and Down's and Turner's syndromes.

The reasons for the increased incidence of Type 1 diabetes in children are relatively unclear. Various explanations have been proposed; for example, genetic factors such as the 'thrifty gene' (Need 1962), the 'thrifty phenotype' (Hales & Barker 1992) theories. More recently, the focus has been on environmental changes that could overload the beta cells, which gave rise to the 'overload hypothesis' and the 'spring harvest hypothesis' in which genetically predisposed children have an accelerated growth rate and increased body fat during spring. Likewise, puberty occurs at a younger age. Various environmental triggers such as the decline in breast feeding, age at which solids are introduced, exposure to foreign antigens early in life that impair the immune system, impact of maternal diet and the 'hygiene hypothesis,' have been implicated (Chapter 1).

Currently an important study, The TRIGIR study, is underway. It involves 2160 newborn infants with first-degree relatives with Type 1 diabetes and lasted for 6–8 months and included. HLA typing was performed on cord blood or heel prick at birth. All mothers are encouraged to breastfeed and two weaning formulas were compared: hydrolysed casein and standard cow's milk. The randomised code will be opened when the last recruited child turns 10 years of age (2017) (Akerblom 2011). The study will provide important information about the protective effect of breast feeding and Type 1 diabetes.

Diabetes is often misdiagnosed or the diagnosis is delayed in developing regions and under-resourced communities in developed countries, where the symptoms might be attributed to malnutrition or starvation because people do not know the signs and symptoms (Kaufman & Riley 2007). As a consequence, morbidity and mortality rates are high and are compounded by lack of equipment and essential medications. The International Diabetes Federation (IDF) insulin for life programme has had a significant impact on the lives and survival of many children in underprivileged countries.

Type 2 diabetes, once rare in children, is increasing (IDF Consultative Section on Diabetes Education 2002; Sinha *et al.* 2002; Alberti *et al.* 2004; Wilmot *et al.* 2010). Up to 45% of newly diagnosed diabetes in children and adolescents is Type 2 (Shaw 2007). Emerging epidemiological data indicate Type 2 diabetes mainly occurs in overweight children from specific ethnic groups particularly African Americans, Hispanics, Asians, Native Americans, Indigenous Australians, and Middle Eastern people (Shaw 2007). The increasing prevalence in Asian countries is linked to the increase in western lifestyles with high fat diets and reduced exercise (Gill 2007).

A recent study points to a link between increasing obesity and high consumption of fructose (American Journal Public Health 2007). Fructose appears to affect fat degradation in the liver by inhibiting PPAR-alpha receptor activity, which is lower in humans than rats, and the leptin signalling system, which accelerates fat oxygenation in the liver and reduces fat synthesis (Gressner *et al* 2007). Insulin resistance and impaired glucose tolerance and other features of the metabolic syndrome are present in 25% of obese children, which puts them at high risk of Type 2 diabetes (Sinha *et al.* 2002).

In addition, high rates of television viewing, an indicator of inactivity, are associated with increased risk of developing diabetes and higher HbA_{1c} (Margeirsdottir *et al.* 2007; Wilmot *et al.* 2012). Other possible causes include maternal obesity and maternal malnutrition during pregnancy and low birth weight (Wei *et al.* 2003) and low birth weight associated with 'catch up growth' (Bhargava *et al.* 2004), see Chapters 1, 4 and 14. These findings led to the theory of the Developmental Origins of Health and Disease (DOHaD) (Yajnik 2007). The Scientific Advisory Committee on Nutrition (SACN) (2011) advised against the early introduction of gluten because of a possible link between feeding gluten-containing foods before 4 months and Type 1 diabetes and coeliac disease. Introducing gluten-containing foods after 4 months and before sis months might reduce these risks. The SACN position statement is currently being revised.

Although the onset of Type 2 diabetes may be less dramatic than Type 1, Type 2 diabetes in children is associated with significant risk of dyslipidaemia, hypertension, and polycystic ovarian syndrome, asthma, and obstructive sleep apnoea (Tait 2008). Cardiovascular disease develops at an early age and is often present at diagnosis (Pinhas-Hamiel 2007) and progression to complications is faster than in children with Type 1 diabetes. Significantly, children and adolescents with Type 2 diabetes may be at higher risk of microvascular disease especially nephropathy than those with Type 1 (Alberti *et al.* 2004; Shaw 2007).

Thus, early identification through comprehensive population health and screening programmes and effective management of Type 2 diabetes in children is imperative to reduce the burden of the disease and the projected health care costs and should include school-based programmes (Weiss & Caprio 2005; Zimmett *et al.* 2007). However, the best screening test to use is unclear (Alberti *et al.* 2004). The IDF recently introduced diagnostic criteria for the metabolic syndrome in children, which is described in Chapter I. It is important to differentiate among Type 1, Type 2 and monogenic diabetes because the therapeutic approaches and education required differ among the three forms. It may be necessary to measure diabetes-associated autoantibodies such as ICA, GAD, IA 2 and IAA to detect underlying genetic abnormalities. HbA_{1c} might be useful but the evidence to support HbA_{1c} as a diagnostic tool is still debated (Craig *et al.* 2009). Measuring fasting insulin and/or c-peptide when the blood glucose is high enough to stimulate insulin release might be useful to diagnose Type 2 diabetes in young people (Craig *et al.* 2009).

Managing children and adolescents with diabetes

The health care needs of children and adolescents change as they grow and develop regardless of diabetes type. Some aspects of care are common to both Type 1 and Type 2 but there are inherent differences in managing Type 1 and Type 2. Multidisciplinary team care involving a paediatric endocrinologist, diabetes educator, dietitian, psychologist, and other experts as indicated is essential to achieving optimal outcomes.

A number of management guidelines and position statements are in current use and should be referred to for specific detailed information. These include:

- National Evidence-Based Clinical Care Guidelines for Type 1 Diabetes in Children, Adolescents and adults (2012) Australian Paediatric Endocrine Group and the Australian Diabetes Society.
- Standards of medical care in diabetes: special considerations for children and adolescents (ADA 2013).
- SIGN (2010).
- Nice Guidelines.
- Clinical Practice Consensus Guidelines (2009) Compendium International Society for Paediatric and Adolescent Diabetes.

Aspects of care that apply to both Type 1 and Type 2 diabetes in children and adolescents

Where possible, education and stabilisation at diagnosis should occur in an ambulatory setting. However, hospitalisation is necessary in ~30% of newly diagnosed Type 1 children (Silverstein *et al.* 2005). If hospitalisation is necessary, for example, in the case of ketoacidosis, the time spent in the hospital should be kept to a minimum. The overall aims of management are to provide an individualised education and management plan to achieve:

- An accurate diagnosis.
- Prevent or delay the onset of diabetes-related complications including short-term complications such as hypoglycaemia and ketoacidosis. Long-term complications are rare before puberty but complication screening typically begins around age 10 or earlier.
- A balanced nutritious diet suitable for the growth and development stage of the child.
- Acceptance of the diabetes by the child and the family.

- Assist the child to gradually take over the self-care tasks.
- Develop an holistic, integrated health plan that includes psychological heath, sexual health, responsible contraception and planned pregnancy suitable to the age and developmental stage of the young person.
- HbA$_{1c}$ should be measured 3–4 monthly and the target should be individualised working towards HbA$_{1c}$ 7.5% without hypoglycaemia.
- Admission to acute care should the need arise.
- Screening for microvascular complications and blood pressure generally commences between 10 and 12 years.
- Smooth transfer to adult care, which includes a structured familiarisation and education process, which should be a collaborative process between paediatric and adult services (SIGN 2010).
- Diabetes service providers and schools/education facilities should work together to ensure the child's diabetes self-care needs can be performed in school and school staff are knowledgeable about managing hypoglycaemia and disk days and have emergency telephone numbers if needed. Some Australian schools have structured gardening and cooking programmes that focus on preventative heath, healthy eating and activity.

Almost all guidelines recommend a knowledgeable and experienced multidisciplinary team provides diabetes care. The child should be involved in developing their diabetes management plan within their capabilities. Disagreements between the family and the child about who is responsible for managing their diabetes and poor adherence are predictors of high HbA$_{1c}$ (Anderson *et al.* 1991). The child's involvement in their self-care gradually increases as they mature and their fine motor and problem-solving and coping skill develop.

Differentiating between Type 1 and Type 2 diabetes at diagnosis is not always straight-forward due to the increasing prevalence of obesity, ketonuria, and diabetic ketoacidosis (DKA) (Svoren & Wolfsdorf 2006). About one third of adolescents with Type 2 diabetes are ketotic and 25% of newly diagnosed people present with DKA. If the diabetes type is not clear it may be advisable to measure islet cell autoantibodies and C-peptide. Table 1.2 in Chapter 1 depicts the main differences between Type 1 and Type 2 diabetes as discussed at the beginning of the chapter.

Regular assessment of general health and diabetes status and how the family is managing is essential because there are major physical, psychological, emotional, spiritual, and social differences among the growth and development stages. Assessing maturity, sensitive supervision and allowing the child to gradually take over specific diabetes self-care tasks according to their capability should be factored into an holistic diabetes plan. The family needs to be involved in developing the care plan and monitoring progress.

Educating teachers and other carers is also important and the child should be involved in these activities if appropriate. Diabetes should not preclude the child from attending school excursions and camps but extra precautions will need to be taken, for example, being able to eat on time. Diabetes camps provide an important learning experience and many children who attended camps when they were young help out on diabetic camps, as they grow older. The peer support children and adolescents receive in camps contributes to psychological well being (ADA 2004).

Preventive care includes regular blood glucose monitoring, complication screening, immunisation according to immunisation schedules and influenza vaccinations during at-risk periods when the child is >6 months as well as screening for other diseases associated with compromised immunity.

Managing Type 1 diabetes

Type 1 usually presents with a sudden onset of symptoms and insulin injections are needed for survival. A well balanced diet and adequate appropriate exercise are also essential. Insulin and dietary requirements can change rapidly, especially in children, due to rapid changes in activity levels and growth. Therefore, consistent acceptable blood glucose levels may be difficult to achieve.

(Silverstein *et al.* 2005) suggests the following insulin doses. The number of doses per day depends on a number of factors; increasingly basal bolus regimens are used for older children and adolescents:

- Newly diagnosed Type 1: initial dose ~0.5–1.0 units/kg/day. Lower doses may be required before puberty. Higher doses may be needed after puberty and in DKA. Infants and toddlers require very small doses. Insulin pens that can deliver 0.5 unit doses are available and should be used where possible. If these pens are not available the insulin may need to be diluted to achieve accurate 1 unit dose increments. Specific diluents are required for specific insulins and can be obtained from the relevant manufacturer. Great care and appropriate parental education is required for accurate dilutions.
- Newly diagnosed Type 1 is often followed by a honeymoon period once the acute metabolic disturbance is reversed. Endogenous insulin production increases for varying periods up to ~12 months. Insulin doses usually need to be reduced to prevent hypoglycaemia. Insulin requirements increase as the honeymoon phase ends and at the onset of puberty.
- During puberty 1.5 units/kg/day are often needed.

Screening for associated autoimmune diseases such as coeliac disease (Chapter 10), and thyroid disease may be required.

A supportive and encouraging family is important if the child is to accept diabetes and eventually take over diabetic self-management. The family in turn needs support, advice and encouragement. Good control is associated with a structured supportive family (Johnson *et al.* 1990; Thompson *et al.* 2001). Families need to provide appropriate supervision and discipline and maintain a family structure that meets the needs of the child and other family members.

Hypoglycaemia can be unpredictable in children whose activity level and intake and consequently insulin needs can vary enormously from day-to-day and within the day. Insulin need also change with exercise and pubertal hormone changes. Hypoglycaemia can be difficult to deal with in young children and can manifest as:

- unaccustomed naughtiness;
- noisy behaviour;
- aggression;
- crying;
- tremulousness.

If it is not recognised and treated promptly the child can become unconscious, which is frightening for the child and those around them (see Chapter 6). Parents often feel safer if they have glucagon available and some also like it to be available at school if the teacher or school nurse is appropriately educated. Nocturnal hypoglycaemia can be particularly difficult to manage. There may not be any significant long-term effects associated with nocturnal hypoglycaemia but it can affect mood the following day. The child maybe irritable on waking and might impair recognition of daytime hypoglycaemia

Table 13.1   Self-management expectations according to age and stage. (a) Metabolic targets need to be appropriate to the age and stage and revised regularly as the child grows and develops; and (b) recommended HbA$_{1c}$ targets.

key	Key milestones	Management considerations
(a) Developmental stage		
Babies <1 year	The parents are responsible for care Significant hypoglycaemia risk due to undeveloped catecholamine response	Family stress Unrecognised hypoglycaemia, coma, seizures Nocturnal hypoglycaemia
1–3 years	The parents are responsible for care Food refusal is common and increases the risk of hypoglycaemia Hypoglycaemia may manifest as temper tantrums	Consistent 'rules' and discipline are important Blood glucose testing is needed to distinguish normal toddler's behaviour from hypoglycaemia
3–7 years	Fine motor skills are developing and while the parents retain responsibility for providing care they should involve the child in their care	Involve the child in self-management
8–11 years	Children are capable of undertaking many diabetes self-management tasks but still require parental guidance and support They may enjoy diabetes camps and teaching their class about diabetes but care must be taken to ensure these activities do not negatively impact on their 'difference' from non-diabetic children	Diagnosis at this age often results in mild depression and depression increases with longer duration of diabetes but is different for girls and boys Depression may be precipitated when the 'honeymoon phase' ends.
Adolescence	Physical, cognitive, and emotional development occurs rapidly Puberty can affect metabolic control Diabetes self-care can inhibit independence Most adolescents should be responsible for their self-care but parental support and guidance are still needed	Poor metabolic control and non-adherence may indicate psychological problems or family conflict Parental support still needed but needs to be tactful
(b) HbA$_{1c}$ targets		
Age range	HbA$_{1c}$ targets	Blood glucose target range
Children <6 years	7.5–8.5%	<6 months, 5–15 mmol/L
6–12 years	<8%	<6 years, 7–12 mmol/L (bedtime)
Adolescents	<7.5%	>12 years, 4–8 mmol/L, 7–10 mmol/L (bedtime)

[a]Australian Clinical Practice Guidelines (2005). But note the imperative to individualise targets.

(Dunger & Hovorka 2007). If hypoglycaemia is severe and frequent diet, exercise, and medication regimen need to be revised and other contributing factors excluded. The parents may learn to use glucagon, see Chapter 6. Table 13.1 depicts the major management strategies according to developmental stage.

The glucagon response might be blunted in adolescents with Type 1 diabetes. Inadequate glucagons response is associated with the duration of diabetes but can occur within a month of diagnosis, which means a key protective mechanism against hypoglycaemia is deficient (EURODIAB 2012). Other factors that can affect hypoglycaemia recognition include environmental factors such as distraction, and genetic makeup, glycaemic control and age.

During adolescence the hormonal surge at puberty can make blood glucose control difficult. Dietary restrictions and the diabetes self-care regimen can be seen as obstacles to fitting in with peer activities and may be neglected. Achieving independence from the family can be difficult if diabetes is diagnosed at this time.

Social pressure and the emphasis on food that is part of the diabetes management regimen can increase the likelihood of eating disorders. Young people with diabetes fear putting on weight and skip meals and run their blood glucose levels high to avoid weight gain (Dunning 1994). Eating disorders are widespread among adolescent girls and diabetic-specific concerns may contribute to their development. The full range of subclinical and clinical eating disorders may be more prevalent in women with diabetes (Colton 2007). Eating disorders in Type 1 diabetes often arises in adolescence and often persists into adulthood (Colton 2007). Colton distinguished between disturbed eating and eating disorders and found girls with an eating disorder had higher HbA_{1c} and BMI but that the HbA_{1c} was not necessarily higher in the presence of disturbed eating. Health professionals need to be sensitive to social pressures and body image issues and the possibility that an eating disturbance might be present. Screening for disturbed eating is essential and referral for specific counselling might be indicated to avoid long-term nutritional problems and other associated risks such as depression. Children with Type 2 diabetes may be at particular risk given the focus on weight loss.

The menarche affects control in girls and thereafter the blood glucose profile often reflects the stages of the menstrual cycle (see Chapter 11). When the child becomes an adolescent contraceptive and pregnancy counselling are vital. Metabolic control often deteriorates partly due to the increase in growth hormone and reduced insulin sensitivity at puberty. Psychosocial issues such as privacy, body image, and independence also have an impact. Negative feedback about the adolescent's metabolic control and 'nagging' about the risk of long-term complications is unlikely to be effective and may actually result in non-attendance.

Polycystic Ovarian Disease (PCOS) is associated with insulin resistance and diabetes and often first manifests at menarche. The effects of unpredictable, heavy menstrual bleeding are disabling and place the young woman at risk of iron deficiency anaemia, and tiredness (Legro & Dunaif 1997). Chronic anovulation increases the risk of endometrial hyperplasia and endometrial cancer. Infertility is a consequence and has a negative impact on the young person's self-concept. Early diagnosis and management is important. PCOS often manifests as excess facial hair and irregular periods, see Chapter 14.

Generally, paediatric depression is serious, common, and persistent. It is the second leading contributor to the global disease burden between ages 15 and 44 and recurs in 70% of affected individuals (World Health Organization (WHO)). It is more common in boys before puberty and in girls after puberty. Mood disorders are associated with high morbidity, concomitant diseases, and risk-taking behaviour such as excess alcohol consumption, smoking, and illegal drug use. Children with diabetes are at particular risk and higher rates of depression have been reported in young people with diabetes than the general population (Blanz 1993) thus regular mental health assessment is essential. Bryden. (2002) reported poor clinical outcomes in approximately one third of young people with diabetes, which highlights the need to identify problems early.

Children from single parent families and families with marital conflict are at increased risk of poor metabolic control (Thompson *et al.* 2001). Family dysfunction, inadequate treatment adherence and unacceptable glycaemic control often go hand-in-hand (Lorenz & Wysocki 1991). Unacceptable glycaemic control carries the risk of admissions to hospital with ketoacidosis and the development of long-term diabetic complications (see Chapter 10). Non-adherence is multifactorial and may be a sign of rebellion or forgetfulness. Aggressive antisocial conduct is more likely to result in poor metabolic control whereas emotional problems tend to lead to better glycaemic control (Bryden *et al.* 2001).

Discrepancies between home blood glucose tests and HbA_{1c} might indicate underlying stress and coping problems. It represents an opportunity to explore factors operating in the young person's life, their feelings about diabetes and the management regimen and their coping mechanisms (Conrad *et al.* 2006). This needs to be undertaken very tactfully using techniques suitable to the child. For example, inviting young children to write a story, poem, or draw a picture about their life with diabetes for the next visit, which can act as the basis for meaningful discussion and/or indicate whether referral for specialist counselling is needed.

An emerging issue that has both positive benefits and negative consequences for young people is their disclosure of personal information on the Internet. Internet support groups can enable young people to anonymously discuss diabetes with peers, access information, and reduce feelings of isolation. However, an analysis of information entered on MySpace revealed that most entries by 16- and 17-year-olds included personally identifiable information, information about personal risk-taking behaviours such as sexual activity and drug and alcohol use, and often included a photograph/s (Moreno *et al.* 2007). Moreno *et al.* did not mention diabetes status but there is no reason to suspect the results would be different.

The transfer from paediatric care to adult specialist care can be very stressful. Neglecting the diabetes self-care, not attending appointments and poor metabolic control is common at this time 991). Tact and understanding are very important if these young people are not to be lost to adequate medical supervision (Rosen *et al.* 2003).

Managing childhood Type 2 diabetes

Many of the management issues discussed for children with Type 1 diabetes apply to children with Type 2 but the medication regimen and nutrition requirements are different. A comprehensive complication assessment should be undertaken at diagnosis and then as indicated, but at least annually.

Diet and exercise are essential aspects of management, even if medicines are needed. Nutrition needs to be suitable to the child's development needs and the need to control weight.

Schwenk (2007) showed an intensive weight management programme consisting of intensive nutrition information, and a structured education programme led to improvements in blood pressure, HDL, and LDL cholesterol, weight loss, and lower BMI compared to controls. However, Schwenk noted the programme was intensive and time consuming. Cost-benefit analysis was not reported.

Medications are often needed to control fasting and postprandial blood glucose and blood lipids if they are not controlled using lifestyle interventions. Metformin is first line therapy and may assist with weight loss (Copeland *et al.* 2005) Weight loss and exercise are central to management but symptoms, weight loss, and persistent hyperglycaemia indicates medications are needed. Insulin (~2 units/kg) may be required initially (Svoren & Wolfsdorf 2006).

The only glucose lowering medicines approved for use in Type 2 diabetes in children are insulin and metformin. The recommended starting dose of metformin for children 10–16 years is 500 mg/day, which can be increased to 500 mg DB with further weekly 500 mg increments to a maximum daily dose of 2000 mg provided there are no contraindications to its use or associated adverse events (Svoren & Wolfsdorf 2006). Alternatively, 500 mg metformin XR can be administered with the evening meal to reduce the gastrointestinal side effects. Bedtime basal insulin such as glargine can be commenced at bedtime if blood glucose is not controlled using metformin.

HbA_{1c} should be measured every 3 months and treatment intensified if blood glucose and HbA_{1c} targets are not achieved.

Education for the child and parents is essential and should include information about hypoglycaemia if insulin or insulin secretagogeus are used (Chapter 5).

Table 13.2 Important medicine-related information children need. Information should be provided using recognised education strategies and quality use of medicines. Quality use of medicines is discussed in Chapter 5.

(1) Children have a right to information about their medicines appropriate to their age, diabetes type, and developmental levels. The information should encompass over-the-counter and can medicines as well as conventional medicines be personalised.

(2) Children are innately curious and want to know about their medicines. Health professionals should provide relevant information to the child as well as their parents.

(3) Children should gradually assume responsibility for their medicines management including keeping a record of the medicines they are taking.

(4) Health professionals, family and carers should set a good example with respect to medicines use including safe use, appropriated storage and disposal, and sharps disposal.

(5) Children should be involved in discussions about participating in clinical trials and be given the opportunity to accept or decline participation.

Medication self-management

Managing medicines is an important aspect of self-care that must gradually be assumed by the child. The transition to assuming responsibility for managing diabetes medicines is a key aspect of most diabetes education programmes. However, adolescents are likely to use a range of other medicines, thus medication management should include age appropriate information about other medicines including over-the-counter and complementary medicines (CAM) as well as diabetes medicines.

Self-initiated over-the-counter medicines use begins early in adolescence: by ~16 years the majority of adolescents have self-prescribed medicines such as analgesics and antipyretics, girls self-prescribe more frequently than boys (Buck 2007). However, adolescent's knowledge about these medicines is often inadequate and, significantly, parental education did not influence medication knowledge.

Medicine education programmes for adults are usually appropriate for children >11 years. A number of medicines education programmes have been developed for younger children (Curry *et al.* 2006; Gardiner & Dvorkin 2006; Federal Drug Administration (FDA) undated). Table 13.2 suggests important information to facilitate the transition to medication self-management.

Other conditions associated with diabetes

A range of conditions associated with diabetes was discussed in Chapter 10 and are relevant to children and adolescents such as liver problems such as NASH, celiac disease, cystic fibrosis-related diabetes. Other rare conditions that can occur in young people with diabetes that require early diagnosis and monitoring include:

- Mauriac syndrome in children with persistently poorly controlled diabetes and is more common in developing countries that do not have access to essential medicines and other products.
- Hypothyroidism due to autoimmune thyroiditis.
- Hyperthyroidism, which is less common than hypothyroidism.
- Lipodystrophy (lipoatrophy and lipohypertrophy), which is less common since human insulin was introduced but does still occur, thus it is important to check insulin injection sites regularly.

- Necrobiosis lipoidica diabeticorum, which typically occurs in the pretibial region.
- Limited joint mobility (LJM), which is an early complication of Type 1 diabetes. It is bilateral and usually painless and occurs in the finger and large joints and the skin usually has a tight waxy appearance. LJM is associated with increased risk of retinopathy, nephropathy and neuropathy.

Management consists of monitoring growth and development, screening for specific conditions such as thyroid function tests and routine examination of joints and radiological examination if indicated. Optimising glycaemic control is essential (Kordonouri *et al.* 2009).

Complementary therapy use in children

Complementary therapy (CAM) use in children is a complex issue. There are benefits and risks depending on the age of the child and the therapy used and their capacity to make an informed choice and understand the consequences of the choice to use or not use CAM. Young children with immature livers, developing central nervous systems and immune systems that increases their susceptibility to adverse medicine events: both conventional and CAM medicines.

CAM cathartic and diuretic medicines may cause electrolyte imbalance and dehydration rapidly in young children. Long-term use may increase the likelihood of acute, chronic, or cumulative adverse effects; others are contraindicated in children (Woolf 2003). However, therapies such as music, massage, yoga, and meditation have significant health benefits. Most parents/children who use CAM do not stop their conventional management regimen but only ~32% inform their conventional health professionals they use CAM. Thus, health professionals should ask about CAM use and the reasons for using specific therapies on a regular basis.

The reported prevalence of CAM use in children generally varies from 2% to 95% depending where the information was collected and the underlying condition being treated (Cranswick & Lim 2006; Picciano 2007; Tsao *et al.* 2007). In Germany, Dannemann *et al.* (2008) found 42% of a sample of children with Type 1 diabetes used at least one CAM modality. Significantly the children did not stop their insulin. Commonly used therapies include:

- vitamin and mineral supplements;
- echinacea for treating common childhood illnesses such as URTI or to boost the immune system;
- massage, with and without essential oils. Massage reduces stress and improves quality in children with Type 1 diabetes and their parents providing the massage (Field *et al.*);
- yoga;
- meditation;
- energy therapies;
- music therapy;
- hypnotherapy.

General reasons for using CAM include to improve well being, reduce stress and anxiety, the assumption that CAM have fewer side effects, and because the parents have an interest in self-care. Particularly risky therapies are:

- ear candles;
- aromatherapy candles;

- essential oils in vapourisers within reach of small children. Ingesting of even small doses of some essential oils, for example, *Eucalyptus* sp. from a vapouriser can cause oral burns and toxicity;
- moxibustion;
- case reports indicate Infacalm drops cause hypoglycaemia, drowsiness, and tachycardia in susceptible children.

More information about CAM can be found in Chapter 19.

Strategies for enhancing adherence during adolescence

Establishing a therapeutic relationship with the young person is essential so they feel comfortable about discussing issues with health professionals.

Young people with and without diabetes engage in risk-taking behaviour including not following medical advice, but no more so than adults (Johnson *et al.* 1990). A management approach that seeks concordance between health professional advice and the young person's behaviour is more likely to be successful (Fleming & Watson 2002).

A range of issues can impact on normal growth and development and some issues have a greater priority than health status for the young person. It is normal adolescent behaviour to think in the short-term, learn from their experience, and experiment. This means that short-term goals are more likely to be effective and can be modified progressively. Young people should be encouraged to discuss their experiences, which can be used as experiential teaching and learning strategies.

Many young people feel vulnerable and this can be exacerbated by diabetes and the need to take on the responsibility for adult roles and diabetes management. Exploring these concerns can help young people acknowledge and deal with them.

Many young people feel frustrated when they 'do all the right things' and their metabolic control is inadequate. This can lead to decreased motivation and feelings of helplessness and hopelessness especially if they do not have a supportive family (Kyngas 2000). Focusing on the positive aspects and small gains and not on 'good' and 'bad' control can take the focus off 'failure'. Striving for diabetes balance is more important than control. Metabolic control will be achieved if the individual's life is in balance.

The lack of a consistent and accessible health service and dealing with new health professionals when moving to adult care can be stressful. Collaboration between paediatric and adult services and a planned transition process can overcome some of these problems (Dunning 1994; Department of Health 2001).

Using multiple strategies and consultation techniques that encourage young people to ask questions is more likely to uncover accurate and meaningful information than the consultation where the young person tells the health professional 'what they want to hear' and the health professional does not pick up on relevant cues that things may not be 'all right'. Adherence issues should be discussed in the context of the young person's lifestyle and goals. Adherence can be enhanced by:

- organising a youth-appropriate service;
- seeing the young person separately from their parents as they mature and begin to take responsibility for their diabetes management;
- addressing the broader issues and life priorities and put diabetes into that context;
- giving clear simple instructions and supporting verbal information with written instructions and the availability of telephone advice;
- utilising family/carers as appropriate;

- considering the type of questions likely to get honest answers, for example, instead of asking 'do you always take your correct dose of insulin?' try 'what dose of insulin suits you best?' (Fleming & Watson 2002).

Nursing responsibilities in hospital

In addition to the care tasks outlined in specific chapters such as Chapter 1 it is important to:

- Document height and weight on percentile charts.
- Test blood glucose 4 times per day and when the child feels symptoms of hyper or hypoglycaemia. Vary testing times so that some tests are performed 2 hours after a meal or after activity. Test at night to detect nocturnal hypoglycaemia. Children managed using insulin pumps require more frequent monitoring.
- Test blood ketones if blood glucose is ~15 mmol/L or the child is acutely ill or has a fever.
- Encourage independence and encourage the child to administer their insulin injections and test their blood glucose. This can be an opportunity to assess technique or for the child to learn these techniques.
- Monitor dietary intake and ensure appropriate dietary review by dietitian.
- Ensure diabetic knowledge is assessed.
- Ensure privacy during procedures.
- Avoid admitting adolescents and children to wards with older people, if possible.

Clinical observation

Enuresis is an unusual presentation of diabetes in children.

Ketoacidosis in children

The management of ketoacidosis is described in Chapter 7. Additional issues specific to children are:

- Cerebral oedema is a very serious medical emergency in children. Monitoring mental status and strict fluid calculations are essential, especially when using IV insulin infusions.
- Headache and/or altered behaviour may indicate impending cerebral oedema. Management includes bolus IV mannitol, nursing with the head of the bed elevated and fluid restriction.
- Sodium bicarbonate is not usually given in childhood DKA because of the risk of hypokalaemia, cerebral acidosis, and changed oxygen affinity of haemoglobin.
- Monitor sodium levels and adjust IV fluid appropriately as the blood glucose falls. Hyponatraemia can herald impending cerebral oedema.

References

ADA (2004) Nephropathy in diabetes. Position statement. *Diabetes Care*, **27** (Suppl. 1), S79–S83.
ADA (2004) Retinopathy in diabetes. Position statement. *Diabetes Care*, **27** (Suppl. 1), S84–S87.
ADA (2009) Diabetes care in the school and day care setting. Position statement. *Diabetes Care*, **27** (Suppl. 1), S122–S128.

ADA (2000) Type 2 diabetes in children and adolescents. Consciences statement. *Diabetes Care*, **23**, 381–389.

ADA (2004) Diabetes care in camps. Position statement. *Diabetes Care*, **27** (Suppl. 1), S129–S131.

Akerblom, H. (2011) The trial to reduce IDDM in the genetically at risk (TRIGIR) study: Recruitment, intervention and follow up. *Diabetologia*, **54** (3), 627–633.

Alberti, G., Zimmet, P, Shaw, J, Bloomgarten Z, Kaufman F, Silink M.*et al.* (2004) The International Diabetes Federation Consensus Workshop. Type 2 diabetes in the young: The evolving epidemic. *Diabetes Care*, **27**, 1798–1811.

American Diabetes Association (ADA) (2013) Standards of medical care in diabetes (position statement) *Diabetes Care*, diabetes **care.diabetes**journals.org/content/36/Supplement_1

Anderson, B., Auslander, W., Jung, K., Miller, P. & Santiago, J. (1991) Assessing family sharing of diabetes responsibilities. *Diabetes Spectrum*, **4** (5), 263–268.

Australian Paediatric Endocrine Group (2005) *The Australian Clinical Practice Guidelines on the Management of Type 1 Diabetes in Children and Adolescents* (www.chw.edu.au/prof/ services/ endocrinology/APEG).

Bhargava, S., Sachdev, H. & Fall, C. (2004) Relation of serial changes in childhood body-mass index to impaired glucose tolerance in young adulthood. *New England Journal of Medicine*, **350**, 865–875.

Blanz, B., Rensch-Riemann, B., Fritz-Sigmund, I. & Schmidt, H. (1993) IDDM is a risk factor for adolescent psychiatric disorders. *Diabetes Care*, **16**, 1579–1587.

Bryden, K. (2002) Turbulent time: The adolescent with Type 1 diabetes. *Journal of Diabetes Nursing*, **6** (3), 83–87.

Bryden, K., Pevelr, R., Stein, A. *et al.* (2001) The clinical and psychological course of diabetes from adolescence to young adulthood: A longitudinal study. *Diabetes Care*, **24**, 1536–1540.

Buck, M. (2007) Self-medication by adolescents. *Paediatric Pharmacology*, **13** (5), 1–4.

Bush, P., Ozias, J., Walson, P. & Ward, R. (1999) Ten guiding principles for teaching children about medicines. *Current Therapeutics*, **21**, 1280–1284.

Colton, P. (2007) Eating disturbance common and persistent in girls with Type 1 diabetes. *Diabetes Care*, **30**, 2861–2862.

Conrad, S. & Gitelmand, S. (2006) If the numbers don't fit … discrepancies between meter glucose readings and haemoglobin A_{1c} reveal stress of living with diabetes. *Clinical Diabetes*, **24**, 45–47.

Craig M, Hattersley A Donaghue K (2009) Definition, epidemiology and classification of diabetes in children and adolescents, *Peadiatric Diabetes*, **10** (Sup 12), 3–12.

Cranswick, N. & Lim, A. (2006) Use of over-the-counter and complementary medicine in children. *Australian Doctor*, 21ˢᵗ July, 25–32.

Copeland, C., Becker, D., Gottschalk, M. & Hale, D. (2005) Type 2 diabetes in children and adolescents: risk factors, diagnosis, and treatment. *Clinical Diabetes*, **23**, 181–185.

Curry, H., Schmer, C. & Ward-Smith, P. (2006) Kid Cards: Teaching children about their medications. *Journal of Paediatric Health Care*, **20**, 414–418.

Dannemann, K., Hecker, W., Haberland, H. *et al.* (2008) Use of complementary and alternative medicine in children with Type 1 diabetes mellitus – Prevalence, patterns of use, costs. *Paediatric Diabetes Online*, http://www.blackwell-synergy.com/doi/abs/10.111/j.1399–5448.2008.00377.x (accessed April 2008).

Department of Health (2001) Diabetes National Service Framework: Standards for Diabetes Services. Department of Health, London.

Dunger, D. & Hovorka, R. (2007) No more nightmares: treatments to prevent nocturnal hypoglycaemia in children. *Diabetes Voice, May Special Issue* **22**–25.

Dunning, P. (1994) Having diabetes: Young adult perspectives. *The Diabetes Educator*, **21** (1), 58–65.

EURODIAB ACE Study Group (2000) Variation and trends in incidence of childhood diabetes in Europe. EURODIAB ACE Study Group. *Lancet*, **355** (9207), 873-6. Erratum in *Lancet* 2000 **356** (9242), 1690.

Federal Drug Administration (FDA) (undated) FDA Center for Drug Evaluation and Research. *Medicines in My Home*. www.fda.gov/medsinmyhome/MIMH_background.htm (accessed December 2007).

Field, T., Morrow, C., Valdeon, C. *et al.* (1997) Massage lowers blood glucose levels in children with diabetes. *Diabetes Spectrum*, **10**, 237–239.

Fleming, T. & Watson, P. (2002) Enhancing compliance in adolescents. *Current Therapeutics*, **43** (3), 14–18.

Gardiner, P. & Dvorkin, L. (2006) Promoting medication adherence in children. *American Family Physician*, **74**, 793–800.

Gill, T. (2007) Young people with diabetes and obesity in Asia: A growing epidemic. *Diabetes Voice*, **52**, 20–22.

Gressner, O., Weiskirchen, R. & Gressner, M. (2007) Evolving concepts of liver fibrogenesis provide new diagnostic and therapeutic options *Comparative Hepatology* **6**, 7 DOI:10.1186/1476-5926-6-7.

Hales, C. & Barker, D. (1992) Type 2 (non-insulin dependent) diabetes mellitus: A thrifty phenotype hypothesis. *Diabetelogia*, **35**, 595–601.

IDF (International Diabetes Federation) Consultative Section on Diabetes Education (2002) International Diabetes Curriculum: Paediatric and Adolescent Module. International Diabetes Federation, Brussels.

International Society for Pediatric and Adolescent Diabetes ISPAD (2000) Consensus Guidelines for the Management of Type 1 Diabetes Mellitus. Zeist, Medical Forum International.

Johnson, S., Freund, A. & Silverstein, J. (1990) Adherence–health status relationships in childhood diabetes. *Health Psychology*, **9**, 606–631.

Kaufman, F. & Riley, P. (2007) Protecting our children worldwide: The first UN-observed World Diabetes Day. *Diabetes Voice*, **52**, 9–12.

Kordonouri, O., Maguire, A., Knip, M. *et al.* (2009) Other complications and associated conditions with diabetes in children and adolescents *Paediatric Diabetes*, **10** (Supp 12) 204–210.

Kyngas, H. (2000) Compliance of adolescents with diabetes. *Journal of Paediatric Nursing*, **15** (4), 260–267.

Legro, R. & Dunaif, A. (1997) Menstrual disorders in insulin resistant states. *Diabetes Spectrum*, **10** (3), 185–190.

Lee, P. (2008) Exploring online pre-admission information for children *Nursing Times.Net* ghttp://www.nuringtimes.net/nursingpractice/critical-zones/childresn's-nursing/explorin   online-pre-admission-for-children1380247.article (accessed October 2012).

Levine, M. & Marcus, M. (1997) Women, diabetes and disordered eating. *Diabetes Spectrum*, **4** (5), 191–195.

Lorenz, R. & Wysocki, T. (1991) Conclusions: Family and childhood diabetes. *Diabetes Spectrum*, **4** (5), 290–292.

Margeirsdottir, H. (2008) Time watching television linked to glucose control in pediatric Type 1 diabetes. *Diabetes Care*, **30**, 1567–1570.

Moreno, M., Parks, M. & Richardson, L. (2007) What are adolescents showing the world about their health risk behaviours in MySpace? *Medscape General Medicine*, **9** (4), 9–15.

Morgan, K., Silverstein, J., Moore, K. *et al.* (3013) Management of newly diagnosed Type 2 diabetes mellitus (t2DM) in children and adolescents. *Paediatrics*, DOI: 10.1542/peds.2012-3494.

Need, J. (1962) Diabetes mellitus: A thrifty genotype rendered detrimental by 'progress.' *American Journal of Human Genetics*, **14**, 353–362.

National Evidence-Based Clinical Care Guidelines for Type 1 Diabetes in Children, Adolescents and Adults (2012) Australian Paediatric Endocrine Group and the Australian Diabetes Society. www.**diabetessociety**.com.au/position-statements.asp.

Picciano, M. (2007) Dietary supplement use among infants, children, and adolescents in the United States, 1999–2002. *Archives Pediatric Adolescent Medicine*, **161**, 978–985.

Pinhas-Hamiel, O. (2007) Complications of Type 2 diabetes in young people – A ticking bomb. *Medical News Today*, 30th May http://www.medicalnewstoday.com/medicalnews.php?newsid=72100&nfid=crss (accessed June 2007).

Rosen D, Blum R, Britto M, Sawyer M, Siegel M. (2003) Transition to adult health care for adolescents and young adults with chronic conditions. *Journal of Adolescent Health*, **33**, 309–11.

Schwenk, T. (2007) Weight management in overweight children. *Journal Watch*, **6** (6), 3.

Scientific Advisory Committee on Nutrition (SACN) (2011) *Joint Statement on timing of introduction of gluten into the infant diet.* http://www.bsna.co.uk/categories/complementary_feedings/news/index- (accessed January 2013).

Shaw, J. (2007) Childhood and adolescent obesity, diabetes and their consequences. *International Diabetes Monitor*, **13** (3), 12–16.

Silverstein J, Klingensmith G, Copeland G et al. (2005) American *Diabetes Association Care of Children and Adolescents With Type 1 Diabetes A statement of the American Diabetes Association Diabetes Care*, **28** (1), 186–212.

Siafarkis, A., Johnston, R., Bulsara, M. *et al.* (2012) Early loss of glucagons response to hypoglycaemia in adolescents with Type 1 diabetes. *Diabetes Care* **35**, 1757–1762.

SIGN (2010) *Scottish Intercollegiate Guideline Network: National Clinical Guideline* SIGN, Edinburgh.

Sinha, R., Fisch, G., Teague, B. *et al.* (2002) Prevalence of impaired glucose intolerance among children and adolescents with marked obesity. *New England Journal of Medicine*, **346**, 802–810.

Soltesz, G. (2007) Diabetes in children: Changing trends in an emerging epidemic. *Diabetes Voice*, **52**, 13–15.

Srinivasan, S. & Donaghue, K. (2007) Paediatric diabetes – Which children can gain insulin independence? *Medical Journal of Australia*, **186** (7), 436–437.

Svoren, B. & Wolfsdorf, J. (2005) Management of diabetes mellitus in children and adolescents. *International Diabetes Monitor*, **18** (95), 9–18.

Tait, A. (2008) Obese children at greater risk for perioperative adverse respiratory events. *Anesthesiology*, **108**, 375–380.

Thompson, S., Auslander, W. & White, N. (2001) Comparison of single-mother families on metabolic control of children with diabetes. *Diabetes Care*, **24** (2), 234–238.

Tsao, J., Meldrum, M., Kim, S., Jacob, M. & Zelter, L. (2007) Treatment preferences for CAM in children with chronic pain. *Evidence Based Complementary and Alternative Medicine*, **4** (3), 364–374.

Wei, J., Sung, F. & Li, C. (2003) Low birth weight and high birth weight infants are both at increased risk to have Type 2 diabetes among schoolchildren in Taiwan. *Diabetes Care*, **26**, 343–348.

Weiss, R. & Caprio, S. (2005) The metabolic consequences of childhood obesity. *Best Practice & Research Clinical Endocrinology & Metabolism*, **19** (3), 405–419.

Wilmot, E., Davies, M., Yates, T. *et al.* (2010) Type 2 diabetes in younger adults: The emerging UK epidemic. *Postgraduate Medical Journal* **86**, 711–718.

Wilmot, E., Edwardson, C., Achana, F. *et al.* (2012) Sedentary time in adults and the association with diabetes, cardiovascular disease and death: A systematic review. *Diabetologia*, DOI 10 1007/s00125-012-2677-z.

Woolf, A. (2003) Herbal remedies and children: Do they work? Are they harmful? *Paediatrics*, **112**, 240–246.

World Health Organization (2004) Mood (affective) disorders (F30–F39). *International Statistical Classification of Diseases and Health Related Problems* 2nd edn. World Health Organization, Geneva.

Yajnik, C. (2007) Growth and nutrition in early life and risk of Type 2 diabetes. *International Diabetes Monitor*, **19** (4), 1–8.

Zimmet, P., Alberti, G., Kaufman, F. *et al.* IDF Consensus Group (2007) The metabolic syndrome in children and adolescents – an IDF consensus report. *Paediatric Diabetes*, **8**, 299–306.

Clinical Practice Consensus Guidelines (2009) Compendium International Society for Paediatric and Adolescent Diabetes. www.ispad.org/sites/default/files/.../ispad_guidelines_2009.

Chapter 14

Women, Pregnancy, and Gestational Diabetes

Key points

- Diabetes affects women through the impact it has during pregnancy and poses a significant threat to both the mother and the child.
- Adverse maternal and foetal outcomes are still common in many parts of the world. Gestational diabetes accounts for 90% of new diagnoses in pregnancy.
- Women with diabetes have particular health issues and care needs. These include pregnancy care, polycystic ovarian syndrome (PCOS), contraception and menopause.
- Good control before and during pregnancy reduces the risks to mother and baby.
- Better outcomes are achieved if the pregnancy is planned and normoglycaemia achieved and maintained before, during, and after pregnancy.
- Insulin is required in Type 2 diabetes during pregnancy and breastfeeding.
- Existing renal disease and retinopathy may deteriorate during pregnancy.
- PCOS is associated with obesity, insulin resistance, GDM, and infertility.

Rationale

Hormonal changes associated with pregnancy, PCOS and menopause affect glucose homeostasis and mental well being. Coordinated care and prepregnancy planning are necessary to ensure optimal outcomes for mother and baby. Planning for an optimal delivery begins in childhood with a healthy lifestyle, health education and sex education as well as prevention messages in high risk families and communities. Diabetes prevention messages and screening and maternal and child health should ideally be integrated into primary health care and general health screening programs. Diagnostic procedures and criteria should be appropriate to the woman's cultural group. In some developing

Care of People with Diabetes: A Manual of Nursing Practice, Fourth Edition. Trisha Dunning.
© 2014 John Wiley & Sons, Ltd. Published 2014 by John Wiley & Sons, Ltd.

countries birth attendants, traditional healers and healthcare workers are primary sources of information and care. Working collaboratively with these people and educating them about diabetes is essential (International Diabetes Federation (IDF) (2009).

Diabetes can develop during pregnancy, gestational diabetes (GDM). Most non-diabetic women are screened for diabetes during pregnancy so GDM can be detected early and blood glucose levels can be controlled to avoid the risks having diabetes places on both mother and baby. Women particularly at risk of GDM are those who: have a history of diabetes in the family, had diabetes during a previous pregnancy, or previously delivered a large baby. There is increasing evidence that maternal hyperglycemia has a lasting legacy for the child and predisposes them to obesity in e and Type 2 diabetes in adolescence and adulthood (IDF 2009).

Polycystic ovarian syndrome

Polycystic ovarian syndrome (PCOS) is common, occurring in 6–10% of women in the reproductive age and 28% of obese women. Seventy five percent of women with PCOS are overweight or obese. PCOS has long term health effects including menstrual irregularities, infertility, gestational diabetes (GDM), impaired glucose tolerance, insulin resistance, Type 2 diabetes, and emotional stress and body image concerns. Thus, screening women with PCOS for these metabolic changes and evidence of diabetes complications and risk factors at diagnosis and regularly thereafter is essential.

The risk factors for PCOS are shown in Figure 14.1. Making the diagnosis is a process of exclusion and consists of taking a careful family and individual history, and measuring relevant hormone levels such as:

- Testosterone (normal <2.4 mmol/L in women).
- Sex hormone binding globulin (SHBG): likely to be low in PCOS (normal range 30–90) and is often secondary to insulin resistance and results in higher levels of free testosterone.
- Free androgen index (FAI): likely to be high in PCOS (normal range 1–5%).

FAI is a more useful measure than testosterone unless the laboratory can test for free testosterone. Pelvic ultrasound may be indicated to determine whether the ovaries are polycystic and whether the endometrium is thickened if the woman has oligo or amenorrhoea (Rotterdam Consensus Workshop 2004; Teede *et al.* 2007). Determining follicle-stimulating hormone (FSH), thyroid stimulating hormone (TSH) and beta human chorionic gonadotrophin (HCG) and prolactin levels may be necessary to exclude other endocrine conditions.

Practice points

(1) Hormone evaluation should be undertaken before prescribing contraceptives.
(2) The risks and benefits of contraceptives should be considered in light of the risks of unplanned pregnancies to the mother and child.
(3) Oral contraceptives can mask the hormonal changes associated with PCOS.
(4) Each woman should be individually assessed for cardiometabolic risk before commencing contraceptives and monitored according to metabolic and weight targets (Damm *et al.* 2005; Yildiz 2008).

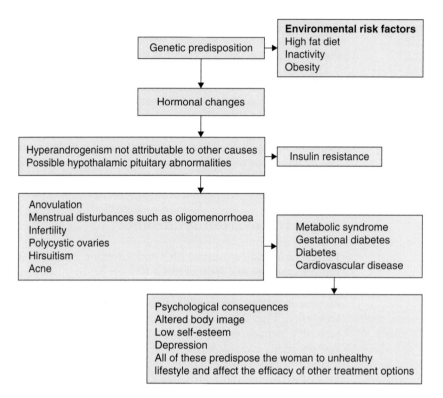

Figure 14.1 Risk factors for polycystic ovarian syndrome and the possible long-term effects. There is still controversy about the diagnostic criteria and several degrees of severity exist. There is no single diagnostic test: diagnosing PCOS is process of exclusion. Diagnostic criteria include National Institute of Health criteria, Rotterdam criteria, and International Androgen Excess Society criteria.

A multidiscipline supportive team approach is important to address the various underlying features of PCOS. Reassurance and education about diet and exercise and weight management aiming to lose 5–10% of weight at diagnosis, the need for regular follow up is important. The PCOS Association of Australia provides useful information about theses issues on its website. In addition, counselling about fertility may be needed. Because PCOS is associated with insulin resistance, and usually obesity, blood glucose and lipids should be checked regularly and an OGTT performed if indicated because fasting glucose is not a reliable diagnostic test in PCOS (Teede *et al.* 2007) (see Chapter 1). Cardiovascular assessment should be undertaken on a regular basis. Advice about diet and exercise (Chapter 4) are essential and psychological counselling may be required (Chapter 15).

Weight loss has been demonstrated in women with PCOS consuming the following diets: Atkins, Ornish, Weight Watchers, Zone, and the CSIRO Total Wellbeing Diet (Moran *et al.* 2003). The woman's food preferences should be considered and the diet should conform to dietary recommendations. A recent study suggests young women consuming Atkins-type diets are at increased risk of cardiovascular disease (CVD) (Pagona *et al.* 2012). A prospective study involving 44000 women predicted Atkins-style diets would be responsible for additional 4 to 5 cases of CVD for every 10 000 women per year, which represents a 28% increase in the incidence of CVD. Women with PCOS often try a range of diets and are already at high risk of CVD, thus sensitive dietary advice is important.

If diet and exercise do not control blood glucose, Metformin may be *added to* the diet and exercise regimen. The commencing dose is 500 mg of slow release Metformin daily increasing to 2 g per day. Experts recommend giving Metformin at night (Teede *et al.* 2007; Alberti *et al.* 2007) and there is evidence to support such a recommendation, but Metformin is not currently approved for night dosing in some countries such as Australia. Metformin helps regulate the menstrual cycle and reduce hirsutism and the progression to diabetes by ~50 in high risk women (Alberti *et al.* 2007; Teede 2007). The role of Metformin in improving fertility is unclear and it is not first-line fertility treatment. Metformin might be more effective in lean women (De Maria 2007). Nevertheless, fertility should be discussed if Metformin is commenced because of the chance of becoming pregnant. Obesity affects fertility independently of PCOS; thus, loosing weight is essential if the woman wants to have a child. Age may also be a factor. Fertility declines from ~28 years and falls dramatically after age 35 and falls again after age 40.

Oral contraceptives (OC) may be indicated to help reduce hirsutism and control menstrual irregularities once other causes of hirsutism are ruled out. For example, low dose combined OCs such as Ethinyl Estradiol 20 μg increases SHBG and reduces free androgen levels. At higher doses OC exacerbate insulin resistance (Meyer *et al.* 2007). Hair removal products or topical antiandrogens such as Vaniqua may be indicated, and cosmetic electrolysis or laser as a last resort. Obesity exacerbates hirsutism so managing weight will help normalise androgen levels. The risks and benefits of all these options need to be carefully discussed with the woman considering her individual needs and risk profile.

Antiandrogens such as spironolactone 50 mg BD or cyproterone acetate 25 mg daily for days 1–10 of the active OC tablets may be prescribed to enhance fertility. These medicines must be taken with the OC to prevent menstrual irregularities and adverse effects in pregnancy. The regimen takes ~6 months to be effective. Women who have more than four cycles of antiandrogens per year are at increased risk of endometrial hyperplasia and endometrial carcinoma. The woman should be monitored regularly for these conditions and plan to have a withdrawal bleed every 2–3 months to reduce these risks.

If endometrial hyperplasia is suspected a transvaginal ultrasound and endometrial biopsy are indicated to confirm the diagnosis especially if prolonged or irregular vaginal bleeding occurs. Hysteroscopy may be needed to determine whether fibroids or polyps are present. Endometrial hyperplasia sometimes resolves spontaneously. If endometrial hyperplasis atypia is present it may progress to endometrial carcinoma, which is induced by oestrogen and has a relatively good prognosis. Treatment depends on the woman. Intrauterine devices are appropriate if contraception is a goal and to control heavy bleeding. High-dose progestins may be indicated to limit endometrial thickening. The ultrasound and/or biopsy should be repeated after 6 months of treatment.

Partners and family need to be involved in explanations about PCOS and its effects, management discussions and education programmes where relevant to enable them to support the woman and understand the associated risks. Achievable goals need to be set in consultation with the woman. The effect of having PCOS, its symptoms, and the impact on fertility can generate significant psychological distress, which exacerbates hormonal imbalance, contributes to the diabetes and cardiovascular risk, and reduces quality of life (Coffey & Mason 2003; Wilhelm *et al.* 2003). Screening tools such as the K10 Profile or Depression Anxiety Stress Scale (DASS) used on a regular basis can help identify the degree and progression of anxiety and depression, are a helpful guide to treatment and can facilitate early referral for counselling (see Chapter 15). Anxiety and depression need to be treated, preferably with non-medicine options, because these conditions affect the success of other treatment measures.

Interestingly, Kim *et al.* (2002) reported lower blood glucose levels and lower odds of developing diabetes in young white and African-American women in the CARDIA study. Insulin levels were higher after adjusting for covariates but the clinical significance of this finding is unknown. Insulin sensitivity was found to decline in women with PCOS treated with triphasic OCs but there were no adverse effects on lipid metabolism (Korytkowski *et al.* 1995). The effects on insulin sensitivity and production might be a consideration in women with the metabolic syndrome, those at risk of GDM, or obese women with Type 2 diabetes, however, more research is needed to clarify the clinical implications.

A recent study suggests pregnant women who take antipsychotic medicines are at increased risk of GDM (Boden *et al.* 2012). The researchers found a two-fold risk of GDM among pregnant women on olanzapine and/or clozapine (n = 169) 338 on other antipsychotics compared with 350 000 controls. It is not clear whether any of the women dad PCOS but the antipsychotic medicine side effects include weight gain, insulin resistance, hyperglycaemia and hyperlipidaemia, which increase the risk of hyperglycaemia (see Chapter 10), especially when the stress of PCOS and pregnancy are added.

Exercise improves mood and fitness. Women with PCOS report significant body image issues, mood disturbances, depression, reduced emotional well being, low quality of life and life satisfaction and a negative impact of PCOS on their sexual self-worth and sexual satisfaction (Janssen *et al.* 2008). Managing symptoms such as hirsutism, obesity, menstrual irregularity and low fertility can significantly improve their emotional and sexual well being. Tailored psychotherapy such as cognitive behavioural therapy or self-help programmes such as *Mood Gym*, and stress management can be beneficial. If medicines are indicated those that reduce PCOS symptoms may be useful. For example, SSRIs to control weight but the woman should be warned that these medicines could affect her sleep.

Pregnancy

Managing diabetes during pregnancy is challenging for the woman concerned and health professionals. Hormones released by the placenta predispose the mother to hyperglycaemia and increase the amount of glucose available to the foetus. Insulin sensitivity increases in the first trimester but insulin resistance develops in the second and third trimesters. The placental glucose transporter, GLUT-1, increases the transplacental glucose flux. The activity of GLUT-4 at the maternal cellular level decreases, which means glucose is not utilised by the mother and high levels cross the placenta where they are utilised by the foetus. This sets the scene for microsomal and foetal abnormalities and makes vaginal delivery difficult (Hollingsworth 1992).

Prepregnancy counselling is essential to limit risks to mother and baby (Coustan 1997; Australasian Diabetes in Pregnancy Society (ADIPS) 2012). Women who attend prepregnancy counselling have significantly lower risk of major foetal abnormalities (Ray *et al.* 2001). Such counselling should be provided to all women with diabetes of reproductive age, for example, at each annual review (ADIPS 2012). Women with Type 2 diabetes and GDM are usually older than those with Type 1, and are often overweight, higher parity, and belong to Ethnic and minority ethnic groups (ADIPS 2012). However, Type 2 diabetes is increasing in prevalence among adolescents and unwanted and unplanned pregnancy rates are high in this age group. In addition women are delaying childbirth, often until the mid-30s or 40s, which carries age-associated risks, and increases the likelihood that diabetes complications will be present and could affect the pregnancy. For example, age appears to be a significant factor in pregnancy-related MI although MI during pregnancy is rare (Karamermer & Ross-Hesselink 2007).

Coordinated multidisciplinary team care that includes as a minimum an obstetrician, endocrinologist, diabetes educator, dietitian, and paeditrician with experience managing diabetes is essential to optimal outcomes. Key management includes strategies to:

- Plan the pregnancy.
- Achieve and maintain HbA_{1c} as close as possible to normal before (<7%), during and after pregnancy as long as hypoglycaemia can be avoided/minimised. Recommended blood glucose targets are:
  - 4–6 mmol/L preprandially;
  - < 8 mmol/L one hour postprandially;
  - < 7 mmol/L 2 hours postprandially;
  - > 6 mmol/L before bed (SIGN 2012).
- Regular blood glucose monitoring is essential to achieving optimal outcomes.
- Commence folate supplements (5 mg daily) and ref the woman for a nutritional review.
- Undertake a comprehensive medication review (see Table 14.1). Stop GLM and commence insulin if the woman has Type 2 diabetes. Optimise the insulin regimen in women with Type 1 diabetes. Insulin analogues confer advantages during pregnancy and may reduce the risk of significant hypoglycaemia. However, not all insulin analogues are approved fro use during pregnancy. CSII appears to be safe. Cease medicines likely to adversely affect the foetus. However, Metformin and sulphonylurea are not associated with increased risk of congenital malformations or early foetal loss but they do cross the placenta and are not recommended in pregnancy (SIGN 2010). Commonly used medicines that *may* be contraindicated in pregnancy include:
- ace inhibitors
- beta blockers
- aspirin
- coumarins
- calcium channel blockers
- ace inhibitors have been associated with congenital malformations.
- Statins due to the risk of foetal malformations. However, hypertension should be prevented. Generally they should not be used while breast feeding.
- NSAIDS
- Caution is required with antidepressants, corticosteroids, and opioids (Gardiner 2002; ADIPS 2012).
- Ask about complementary medicine/therapy (CAM) use. Women frequently use CAM during pregnancy, particularly supplements such as raspberry leaf, ginger and chamomile tea (Foster *et al.* 2006). They also use massage and essential oils. Women who use CAM are generally well-informed and likely to take proactive self-care, be well educated, non-smokers and primiparous. The proportion of pregnant women with diabetes using CAM is unknown, but CAM use is high in the general diabetic population. While there are many benefits, there are also risks especially in the first trimester, and women with renal and liver disease; see Chapters 8 and 10. Some women elect to use complementary approaches (CAM) to pain management during labour or supplement conventional pain management strategies with CAM. Tournaire & Theau-Yonneau (2007). Undertook a systematic review of randomised controlled trials, which indicated pain was reduced and women receiving acupuncture and those receiving hydrotherapy required less analgesia. Women were not dissatisfied with conventional pain relief and had different expectations of pain management from health professionals. Strategies such as massage with or without essential oils, which reduce fear also have positive benefits including reducing lower back pain (Alaire 2001). Combination or single herbal medicines are sometimes used to manage pain,

Table 14.1 Medication management during pregnancy. A comprehensive medication review should be undertaken regularly in all people with diabetes, when planning a pregnancy and when the woman becomes pregnant. See also Chapter 5.

Medication	Management	Potential adverse events
Insulin in Type 1 and Type 2 diabetes	Dose should be titrated regularly according to blood glucose monitoring pattern to achieve targets and avoid hypoglycaemia. Insulin aspart has been shown to be safe to mother and foetus in Type 1 diabetes (Hod *et al.* 2007) and achieving postprandial blood glucose control (Pettitt *et al.* 2007). Glargine has been associated with mitogenic activity and should be used with caution in pregnancy (Hirsch 2005) (see Chapter 14: Cancer). Women with Type 2 diabetes may need education about managing insulin and hypoglycaemia as well as reassurance.	Hypoglycaemia, especially nocturnal hypoglycaemia during 6–18 weeks gestation. Significant repeated hypoglycaemia should be investigated to ensure there are no underlying disease processes and foetal growth and development monitored. Death, although rare, does occur (Ter Braak *et al.* 2002). Weight gain. The low risk of cancer associated with Glargine should be discussed with the woman.
Oral glucose lowering agents (OHA) in Type 2 diabetes	Metformin The overall individual risks need to be considered just those associated with pregnancy. Metformin may be indicated in severe insulin resistance (Simmons *et al.* 2004). There is limited information about dose adjustment during pregnancy. Sulphonylureas Sulphonylureas cross the placenta, but second generation cross to a lesser extent: glipizide 6.6% and glyburide 3.9% (Feig *et al.* 2007). Thiazolidinediones (TZD) Rosiglitazone crosses the placenta especially after 10 weeks gestation.	A number of studies suggest OHAs do not increase the risk of foetal malformation (Gutzin *et al.* 2003) and the concentration in breast milk is low (Gilbert *et al.* 2006). Australasian Diabetes in Pregnancy Study Group (ADIPS 2005) suggested the potential harm from Metformin use in pregnancy is outweighed by the benefits. However, long-term data are not available thus, caution is recommended. The product prescribing recommends changing to insulin during pregnancy. Feig *et al.* (2007) found no evidence of foetal abnormalities in animal or human studies if the medicines were used in recommended doses but the studies were small and short term and these medicines cannot be recommended for use in pregnancy. When a woman with Type 2 diabetes becomes pregnant she should be referred urgently to an endocrinologist and OHAs continued until the transfer to insulin to avoid the risk of hyperglycaemia to the foetus (ADIPS 2005).
Antihypertensive agents	ACE inhibitors should be ceased during pregnancy. Methyldopa, Oxprenolol, Clonidine, Labetolol, Prazosin and Nifedipine can be continued safely (Australasian Society for the Study of Hypertension in Pregnancy 2005). The effects of angiotensin 2 blocker is not known	ACE represent a threat to the foetus in the 3rd trimester and their safety is not established in the first trimester.
Lipid lowering agents		Statins have been associated with foetal abnormalities and are contraindicated in pregnancy (Edison & Muenke 2004).
Any other medicine	Check the prescribing information before using.	

for example, motherwort. Women sometimes use herbal medicines during the last 4–5 weeks of pregnancy to prepare the cervix and facilitate delivery, for example raspberry leaf in tablet form and was found to shorten the second stage of labour and fewer women required forceps deliveries (Simpson *et al.* 2001). CAM use prior to and during labour should be discussed with the obstetrician and/or midwife. Thus, CAM use should be assessed at regular intervals throughout pregnancy.

- Undertake a comprehensive diabetes complication and manage existing disease before pregnancy. For example, retinopathy requiring laser therapy, cardiovascular disease. The eyes should be examined through dilated pupils. Women should be aware that pre-existing retinopathy could progress during pregnancy. Pre-existing cardiovascular disease can be exacerbated by pregnancy due to haemodynamic changes and increased cardiac output. Delivery places extra demand on the heart (Karamermer & Ross-Hesselink 2007). Significant coronary artery stenosis should ideally be treated prior to pregnancy. The haemodynamic changes gradually return to normal in 3–6 months (Karamermer & Ross-Hesselink 2007). Kidney function should be checked because women with microalbuminuria at risk of pre-eclampsia and microalbuminuria may progress during pregnancy if significant renal impairment is present and require dialysis (Biesenbach *et al.* 1992; Rossing *et al.* 2004); see Chapter 8. Some experts regard significant renal impairment to be a contraindication to pregnancy (ADIPS 2012) particularly given a third of women with severe renal impairment die within ~16 years (Rossing *et al.* 2004). Identify autonomic neuropathy-associated conditions such as gastroparesis, hypoglycaemic unawareness and orthostatic hypotension, which make management more difficult, are distressing for the woman and her family and may put her safety and/or life at risk. Autonomic neuropathy may predispose the mother to intractable vomiting and precipitate metabolic disturbances such as ketoacidosis.
- Assess general health and psychological wellbeing. For example detect the presence of comorbidities such as thyroid and coeliac disease in women with Type 1 diabetes and CVD in Type 2 diabetes, which could complicate the pregnancy.
- Undertake an education review of general diabetes knowledge and provide specific pregnancy and childbirth information. Revise home management of emergencies such as sick days/hyperglycaemia and morning sickness.
- Encourage women who smoke to quit and limit alcohol consumption.
- Perform an ultrasound at 18–20 weeks and if necessary the ultrasound should be repeated to check foetal cardiac status at 24 weeks and foetal growth at 28–30 weeks and again at 34–36 weeks.
- Encourage the woman to eat a healthy well-balanced low GI diet to ensure optimal nutrition for herself and the developing foetus. The carbohydrates need to be spread over the day if problems occur. Foods likely to cause listeriosis should be avoided. Dietitian advice is advisable. Listeriosis can be transmitted from the mother to the foetus and cause miscarriage, stillbirth, premature delivery or a very ill baby at birth.
- Encourage participation in regular exercise such as 'Preggie Bellies' helps blood glucose control, general fitness, and well being and mental health.
- Encourage participation in childbirth classes.
- Develop and document a plan for managing insulin during delivery and in the immediate post partum period.
- Develop a plan for reviewing the mother's glycaemic control after discharge and ensuring the woman has adequate support at home.
- Foster mother–child bonding by providing woman-centred holistic care and supporting the woman and her family to adjust to parenthood. Monitoring for the 'three day blues' and postnatal depression is essential. For example, Rasmussen *et al.* (2007) found women with Type 1 diabetes were significantly stressed about the baby's safety

if they had a 'hypo' and relied on their mothers and husbands for support. Mutual mother/daughter guilt feelings emerged (the guilt dynamic) where daughters felt guilty about the impact their diabetes had on their mother's lives and mothers felt guilty because their daughters developed diabetes and they could not prevent it. Chapter 15 describes psychological therapy. In addition, many small studies indicate massage, with and without essential oils, reduces stress, improves sleep for both the mother and baby, facilitates bonding and is safe (Bongaard 2007). Thus, massage may be a useful non-medicine option in high-risk groups or could be used in combination with other therapies (Bongaard 2007).

- Specific care of the mother and baby during labour and delivery are specialty areas and outside the scope of this book. Most women should deliver at term and vaginally unless there are medical or obstetric reasons for earlier delivery/Caesarian section. Usually blood glucose is measure every 1–2 hours and usual diet and insulin dose maintained. If a Caesarian section is needed, the procedure should be scheduled for the morning if possible. The dose of long-acting insulin on the evening prior to the surgery may need to be reduced to reduce the risk of hypoglycaemia after delivery. Women with Type 1 diabetes may need an insulin/glucose infusion.
- Women are encouraged to breast feed. Strategies to reduce hypoglycaemia during breastfeeding include having a snack before or while feeding, avoiding caffeine, drinking plenty of water, and having glucose close by to treat hypoglycaemia early if it occurs. Insulin is not contraindicated in breastfeeding.
- Discuss contraception plans prior to discharge.

Comprehensive assessment should be undertaken 1–4 weekly during the first 30 weeks of pregnancy and then weekly until delivery. Routine foetal monitoring should occur and an ultrasound performed to ensure the estimated date of delivery is accurate and develop the delivery plan. In most cases the women will be able to have a normal vaginal delivery unless there are obstetric complications.

Complications of pregnancy

Complications can be reduced by careful monitoring and proactively managing the pregnancy especially controlling blood glucose and other risk factors. The following maternal complications are possible:

- Early: miscarriage, foetal abnormalities, and difficulty performing ultrasound.
- Hypertension is common and manifests as a range of conditions from mild hypertension to pre-eclampsia superimposed on chronic hypertension and occurs in 10–22% of pregnancies (Donovan 2012). Hypertension increases the risk of adverse outcomes for mother and baby and increase the possibility that labour will need to be induced or Caesarian section will be required because of conditions such as macrosomia, shoulder dystocia. Increased risk of perioperative complications if surgery is required. Some antihypertensive medicines are not recommended during pregnancy including ACE inhibitors and ARB and diuretics, BETA blockers and calcium challenge antagonists except Nifedipine should be avoided (Donovan 2012).
- Hypoglycaemia can have serious consequences in women having epidural anaesthesia because the usual counter-regulatory response is blocked and because pregnant women are more prone to hypoglycaemia. Hypoglycaemia can retard reversal of hypotension in these situations (Marx *et al.* 1987). However, maternal glucose is often higher during Caesarian section than vaginal delivery (Andersen *et al.* 1998).
- Postpartum: maternal haemorrhage, infection, thrombosis, hypoglycaemia.

- Deterioration in existing diabetes complication especially renal disease and retinopathy and cardiovascular status. Cardiovascular disease is encountered more frequently because women ore older when they begin their families, a family history of cardiac disease, and have often have diabetes for >10 years. In addition, obesity is more common and smoking increases the risk. An ECG should be performed if chest discomfort develops especially if the woman has known cardiovascular risk factors (Karamermer & Ross-Hesselink 2007). Indications of heart disease include:
  - serious or progressive dyspnoea (mild dyspnoea is common);
  - syncope on exertion;
  - chest pain/discomfort associated with exertion.

The maternal death rate is comparable to non-diabetic women when care is delivered by a qualified, collaborative multidisciplinary team, ~0.5% of pregnancies in the UK (Chief Medical Officer's Report 2000).

Effects of diabetes on the baby

Consequences of maternal hyperglycaemia for the foetus include macrosomia, foetal distress, and birth injuries, which are largely preventable by good obstetric management and controlling maternal blood glucose levels. After delivery the baby may develop hypoglycaemia, hypothermia, hypocalcaemia, transient cardiomyopathy or other problems depending on the intrauterine conditions during pregnancy, delivery, and gestational age. The baby will need intensive monitoring initially, which might affect the bonding process.

Neonatal hypoglycaemia, defined as blood glucose <2.6 mmol/L up to 72 hours after birth, can cause significant morbidity and death if it is not recognised and treated effectively (Western Australian Center for Evidence Based Nursing and Midwifery 2006). The estimated incidence of newborn hypoglycaemia is between 1 and 5 per 1000 live births but may be up to 30% in at-risk infants (Hewitt *et al.* 2005). Hypoglycaemia is often present at birth and is usually transient in babies of non-diabetic mothers. Infants most at risk are:

- <2 kg or >4 kg at birth;
- born before 37 weeks gestation;
- <10th percentile for weight (small for gestational age);
- >90th percentile for weight (large for gestational age);
- retarded uterine growth;
- born to mother with diabetes or GDM;
- those with sepsis effectively (World Health Organization (WHO 1997; Western Australian Center for Evidence Based Nursing and Midwifery 2006).

The maternal and baby's blood glucose levels correlate at birth. Thus, the maternal blood glucose level is the most significant determinant of neonatal hypoglycaemia (Andersen *et al.* 1998). The signs of hypoglycaemia in the neonate are often non-specific and include high pitched crying, hypothermia and poor temperature control, sweating, refusing to feed or poor sucking, exaggerated Moro reflex, irritability, hypotonia, tachyapnoea, tachycardia, cyanosis, and lethargy. All of these signs also occur in other conditions.

Traditionally, hypoglycaemia is diagnosed in the presence of Whipple's Triad: the presence of characteristic clinical signs of low blood glucose, low blood glucose, resolution of the signs once euglycaemia is re-established. However, the symptoms are unreliable in neonates, as can be seen from the preceding list. Having a high level of suspicion and performing a blood glucose test are essential. Once hypoglycaemia is corrected, babies are usually able to maintain blood glucose levels with normal breastfeeding on demand. Supplemental formula feeds may be required in the first 48 hours. Babies need to be kept warm and closely monitored in the neonatal nursery until they are stable.

Longer term effects of maternal hyperglycaemia on the child

Childhood obesity is increasing in many countries especially in ethnic minorities; see Chapter 1. The factors contributing to childhood obesity and associated consequences (insulin resistance, Type 2 diabetes, and diabetic complications) are debated. Genetic and environmental factors play a role (Dornhorst 2003) including the intrauterine environment during pregnancy, which has lasting effects on the child, originally called the Baker Hypothesis and now referred to as the foetal origins hypothesis or the Developmental Origins of Ault Health and Disease (DOHaD) (Armitage *et al.* 2008). Put simply, the hypothesis states 'exposure to an unfavorable environment during development (either in utero or in the early postnatal period) programmes changes in foetal or neonatal development such that the individual is then at greater risk of developing adulthood disease (Armitage *et al.* 2008).

The foetus adapts structurally and functionally to reduced availability of essential nutrients. That is, under intrauterine 'famine' conditions available glucose is diverted to vital organs such as the brain and away from less immediately vital organs such as the pancreas. Insulin resistance develops in peripheral tissues to ensure a constant supply to vital organs and growth (birth weight) is retarded. The combination of reduced beta cell mass and pre-programming insulin-sensitive tissue to be insulin-resistant confers the risk of future diabetes on susceptible individuals (Barker *et al.* 1993). Low birth weight may be due to inadequate maternal intake and/or placental dysfunction. The association between Type 2 diabetes and low birth weight has been demonstrated in a number of population-based studies; however, the risk in developed countries with an adequate food supply is low (Boyko 2000) but may be higher in less affluent countries..

High birth weight is also associated with future risk of impaired glucose tolerance and Type 2 diabetes (Pettitt *et al.* (2007), which is likely to be a significant factor as the number of overweight women giving birth increases and they deliver higher birth weight babies. High birth weight is primarily due to maternal hyperglycaemia. However, starvation and under nutrition also predispose the child to poor health outcomes.

Memory deficits in childhood have also been attributed to poorly controlled maternal diabetes during pregnancy (De Boer 2007). De Boer suggested inadequate levels of iron and oxygen during development of the hippocampus (memory centre) *in utero* contributed to the deficits, which were significant by age three and a half. She suggested available iron was used to manufacture haemoglobin and diverted away from the hippocampus, which is a metabolically active part of the brain that requires a lot of iron during prenatal neuronal development. The longer term implications of De Boer's study are unknown and the research is ongoing. Significantly, the deficits were only noticeable on difficult memory tasks. The findings do underscore the importance of prenatal iron supplements and planning pregnancies.

Gestational diabetes

Gestational diabetes (GDM) refers to carbohydrate intolerance of variable severity that first appears during pregnancy (Rice *et al.* 2012). GDM is the most common metabolic complication of pregnancy. Insulin resistance and hyperglycaemia develop as a result of the hormones produced by the placenta and declining beta cell function. The hormones oestradiol, cortisol and human placental lactogen rise during pregnancy to ensure that the foetus receives sufficient glucose to grow and develop normally. As a consequence, the mother's cells become more resistant to insulin and the mother compensates by producing more insulin and using fat stores to produce energy for her own needs. GDM may in fact represent part of the continuum towards Type 2 diabetes.

It is recommended that all pregnant women be screened for diabetes between 24 and 28 weeks gestation, the time the placenta begins to produce large quantities of diabetogenic hormones, using a 75 gram glucose load. (ADIPS 2012). The OGTT should be performed in the morning under test conditions after an 8 hour overnight fast. The IADPSG Consensus Panel (2010) recommended the following diagnostic criteria: Fasting venous glucose ≥ 5.1–6.9 mmol/L, and two-hour venous glucose ≥ 8.5 mmol/L. The diagnosis is established if one or more of the three glucose levels are abnormal. These levels were chosen because they are associated with an odds ratio of 1.75 for adverse outcomes compared with mean glucose levels in the HAPO study (HAPO Collaborative 2008). Overt diabetes is present if the fasting glucose is ≥7.0 mmol/L or a random or two hour glucose is ≥ 11.1 mmol/L (ADIPS 2012).

Women who do not meet the diagnostic criteria for GDM may still have babies with glucose-related macrosomia, respiratory distress, hyperbiluribinaemia, and hypoglycaemia and require admission to neonatal intensive care. Adverse pregnancy outcome such as stillbirth, Caesarian section, and pre-eclampsia can also occur.

Usually the blood glucose returns to normal after the baby is delivered. However, approximately 40% of women with gestational diabetes develop Type 2 diabetes in later life. In addition, the baby is at increased risk of obesity and Type 2 diabetes. In most cases the OGTT is repeated 6–8 weeks after delivery and then on regular basis, for example, yearly in at risk women, although many women do not return for follow up. A National Gestational Diabetes Register was established in Australia in 2011 as a strategy to encourage women to have follow up screening. Registration is voluntary. Women who elect to join the Register and their nominated doctor are sent reminders to have their glucose checked.

A recent study of women with GDM in Sweden between 1995 and 2005 (*n* = 385) were tested for beta cell autoantibody markers to determine their risk of developing Type 1 diabetes (Nilsson *et al.* 2009). Six per cent tested positive for at least one islet cell antibody: ICA, GAD or IA-2A. These women were followed and autoantibody levels reanalysed. An OGGT was performed in women who did not develop diabetes. Fifty per cent of the autoantibody positive women developed Type 1 diabetes and 21% had IFG or IGT, but none had developed Type 2 diabetes. The overall sample size in the study was small, but autoantibody testing may be indicated in some women who develop GDM.

Risk factors for gestational diabetes?

Gestational diabetes can occur in any pregnancy, however, those women at highest risk are categorised as:

- Being obese >12% of ideal bodyweight and/or BMI > 35 kg/m2.and having other features of the metabolic syndrome, see Section 1.6.
  - previous GDM;
  - ethnicity e.g. Indian, Aboriginal, Pacific Islander, Maori, Middle Eastern and African women;
  - maternal age > 40 years, especially if a first degree relative has diabetes;

○ previous large baby >4500 grams at birth;
○ PCOS;
○ On diabetogenic medicines such as corticostemroids and antipsychotics (ADIPS 2012).

Managing gestational diabetes

The following capillary self-monitoring blood glucose targets are generally accepted. However, the blood glucose patterns and the factors that affect blood glucose must be interpreted when making management decisions

- fasting ≤ 5.0 mmol/L;
- one hour post prandial ≤ 7.4 mol/L;
- two hours post prandial ≤ 6.7 mmol/L (ADIPS 2012).

Diet and exercise are first line treatment of GDM to control maternal blood glucose and supply essential nutrients for normal foetal growth and development. Generally low GI foods are recommended where 40–50% calories come from complex high fibre carbohydrate, 20% from protein and 30–40% from unsaturated fats distributed evenly throughout the day. Nutrition counselling by a dietitian is recommended. Insulin is indicated if the blood glucose targets cannot be met.

Calorie restriction can predispose the woman and the foetus to ketonaemia and reduce psychomotor development and IQ between the 3rd and 9th year of age in the child especially during the second and third trimesters (Rizzo *et al.* 1995). Pregnant women who remain active have a 56% lower risk of developing glucose intolerance and GDM than inactive women (Zhang *et al.* 2006) and lower risk of Type 2 diabetes in the longer term (Ceysens *et al.* 2006). There are no data for optimal weight gain during pregnancy (Metzger *et al.* 2007). The Fifth International Workshop-Conference on GDM (2003) recommended a relatively small weigh increase during pregnancy: ~7 kg for obese women and up to 18 kg in underweight women.

Women at risk of GDM are advised to monitor their fasting and 2-hour postprandial blood glucose levels after each meal although there is no objective evidence to support the recommended frequency. CGM may be used to obtain a blood glucose pattern in some women; see Chapter 3.

Insulin will be required during pregnancy if blood glucose cannot be controlled using diet and exercise, generally when the fasting glucose is >5.0 mmol/L on three consecutive occasions but the duration of time on diet/exercise therapy before commencing insulin is unknown. Buchanan *et al.* (1994) recommended using insulin if the foetal abdominal circumference is >75th percentile for gestational age on ultrasound. However, a limitation of this method is that it provides a 'snapshot' rather monitoring continuous longitudinal foetal growth and should not be used alone especially given foetal macrosomia is related to maternal blood glucose levels. Insulin analogues are generally used; see Chapter 5 and the starting dose is calculated according to the woman's weight generally ~0.8 units/kg (non-obese), 0.9–1.0 units/kg (overweight and obese respectively).

Oral glucose lowering medicines (GLMs) are contraindicated because they cross the placenta and cause neonatal hypoglycaemia and may have other unknown effects. However, Metformin is used in Europe and South Africa and glibenclamide in South Africa without any reported foetal or maternal adverse outcomes. Although most other countries do not recommend OHA use during pregnancy (Metzger *et al.* 2007) the Metformin in Gestational Diabetes (MiG) (Rowan 2007) set up to compare Metformin with insulin on perinatal outcomes suggests Metformin is safe in the short term but may be contraindicated if the baby is small, or if the mother has pulmonary oedema or sepsis due to the risk of lactic acidosis; see Chapter 7. Metformin reduces absorption of vitamin B$_{12}$ but this can be overcome by supplementing with calcium.

Insulin is given as required during labour. Some obstetric units use insulin infusions to control hyperglycaemia, which may be exacerbated by the pain and stress of labour. Frequent blood glucose monitoring is required because insulin requirements fall dramatically after delivery and maternal hypoglycaemia is possible. The baby is prone to hypoglycaemia after delivery and should be monitored closely for 24 hours as indicated in the preceding section.

Encourage breastfeeding. Breastfeeding provides essential nutrition and immunity for the baby. It decreases the risk of obesity and Type 2 diabetes in later life in babies of women who develop GDM. Some studies also suggest cow's milk and gluten-containing solid foods should not be introduced before three months of age. Exposure to cow's milk protein may be a risk factor for Type 1 diabetes in children with a dysfunctional gut immune system (Luopajärvi *et al.* 2008). Cow's milk contains different variations of the milk protein casein (A1 or A2) depending on the breed of cattle. Breeds that produce A1 protein in their milk are more common in Europe. Consumption of A1 milk is associated with Type 1 diabetes (Laugesen & Elliott 2003). Likewise, gluten is a risk factor for Type 1 diabetes-associated autoimmunity in children with a genetic risk of Type 1 diabetes (Ziegler *et al.* 2003). The UNICEF infant feeding guidelines recommend women breastfeed exclusively for six months, introducing solid foods after six months but to continue breastfeeding for up to two years of age.

Type 1 diabetes

As stated, planning the pregnancy and achieving optimal health before becoming pregnant significantly improves outcomes. Insulin requirements vary throughout the pregnancy and frequent blood glucose monitoring is essential so doses can be adjusted appropriately.

The specific insulin dose depends on individual characteristics. Overweight women may be less sensitive to insulin and may require larger doses than lean women. NovoRapid is approved for use in pregnancy. There do not appear to be any safety issues using the other insulin analogues in pregnancy but clinical experience with Apidra and Detemir is not as extensive with the other analogues (Nankervis 2008 oral presentation).

Blood glucose testing before and one hour after each meal is ideal to help titrate insulin doses as needed. Insulin requirements usually increases by ~20% in the first 5–6 weeks due to increased levels of progesterone and continues to rise slowly to weeks 9–11 at which time the placenta begins to produce progesterone and ovarian production ceases (Jovanovic 2004).

Progesterone levels may decline temporarily during the switch and consequently insulin requirements can drop especially in lean insulin-sensitive women. Hypoglycaemia risk increases. It may be necessary to perform 3 AM blood glucose tests to determine whether hypoglycaemia occurs during the night. Progesterone levels increase again after ~8–10 days and insulin requirements begin to increase and continue to do so during each trimester. At term when contractions begin insulin requirements drop because the available glucose is utilised to support uterine contractions. Three AM blood glucose testing may be required again at this time.

After delivery insulin requirements generally drop significantly and only very low doses may be needed in the first 24–48 hours and eventually return to prepregnancy requirements. However, breastfeeding women usually require less long acting insulin because blood glucose is used to produce milk, but they may need more short-acting insulin at mealtimes. Hyperglycaemia may mean extra lactose in breast milk and cause problems for the baby such as diarrhoea and putting on excess weight.

Women with Type 1 diabetes may have hypertension as a consequence of nephropathy or hypertension may develop as a consequence of the pregnancy (American Diabetes Association 2013 Blood pressure must be carefully monitored and controlled to reduce the risk of pre-eclampsia, progression of renal disease and retinopathy. Medicines management can be complication because ACE inhibitors, beta blocking agents and diuretics are generally contraindicated.

Type 2 diabetes

Women with Type 2 diabetes and hyperglycaemia may be commenced on insulin prior to conceiving to optimise blood glucose levels and improve pregnancy outcomes.

Women with Type 2 diabetes are usually commenced on insulin during pregnancy. As with Type 1 diabetes insulin requirements slowly increase over the course of the pregnancy. However, the typical temporary drop seen ~9–11 weeks in women with Type 1 diabetes may not occur because women with Type 2 diabetes are generally insulin resistant. Insulin requirements are affected by hormone levels but also by arbohydrate intake and activity levels.

Women with Type 2 diabetes should monitor their blood glucose with the same frequency as those with Type 1 but are generally less prone to nocturnal hypoglycaemia.

After delivery women who were treated with diet and exercise may be able to resume that regimen but insulin is recommended if the woman decides to breast feed (ADIPS 2005). OHAs can be used but Metformin is present in breast milk and the baby *may* develop hypoglycaemaia. Therefore, regular blood glucose testing may be needed, but could be stressful for the parents.

Practice points

(1) Some women worry about whether injecting insulin into the abdomen can cause or exacerbate stretch marks.
(2) Some women worry about damaging their baby by injecting insulin into the abdomen.
(3) There is no evidence that insulin causes stretch marks and the needles are not long enough to penetrate into the uterus and damage the baby.
(4) It may be difficult to pinch up a fold of skin during late pregnancy as the skin stretches and tightens. It may be necessary to inject into other sites such as the side of the abdomen or thighs.

Menopause and diabetes

Menopause is a normal life stage for all women as the ability to bear a child ends and levels of oestrogen and progesterone gradually decline. Small amounts of oestrogen are usually still produced. Menopause is complete when menstruation does not occur for 12 months around 51 years of age although women with Type 1 diabetes may experience menopause at an earlier age. However, overweight women with Type 2 diabetes may go through menopause later because oestrogen levels do not decline as rapidly in overweight women. Women are living longer, thus they spend a considerable proportion of their lives in the post menopausal stage. Older women may develop diabetes as discussed in Chapter 12.

Signs and symptoms of menopause

Some of the symptoms associated with menopause may be associated with normal ageing, others are due to hormonal fluctuations. The signs and symptoms include:

- mood swings, irritability, anxiety, and depression;
- difficulty remembering things;
- increased premenstrual tension;
- heavier or lighter menstrual flow;
- hot flushes;
- changed sexual functioning such as lower libido, vaginal dryness, and recurrent candidia infections;
- susceptibility to UTI;
- fluctuating and unpredictable blood glucose levels, which adds to the distress associated with menopause. some women with Type 1 diabetes experience more frequent hypoglycaemia. unexplained hypoglycaemia may be one of the first signs of menopause;
- sleep disturbance due to hot flushes and/or nocturnal hypoglycaemia;
- weight gain, especially in Type 2 diabetes, which may be associated with reduced activity and may lead to hyperglycaemia;
- chronic back and joint pain, which can be exacerbated by being overweight.

Managing the menopause

Maintaining a healthy active lifestyle is important for all women. A dietary review may be helpful to ensure adequate nutrition is maintained and limit the risk of common nutritional deficiencies such as calcium and vitamin D and the risk of osteoporosis and fractures. A diet rich in phytoestrogens such as soy products and legumes helps maintain hormonal balance. Limiting alcohol and caffeine helps control hot flushes. A healthy diet and regular exercise control weight and reduces strain on joints, which reduces back pain a well as improving blood glucose utilisation as well as reducing cardiovascular and osteoporosis risk, and improving mental wellbeing.

Regular blood glucose monitoring is important to distinguish menopausal symptoms such as sweating from hypoglycaemia and to guide OHA/insulin dose adjustment. Some overnight testing may be necessary.

A medication review is advisable. Medications, particularly OHA and insulin doses, may need to be adjusted. A through complication assessment is advisable. The risk of cardiovascular disease increases thus lipid lowering and antihypertensive agents may be needed, if they are not already prescribed.

Hormone replacement therapy (HRT) may improve glycaemic control and lipid levels, depending on the preparations used, and improve cardiovascular risk in younger postmenopausal women (Khoo & Mahesh 2005). Several cardiovascular events are reduced by 34–45% in women aged 50–59 on HRT and with longer use but not those >60 years (Hodis & Mack 2008). However, HRT should not be prescribed to prevent cardiovascular disease. Diet and exercise, lipid lowering medicines especially statins, and aspirin may be needed in women with cardiovascular risk factors, but fenofibrate may be contraindicated because of the risk of venous embolism. HRT is increasingly being known as menopausal hormone therapy (MHT) (National Center for Complementary and Alternative Medicine 2008).

The individual benefits and risks need to be considered and carefully explained to the woman. Younger recently menopausal women have fewer risks than older postmenopausal women. Possible adverse events include stroke, venous thrombosis, and breast cancer, but the relative risks are low if HRT is commenced within 5 years of menopause (WHI study 2002).

HRT may be useful in younger post menopausal women with Type 1 diabetes to prevent osteoporosis, but should be used at the lowest effective dose. Long-term HRT to prevent osteoporosis is not advisable but HRT does have a role in managing menopausal symptoms in the short term (Australian Drug Evaluation Committee 2003). Bisphosphonates may be an alternative if HRT is contraindicated (Khoo & Mahesh 2005).

Antibiotics and antifungal agents may be needed to manage UTIs and candida infections but general hygiene, passing urine after sexual intercourse, wearing cotton underwear, eating a healthy diet, and controlling hyperglycaemia are important preventative measures. Cranberry preparations prevent UTIs but may be contraindicated with some medications likely to cause bleeding.

Contraception options for women with diabetes

Planned pregnancy is vital in women with diabetes thus contraceptive advice is essential. Women with diabetes need specific advice about their contraception options from a qualified expert. The same range of contraceptive methods available to non-diabetic women is available to and is suitable for women with diabetes and the same risks and benefits apply (Broecker & Lykens 2011; Damm *et al.* 2005). However, the risks and benefits of each contraceptive option should be discussed with individual woman with diabetes because extra precautions may apply: for example, women with hypertension, those at risk of embolism, and those with microvascular disease and cardiovascular disease. These risks associated with contraceptives may be greater in women with Type 2 diabetes (Damm *et al.* 2005). Thus, the benefits and risks need to be carefully considered for each individual woman and include the risk of obesity, cardiovascular disease, renal impairment and retinopathy (Broecker & Lykens 2011).

Important but often overlooked risks are the risks of becoming pregnant and pregnancy-related complications. These risks should be included in the discussion. Each woman should receive accurate information about the available contraceptive choices and the partners should be involved in discussions where relevant and possible. Information about safe sex is also important to protect from unwanted pregnancy and sexually transmitted infections (STI). The best way to reduce STIs is to use a barrier method such as male and female condoms and dams. These methods can be used during oral, vaginal and anal sex.

Commonly used contraceptive methods include (Better Health Channel 2012):
- Physical barrier methods include male and female condoms and diaphragms, which are effective contraceptive measure if used correctly, but pregnancy can occur if they are not used correctly. Diaphragms must be left in place for at least six hours after intercourse. Barrier methods are safe for women with diabetes.
- Intrauterine devices (IUD). An IUD is a small plastic device with copper or hormones (Mirena) added, which is placed into the uterus. The IUD can sty in place for 5–10 years depending on the type of device but can be removed if the woman wants to become pregnant or experiences problems. IUDs are effective contraceptives and are

safe for most women with diabetes but hormone-containing IUDs can have a small effect on the hormones that control the menstrual cycle. Copper IUDs are associated with heavier periods.

- Hormonal contraceptives:
  - Oral tablets (OC) and vaginal rings, which are highly effective if used correctly. There are many types of OC with different hormone combinations. While they can be used by women with diabetes, they are not recommended for women at risk or cardiovascular disease and those who smoke. The mini pill only contains synthetic progesterone and is suitable for women who experience side effects from oestrogen or women when oestrogen-containing OCs are contraindicated. Hormone contraceptive patches are a useful alternative for some women. Vaginal rings contain similar hormones to the combined pill. The ring is inserted into the vagina and stays in place for three weeks after which time it is removed and another ring inserted after a week.
  - implants and injections, what are very effective; however, they cause side effects. These methods include: implanon, which is implanted under the skin and lasts for three years. Depo-Provera/Depo_Ralovera are injectable contraceptives that contain progestogen and are effective for 13–14 weeks. Progestin only contraceptive methods should be avoided while breastfeeding or used with caution (Damm *et al.* 2012).
- Sterilisation, which is mostly a permanent surgical method of achieving contraception. Two methods are available for women: tubal ligation, which is performed under general anaesthetic, and Essure, which involves inserting small coils into the fallopian tubes under local anaesthetic. Male sterilisation, vasectomy, can be reversed.
- Natural methods, which include the Billing's method and withdrawing the penis from the vagina before ejaculating, but these methods often result in pregnancy
- Emergency contraception (EC) might be required and is safe for women with diabetes. Emergency contraception involves taking an OC containing progestogen, as soon as possible after intercourse and is best taken within 72 hours but it can be taken up to 120 hours after unprotected sex. Emergency contraception pills prevent 85% of expected pregnancies if taken within the prescribed time following intercourse. EC can be considered in high risk women with diabetes providing the woman and her partner are fully informed and prepared to accept the decision without knowing whether they are pregnant or not.

Concerns have been raised about the effects of OCs on glucose and fat metabolism, which could exacerbate cardiovascular risks. However, several studies suggest OCs do not adversely affect blood glucose or lipid levels, or exacerbate retinopathy or hypertension (Kaunitz 2002) including in women with previous GDM. Other research suggests high-dose combined OC has a small beneficial effect on glucose homeostasis and lipid metabolism, whereas progesterone only OC improves lipid metabolism (Visser *et al.* 2006). The risks of vascular complications, retinopathy and rates of thrombolism appear to be low, but progesterone-only preparations cause more irregular bleeding. All methods are effective contraceptives.

Combination OCs, monthly contraceptive injections, vaginal rings and patches appear to be appropriate for women with diabetes <35 years (Kaunitz 2002). These methods might be contraindicated in older women and those with hypertension, and/or micro and macrovascular disease. For these women IUDs including progesterone-releasing mirena, progesterone only mini pills, or depot progesterone, for example, Depot Provera injections or implanon implants may be viable alternatives (Kaunitz 2002).

Trials are currently underway in seven countries, including Australia, to determine the safety and effectiveness of an injectable hormone-based male contraceptive. The contraceptive contains testosterone and progestogen. Other studies have investigated a combination of implanted testosterone and injected progestogen, which did not result in any pregnancies in the men's female partners or affect the men's energy and libido. These studies appear promising but male contraception is not yet available in Australia.

> **Practice points**
> - Contraception is an essential aspect of sexual health (see Chapter 11).
> - Contraception appropriateness must be considered fort eh individual women considering her risks and the likely benefits. These include the considering the risks of STI and unwanted pregnancies.
> - Appropriate contraception choices are likely to change over the lifespan and should be regularly assessed as part of a medicines review and/or complication screening processes.
> - Discussions about contraception options should involve both partners where practical but the decision to include the partner rest with the woman concerned.
> - The woman (and her partner) should be given individualised information about the risks and benefits of each contraceptive option so she can make an informed decision.

Complementary approaches to managing the menopause

Many women began using CAM to manage menopausal symptoms in 2002 when the findings from the Women's Health Initiative study were released, which questioned the long-term safety of HRT use. At the time many women stopped using HRT and many tried CAM alternatives. The value of using CAM to manage menopausal symptoms is still debated and the long-term benefits of CAM hormone replacement medicines to prevent osteoporosis are unknown. Conventional hormone replacement medicines significantly reduce menopausal symptoms and osteoporotic fractures. Many research trials focus on managing hot flushes and preventing osteoporosis, however, CAM practitioners focus on managing the transition to and through menopause, rather then treating isolated symptoms.

For this and other reasons, CAM therapies continue to be popular with many menopausal women who fear the risks associated with conventional HRT. Australian women of menopausal age are high CAM users (MacLaren *et al.* 2001). Popular CAM menopausal treatments include phytoestrogens, herbal medicines, acupuncture, homeopathy, acupuncture, massage and essential oils, and wild yam cream. Although research shows conflicting results about the benefits of CAM for managing menopausal symptoms they are widely used.

Phytoestrogens

Phytoestrogens are naturally occurring plant compounds, which have a similar chemical composition to but lower potency than oestrogen. Phytoestrogens act at oestrogen receptor sites and may reduce menopausal symptoms but it is not clear whether the effects are due to phytoestrogens or other products in particular foods. Phytoestrogens reduce cholesterol and may have a place in managing cardiovascular risk. They may also improve cognition and increase bone mass. There are three main phytoestrogens:

(1) isoflavones: found in soy products and beans, for example, lima beans and lentils;
(2) lignans: found in fruit, vegetables, grains and seeds such as linseed and flaxseed;
(3) coumestans: found in sprouted seeds such as alfalfa.

Phytoestrogen should be used with caution by women using medicines that contain oestrogen for example, OCs, HRT, and some cancer medicines, for example, selective oestrogen receptor modulators such as tamoxifen, and women at risk of breast, uterine or ovarian cancer, endometriosis or uterine fibroids. Women in these categories should seek expert advice rather than self-prescribing.

Herbal medicines

If women choose to use CAM medicines to manage the menopause they should be clear about their therapy goals and seek the advice of a qualified practitioner. CAM medicines are usually used to manage the symptoms of menopause such as hot flushes, to improve sleep, and maintain wellbeing. Commonly used medicines include:

- *Hypericum perforatum* (St John's Wort), which effectively reduces anxiety and mild to moderate depression (Ernst 1995).
- Vitus Agnus Castus (Chaste tree) is reputed to be a hormone regulator but is only useful if other hormones are not being used. It can interact with oral contraceptives and HRT
- *Onothera biennis* (evening primrose) oil, which has limited evidence to support an effect.
- *Cimicifuga racemosa* (black cohosh), to reduce symptoms including hot flushes. It is a key ingredient in medicines such as remifemin, which has been shown to reduce LH without affecting FH (Duker 1991). Some studies have not shown any reduction in hot flushes (Newtown *et al.* 2006). There have been case reports of liver damage and hepatitis but no causal association has been proven. However, preparations containing black cohosh may be contraindicated in women at risk of these conditions. Generally it should not be used longer than 6 months or during pregnancy and lactation.
- *Angelica sinensis* (dong quai) there is limited evidence that dong quai reduces hot flushes. It interacts with warfarin and may be contraindicated in women using warfarin or the effects on the INR monitored carefully.
- *Panax ginseng or P. quinquefolius* (ginseng), which may be useful to improve mood, general well being, and sleep. It does not improve hot flushes. Ginseng has hypoglycaemic properties and may represent a hypoglycaemia risk. However, blood glucose levels are often higher during menopause and the glucose lowering effect may be a beneficial interaction.
- *Piper methysticum* (kava) reduces anxiety but has been linked to liver damage. Therefore, kava may be contraindicated in women with existing lover disease or those at risk of liver disease.
- *Trifolium pratense* (red clover) red clover contains phytoestrogens and is a key ingredient in CAM medicines such as promensil. Some women report overall benefits but there is limited evidence that it reduces hot flushing.
- Dehydroepiandrosterone (DHEA) occurs naturally in many foods and is often taken as a dietary supplement. DHEA is converted to oestrogen and testosterone in the body. It may reduce the frequency and intensity of hot flushes and improve sexual

arousal. Significantly, endogenous DHEA levels decline with age and many people use DHEA supplements to reduce age-associated symptoms as well as menopause. It may increase the risk of breast and prostate cancer but evidence is lacking. DHEA is sometimes added to bioidentical hormonal compounds such as Biest and Triest, which increased in popularity after the release of the results of the WHI study, which suggested HRT was linked with increased risk of breast cancer (Rossouw *et al.* 2002).

- Progesterone creams are available on prescription; some formulations contain oestrogen and testosterone. Progesterone declines after menopause due to declining oestrogen levels. However there is little evidence that progesterone creams reduce menopausal symptoms or improve osteoporosis risk. Only a small amount of progesterone is absorbed form topically applied formulations. *Dioscorea villosa* (wild yam) cream does not contain progesterone although it was originally marketed in this way because it contains diosgenin, an oestrogen-like compound. Wild yam is an antispasmodic and gentle liver tonic and CAM practitioners prescribe it for these indications. Progesterone used in conventional pessaries, OCPs and suppositories is synthesised from diosgenin. However, specific enzymes are required to produce progesterone from diosgenin and these enzymes are not present in the human body. Traditionally, wild yam was taken orally rather than cream but the cream formulation is a popular self-prescribed menopausal treatment. Progesterone is mainly prescribed to protect the lining of the uterus in women who use oestrogen. Substituting progesterone creams especially wild yam for the progesterone component of combined HRT can increase the risk of endometrial cancer.

Practice points

(1) Women who elect to use CAM to manage menopausal symptoms should do so under the management of a suitably qualified practitioner.
(2) They should advise all their conventional health practitioners that if they use CAM.
(3) More research is needed into the benefits of most CAM for managing menopausal symptoms.
(4) CAM medicines used to manage menopausal symptoms can interact with conventional medicines.
(5) Pregnant women need to seek expert advice about using CAM especially CAM medicines and especially in the first trimester.

References

Allaire, A. (2001) Complementary and alternative medicine in labour and delivery suite. *Clinical Obstetrics and Gynaecology*, **44**, 681–691.

Alberti, G., Zimmet, P. & Shaw, J. (2007) International Diabetes Federation Consensus on Type 2 diabetes. *Diabetic Medicine*, **24**, 451–463.

Andersen, O., Hertel, J., Schmolker, L. & Kuhl, C. (1998) Influence of the maternal plasma glucose concentration at delivery on the risk of hypoglycaemia in infants of insulin-dependent diabetic mothers. *Acta Paediatrica*, **74**, 268–273.

American Medical Association (AMA) (2013) Standards of Medical Care care.diabetesjournals.org/content/36/Supplement_1/S11.full (accessed March 2013).

Armitage, J., Poston, L. & Taylor, P. (2008) Developmental origins of obesity and the metabolic syndrome: The role of maternal obesity. *Front Hormonal Research* **36**, 73 –84.

ADIPS (Australasian Diabetes in Pregnancy Society) (2005) Consensus guidelines for the management of Type 1 and Type 2 diabetes in relation to pregnancy *Medical Journal of Australia* **183** (7), 373 –377.

ADIPS (2012) ADIPS *consensus guidelines for the testing and diagnosis of gestational mellitus in Australia*. ADIPS.

Australian Drug Evaluation Committee (ADEC) (2003) *Update to ADEC statement on use of hormone replacement therapy*. ADEA 17th October http://www.tga.health.gov/au/docs/html/hrtadec2.htm (accessed December 2007).

Barker, D., Gluckman, P., Godfrey, K. et al. (1993) Fetal nutrition and cardiovascular disease in adult life. *Lancet*, 341(8850), 938–941

Better Health Channel (2012) *Contraception choices fact sheet*. http://www.betterhealth.vic.gov.au (accessed December 2012).

Biesenbach, G., Stoger, H. & Zazgornik, J. (1992) Influence of pregnancy on progression of diabetic nephropathy and subsequent requirement for renal replacement therapy in female type I diabetic patients with impaired renal function. *Nephrology Dialysis Transplant*, 7, 105–109.

Boden, R., Lundgren, M., Brandt, L., Reutfors, J. & Kieler, H. (2012) Antipsychotics during pregnancy. *American Medical Archives of General Psychiatry* **69** (7), 715–721.

Bongaard, B. (2007) Is massage beneficial for pregnant women? *Alternative Medicine Alert*, **10** (12), 133–136.

Boyko, E. (2000) Proportion of type 2 diabetes cases resulting from impaired fetal growth. *Diabetes Care*, **23**, 1260-1264.

Broecher, J. & Lykens, J. (2011) Contraception options for women with diabetes mellitus: An evidence-based guide to safety and counseling American Diabetes Association. *DOS Against Diabetes* **April,** 11 – 18.

Buchanan, T., Kjos, S. & Montoro, M. (1994) Use of foetal ultrasounds to select metabolic therapy for pregnancies complicated by mild gestational diabetes. *Diabetes Care*, 17, 275–283.

Ceysens, G., Rouiller, D. & Boulvain, M. (2006) Exercise for diabetic pregnant women. *Cochrane Database of Systematic Reviews*, Rev CD004225.

Chief Medical Officer (2000) *The Report on the Confidential Enquiries into Maternal Deaths 1997–1999*. Her Majesty's Stationery Office, London.

Coffey, S. & Mason, H. (2003) The effect of polycystic ovary syndrome on health-related quality of life. *Gynecology and Endocrinology*, 17 (5), 379–86.

Coustan, D. (1997) Is preconception counselling for women with diabetes cost-effective? *Diabetes Spectrum*, **10** (3), 1195–2000.

Damm, P., Mathiesen, E., Clausen, D. & Petersen, K. (2005) *Metabolic syndrome and related disorders: Contraception for women with diabetes mellitus*. http://www.liebertonline.com/doi: 10. 1089/met.2005.3.244 (accessed February 2008).

DeBoer, T. (2007) Maternal diabetes linked to infant memory problems. *Child Neurology*, 47, 525.

DeMaria, E. (2007) Bariatric surgery for morbid obesity. *New England Journal of Medicine*, **356**, 2176–2183.

Donovan, P. (2012) Hypertensive disorders of pregnancy *Australian Prescriber*, 35, 47–50.

Dornhorst, A. (2003) Maternal hyperglycaemia – Food for thought. *Practical Diabetes International*, **20** (8), 283–289.

Dornhorst, A., Paterson, C. & Nicholls, J. (1992) High prevalence of gestational diabetes in women from ethnic minority groups. *Diabetec Medicine*, **9**, 820–825.

Duker, E. (1991) Effects of extracts from *Cimicifuga racemosa* on gonadotropin release in menopausal women and ovariectomised rats. *Plana Medica*, **57**, 420–424.

Edison, R., and Muenke, M. (2004) Central nervous system and limb anomalies in case reports of first trimester statin exposure. *New England Journal of Medicine*, 350, 1579–1582.

Ernst, E. (1995) St John's Wort, an antidepressant? A systematic criteria-based review. *Phytomedicine*, **2** (1), 67–71.

Feig, D., Briggs, G. & Koren, G. (2007) Oral antidiabetic agents in pregnancy and lactation: A paradigm shift? *Annals of Pharmacotherapy*, **41**(7), 1174–1180.

Forster, D., Denning, A., Wills, G., Bolger, M. & McCarthy, E. (2006) Herbal medicine use during pregnancy in a group of Australian women. *BMC Pregnancy and Childbirth*, 6, 21.

Gardiner, S. (2002) Drugs in pregnancy. *Current Therapeutics*, **October,** 31–33.

Gilbert, C., Valois, M. & Koren, G. (2006) Pregnancy outcome after first-trimester exposure to Metformin: A meta-analysis *Fertility and Sterility*, **86** (3), 658–663.

Gutzin, S., Kozer, E. & Mcgee, L. (2003) The safety of oral hypoglycaemic agents in the first trimester of pregnancy: A meta-analysis. *Canadian Journal of Clinical Pharmacology*, **10**, 179–183.

HAPO Collaborative Research Group (2008) Hyperglycaemia and adverse pregnancy outcomes. *The New England Journal of Medicine* **358**, 1991–2002.

Hewitt, V., Robertson, R. & Haddow, G. (2005) Nursing and midwifery management of hypoglycaemia in healthy term neonates: A systematic review. *Journal of Evidence Based Healthcare*, **3** (7), 169–205.

Hirsch, I. (2005) Insulin analogues. *New England Journal of Medicine*, **352**, 174–183.

Hod, M., Damm, P., Kaaja, R., *et al.* (2007) Foetal and perinatal outcomes in Type 1 diabetes pregnancy: A randomized study comparing insulin as part with human insulin in 322 subjects. *American Journal of Obstetrics & Gynaecology*, **198** (2), 186 and 1–7.

Hodis, H. & Mack, W. (2008) The beneficial effect of hormone replacement therapy on mortality and coronary heart disease in younger versus older postmenopausal women. *Medscape Obstetrics/ Gynaecology & Womens' Health*, http:www.medscape.com/viewarticle/569935?src=mp (accessed March 2008).

Hoffman, L., Nolan, C., Wilson, D., Oats, J. & Simmons, D. (1998) Gestational diabetes mellitus – Management guidelines. *Medical Journal of Australia*, **169**, 93–97.

Hollingsworth, D. (1992) *Pregnancy, Diabetes and Birth*. Philadlephia USA Williams & Wilkins.

International Association of Diabetes and Pregnancy (IADSP) consensus panel (2010) IADSP group's recommendations on the diagnosis and classification of hyperglycaemia in pregnancy. *Diabetes Care* **33**, 676–682.

International Diabetes Federation (IDF) (2009) *Policy briefing – diabetes in pregnancy: Protecting maternal health*. IDF, Brussels www.idf.org (accessed October 2012).

Janssen, O., Hahn, S., Tan, S., Benson, S. & Elsenbruch, S. (2008) Mood and sexual function in polycystic ovary syndrome. *Seminars in Reproductive Medicine*, **26** (1), 45–52.

Jovanovic, J. (2004) Answers to questions about pregnancy and diabetes. *Diabetic Mommy* http://www.diabeticmommy.com/sp-pregnancy-diabetes-bd-faq-answers.html (accessed November 2007).

Karamermer, Y. & Ross-Hesselink, J. (2007) Coronary heart disease and pregnancy. *Future Cardiology*, **3** (5), 559–567.

Kaunitz, A. (2002) Contraception for women with diabetes. *Medscape Obstetrics and Gynaecology & Women's Health*, **7** (2), (Posted 12. 9. 2002) (accessed February 2008).

Kim, C., Siscovick, D., Sidney, S., *et al.* (2002) Oral contraceptive use and association with glucose, insulin and diabetes in young adult women: The CARDIA study. *Diabetes Care*, **25** (6), 1027–1032.

Korytkowski, M., Mokan, M., Horowitz, M. & Berga, S. (1995) Metabolic effects of oral contraceptives in women with polycystic ovary syndrome. *Journal of Clinical Endocrinology and Metabolism*, **80**, 3327–3334.

Khoo, C. & Mahesh, P. (2005) Diabetes and the menopause. *Journal British Menopause Society*, **11** (1), 6–11.

Marx, G., Domurat, M. & Costin, M. (1987) Potential hazard of hypoglycaemia in the parturient. *Canadian Journal of Anaesthesiology*, **34** (4), 400–402.

Laugesen, M. & Elliott, R. (2003) Ischaemic heart disease, Type 1 diabetes, and cow milk A1 beta-casein. *New Zealand Journal of Medicine*, **116**, 1168.

Luopajärvi, K., Savilahti, E., Virtanen, S. M. *et al.* (2008) Enhanced levels of cow's milk antibodies in infancy in children who develop type 1 diabetes later in childhood. *Pediatric Diabetes*, **9** (5), 434–41

MacLaren, A., & Woods, N. F. (2001). Midlife women making hormone therapy decisions. *Women's Health Issues*, **11** (3), 216–230.

Menato, G., Bo, S., Signorlie, A., *et al.* (2008) Current management of gestational diabetes mellitus. *Expert Review of Obstetrics and Gynaecology*, **3** (1), 73–91.

Metzger, E., Buchanan, T. & Coulstan, D. (2007) Summary and recommendations of the fifth International Workshop – Conference on Gestational Diabetes Mellitus. *Diabetes Care*, **30**, S251–S260.

Meyer, C., McGrath, B. & Teede, H. (2007) Effects of medical therapy on insulin resistance and the cardiovascular system in polycystic ovarian syndrome. *Diabetes Care*, **30**, 471–478.

Moran, I., Noakes, M. & Clifton, P. (2003) Dietary composition in restoring reproductive and metabolic physiology in overweight women with polycystic ovarian syndrome. *Journal Clinical Endocrinology and Metabolism*, **88**, 812–819.

Nankervis, A. (2008) Practical management of diabetes in pregnancy. Sanofi-Aventis Seminar April, Melbourne.

National Center for Complementary and Alternative Medicine (NCCAM) (2008)Menopausal Symptoms and complementary health practices nccam.nih.gov/health/menopause/menopausesymptoms (accessed December 2012).

National Women's Health Information Center (2006) *Menopause and menopause treatments*. http://nccam.nih.gov/health/menopauseandcam (accessed February 2008).

Nilsson, A., Lagerquist, E., Lynch, K. *et al.* (2009) Temporal Variation of *Ljungan Virus* Antibody Levels in Relation to Islet Autoantibodies and Possible Correlation to Childhood Type 1 Diabetes *The Open Pediatric Medicine Journal*, 3, 61–66

Newton, K., Reed, S. & Lacroix, A. (2006) Treatment of vasomotor symptoms of menopause with black cohosh, multibotanicals, soy, hormone therapy, or placebo. *Annals of Internal Medicine*, 145 (12), 869–879.

Oakley, C. (1992) Care of gestational diabetes mellitus. *Diabetes Care*, 1, 6–8.

Pagona, L., Sandin, S., Lof M, *et al.* (2012) Low carbohydrate-high protein diet and incidence of cardiovascular disease in Swedish women: Prospective cohort study. *British Medical Journal*, June DOI; 10.1136/bmj.e4026.

Pettitt D, Jovanovic, L. (2007) Low birth weight as a risk factor for gestational diabetes, diabetes, and impaired glucose tolerance during pregnancy. *Diabetes Care*. 10 (2):S147–S149.

Polycystic Ovarian Syndrome Association of Australia. www.posa.asn.au (accessed March 2008).

Rasmussen B, O'Connell B, Dunning T. (2007) Young women with diabetes using internet communication to create stability during life transitions. *Journal of Clinical Nursing* 1365:17–24.

Ray, J., O'Brien, T. & Chan, W. (2001) Preconception care and the risk of congenital abnormalities in the offspring of women with diabetes mellitus: A meta-analysis. *Quality Journal of Medicine*, 94, 435–444.

Rice, G., Illanes, S. & Mitchell, M. (2012) Gestational diabetes mellitus; A positive predictor of Type 2 diabetes? *International Journal of Endocrinology*, my DOI: 10.1135-2012/721653.

Rizzo, T., Dooley, S., Metzger, B. *et al.* (1995) Prenatal and perinatal influences on long term psychomotor development in offspring of diabetic mothers. *American Journal of Obstetrics and Gynaecology*, 173 (6), 1753–1758.

Ross, G. (2002) How to plan a healthy pregnancy. *Diabetes Conquest*, **Autumn**, 28.

Rossouw, J., Anderson, G. & Prentice, R. (2002) Writing Group for the Women's Health Initiative Investigators. Risks and benefits of oestrogen plus progestin in healthy menopausal women: Principal results from the Women's Health Initiative randomized controlled trial. *Journal American Medical Association*, 288 (3), 321–333.

Rotterdam ESHRE/ASRM Sponsored PCOS Consensus Workshop Group(2004) Revised 2003 consensus on diagnostic criteria and long term health risks related to Polycystic Ovarian Syndrome. *Fertility and Sterility*, 81, 19–25.

Rossing, K., Jacobsen, P., Hommel, E. *et al.* (2002): Pregnancy and progression of diabetic nephropathy. *Diabetologia*, 45, 36–41.

Rowan, J. (2007) A trial in progress: Treatment with Metformin compared with insulin in the Metformin in gestational diabetes study (MiG). *Diabetes Care*, 30, S214–S219.

SIGN (2010) Scottish Intercollegiate Guidelines Network. SIGN, Edinburgh.

Simmons, D., Walters, J., Rowan, J. & McIntyre, D. (2004) Metformin therapy and diabetes in pregnancy. *Medical Journal of Australia*, 180, 462–464.

Simpson, M., Parsons, M., Greenwood, J. & Wade, K. (2001) Raspberry leaf in pregnancy: Its safety and efficacy in labour. *Journal of Midwifery and Women's Health*, 46, 51–59.

Teede, H., Hutchison, S. & Zoungas, S. (2007) The management of insulin resistance in polycystic ovarian syndrome. *Trends in Endocrinology and Metabolism*, 18, 273–279.

Ter Braak, E., Evers, I., Erkelens, W. & Visser G. (2002) Maternal hypoglycaemia during pregnancy in Type 1 diabetes: Maternal and foetal consequences. *Diabetes Metabolism Research Reviews*, 18, 96–105.

The Australasian Diabetes in Pregnancy Society (2005) Consensus guidelines for the management of Type 1 and Type 2 diabetes in relation to pregnancy. *Medical Journal of Australia*, 183 (7), 373–377.

The Australasian Society for the Study of Hypertension in Pregnancy Consensus Statement. *The Detection, Investigation and Management of Hypertension in Pregnancy: Executive Summary*. http://www.racp.edu.au/asshp/asshp.pdf (accessed December 2007).

Tournaire, M. &, Theau-Yonneau, A. (2007) Complementary and alternative approaches to pain relief during labour. *Evidence Based Complementary and Alternative Medicine*, 4 (4), 409–417.

Visser, J., Snel, M. & Van Vilet, T. (2006) Hormonal versus non-hormonal contraceptives in women with diabetes mellitus Type 1 and 2. *Cochrane Database of Systematic Reviews*, 18 (4), cd003990.

Western Australian Center for Evidence Based Nursing and Midwifery (2006) Management of asymptomatic hypoglycaemia in health term neonates for nurses and midwives. *Best Practice*, 10 (1), 1–4.

World Health Organization (WHO) (1997) *Hypoglycaemia in the Newborn*. WHO, Geneva.

Women's Health Initiative (WHI) Writing Group for the WHI investigators (2002) Risks and benefits of HRT. *Journal of the American Medical Association*, **288**, 321–333.

UNICEF. http://www.unicef.org (accessed November 2012).

Wilhelm, K., Mitchell, P., Slade, T., Brownhill, S. & Andrews, G. (2003) Prevalence and correlates of DSM-IV major depression in an Australian national survey. *Journal Affective Disorders*, **75**, 155–162.

Yildiz, B. (2008) Oral contraception in women with polycystic ovary syndrome. *Seminars in Reproductive Health*, **26** (1), 111–120.

Zhang, C., Solomon, C., Manson, J. & Hu, F. (2006) A prospective study of pregravid physical activity and sedentary behaviours in relation to the risk of gestational diabetes mellitus. *Archives of Internal Medicine*, **166**, 543–548.

Ziegler, A. G. , Schmid, S., Huber, D., Hummel, M. & Bonifacio, E. (2003) Early infant feeding and risk of developing type 1 diabetes-associated autoantibodies. *Journal American Medical Association*, **290** (13),1721–1728.

Chapter 15
Psychological and Quality of Life Issues Related to Having Diabetes

Key points

- The focus of an individualised diabetes management plan should be on achieving a balanced life rather than 'metabolic/diabetes control.' Achieving life balance is an ongoing process of adaptation to life circumstances.
- Assessing psychological well-being and the individual's social situation and explanatory models should be undertaken at diagnosis and regularly thereafter as an essential part of the diabetes care plan. Assessments should take account of life transitions and their effect on the individual's psychological, spiritual and physical well being.
- Inadequate self-management, including medicine self-management, could be a trigger to screen for depression, diabetes-related distress or anxiety, include changes in health status e.g. the development of a diabetes complication, the end of the 'honeymoon period' in Type 1 diabetes, commencing insulin in Type 2 diabetes, eating disorders and cognitive impairment.
- Appropriate support is essential to achieving optimal balance and diabetes and general health outcomes.
- An effective therapeutic relationship with heath professionals is as important as other management strategies.
- Every individual and relevant others when indicated should be involved in developing their diabetes management plan and monitoring the effectiveness of the plan.
- Most quality of life research indicates people with diabetes have worse quality of life than people without diabetes.
- Quality of life is individual, complex, and multifactorial and encompasses life priorities, which might change according to life circumstances.
- Labels such as 'non-compliant' or 'diabetic' are judgmental and should be avoided where possible (Diabetes Australia 2011).

Care of People with Diabetes: A Manual of Nursing Practice, Fourth Edition. Trisha Dunning.
© 2014 John Wiley & Sons, Ltd. Published 2014 by John Wiley & Sons, Ltd.

Rationale

Each person with diabetes is unique. People with diabetes focus on being well and living a normal life; thus, they strive to achieve their definition of life balance, which may be significantly different from health professional's view of what is important. Achieving a balanced lifestyle and good quality of life is essential to the physical, spiritual and psychological well being of people with diabetes. Depression is more common in people with diabetes and can impact on their self-care and long-term health outcomes. Health professionals are often preoccupied with metabolic control. Changing the focus to achieving balance is more likely to assist the person to achieve optimal metabolic control for their particular circumstances and social situations. Achieving such balance and undertaking diabetes self-care for a lifetime is hard, relentless work.

Appropriate assessment tools should be used to assess adherence, psychological well being and the outcomes of self-care. Many studies use HbA_{1c} as the primary outcome measure of education/psychological interventions, yet self-care and adherence are some of the *mediators* of HbA_{1c}; thus, HbA_{1c} is not an appropriate primary outcome measure (SIGN 2010). Likewise, health professional performance as a mediator is rarely measured, except using ubiquitous 'patient satisfaction surveys' that do not encompass highly relevant mediators such as knowledge, beliefs, congruence, ability to develop a therapeutic relationship and cultural competence (Dunning 2013a).

Introduction

People with diabetes are at increased risk of developing various degrees of psychological distress and psychological disorders including depression and eating disorders (Rubin & Peyrot 2001, SIGN 2010; American Diabetes Association 2011). Australians with Type 2 diabetes report lower levels of health satisfaction in all domains and experience moderate to severe symptoms of depression and distress, especially adults with Type 1 and insulin-treated Type 2, who felt they had less control over their diabetes The most commonly reported problem overall was worrying about the future (MILES 2011).

This chapter presents a brief outline of the complex, multifactorial psychological and quality of life aspects of being diagnosed and living with diabetes. A range of factors affect psychological and spiritual well being and impact on health outcomes and encompass social, individual and health professional factors (SIGN 2010; American Diabetes Association (ADA) 2011). Such factors include but are not limited to the following:

Social factors include
- cultural beliefs and customs;
- general and diabetes-related attitudes and beliefs;
- family functioning including family roles, conflict, inadequate communication skills and lack of cohesiveness;
- social circumstances including resources;
- religion.

Individual factors include
- general and diabetes-related attitudes and beliefs;
- perceptions of the severity of diabetes;
- general health, which changes over time and in different circumstances where they are situated in their personal life journey and their diabetes journey;
- physical and cognitive capacity including health literacy and numeracy;
- availability and quality of support;

- available financial, emotional and social resources;
- psychiatric history;
- age.

Health professional factors

Health professionals can hinder or facilitate effective self-care and well being. Some health professional-related factors are the same as for individuals with diabetes, others are different. Health professional factors include:

- Knowledge and competence in a range of areas.
- Clinical inertia, which can be considered the health professional equivalent of non-adherence. For example, older physicians are less likely to initiate new medicines and follow guidelines (Tung 2011). The same may be true of other health professional groups.
- Ability to look beyond diabetes and considering all the factors that could be operating at the time.
- Interpersonal communication skills, especially the key skills of listening and being truly present in an encounter (Dunning 2013).
- Beliefs and attitudes including about the severity of diabetes and. The unspoken, untrue implication that Type 1 diabetes is more serious than Type 2.
- Personal health and well-being including whether they have diabetes and the type of diabetes and where they are situated in their personal life journey and their diabetes journey.
- Setting an appropriate/inappropriate example e.g. people with diabetes find it difficult to follow 'lifestyle advice' from health professionals who smoke, are overweight, and/or physically inactive because they do not 'practice what they preach.'
- Knowing when to refer and individual.
- Available resources.

Symptoms associated with hyperglycaemia, hypoglycaemia and the focus on diet can mask signs of psychological distress and eating disorders. If present, psychological disorders can interfere with self-care, medicine adherence and exacerbate hyperglycaemia, thus setting up a vicious cycle. Improving depression results in improved glycaemic control (SIGN 2010). Depression is often undetected in older people and is often considered to be part of normal ageing. Approximately 15% of older community dwelling older people experience depressive symptoms and at least 24% of people with diabetes of all ages are depressed (Goldney & Phillips 2004) the incidence rises sharply in older people living in residential facilities (Chapter12). In Australia, the second highest suicide rate occurs in men >85.

The decision to take control of diabetes and undertake self-care is vital Hernandez (1995). Hernandez found people with Type 1 diabetes were initially concerned with being normal and adopted a passive role in their care. The decision to assume control often occurred at a turning point in their lives. The impetus for assuming control include feeling betrayed by or not listened to by health professionals, realising that adhering to management regimens would not automatically prevent complications, and health professionals accusing them of 'cheating' when their blood glucose levels were unstable (Patterson & Sloan 1994). Life and other events may impact on an individual's willingness and ability to perform self-care because of work, religious, cultural, social, and health-related issues. These include:

- Knowing their body and being able to differentiate normal from abnormal. Currently, most diabetes education and management programmes focus on the abnormal or assume all people respond the same way, the way the 'average person' responds. People gradually learn to recognise and respond to abnormal body cues e.g. to hypoglycaemia. However, diabetes complications such as autonomic neuropathy result in changes and the individual no loner experiences the familiar cues, which can be terrifying. Likewise, Type 2 diabetes often presents with few symptoms and/or serious complications can be asymptomatic, which affect individual's perception of diabetes and it severity.

- Knowing how to manage diabetes and having the physical and mental capability and financial and other resources to manage the self-care tasks and problem-solve in a range of situations, especially when they are experienced for the first time.
- Having supportive, constructive relationships in place with family/carers/friends and health professionals.
- Positive attitudes, resilience and adaptive coping mechanisms.
- Health professionals knowing the person with diabetes in order to understand their feelings about diabetes, the lessons they learned from living with diabetes, their explanatory models, and the way they undertake self-care.

Psychological adaptation and maintaining a good quality of life is dependent on the individual's degree of resilience. Resilience refers to the ability to overcome adversity and not only to rise above it, but also to thrive. It has its foundation in belonging, life meaning and expectations and happiness. Resilience is at the heart of spirituality, social cohesion, and empowerment (Dunning 2013b). Chronic conditions such as diabetes have a major impact on an individual's life plan, their partner, families, and other relationships. Acquiring coping skills and being resilient have positive effects on emotional well being and, therefore, on physical outcomes. Coping with diabetes is an issue for some people. Coping issues for young people with Type 1 diabetes encompass:

- being expected to cope
- being expected to cope all the time;
- being seen to cope by others;
- having to cope for the rest of their lives;
- having no respite from coping with diabetes (Dunning 1994).

These issues are important across the lifespan as people with diabetes face life and diabetes-related challenges. Many factors influence how a person reacts to and accepts the diagnosis of diabetes and assumes responsibility for self-care. Reactions to the diagnosis of diabetes are unique to the individual concerned; however, several common reactions have been documented. They include: anger, guilt, fear, helplessness, confusion, relief and denial. Appreciating some of the issues and reactions involved will enable clinicians to better understand the complexity of living with diabetes and enable them to help the individual set achievable goals, develop appropriate coping strategies and plan appropriate self-care (Skinner 2013).

A period of grief and denial is normal. Figure 15.1 shows one model of the 'diabetic grief cycle' loosely based on Helen Kubler Ross' work, associated with death and dying. Lack of knowledge and/or inaccurate knowledge about diabetes, often produces stress and anxiety. The invisible nature of the condition: as indicated; Type 2 diabetes and most diabetic complications are often present without symptoms e.g. MI, UTI and retinopathy are silent, can lead to disbelief and denial of the diagnosis. Denial is an appropriate coping mechanism *early* in the course of the disease and enables people to maintain a positive attitude and come to terms with their altered health status.

Adequate time must be allowed for the person to grieve for their perceived losses, for example, loss of spontaneity, lifestyle, having to plan ahead, loss of the respect and

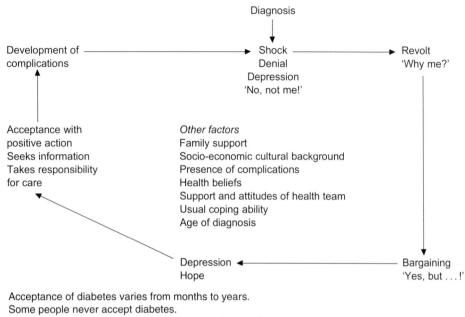

Diagnosis

Development of ——————————————→ Shock ——————————————→ Revolt
complications   Denial   'Why me?'
                                     Depression
                                     'No, not me!'

Acceptance with   *Other factors*
positive action   Family support
Seeks information   Socio-economic cultural background
Takes responsibility   Presence of complications
for care   Health beliefs
                                Support and attitudes of health team
                                Usual coping ability
                                Age of diagnosis

Depression ←——————————————— Bargaining
Hope   'Yes, but ...!'

Acceptance of diabetes varies from months to years.
Some people never accept diabetes.
The development of complications means another readjustment.

Figure 15.1   Model of the diabetic grief cycle.

love of the people they value ((Funnell 2006) and changed body image. However, prolonged denial can inhibit appropriate self-care, cause people to ignore warning signs of other problems and lead to non-attendance at scheduled medical appointments or investigative procedures and/or not seeking advice about health problems, which increases the risk of adverse health outcomes and diabetes complications. Denial can continue for longer than 5 years after the initial diagnosis in people with Type 1 diabetes (Gardiner 1997). Inadequate self-care could also indicate burnout from the unremitting demands of living with diabetes and lead to frequent use of health services by some people with diabetes. Frequent presentations to hospital or emergency departments could be a trigger to health professionals to refer the individual for counselling.

Accepting diabetes involves dealing with some or all of the following:

- mental and physical pain;
- hospitalisation or frequent outpatient or doctor visits;
- the health system, including health professional's beliefs and attitudes, and often hospitals and emergency services;
- lifelong treatment;
- body image changes, which can be positive or negative;
- friends/family relationships;
- fluctuating blood glucose levels;
- emotional stability;
- loss of independence;
- societal attitudes and expectations and discrimination, especially in some countries.

The tasks required to maintain acceptable blood glucose control are tedious and sometimes painful. There are financial costs involved, which can be a burden for some people (insulin, testing equipment, doctors' visits, increased insurance premiums), which add to the stress associated with having a disease they did not want in the first place.

Clinical observations

- There are no holidays from diabetes for the person with diabetes.
- The individual has to live with diabetes 365 days a year 24-hours a day, every day for the rest of their life.
- Some migrant groups 'take holidays' from diabetes when they visit relatives in their home countries. The 'holiday' often includes not taking medicines as pre-scribed, using complementary medicines and other complementary therapies, over eating because it is socially expected and not testing their blood glucose.

Managing a chronic illness means straddling two paradigms—the biomedical and the psychosocial, neither adequately address spirituality; they all need to be integrated in order to achieve optimal health outcomes. An individual's path through life is influenced by life trajectories and turning points and these include the diagnosis of diabetes, expectations of treatment, and social support. Helping an individual define their life trajectory and identify turning points is part of holistic care (Dunning 2013b).

In the context of this book, spirituality refers to the dimension of self that enables the individual to find meaning and purpose in life. Spirituality can be a motivating force that enables the individual to transcend life's trials such as the diagnosis of diabetes (Parsian & Dunning 2008). Hodges (2002) described four dimensions of spirituality, which each play a role in the incidence and degree of happiness or depression an individual experiences:

(1) finding meaning of and in life;
(2) intrinsic values;
(3) transcendence;
(4) spiritual community.

Interestingly, Wolpert (2006) described depression as 'soul loss.' Parsian and Dunning (2008) found a significant association among spirituality, being female, higher education, and duration of diabetes (>10 years) and lower HbA_{1c} and higher self-concept in young adults with diabetes when they developed and validated a tool to measure spirituality. Significantly, participants in the study did not consider religion and spirituality to be the same thing and only two spiritual respondents used religious practices, mostly prayer, to help them cope. Over the past 10 years research has demonstrated a link between being affiliated with a religious group and better physical and mental health outcomes although the association is not clear and may have a cultural element (UK Mental Health Foundation 2006; Gilbert 2007).

Diabetes has a 'bad reputation' in the community accompanied by many myths, or more correctly misinformation, for example 'eating sugar causes diabetes', and Type 2 diabetes is a mild form of the disease. Such misinformation must be discussed and dispelled because it can be associated with self-blame and guilt feelings. In addition, social pressures and ignorance often cause frustration and contribute to denial of the diabetes and failure to follow medical advice. For example, pressure from friend and relatives who say 'a little piece of cake won't hurt you' can be confusing for people with Type 1 and Type 2 diabetes. In some cultures diabetes changes the individual's 'value' and compromises their acceptance in society, acceptability as a marriage partner and compromises their job prospects. Diabetes might be denied or hidden.

Depression

The World Health Organization predicted that depression will be the second major health issue by 2020. In Australia 5.8% of adults experience a depressive disorder (Andrews *et al.* 1999) and depression accounts for 8% of the non-fatal disease burden. People with diabetes have a higher incidence of depression than the general public and the depression often precedes the diagnosis of diabetes. Depression may be an independent risk factor for diabetes (Rubin & Peyrot 2001. However, the mechanism linking diabetes and depression and whether depression precedes diabetes or diabetes leads to depression is unclear (Eaton *et al.* 1996; Peyrot 1997; Carnethon *et al.* 2003). Lustman (1997) suggested depression and hopelessness arise from having a chronic disease.

Likewise, it is not clear whether depression increases the risk of diabetes *per se* or through the associated lifestyle risk factors such as poor diet, smoking and inactivity. Carnethon *et al.* (2003) found depression was associated with lower than high school education in a cohort from the NHANES 1 study (*n* = 6910): low education was an independent of risk factor for developing diabetes. Carnethon *et al.* (2003) suggested causal mechanisms for the link could include genetic predisposition, inflammation and activation of the hypothalamic–pituitary–adrenal axis. These factors are similar to those proposed for the association among diabetes, cardiovascular diseases and depression; see Chapter 8.

Depression could be a component of the insulin resistance syndrome (see Chapter 1). People who are depressed are less likely to perform adequate preventative health self-care, more likely to present to the emergency department, require specialist intervention and exhibit lowered self-worth and physical functioning (Ciechanowski *et al.* 2000). The course of depression in people with diabetes is chronic and severe and depressive episodes may be particularly severe because of the hyperglycaemia and the neuroendocrine response (Rubin & Peyrot 2001) and the presence of microvascular and macrovascular complications. Thus, depression is associated with increased health care costs (Egede *et al.* 2002; SIGN 2010; ADA 2011).

Cavan *et al.* (2001) suggested the reasons people with diabetes become depressed might be:

- the heavy disease burden;
- the strain diabetes places on relationships, especially family relationships, and especially in some cultures;
- the stigma associated with diabetes in the family and the community;
- shock and guilt at the diagnosis that are not adequately addressed and resolved;
- the uncertainty of the future;
- loss of control;
- past and current negative experiences with health professionals.

The perceived severity of diabetes affects the person's mental status. Type 2 diabetes has traditionally been considered to be less serious than Type 1 diabetes especially where it is treated without medications, even though Type 2 diabetes is a progressive disease of beta cell failure and complicaions are frequently present at diagnosis. Health professional messages that diabetes is not serious can lead to false hope, and depression and stress occur when medicines, especially insulin, is required (Dunning & Martin 1997,

1999; MILES 2011). Considering the silent, insidious nature of Type 2 diabetes and the frequency with which complications are present at diagnosis, diabetes is hardly 'nothing to worry about.'

Symptoms of depression

The presence of five or more of the following signs every day for >2 weeks are suggestive of depression and should be formally assessed (US National Institute of Mental Health 2002):

- persistent low mood, feeling sad, hopeless, anxious or empty;
- pessimism;
- feeling guilty, worthless or helpless, loss of interest in usual activities such as work, hobbies, and sexual relationships;
- low energy, fatigue;
- difficulty concentrating, remembering, making decisions;
- insomnia, waking early, oversleeping;
- appetite and/or weight changes;
- suicidal thoughts or attempts to commit suicide or dwelling on death;
- irritability.

In addition, depression is characterised by reduced confidence and neglect of self-care in people with diabetes. However, not all people who neglect their self-care are depressed and assumptions must always be checked (Lustman *et al*. 1996; SIGN 2010).

Maintaining mental health and managing depression

'The effectiveness of interventions depends on the context in which it is delivered' (Wilson & Holt 2001). The way the health professional interacts with people with diabetes and delivers care may be more important than the care itself (Balint 1955). While Balint's study is old, its message is still relevant today and many Balint Groups have been established especially in the US to help health professionals become more effective carers. Managing depression and diabetes is complex. Complexity theories suggest all the circumstances that influence behaviour must be considered (Lancaster 2000), which is certainly true of diabetes and depression, where individuals:

- Operate within self-adjusting biochemical, cellular, physiological, social, cultural and religious systems and where a change in one will result in a change in the others.
- Illness and wellness are part of a continuum, are dynamic and arise from an interaction among these factors.
- Physical and psychological health can only be maintained using an holistic model of care that incorporates all of these aspects.

Effective management strategies include:

- Counselling strategies such as cognitive behavioural therapy (CBT), interpersonal therapy, motivational interviewing, acceptance and commitment therapy, goal setting and guided self-determination reduce self-defeating thought patterns and negative behaviours and improve adherence with management regimens. Clinicians can use counselling strategies in routine care. For example, Elley *et al*. (2003) showed counselling in general practice effectively increased physical activity and improved quality of life over 12 months. In a second study (Elley *et al.* 2007) found a personalised approach focusing on barriers and facilitators to physical activity, internal motivators, recognising time, physical and psychological limitations and spiritual benefits as well as the role of significant others, was important. CBT requires the individual to be able to think rationally and actively participate in their management. Usually, a close working relationship with the therapist is needed and it may take months for the individual to change unhealthy thought/behaviour patterns (Better Health Channel 2007).

- Coping strategies including problem-focused coping to deal with or prevent problems and emotion-focused coping to deal with negative emotions (Peyrot & Rubin 2007).
- Enhancing diabetes-specific self-efficacy, which involves encouraging realistic expectations and enhancing motivation by helping people identify their successes and encouraging optimism and realistic expectations. For example, motivational interviewing (Rollnick *et al.* 1999). High self-efficacy is associated with lower rates of depression (Steunenberg *et al.* 2007) and spirituality (Parsian & Dunning 2008).
- Improving metabolic control to relieve the effects of hyperglycaemia and fear of hypoglycaemia on mood and quality of life.
- Interactive behaviour change technology (IBCT), which includes PDAs, patient-centred Internet websites, on-line peer support groups, brain training websites, coaching telephone calls, DVDs, audiotapes, touch screen kiosks designed to help people maintain independence, can help people improve their diabetes self-care and monitor change (Piette 2007). IGCT can also be useful to support informal caregivers and promote activity, for example, pedometers can help people engage in physical activity. People search the Internet for information about depression more than any other condition (Taylor 1999). The Internet enables people to remain anonymous, which is important to some people (Rasmussen *et al.* 2007a). People need advice about how to assess the veracity of websites because the information is often of low quality, may be misleading and can do more harm than good. Griffiths & Christensen (2002) undertook a cross-sectional study of 15 Australian depression Internet sites in November and December 2001 and found the quality of the content of many sites was poor (the author undertook a quick assessment in late 2012 with similar results). Sites receiving the highest rating were beyond Blue, BluePages, CRUIAD and InfraPsych. However, information technologies do not take the place of human contact and are more effective when combined with human contact (Piette 2007).
- Positive psychology.
- Complementary therapies (CAM) and self-help programmes. CAM with the best evidence for effectiveness in depression are *Hypericum perforatum* for mild–to-moderate depression, exercise, bibliotherapy involving CBT and light therapy for winter depression. There is limited evidence to support acupuncture, light therapy for SAD syndrome, massage, relaxation therapies, SAM-e, folate and yoga breathing exercises (Jorm *et al.* 2002). CAM medicines should be used under the supervision of a qualified practitioner and health professionals and people with diabetes should be aware of possible adverse events associated with CAM use (Chapter 19).
- Identifying and treating underlying physical disorders that contribute to psychological distress and depression such as hypothyroidism and underlying psychiatric disorders, and referring the individual to appropriate mental health services as soon as possible. Counselling and/or antidepressant medicines may be needed. Antidepressant medicines such as serotonin reuptake inhibitors are commonly used and are effective in people with diabetes (Rubin & Peyrot 1994; SIGN 2010) However, tyicyclic antidepressants and atypical antipsychotic medicines contribute to hyperglycaemia

(Lustman *et al.* 2006) see Chapter 10. The individual's previous experience with anti-depressant medicines and the likely side effects need to be considered. As indicated, depression is a chronic condition and regular monitoring is essential and needs to be incorporated into routine care including in the acute care setting

Recently, an Australian model of collaborative care, TrueBlue, that used existing clinical software and practice nurses as case managers demonstrated improved depression and treatment intensification that was sustained over the 12 months of the intervention. In addition, the 10-year cardiovascular disease risk was reduced (Morgan *et al.* 2013).

Screening for psychological distress and depression

A range of screening tools is used and have advantages and disadvantages and varying degrees of validity in some settings. Not all are suitable for clinical monitoring because for their complexity and length; some tools cannot be used without permission and some copyright holders require potential users to sign an agreement and pay to use the tools. Commonly used tools include:

- Beck Depression Inventory (BDI).
- Brief Case Finding for Depression (BCD).
- Brief Illness Perceptions Questionnaire (BIPQ).
- Caregiver Strain Index (CSI).
- Center for Epidemiological Studies Depression Scale (CES-D).
- Depression Anxiety Stress Scale (DASS).
- Diagnostic and Statistical Manual of Mental Disorders (DSM-1V 1994).
- Diabetes Family Support and Conflict Scale (DFSC).
- Diabetes Self-care Inventory (DSCI) and The Diabetes Self-Care Inventory-revised (DSCI–revised).
- Diabetes Health Profile.
- Diabetes-Specific Quality of Life.
- Geriatric Depression Score.
- Hospital Anxiety and Depression Scale (HADS).
- K-10 Profile.
- Patient Health Questionnaire (PHQ-9).
- Partners in Health Care (PIH).
- Personal Well being Index (PWI).
- Problem Areas in Diabetes (PAID).
- Quality of Life Questionnaire (QoL-Q).
- Wellbeing Enquiry for Diabetes.
- World Health Organization Well Being Index (WHO-5) especially in older people (Bonsignore *et al.* 2001).

In order to help people discuss mental health problems health professionals need to mindful of the burden diabetes imposes on people's lives and ask good questions that aim to elicit a specific response, for example, ' what is the hardest thing about living with diabetes for you at the moment?' to identify the key issue to be addressed. Focus on successes and support the individual's problem-solving skills, for example, 'How do you think you can manage that?' Involve the family and significant others if relevant and with the individual's permission (Speight & Singh 2013) and help them develop emotional resilience and optimism, which are key aspect of empowerment. Importantly, health professionals do not empower people with diabetes; but they can help the individual become self empowered as part of their spiritual journey of becoming.

Antipsychotic medicines and diabetes

Second generation antipsychotic medications effectively treat a range of psychiatric disorders and offer many benefits over older medications such as chlorpromazine and haloperidol (Wirshing *et al*. 2002; deVane 2007). However, they do have significant side effects, namely rapid weight gain, hyperlipidaemia and insulin resistance, that can affect metabolic control and increase the cardiovascular risk in people with established diabetes and cause hyperglycaemia in non-diabetics; however, there is considerable variability in responses among individuals receiving the same medication.

A consensus panel of experts from the American Diabetes Association, American Psychiatric Association, the American Association of Clinical Endocrinologists and the North American Association for the study of Obesity (2004) recommended:

- Assessing weight, blood glucose, lipids and blood pressure before starting antipsychotic medicines or as soon as possible after.
- Actively managing these conditions, if present.
- If weight increases by >5%, consider changing to another antipsychotic less likely to cause metabolic effects.
- Antipsychotics listed in order of those with the most to the least metabolic effects are: Olanzapine, Quetiapine, Risperidone, Ziprasidone, Aripiprazole. These medicines all cause weight gain.
- Institute lifestyle modification to mange weight if possible, which will involve helping the person adhere to advice.

However, people often do not comply with their antipsychotic medicines for various reasons including the fact they stifle creativity. For example, the author belongs to a creative writing group in her hometown, which meets monthly to attend various writing-related activities and read and critique each others' work. At least five members (n = 20) have disclosed they were prescribed antipsychotic medicines for various reasons and all stated they omit or reduce their medicine doses to maintain a degree mania, which fuels their creativity. Four of the five developed diabetes and significant weight gain after starting on antipsychotic medicines.

Type 1 diabetes

Diabetes diagnosed in childhood can produce enormous guilt and anxiety for the child and the parents (Rasmussen *et al*. 2007b). Marital strife is not uncommon and is often exacerbated by the diabetes. The parents must learn how to care for the child at the same time as coping with their own feelings. Inflicting pain on a child (injections, blood tests) is very difficult to do, and such tasks often fall to the mother.

As the child matures and develops they need to assume responsibility for their diabetes self-care. It can be extremely difficult for the parents to 'let go,' and, therefore, for the child to achieve independence. Other children in the family may feel deprived of attention. Sweets, the traditional reward for good behaviour, are often withdrawn and may be seen as a punishment.

Some childhood behaviour such as irritability and awkwardness can be difficult to distinguish from hypoglycaemia, making hypoglycaemia management difficult.

Hypoglycaemia itself is feared and hated by children and parents and mostly under-rated by healthcare staff. It is not unknown for people to deliberately run their blood glucose levels high to avoid hypoglycaemia (Dunning 1994) (Chapter 6). Parents with diabetes may have concerns about passing diabetes to their own children in the future. Support, encouragement and referral for counselling, if necessary, are vital aspects of diabetes care.

Diabetes is the perfect disease for manipulating others and gaining attention. Withholding insulin can result in ketoacidosis, which mobilises the family, friends and health resources. Hypoglycaemia can have the same effect. Repeated admissions for hypoglycaemia or DKA need to be investigated carefully and diplomatically.

An individual's response to the diagnosis of diabetes depends on their overall psycho-logical and social adjustment and the availability of structured family support. Fitting diabetes into family life can be difficult and changes with duration of diabetes and the intensity of the treatment regimen (Gardiner 1997). Likewise, major life transitions such as leaving home, starting a new job, going to university and having a child require readaption (Rasmussen *et al.* 2007b).

The *Australian National Diabetes Strategy and Implementation Plan* (Diabetes Australia 1998) identified some issues specific to people with Type 1 diabetes, which still apply. They are:

- Dependency, for example, during severe hypoglycaemia and fears of being dependent should they develop complications such as blindness.
- Loss of control, either in the short term, e.g. during hypoglycaemia or in the long term.
- Public confusion about the difference between Type 1 and Type 2 diabetes. This confusion extends to health professionals as the following quote from a referral for diabetes education indicates: 'He used to have Type 2 but the doctor started him on insulin yesterday and he is now Type 1. Needs education.'
- Who to tell about their diabetes at work – workmates, friends.
- Restrictions, for example, some sporting activities, jobs, and hassles getting a driver's license.

Note also the cultural issues that affect survival as well as psychological well being in some cultures discussed earlier in the chapter.

Type 2 diabetes

The diagnosis of diabetes in later life means the person may need to change behaviours developed over years. Eating patterns often have to be modified. Restrictions are often resented with resultant anger, denial or neglect. Alternatively, the patient may meticu-lously follow the management plan. Knowledge about possible diabetic complications or the development of complications leads to stress, which in turn contributes to ele-vated blood glucose levels. Relationships may be disrupted as in Type 1 diabetes, with families/spouses becoming overprotective, resulting in over dependence or rebellious-ness. People tend to cope better and manage the self-care tasks more easily if the family is supportive yet allows independence.

Over half of the people with Type 2 diabetes on insulin report reduced quality of life. Insulin has a negative impact, which is greater in younger people with a long duration of diabetes from non-English-speaking backgrounds (Rubin 2000; Davis *et al.* 2001, MILES 2011). Men with Type 2 diabetes self-report depression, disempowerment and perceived loss of control (Tun *et al.* 1990). Hopelessness and depression may be the result of the misapprehension that insulin indicates severe disease. Support and explaining the likely progression to insulin are required early in the course of the disease e.g. at or soon after diagnosis.

Thoolen (2006) in the Netherlands found people with Type 2 diabetes experience little diabetes-related anxiety, do not regard diabetes as a serious disease and have high self-efficacy and low levels of self-care in the early years after diagnosis (n = 196). People who had been diagnosed for >2–3 years were more likely to consider diabetes to be threatening to their health. Patients on intensive treatment reported higher levels of stress and lower self-efficacy. Like other studies, Thoolen's study emphasises the importance of taking a thorough history and considering individual and cultural factors and reactions.

The DAWN study (Funnell 2006) (*n* = 3432, Type 2 and 1672, Type 1) demonstrated that diabetes is associated with a number of physical and psychological symptoms such as shock and disbelief 35–55%, anxiety 38% Type 1 and 19% Type 2. Of these, 51% were concerned about hypoglycaemia, 48% about weight change especially Type 2, and the disease getting worse 34%. Despite these concerns many were relieved to have a diagnosis. In the Australian cohort 75% were optimistic about the future, ~25% said they felt burnt out by diabetes and <40% were tired of complying with diabetes self-care. Most agreed diabetes did not prevent them from doing what they wanted to do.

Fifty-two per cent of people with Type 2 not on insulin worried about having to commence insulin and only 10% thought insulin would help control their diabetes. Li *et al.* (2008) found a higher rate of major depression in people with Type 2 diabetes on insulin than those with Type 2 not using insulin and those with Type 1 diabetes. These studies suggest insulin has a negative impact on people with Type 2 diabetes despite the clinical observation that many report feeling better once they commence insulin and their control improves. Very similar findings emerged in Australia in the MILES study (MILES 2011).

Compliance/adherence/concordance

These terms are judgmental, prejudiced and pervasively negative in nature. They are labels best avoided in relation to diabetes self-care tasks (Diabetes Australia Position Statement on Language 2011). Failure to comply with one self-care task does not necessarily indicate complete neglect of the diabetes. In fact, forgetting and omitting aspects of care is probably 'normal' behaviour and obsessive attention to routine can indicate underlying fear and anxiety that could be diabetes-related.

It is important to establish why a particular behaviour is neglected. Reasons include:

- Unreal expectations on the part of health professionals resulting from lack of knowledge about the person's goals, capabilities and social situation.
- Setting health professional rather than patient goals.
- Lack of knowledge of what is required.
- Low literacy and numeracy.
- Lack of understanding as a result of poor communication, inadequate information or inappropriate information e.g. with respect to culture, age, the particular environment in which the person lives; see Chapter 16.
- Changes in the colour, size or shape of medicines e.g. when given generic medicines instead of non-generic medicines (Kesselheim *et al.* 2012)
- Inadequate support from family/friends and the healthcare team (see Chapter 20).
- Health beliefs and attitudes of the patient, family and health professionals.
- Functional limitations such as low vision and diminished fine motor skills.

- Patient 'burnout'.
- Financial and other resource difficulties.

These factors represent the human side of diabetes.

Psychological distress and cardiovascular disease

The effect of negative emotions on physical functioning is not new. William Harvey noted that mental distress affected the heart and impaired its function in 1628. Sound evidence for the link between emotions and cardiovascular disease, particularly myocardial infarction (MI) and stroke, has emerged in the last ten years and the risk appears to be comparable to those of other known risk factors such as smoking.

Although the course of chronic heart disease and depression fluctuate, negative emotions have cumulative pathophysiological effects. Diabetes is also linked to higher rates of depression than the general population and cardiovascular disease is a major long-term diabetes complication. The emotional impact people with diabetes attribute to MI and to diabetes changes with the longer duration of time after the acute MI. In the initial stages surviving the MI is the major concern; by 3–4 months concerns about diabetes begin to re-emerge and predominate by 6 months (Gujadhur & Dunning 2003).

Depression may contribute to physical damage by activating key neurohormonal systems as well as other mechanisms (Yusef *et al.* 2004; Everson-Rose & Lewis 2005; Rozanski *et al.* 2005). Yusuf *et al.* (2004) showed psychological distress was associated with a 2.5-fold greater risk of acute MI than hypertension, abdominal obesity, diabetes (i.e. the metabolic syndrome; see Chapter 1), and other risk factors in the INTERHEART study (*n* = 29 972 in 52 countries). The association is evident in a number of other studies (Joost *et al.* 2004; Lett *et al.* 2004; Rozanski *et al.* 2005). Janszky *et al.* (2007) found admission for depression is associated with increased risk of MI, independent of other risk factors, but the mechanism remains unclear.

Lett *et al.* (2004) suggested depression could be a marker of a broader issue encompassing a range of factors such as:

- negative affect
- vital exhaustion
- limited social support
- personality factors
- anger
- hostility
- negative emotions
- anxiety.

Depression and negative affect appear to predict increased risk of cardiovascular disease (Frasure-Smith & Lesperance 2003). Significantly, optimistic individuals have lower risk of cardiovascular disease than pessimists when other risk factors were controlled for (Kubzansky & Thurston 2007; Giltay *et al.* 2006). Many researchers and clinicians note that people with heart disease have high rates of depression ranging between 40 and 65% (Januzzi *et al.* 2000). However, 53% of people have a history of depression prior to having an MI, which suggests depression precedes the MI (Rafinelle *et al.* 2005; Glassman & Miller 2007).

The effect of negative emotions on cardiovascular disease is currently being explored, for example, specific biomarkers, genetic predisposition, and psychological resilience. Negative emotions may have direct physiological effects by stimulating the hypothalamic-pituitary–adrenocortical axis, affecting the immune response, and contributing to inflammation. Psychological distress also affects self-care behaviours, in that highly stressed individuals often smoke, drink excess amounts of alcohol, do not exercise or eat inappropriate foods, neglect self-care and do not adhere to health care regimens including medicines. Psychological distress occurs on a continuum ranging from normal to pathological (eustress to distress).

However, the cognitive, behavioural and biological components of psychological distress are the same regardless of where the individual is on the distress continuum. Pathological psychological distress is characterised by intense emotions. There appears to be a dose-dependent relationship between the level of emotion and the degree of risk for cardiovascular disease (Kubzansky 2007).

Holistic diabetes assessment and successful depression management programmes encompass mental health and well being and may include using depression screening tools (Callahan *et al.* 1994). Despite the success of programmes such as Hospital Admission Risk Programs (HARP) in Australia, clinical practice guidelines for managing pre-event and psychosocial cardiac risk factors are lacking. Psychosocial and behavioural risk factors are not closely inter-related and structured integrated management systems are needed and are part of an emerging field of health care: behavioural cardiology (Rozanski *et al.* 2005).

What people with diabetes require from health professionals

- To be treated as 'normal.'
- To be involved in developing their diabetes care plan and monitoring procedures.
- To be treated as a person, not 'a diabetic'.
- To be trusted, accepted and not judged.
- To be listened to and have their experience and knowledge of diabetes recognised, valued, and used when planning their self-care including when they are in hospital.
- To know how and where to obtain advice and be able to obtain it when they need it (now!).

Supportive encouragement and focusing on positive achievements are far more helpful than 'shame and blame'. Achievable goals should be negotiated with the individual because their expectations/goals will be met rather than health professionals' goals. It is important to recognise that managing diabetes is never easy. Using terms such as 'good' and 'bad' when referring to blood glucose levels are judgemental terms. Substitute 'high' and 'low' or 'out of your target range'. Some people resent being called 'a diabetic'. It is preferable to say 'a person with diabetes' (Diabetes Australia 2011; Speight & Singh 2013).

Some people express concern about being admitted to hospital, over and above the usual reactions to illness/hospitalisation. They feel abnormal by being singled out for special meals and having labels such as 'diabetic diet' attached to their documentation. They often feel incompetent when they have been caring for their diabetes for years when staff do not believe they are 'hypo' when they ask for glucose or eat sweets or when they are capable of testing their blood glucose and administer their own insulin injections but are not permitted to do so while they are in hospital. Some people feel they have failed or health professionals blame them if they are admitted to hospital with a diabetic complication. They 'should have known better' and 'taken more care of their diabetes'. People become frustrated in such circumstances and, as one person said 'staff bugger it (diabetes management) up in hospital' (Savage *et al.* 2012). Continuous negative feedback only reinforces that the person is not coping and learned helplessness can result.

Quality of life

Quality of life (QOL) is a highly subjective and multidimensional concept concerned with cognitive status, satisfaction and emotional happiness (Cox & Gonder-Frederick 1992). It has become a major issue in behavioural diabetes research. Poor quality of life is associated with neglected self-care and may predict an individual's capacity for self-care. According to life mission theory people lower their QOL when they are in crisis to survive and adapt. QOL can be increased when the person has the resources to heal (Ventegodt *et al.* 2003). Healing encompasses 'salutogenesis' (Antonovsky 1987) where the individual develops a 'sense of coherence' and develops personally, or in modern terminology, becomes empowered.

The person enters an holistic state of healing when:

- The individual and their health professionals have similar life perspectives and the intent of the health professional is to help the person understand him/herself and take responsibility for their life, and in this case, diabetes.
- They are in a safe environment.
- They have the personal resources.
- They have the will to understand and overcome the crisis and let go of negative emotions and behaviours.
- The individual and their health professionals have healing intent. There is sufficient holding. Holding is a five-fold process that involves acknowledging the patient and giving them respect, trust, care, and acceptance (Ventegodt *et al.* 2003; Dunning 2013a).

There are four categories of determinants of QOL:

(1) Medical: diabetes type, treatment regimen, level of metabolic control and presence of complications. The severity of complications reduces QoL.
(2) Cognitive: acute and chronic blood glucose control and neuropsychological changes can reduce quality of life for the person with diabetes and their family. The effect of depression on QOL is greater than the effect of diabetes and is additive to other factors (Goldney & Phillips 2004).
(3) Attitudinal: self-efficacy, locus of control and social support. People with good support have better quality of life and less depression. Empowerment strategies and improving an individual's sense of being in control improve their quality of life. This includes considering spirituality, an integral aspect of empowerment.
(4) Demographic: gender, education level, ethnicity and age. Men report better QOL than women and young people report better QOL than old people. Higher education is associated with better quality of life.

Measuring quality of life

Most people understand what is meant by 'quality of life' but it is a difficult concept to measure. A number of tools have been developed that measure the general aspects of QOL and are widely used n research because they can compare participants with each other. Diabetes-specific QOL are available. These tools include generic Health-Related Quality of Life, Short Form 36 (SF-36), the Diabetes Specific Quality of Life and the Symptoms Check List, and the DCCT QOL tool (Bradley & Gamsu 1994) see the previous list. Sometimes a number of tools are used together.

Some of these tools are simple to use and are, or could be incorporated into the routine diabetes assessments. However, it is important to realise that, although these tools are validated and widely used, they, may not indicate an *individual's* specific QOL. Patient-generated quality of life measures developed specifically by the individual may be useful to monitor the QOL issues relevant to the individual (Jenkinson & McGee 1998). The process consists of asking the individual to nominate their top 3–5 QOL issues, then developing a Likert scale on which the individual rates each issue. The author prefers to us a three point Liker scale ranging from high, don't know unsure to poor because it is easier for people to make choices and still enable them to choose a 'don't know' option if they choose. Significantly, in the authors practice pets and being with family consistently rate high as important QOL issues for a wide range of people. The tool can be administered as part of complication screening, when health status changes and during major life transitions.

Measuring quality of life may be useful to plan holistic nursing care and address issues of empowerment. It is important to consider individual meaning of quality of life and to ask about these individual issues as well as global issues.

Guidelines to encourage mental and physical well being

- Recognise that psychological issues affect metabolic control and need to be addressed in order to maintain quality of life and effective diabetes self-care.
- Provide supportive education and advice, when it is required and tailor education to the individual's needs. An empowerment model of care and an holistic approach are more appropriate for chronic diseases such as diabetes where frequent visits to health professionals are required. Empowerment models seek to involve the individual in decisions about their management and to establish a therapeutic relationship with the individual; see Chapter 16.
- Improve communication. Provide an appropriate environment for consultations, plan for continuity of care including discharge planning, ask open questions and give the individual the opportunity to ask questions. Ask person-focused questions such as 'What are your concerns today?' put the focus on the individual in contrast to 'What can *I* do for you today?'
- Address complications honestly but optimistically. Foster self-esteem and coping skills. In hospital this may mean allowing the person with diabetes to perform their own blood glucose tests and administer their own medications.
- Offer options and help with goal setting.
- Give the message that diabetes is a serious disease and focus on the benefits of good control rather than what will happen if control is poor.
- Focus on the person not their diabetes or metabolic control.
- Acknowledge that it is difficult to live with diabetes.
- Monitor psychological well being as well as physical status (Bradley & Gamsu 1994).

References

American Diabetes Association, American Psychiatric Association, American Association of Clinical Endocrinologists and the North American Association for the Study of Obesity (2004) Consensus development conference on antipsychotic drugs and obesity and diabetes. *Diabetes Care*, 27, 596–601.

American Diabetes Association (ADA) (2011) Standards of medical care in diabetes. *Diabetes Care*, 24, Suppl 1, S–561.

American Psychiatric Association (1994) *Diagnostic and Statistical Manual of Mental Disorders*, 4th edn. American Psychiatric Association, Washington, DC.

Andrews, G., Hall, W., Teeson, M. & Henderson, S. (1999) *The Mental Health of Australians*. Mental Health Branch, Commonwealth Department of Health and Aged Care, Canberra.

Antonovsky, A. (1987) *Unravelling the Mystery of Health: How People Manage Stress and Stay Well.* Jossey-Bass, San Francisco.

Balint, M. (1955) The doctor, his patient and the illness. *Lancet*, 1:683–688.

Better Health Channel (2007) *Cognitive Behaviour Therapy*. http://www.betterhealth.vic.gov.au/bhcv2/bhcarticles.nsf/pages/Cognitive_Behaviour (accessed December 2007).

Bradley, C. & Gamsu, D. (1994) Guidelines for encouraging psychological wellbeing. *Diabetic Medicine*, 11, 510–516.

Bonsignore, M., Barkow, K., Jessen, F. & Huen, R. (2001) Validity of the five-item WHO Well-Being Index (WHO-5) in an elderly population. *European Archives of Psychiatry Clinical Neuroscience*, 251, (Suppl. 2), 1127–1131.

Callahan, C., Hendrie, H., Dittus, R. *et al.* (1994) Improving treatment of late life depression in primary care: A randomized clinical trial. *Journal of the American Geriatric Society*, 42, 839–846.

Carnethon, M., Kinder, L., Fair, J., Stafford, R. & Fortmann, S. (2003) Symptoms of depression as a risk factor for incident diabetes: Findings from the National Health Nutrition Examination Epidemiologic Follow-up Study. *American Journal of Epidemiology*, 158, 416–423.

Cavan, D., Fosbury, J. & Tigwell, P. (2001) Psychology in diabetes – Why bother? *Practical Diabetes International*, 18 (7), 228–229.

Ciechanowski, P., Katon, W. & Russo, W. (2000) Impact of depressive symptoms on adherence, function and costs. *Archives of Internal Medicine*, 160, 3278–3285.

Cox, D. & Gonder-Frederick, L. (1992) Major developments in behavioural diabetes research. *Journal of Consulting Clinical Psychologists*, 60, 628–638.

Davis, T., Clifford, R. & Davis, W. (2001) Effect of insulin therapy on quality of life in Type 2 diabetes mellitus – The Fremantle diabetes study. *Diabetes Research and Clinical Practice*, 52, 63–67.

Diabetes Australia (DA) (1998) *Australian National Diabetes Strategy and Implementation Plan*. Diabetes Australia, Canberra.

Diabetes Australia (DA) (2011) *A New Language for Diabetes: Improving Communication With and About People With Diabetes*. DA, Canberra.

Diabetes Control and Complications Trial Research Group (1993) Influence of intensive diabetes treatment on quality of life outcomes in the DCCT. *Diabetes Care*, 19, 195–203.

Dunning, P. (1994) Having diabetes: Young adult perspectives. *The Diabetes Educator*, 21 (1), 58–65.

Dunning, P. & Martin, M. (1997) Using a focus group to explore perceptions of diabetes severity. *Practical Diabetes International*, 14 (7), 185–188.

Dunning, P. & Martin, M. (1999) Health professional's perceptions of the seriousness of diabetes. *Practical Diabetes International*, 16 (3), 73–77.

Dunning, T. (2013a) The teacher: Moving from good to exceptional, Chapter 5 in *Diabetes Education: Art, Science and Evidence* (ed. Dunning, T.). Wiley Blackwell, Oxford pp. 62–77.

Dunning, T. (2013b) Turning points and transitions: Crises and opportunities, in *Diabetes Education: Art, Science and Evidence* (ed. Dunning, T.). Wiley Blackwell, Oxford pp.117–132.

Eaton, W., Armenian, H. & Gallo, J. (1996) Depression and risk for onset Type 11 diabetes: A prospective population based study. *Diabetes Care*, 19, 1097–1102.

Elley, C., Kerse, N., Arroll, B. & Robinson, E. (2003) Effectiveness of counselling patients on physical activity in general practice: A cluster randomised trial. *British Medical Journal*, 326 (pp. 1–6 downloaded December 2007).

Elley, C., Dean, S. & Kerse, N. (2007) Physical activity promotion in general practice. *Australian Family Physician*, 38 (12), 1061–1064.

Egede, L., Zheng, D. & Simpson, K. (2002) Comorbid depression is associated with increased health care use and expenditure in individuals with diabetes. *Diabetes Care*, 25 (3), 464–470.

Everson-Rose, S. & Lewis, T. (2005) Psychosocial factors and cardiovascular diseases. *Annual Review of Public Health*, 26, 469–500.

Frasure-Smith, N. & Lesperance, F. (2003) Depression and other psychological risks following myocardial infarction. *Archives of General Psychiatry*, 60, 627–636.

Funnell, M. (2006) Diabetes attitudes and wishes and needs (DAWN) study. *Clinical Diabetes*, 24, 154–155.

Gardiner, P. (1997) Social and psychological implications of diabetes mellitus for a group of adolescents. *Practical Diabetes International*, 14 (2), 43–46.

Gilbert, P. (2007) Spirituality and mental health: A very preliminary overview. *Current Opinions in Psychiatry*, 20 (6), 594–598.

Glassman A, Miller G. (2007) Where there is depression, there is inflammation…sometimes! *Biological Psychiatry*, 62, 280–281.

Giltay, E., Kamphuis, M., Kalmijn, S., Zitman, F. & Kromhout, D. (2006) Dispositional optimism and the risk of cardiovascular death: The Zutphen Elderly Study. *Archives of Internal Medicine*, 166, 431–436.

Griffiths, K. & Christensen, H. (2002) The quality and accessibility of Australian depression sites on the World Wide Web. *Medical Journal of Australia*, 176, S97–S104.

Goldney, R. & Phillips, P. (2004) Diabetes, depression and quality of life. *Diabetes Care*, **27** (5), 1066–1070.

Gujadhur, A., Dunning, T. & Alford, F. (2003) Metabolic and cardiac outcomes after acute myocardial infarction. *Journal of Diabetes Nursing*, **7** (6), 208–212.

Hernandez, A. (1995) The experience of living with insulin-dependent diabetes: lessons for the diabetes educator. *Diabetes Educator*, **21**, 33–37.

Hodges, S. (2002) Mental health, depressions and dimensions of spirituality and religion. *Journal of Adult Development*, **9**, 109–115.

Janszky, I., Ahlbom, A., Hallqvist, J. & Ahnve, S. (2007) Hospitalization for depression is associated with an increased risk for myocardial infarction not explained by lifestyle, lipids, coagulation, and inflammation: The SHEEP Study. *Biological Psychiatry*, **62**, 25–32.

Jenkinson, C. & McGee, H. (1998) *Health Status Measurement*. Radcliff Medical Press, Oxford.

Joost, P., van Melle, M., Jonge, P., *et al.* (2004) Prognostic association of depression following myocardial infarction with mortality and cardiovascular events: A meta-analysis. *Psychosomatic Medicine*, **66**, 814–822.

Jorm, A., Christensen, H., Griffiths, K. & Rodgers, B. (2002) Effectiveness of complementary and self-help treatments for depression. *Medical Journal of Australia*, **176**, S84–S96.

Kesselheim, A., Misono, A., Shank, W. *et al.* (2012) Variations in pill appearance of antiepileptic drugs and the risk on nonadherence. http://archinte.jamanetwork.com (accessed December 2012).

Kubzansky, D & Thurston, C. (2007) Emotional vitality and incident coronary heart disease: benefits of healthy psychological functioning. *Archives of General Psychiatry*, **64**, 1393–1401.

Kubzansky, L. (2007) Sick at heart: The pathophysiology of negative emotions. *Cleveland Clinic Journal of Medicine*, **74** (Suppl. 1), S67–S72.

Lancaster, T. (2000) Effectiveness of interventions to help people stop smoking. *British Medical Journal*, **321**, 355–358.

Lett, H., Blumenthal, J., Babyak, M. *et al.* (2004) Depression as a risk factor for coronary artery disease: Evidence, mechanisms, and treatment. *Psychosomatic Medicine*, **66**, 305–315.

Li, C. (2008) Depression common among adults with diabetes. *Diabetes Care*, **31**, 105–107.

Lustman, P. (1997) The course of major depression in diabetes. *Diabetes Care*, **59**, 24–31.

Lustman, P., Griffith, L. & Clouse, R. (1996) Recognising and managing depression in patients with diabetes, in *Practical Psychology for Clinicians* (eds B. Anderson & R. Rubin). American Diabetes Association, Alexandria Virginia , pp. 143–152.

Lustman, P., Clouse, R., Nix, B. *et al.* (2006) Sertaline for prevention of depression recurrence in diabetes mellitus: A randomized trial. *Diabetes Care* **6** (3), 521–529.

MILES (2011) Diabetes Miles Study – Australia *www.diabetesaustralia.com.au/.../12.05.16%20Diabetes%20MILES%20Report.pdf* (accessed October 2012).

Morgan, M., Coates, M., Dunbar, J. *et al.* (2013) The TrueBlue model of collaborative care using practice nurses as case managers foe depression alongside diabetes or heart disease: A randomized trial. *British Medical Journal*, DOI: 10.1136/bmjopen-2012-002171.

National Institute of Mental Health (NIMH) (2002) *Depression and Diabetes*. NIMH, Bethesda, Maryland USA.

Parsian, N. & Dunning, T. (2008) Spirituality and coping in young adults with diabetes. *Diabetes Research and Clinical Practice*, **79** (S1), S121.

Patterson, B. & Sloan, J. (1994) A phenomenological study of the decision-making experience of individuals with long standing diabetes. *Canadian Journal of Diabetes Care*, **18**, 10–19.

Patterson, B., Thorn, S. & Dewis, M. (1998) Adapting to and managing diabetes. *Journal of Nursing Scholarship*, **30** (1), 57–61.

Piette, J. (2007) Interactive behaviour change technology to support diabetes self-management: Where do we stand? *Diabetes Care*, **30** (10), 2425–2432.

Peyrot, M. (1997) Levels and risks of depression and anxiety symptomatology among diabetic adults. *Diabetes Care*, **20**, 585–590.

Peyrot, M. & Rubin, R. (2007). Behavioural and psychosocial interventions in diabetes. *Diabetes Care*, **30** (10): 2433–2440.

Rasmussen, B., O'Connell, B. & Dunning, T. (2007a) Young women with diabetes: using Internet communication to create stability during life transitions. *Journal of Clinical Nursing*, **1365**, 17–24.

Rasmussen, B., O'Connell, B. & Dunning, T. (2007b) Young women with Type 1 diabetes' management of turning points and transition. *Qualitative Health Research*, **17** (3), 300–310.

Rollnick, S., Mason, P. & Butler, C. (1999) *Health Behaviour Change: A Guide for Practitioners*. Churchill Livingstone, Edinburgh, UK.

Rozanski, A., Blumenthal, J., Davidson, K., Saab, P. & Kubzansky, L. (2005) The epidemiology, pathophysiology, and management of psychosocial risk factors in cardiac practice: The emerging field of behavioural cardiology. *Journal of the American College of Cardiology*, **45** (5), 637–651.

Rubin, R. (2000) Diabetes and quality of life. From research to practice. *Diabetes Spectrum*, **13** (1):21–23.

Rubin, R. & Peyrot, M. (1994) Implications of the DCCT: Looking beyond tight control. *Diabetes Care*, **17**, 235–236.

Rubin, R. & Peyrot, M. (2001) Psychological issues and treatments for people with diabetes. *Journal of Clinical Psychology*, **57** (4), 457–478.

Savage S, Dunning T, Duggan N, Martin P. (2012) The experiences and care preferences of people with diabetes at the end of life. *Journal of Hospice and Palliative Care*, **14** (4), 293–302.

SIGN Scottish Intercollegiate Guidelines Network (2010) *Management of Diabetes: A National Guideline*, SIGN, Edinburgh, UK.

Skinner T. (2013) Making choices: Settting goals, Chapter 4 in *Diabetes Education: Art, Science and Evidence* (ed. Dunning T). Wiley Blackwell, Oxford, pp. 49–61.

Speight, J. & Singh, H. (2013) The journey of the person with diabetes, Chapter 21 in *Diabetes Education: Art, Science and Evidence* (ed. Dunning T). Wiley Blackwell, Oxford pp.12–24.

Spitzer, R., Kroenke, K. & Williams, J. (1999) The Patient Health Questionnaire Primary Care Study Group; Validation and utility of a self-report version of the PRIME-MD: The PHQ Primary Care Study. *Journal of the American Medical Association*, **282**, 1737–1744.

Steunenberg, B., Beckman, A., Deeg, D., Bremmer, M. & Kerkhof, A. (2007) Mastery and neuroticism predict recovery from depression in later life. *American Journal of Geriatric Psychiatry*, **15**, 234–242.

Taylor, H. (2001) Explosive growth of 'cyberchrondriacs' continues (The Harris Poll #47), 5 August http://www.harrisinteractive.com/harris_poll/index.asp?PD=117 (accessed January 2007).

Thoolen, B. (2006) Early intensive treatment can negatively affect stress and outcome. *Diabetes Care*, **29**, 2257–2262.

Tun, P., Nathan, D. & Perlminter, L. (1990) Cognitive and affective disorders in elderly diabetics. *Clinical Geriatric Medicine*, **6**, 731–746.

Tung A. (2011) The mystery of guideline non-compliance: Why don't doctors do the right thing? *Anaesthesiology* **53**, 1–9.

UK Mental health Foundation (2006) Making space for spirituality: making space to support service users www.mentalhealth.org.uk/content/assets/PDF/.../making_space.pdf (accessed October 2012).

deVane, L. (2007) *Antipsychotics and Diabetes*. http://www.medscape.com.viewarticle/ 558874?src = mp (posted 28.6. 2007, accessed August 2007).

Ventegodt, S., Andersen, N. & Merrick, J. (2003) Holistic medicine 111: The holistic process theory of healing. *The Scientific World Journal*, **3**, 1138–1146.

Wilson, T. & Holt, T. (2001) Complexity science: Complexity and clinical care. *British Medical Journal*, **323** (7314), 685–688.

Wirshing, D., Boyd, J., Meng, L. *et al.* (2002) The effects of novel antipsychotics on glucose and lipid levels. *Journal of Clinical Psychiatry*, **63** (10), 856–865.

Wolpert, L. (2006) Malignant Sadness: *The Anatomy of Depression*, 3rd edn. Faber & Faber, London.

Yusef, S., Hawken, S. & Ounpuu, S. (2004) Effect of potentially modifiable risk factors associated with myocardial infarction in 52 countries (the INTERHEART study): Case controlled study. *Lancet*, **364**, 937–952.

Further reading

Beck, A. & Beamesderfer, A. (1974) Assessment of depression: The depression inventory. *Medical Problems in Psychopharmacotherapy*, 7, 151–169.

Johnson, S. (1980) Psychosocial factors in juvenile diabetes. *Journal of Health Psychology*, **9**, 737–749.

Lustman, P., Griffith, L., Freedland, K., Kissel, S. & Close, R. (1998) Cognitive behaviour therapy for depression in Type 2 diabetes mellitus: A randomized controlled trial. *Annals of Internal Medicine*, **129**, 613–621.

Raymond, M. (1992) *The Human Side of Diabetes: Beyond Doctors, Diet, Drugs*. Noble Press, Chicago.

Radloff, S. (1977) The CES-D scale: A self-report depression scale for research in the general population. *Applied Psychiatric Measurement*, **3**, 151–401.

Rafinelle, C. (2005) Depression, stress and the risk of heart disease. *Psychiatric Times*, **22**, 11.

Chapter 16
Diabetes Education

I never teach my students – I only try to provide the conditions in which they can learn.

Albert Einstein

Key points

- Teaching and learning is an interconnected process that depends on effective communication and a caring relationship.
- Establishing a caring (therapeutic) partnership with the person with diabetes is very important. The focus of diabetes education should be on helping the person with diabetes become an empowered active participant in their care, but remember, few people are actually disempowered.
- Health literacy is an important consideration. Written information or in other media suitable to the individual's, reading capability, age, culture, life stage and the current context should be provided to support verbal information.
- Diabetes self-care knowledge and capability should be assessed regularly.
- Improving self-care may have a greater impact on outcomes than medical strategies.
- All health professionals caring for the person with diabetes must provide consistent information.
- Establishing how a people learn is important in order to teach them appropriately and enhance their learning.
- Health professionals must reflect in and on their performance to enhance their effectiveness as practitioners
- Significant others should be included in the education where relevant.
- People report better health care experiences when they are actively engaged.

Care of People with Diabetes: A Manual of Nursing Practice, Fourth Edition. Trisha Dunning.
© 2014 John Wiley & Sons, Ltd. Published 2014 by John Wiley & Sons, Ltd.

Rationale

Diabetes education is the cornerstone of diabetes management and is a lifelong, ongoing process. Person-centred education that supports personal empowerment and autonomy and enhances self-care capacity is the most effective teaching method. A balanced therapeutic relationship between the person and their health professional carers is more likely to achieve person-centred education. Collaboration and communication and being truly present in the encounter (Dunning 2013, 62–76) are core elements of teaching and learning. Teaching and learning is an integrated process predicated on knowing the person with diabetes' story and explanatory models and understanding that people with diabetes' and health professionals' perceptions of diabetes, self-care, medicines, risks and benefits and goals are likely to be different (Schwarz *et al.* 2012).

Introduction

Diabetes education is an integral part of managing diabetes. The overall goal of diabetes education is to assist the person to:

- learn about and understand 'diabetes;'
- make informed choices relevant to their personal situation and the relative risks and benefits for them using the best available evidence;
- successfully integrate diabetes into their self-concept;
- incorporate diabetes management tasks into their daily lives and achieve a balanced lifestyle;
- develop effective coping strategies and problem-solving skills;
- perform diabetes self-care;
- successfully negotiate life transitions and turning points;
- achieve optimum metabolic control.

To achieve these goals people with diabetes need to make constant adjustments, especially when negotiating key life transitions (Rasmussen *et al.* 2007; Jutterstrom *et al.* 2012; Dunning 2013, 117–131). Thus, the simple term 'diabetes self-care' encompasses very complex, inter-related factors that affect each other and consequently the outcome. It is also required for life, or as one lady with diabetes told the author 'a life sentence.'

Health professionals aim to deliver holistic person/patient-centred diabetes care. As indicated in the preface, I choose to use the term 'patient' as 'well as person with diabetes' in this book. Some people with diabetes object to being referred to as patients but in my experience the majority of people refer to themselves as patients and/or diabetics, but that could be because health professionals use such words. Significantly, language and particular words affect people differently, many words health professionals use are judgemental; for example, 'non-compliant,' 'non-adherent,' and 'failed to attend.' Speight *et al.* (2012) developed a position statement concerning word usage on behalf of Diabetes Australia as one strategy to help heath professionals improve the way they communicate with and about people with diabetes.

Significantly, the International Alliance of Patient Organisations (IAPO 2005) uses the term 'patients'.

IAPO recognised that patients,' families' and carers' needs and priorities differ among countries and diseases, and described five key principles of patient-centred care:

(1) Respect for patients' unique needs, preferences, values, autonomy, and independence.
(2) Patients have a right and a responsibility to participate as equal partners in health care decisions that affect their lives to the level of their ability and choice. In fact people who are actively engaged in health care decisions report greater satisfaction with care (Alstoni et al 2012).
(3) They have a right to be involved in developing health care policy at all levels to ensure policies are designed with the patient at the centre of care and address access issues.
(4) Health care must consider emotional and non-health factors that affect health such as the social situation, education and employment, and patients must have access to healthcare services relevant to their condition.
(5) 'Accurate, relevant and comprehensive information is essential' to enable people to make informed decisions about their health care options and the benefits and risks of specific treatment to them. Information must be in a format suitable to the individual's age, literacy level, gender, culture, and health care needs (IAPO 2005).

Holistic patient-centred education and care is consistent with these principles and has a core aim of preventing disease and/or disease progression and promoting positive health to achieve the best possible outcomes. Patient education describes the theory and skills the individual needs to learn and encompasses establishing goals to be achieved and conditions in which learning can take place (Redman 2001). Thus, diabetes education is a planned, interactive process using a combination of methods to help people learn relevant information and develop and maintain appropriate health behaviours. Significantly, people who learn to and effectively manage their health and make appropriate lifestyle choices use fewer resources and make more effective use of available resources (Tankova *et al.* 2001).

Standardised patient education and self-management are important frameworks in which the IAPO principles can be applied. However, some frameworks may be limited in their effectiveness because they rely on traditional teaching methods, primary and tertiary care is not well-integrated, and the programmes and services often only reach a small number of people (Wagner *et al.* 2002) although modern communication processes using video, Skype, email, smart phones and other electronic media make it possible to reach a wider audience. Effective chronic disease management consists of:

• Delivering care according to evidence-based guidelines and protocols. Designing services and education programmes to suit the target audience, which might be an individual, a small group or a population. It is possible to apply the principles of holist education and care in all these settings.
• Managing medicines according to quality use of medicines principles (Chapter 5) and pharmacovigilance, which includes monitoring medicine effects and use.
• Well-designed services and practices such as appointment systems, follow up procedures, referral processes, Alert systems, and education programmes suitable to the needs of the target population.
• A focus on prevention and supporting people to self-manage and make relevant behaviour changes by using education methods that facilitate problem-solving and empowerment (Anderson *et al.* 2002; Anderson & Funnell 2005). Ideally a process for identifying people who do not meet targets is part of the process.
• Ensuring health professionals are educated, competent and supported to undertake their roles, that they function in a complementary, collaborative team, and there are clear links among service providers and resources. Health professionals may need training in health coaching methods and, as stated, must be reflective practitioners. In

addition, health professionals have a responsibility to take care of their own health and well being.

- Education programmes that meet the needs of the relevant population and provide opportunities for continuing education for patients and health professionals. A recent review of >30 randomised controlled trials of diabetes education found only half the education interventions included behavioural components (setting goals, counselling techniques or problem-solving), only one third assessed psychosocial factors (beliefs, self-efficacy, mastery, or locus of control), and significant improvements in knowledge was only demonstrated in one-fifth of the studies (Knight & Donan 2006). It is not clear whether people with diabetes were involved in designing the programmes included in the review, but that seems unlikely, given the results. These findings suggest most current diabetes education programmes may not be holistic or person-centred, and continue to 'do things for/to people' instead of 'with them,' despite the rhetoric.
- Performing accurate clinical and investigative procedures and considering each piece of clinical information as part of the whole body of information rather than as isolated 'facts.'
- Generating, documenting and communicating appropriate information including chronic disease registers, referral systems, patient reminders, outcome monitoring and care planning.
- Undertaking continuous quality improvement and audit processes that include patients in the design as well as the evaluation; not only as the subject of the evaluation. Health professional performance should be measured as part of the evaluation process and encompasses more than 'patient satisfaction surveys' (Dunning 2010).

Generally, the diabetes education literature focuses on the person with diabetes. However, to be an effective teacher, the educator must undertake reflective practice and consider their own learning style, teaching style, communication style, beliefs and attitudes, health status, knowledge and competence, and how they affect the way the health professional interacts with other people. In addition, health professionals need to understand how the person's life environment and the teaching environment can facilitate or be barriers to learning, behaviour change, and/or self-care. Thus, patient-centred education and care means really understanding people. Generally, peoples' teaching style reflects their preferred learning style, but may not suit the learner. A learning style self-assessment tool can be found on http://www.idpride. net/learning-style-test.html (accessed October 2012).

Clinical observation

A Finnish equestrienne, who won four Olympic gold medals, was asked: 'what needs to change if things are not working, you are not winning, the horse or the rider? She replied: 'the horse takes his cue from the rider. The *rider* has to change and work with the horse to help him achieve to the best of his ability – that's winning, even if you don't win.' (Interview during Equitana Australia January 2nd 2013).

Learning styles

Learning is 'a natural, evolving process originating within the learner and growing from the learner's need to interact with their environment' (MacKeracher 1996). Thus, the learner, not the teacher, is in control of what the learner learns. Learning can occur through experience (experiential) or as a planned process. People learning different ways (learning style) and the learning style may change over the person's life course; just as teaching styles often change through experience and ongoing learning. Learning style refers to the way an individual processes and uses information. Learning involves using the senses: sight, speech, hearing, and can be active or passive. Usually people use a mixture of learning styles and learn different things in different ways and children learn differently from adults. Table 16.1 is a composite overview of learning styles and teaching methods appropriate to each learning style. The table clearly shows that learning is a process not merely an outcome (Kolb 1984). Kolb described four learning styles:

(1) divergent – emphasises feeling rather than thinking;
(2) assimulative – values facts and thinking over feeling;
(3) convergent – like to apply information and hands-on activities;
(4) accommodative – learn by trial and error/problem-solving.

Other authors have also described learning theories and learning styles and the cognitive processes and physical factors that affect learning and memory, for example:

- Neurolinguistic programming (NLP) (Auditory, kinesthetic, and visual)
- Multiple Intelligence model that consists of eight domains.
- Making connections (Dunning 2013a, 28–40).

A simple self-complete tool that can help health professionals identify an individual's learning style is shown in Table 16.2.

Table 16.1 Learning styles and some teaching strategies that can be used to facilitate learning. People participating in group education programmes are likely to learn in different ways. Therefore, a range of teaching strategies should be used. An individual's preference for one category may be mild, moderate or strong but generally a balance of styles results in more effective learning.

Learning style	Learning process	Teaching strategy
Active	Retain information by doing something active. Like learning in groups. Retain information better if they understand how to apply it.	Teach in group settings. Incorporate activities such as demonstrations and return demonstrations. Use problem-based learning, Conversation maps™, the Felt Man, and similar tools and peer education.
Reflective	Prefer to think about things before they act. Prefer working alone.	Incorporate time for review and reflection. Provide short summaries of important information. Invite feedback. Use decision aid tools such as the Mayo Clinic Diabetes Medication Choice decision aid cards (2009).
Sensing	Like learning facts and solving problems using established methods. Like details and are good at memorising facts but may do this and not understand the information. Like hands-on activities. Dislike complications and surprises. Do not like being asked about information that was not covered in education programmes. Practical and careful and like information to be connected to 'the real world'	Show how the information relates to their personal situation and the 'real world' in general. Use specific examples from the individual's experience. For example, 'You do not eat breakfast but now you are taking insulin at breakfast time you are at risk of having a hypo. How can we reduce the risk or prevent you from having a hypo?'

(Continued)

Table 16.1 Continued.

Learning style	Learning process	Teaching strategy
Intuitive	Like to discover possibilities and relationships Like innovation. Are bored by repetition Are good at understanding new concepts Usually comfortable with abstract images and statistical information Are innovative and work quickly but may miss important details and make careless mistakes.	Link theories to facts. Use practical and actual examples using simple facts and figures and graphs.
Visual	Remember best when they see pictures, diagrams, flow charts, films, and demonstrations.	Use visual and verbal information Incorporate concept and mind maps and/or conversation amps in the teaching. Colour code information for example, 'yellow insulin' or 'purple insulin' to refer to the package colour.
Verbal	Learn best by listening to words.	Use verbal teaching. Give the person tapes to take home. Encourage people to participate and share their stories e.g. in peer education and group learning.
Sequential	Learn best if a logical step wise or staged approach is used. May not fully understand the material unless they use it. May know a lot about specific topics but have trouble relating them to other aspects of the same subject or to different subjects,	Provide logical material where each piece of information follows the preceding information Do not move randomly from topic to topic. Give them 'homework' so they can use the information and develop their global learning skills. Explain how the information relates to other information.
Global	Learn large amounts of information without seeing connections and suddenly make the connection. May solve complex problems quickly or find innovative ways of doing things once they understand the information. May have problems explaining how they did it.	Paint the big picture first. Explain how topics relate to other topics. And to information the person already knows and their experiences.

*Decision aids are information documents designed to help people make decisions about their management options. Decision aids are usually used with education and/or counselling. When used in conjunction with counseling they improve the quality of people's decisions and reduce under use and over use of services (O'Connor *et al.* 2003). Decision aids provide balanced, personalised information about options in enough detail to help them make an informed decision. They are not 'standard diabetes education information' available from pharmaceutical companies and diabetes associations, but can be used with such information.

Table 16.2 A simple tool that can be used to estimate an individual's dominant learning style. It is not comprehensive but can be easily and quickly incorporated into routine education and care.

> *Please put a number in the boxes in the order that best describes how you learn new important information from number 1 to 9. Number 1 is the way you learn best. If you choose the 'other' option please briefly describe how you learn new information.*

- ☐ Read printed information such as books and pamphlets with a lot of words.
- ☐ Read printed information with lots of pictures and diagrams or see models of things.
- ☐ Watch videos.
- ☐ Listen to an audiotape or a lecture.
- ☐ Have somebody show you how to do a task such as testing blood glucose
- ☐ Talk with other people who have similar problems:
  - In a group
  - In an Internet chat room
  - Individual informal discussion

- ☐ Practice using equipment such as injecting insulin or cooking food.
- ☐ Other, please describe:..
  ....

Another method is to ask the individual how he or she became competent at a hobby or task they perform regularly.

Education and other theories/models

Key education and behaviour theories that can be applied to diabetes education include:

- The Health Belief Model, which can suggest best content, topics and information sequencing.
- Self-efficacy, the education should build confidence, for example, by ensuring people achieve successes however small and that these are acknowledged.
- Locus of control; if people feel they are not in control they may require more support, for example, coaching and carer/family support.
- Cognitive Dissonance Theory; design interventions that make people feel unhappy or dissatisfied with their current behaviour and reinforce to prevent relapse.
- Diffusion Theory; ensure the intervention is consistent with the individual's belief system and values.
- Stages of Change; design strategies that fit the individual stages and where the individual is at each stage.
- Narrative Medicine, which recommends every meeting with a patient, should be treated as the first so that nothing is taken for granted and people are enabled to tell their stories and the health professional seeks meaning in the stories and clarifies their assumptions with the individual. Health professionals have their own stories, some have diabetes stories that need to be acknowledged but should not take priority and may or may not be disclosed (Bert 2011). Person-centred care is at the heart of Narrative Medicine.
- Adult education theories; use existing knowledge and problem-solving techniques. A range of other theories can be incorporated into the theories/models listed or used as the basis to develops education programmes such as motivational interviewing, tipping points (O'Connor *et al.* 2007), nudging (Dunning 2013b, 62–76) and art and drama (Assal & Assal 2013, 98–111).

Diabetes education is a lifelong process and information needs change as health status changes, new technology and medicines become available, and new models of car and service delivery emerge. Significantly, there is a poor correlation between knowledge and behaviour. Scare tactics and negative information lower mental and emotional well being and might lead to denial and/or non-adherence (Knight & Donan 2006).

On a practical level, diabetes education is often divided into:

- Survival skills—the initial information necessary to begin the self-care journey and be safe at home (described later in the chapter). Given the increasing prevalence of diabetes, survival skills should actually commence before diagnosis and target at risk populations or the whole population. For example, programmes developed by the National Public Health Institute in Helsinki (2007) designed to be delivered in primary care achieved reductions in three key diabetes and cardiovascular risk factors: BMI, waist circumference, and diastolic blood pressure after one year. People who achieved reductions in four or more risk factors had a lower risk of developing diabetes. These findings suggest diabetes educators need to take a population based approach to diabetes education as well as providing individual education and management.
- Basic knowledge—information that builds on survival information and enables the individual to understand diabetes and its management and their role in diabetes

management generally, and self-care in particular. A lot of such information is acquired through trial and error.

- Ongoing education—the continued acquisition of new information, including changes in technology and management practices as they emerge. A key aspect of delivering new information is helping the individual decide how it applies to them. That is, the information must be personalised to their particular life context.

Acquiring survival skills and undertaking relevant diabetes self-management usually requires changes in established behaviours. Understanding the individual's readiness to make relevant changes and identifying their personal barriers to change is central to behavioural change interventions. Several models have been developed that attempt to describe the behaviour change processes. These include:

- The Health Belief Model (HBM) (Becker & Maiman 1975).
- Social Learning Theory (SLT) (Bandura 1986).
- Theory of Reasoned Action and Planned Behaviour (TRA) (Ajzen & Fishbein 1980).
- The Transtheoretical Model of Change (Stages of Change) (SOC) (Prochaska & DiClemente 1983).
- Empowerment Model (Funnell & Anderson 2000).
- Coaching models such as the Health Care Australia Coaching Model (Linder *et al.* 2003; Gale 2007) that are based on positive psychology and focus on helping people form the intention to change and supporting them to make and sustain changes. This is different from telephone or Internet coaching models that aim to help individuals achieve management targets. For example, by prompting them to have various tests or recommending that they ask their doctor about treatment changes (Vale *et al.* 2003; Young *et al.* 2007). Peer Coaching has become more widely used in recent years as evidence for its benefit emerges.)
- The Ecological Model, which focuses on identifying key resources and supporting self-management grounds diabetes self-management in the context of the individual's social and environmental situation (Fisher *et al.* 2005). It enables the individual's skills and choices to be integrated with the services and support they receive from their social environment, which includes family and friends, health services, and wider community services. The ecological approach determines the impact various factors in the individual's environment have on their self-care ability. The Chronic Care Model and its derivatives is an example of the ecological Model (Wagner 1996).
- Complementary medicine (CAM) and Integrative Models (Phelps & Hassad 2011) focus on finding the 'doctor within' and enhancing the individual's innate capacity for healing. CAM models suggest health professionals are most effective when ' we give they doctor who resides in each patient a chance to go to work'. (Schweitzer, in Cousins 2005, p. 78; Dunning 2013). Self-empowerment is at the heart of Schweitzer's statement. Narrative medicine underpins these models.

Increasingly, business models are being applied to health care, including diabetes education. In particular, marketing strategies and understanding how people make decisions (consumer decision journey) is relevant to diabetes education consultations. Edelman (2012) highlighted the fact that a consumer's journey is complex and iterative through and beyond purchasing a product. Edelman developed a five-point model to highlight the important components of the purchasing journey:

(1) Consider: what products, brands, prices people have in mind when they think about buying a product.
(2) Evaluate: consumers collect information from a range of sources including electronic to narrow their choices (and often purchase on line).
(3) Buy: decide what brand to buy and buy it.
(4) Post purchase: reflect on the buying experience. Their reflections will influence subsequent purchases.
(5) Advocate: consumers tell other people about the product, brand and purchasing experiences. We witness may prominent people advertising products in the media including diabetes products.

Practice point

Reflect on how Edelman's model could be applied to diabetes education. In addition, think about the power of marketing and advertising and how it creates expectations. How could diabetes educators use marketing strategies in diabetes education programmes?

There are several common elements among these models: individual behaviours result from perceived benefit of and perceived barriers to change (HBM); expected outcomes and readiness to make changes (SOC); self-efficacy and perceived ability to control the behaviour (SCT); perceptions of social and cultural norms (TRA, Ecological Model); individual innate capacity (doctor within) (CAM). Coaching involves helping people identify ways of changing (pathway thinking). In addition, these models all rely on understanding people with diabetes' explanatory models for diabetes and a range of other things, their lived experience of diabetes, and how they negotiate complicated health care systems and the associated contradictory language, focus on 'control', discipline, regular surveillance by a range of health professionals, and the need to assume a great deal of responsibility for diabetes care to the individual. Effective components of diabetes management programs are: high frequency of contact with the person with diabetes, the relationship between the individual and health professionals and the person's ability to adjust treatment with or without health professional approval (Pimouguet *et al.* 2010).

Health professionals need to understand the multiplicity of factors that influence people's explanatory models, including their own influence. For example, Type 2 diabetes is frequently described as a 'lifestyle disease,' which has a hidden subtext, for example, self-induced disease and blame, media advertising promotes foods such as 'guilt-free chocolate.' The 'voice' in which health professionals seek or deliver information as well as the actual words they use, affect learning. Three health professional voices have been described:

- the 'doctor' voice used when the health professional is seeking information from the patient;
- the 'educator' voice used when imparting information to the patient;
- the 'fellow human' voice used when encouraging and supporting people.

People with diabetes are more likely to respond to the fellow human voice. They often try to reduce the judgmental connotations inherent within words by developing their own explanations for diabetes (Dunning 2013a, 78–95).

Communication – the central element of effective teaching and learning

Effective communication is central to teaching and learning and the person's role in health-related decision-making. Communication means many things. In the context of diabetes education it is the art of asking good questions and *listening* to the answers.

Research consistently demonstrates low patient-health professional concordance about management decisions (Heisler *et al.* 2003; Parkin & Skinner 2003; Skinner *et al.* 2007; Schwarz *et al.* 2012), which health professionals frequently attributed to patients not recalling the content of the consultation. However, Skinner *et al.* (2007) demonstrated that both patient and health professional recall is poor. Significantly, Skinner *et al.* found some decisions patients and health professionals recalled were not evident in recordings of their conversations and there were discrepancies between the details even when both groups recalled the general topics discussed.

Parkin & Skinner (2003) found patients were more likely to recall talking about diet and less likely to recall discussing moods or emotions. Conversely, health professionals were more likely to recall discussing mood and emotions. Parkin & Skinner found complete disagreement between patients and health professionals in 19.6% of encounters and about decisions made 20.7% of the time. That is, the 'the two parties seem to recall different consultations'. Patients may forget a great deal of what they are told, but it appears health professionals forget a great deal about what they say.

Likewise, Rushford *et al.* (2007) found women hospitalised with a cardiac condition recalled receiving information about medication, smoking cessation, and exercise but very few recalled receiving information about resuming gardening, sexual activity, and driving. Obese inactive women only recalled a limited amount of information about diet and activity and only some women with diabetes recalled receiving information about medicines. Older women were least likely to recall advice.

Recent studies of people in hospital show > 60% could not name the doctor in charge; 58% did not know why they were in hospital, 67% were prescribed a new medicine but 25% of these did not know they were given a new medicine, 38% did not know they were scheduled for an investigative test on the day the test was scheduled (Wilkins 2012). Similar discrepancies occur in primary care where patients report being interrupted by their doctors within the first 18 seconds when the person begins to talk, doctors underestimate the individual's desire for information, 50% report they are not asked whether they have any questions and 50% leave the consultation unsure about what they are expected to do (Alston *et al.* 2012). These facts suggest there is considerable miscommunication within clinical encounters that represent significant missed opportunities for engaging with patients.

The reasons for these discrepancies are not clear. However, the more people are told the more they forget and they tend to recall what they were told first and/or consider important to them, best. These findings suggest there are many barriers to effective communication, many of which are common to patients and health professionals (see Table 16.1).

Specific strategies to enhance education and promote behaviour change include:

- Asking;
  - Does the person have the knowledge and skills to manage their diabetes to best of their ability (including health literacy and numeracy)?
  - Does the person have access to and/or can he or she identify and use relevant resources and support appropriately?
  - Is the individual satisfied with his or her life at the moment? (Schulman-Green *et al.* 2012).

- Having the individual write down their goals, a strategy used in health coaching, to encourage people to own the decision and to remind them of their behaviour change goals.
- Written or verbal contracts between patients and health professionals, patients and carers, or health professionals and carers where one or both parties commit to undertaking behaviours. There is little evidence that contracts improve adherence or achieve behaviour change (Bosch-Capblanch *et al.* 2007).
- Blood glucose awareness training (BGATT) has consistently demonstrated improved hypoglycaemia awareness (ability to detect hypoglycaemia) and fewer episodes of severe hypoglycaemia during driving (Cox *et al.* 2006). It was developed for people with Type 1 diabetes but there is no reason it should not be appropriate to Type 2. BGATT was recently made available on the Internet for health professionals and people with diabetes.
- Adopting a 'tell back-collaborative inquiry' approach (Kemp *et al.* 2008). Many people leave health professionals with limited understanding about what occurred in the encounter. Such misunderstanding is associated with high risk of adverse outcomes. Kemp *et al.* used two video scenarios to assess how people like to receive information. One video showed a doctor explaining a medical condition and its management using three types of inquiry: yes–no (commonly used in health settings), tell back directive (health professional-centred), and tell back collaborative (patient- centred and had elements to address patient's feelings). Not surprisingly, people preferred the tell back collaborative approach. Significantly, the Kalamazoo Consensus Statement developed by communication experts recommends checking for understanding as a core element of communication. Interestingly, Kemp *et al.* (2008) identified only one article, published long before the explosion of patient-centred models, in an extensive literature review that recommended checking for patient understanding (Bertakis 1977). Bertakis reported improved information retention and satisfaction with management.

Thus, an empowering education model that encompasses a 'tell back' collaborative approach enables the individual's explanatory model for diabetes and their personal health care needs to be heard, and provides opportunities to negotiate and agree on compromises. Education encounters are often emotional as well as cognitive and rational, and involve reflection and action. Sometimes people have to make difficult management decisions several times a day, which can be stressful and emotionally exhausting. The ecomap and genomap shown in Chapter 2 could help health professionals understand an individual's social environment.

The following issues need to be considered when designing an empowering education encounter:

- Education alone will not change behaviour (World Health Organization (WHO) (2003; Knight & Donan 2006). For example, 28% of people with Type 1 diabetes do not have their insulin prescriptions filled or inject the prescribed doses (Morris *et al.* 1997); only one-third of people with Type 2 on monotherapy obtain at least 80% of their prescribed medicines (Donan *et al.* 2002), only follow dietary recommendations 50% of the time (Toobert *et al.* 2000); and only 30% who take out gym membership attend the gym. Likewise, the Internet increases knowledge but does not necessarily change behaviour (Cochrane Library 2004).
- The individual's feelings, beliefs and diabetes explanatory models affect their health care behaviours.
- Psychosocial situation and key relationships.
- Education and literacy level.
- Coping style.

- Ability to make informed decisions (the person with diabetes AND health professionals). Thus, education programmes must have the infrastructure to support the quality of clinical decision-making (O'Connor *et al.* 2003 & 2007; Alston *et al.* 2012). There is a growing number of diabetes-related clinical decision aids and guidelines that can be obtained from libraries such as the Cochrane Collaboration, Foundation for Informed decision Making, and the Mayo Clinic. It is interesting that, although key diabetes management guidelines are derived from the same evidence, they often make slightly different recommendations such as treatment targets. The International Patient Decision Aid Standards (IPDAS) Collaboration developed quality criteria concerning essential content, the development process and evaluation processes that can be used to develop diabetes education material, especially when patient decision-making ability is an essential component of care.
- Learning and teaching styles and methods.
- Goals for the session and future life goals.
- Ability to undertake self-care behaviours.
- Satisfaction with the service.

Although current diabetes management and education care models focus on people with diabetes being active participants in their care, and health outcomes are better if the person actively participates, people are not informed about all their options, including the risks and benefits; they are informed about the option the health professional recommends (Alston *et al.* 2012). People, especially those with chronic diseases, want coordinated care, yet only 50% report they receive it (Alston *et al.* 2012).

People's actual role in and preferences concerning health care decision-making is complex. Some people prefer to leave medical decisions to their doctors. Arora *et al.* (2000) found 58% of patients preferred their doctors to make medical decisions. There was a significant association between older age, lower education and income levels, and male gender and preference for doctor-driven decisions. People with severe cardiac disease and serious diabetes were more likely to adopt a passive role. In contrast, those with clinical or symptomatic depression were more likely to take an active role. People with the lowest coping skills and those who placed a higher value on their health were more likely to leave decisions to their health professionals. Many people who choose to use complementary therapies prefer to be active participants in their care (Dunning 2007).

Teaching: an art and a process

Teaching is a communication process involving planning, implementing and evaluating information to be learned. Teaching can be delivered individually or in groups and involves:

- Creating an environment in which learning can occur. This includes establishing a relationship with the person and finding their 'doctor within'.
- Assessing learning needs and learning style or styles. The learning needs are used to set goals and plan the teaching. Assessment is an essential first step because patients and health professionals have different ideas about what is important (Woodcock & Kinmouth 2001). Barriers and facilitators to learning and being able to use the information can be identified and the teaching can build on past experience, existing knowledge, and address misconceptions.
- Prioritising learning needs.
- Setting goals with the individual or group to be achieved that are agreed with the individual or group and are achievable and measurable (Skinner 2013, 49–61).

- Identifying the teaching method most likely to enhance learning and the materials needed to deliver the teaching. This can be as simple as a stick to draw in the sand with or as complex as a sophisticated lecture room. In group settings, a range of teaching strategies need to be used to accommodate different learning styles.
- Delivering the teaching using strategies most likely to facilitate learning.
- Having the insight to 'Seize the day' and teach at a teachable moments as the movie *The Dead Poet's Society* portrayed so poignantly.
- Evaluating the outcome. Evaluation is an essential aspect of quality improvement and should not only focus on patient outcomes (knowledge and behaviour). Teacher performance and the overall teaching programme should also be evaluated. There are different forms of evaluation depending on the purpose of the evaluation see recommended reading at the end of the chapter. When planning the evaluation, the data collection process and validity of any tools used need to be considered.

Thus, there is considerable overlap among teaching, storytelling, and counselling. In the context of diabetes education where the underlying goal is often to achieve and/or maintain behaviour change, the teacher must find the most effective way to invite the individual to see themselves and their role in a different way and find ways to help the individual help themselves. Thus, education is a sophisticated form of marketing. It is a challenge selling the product 'diabetes', with all that entails and the meanings the word holds for individuals and society, to a usually reluctant buyer.

Self-care can be facilitated by co-coordinating self-management activities, recognising that different self-management tasks vary in importance to individuals and at different times in an individual's life, ensuring open, and honest communication with people with diabetes to co-create management plans (Schulman-Green *et al.* 2012). Health professional training in how to deliver patient-centred education and care may improve performance and patient satisfaction and active engagement in their care (Lewin *et al.* 2001).

Diabetes education can be delivered individually and is equally effective delivered in groups including initiating insulin (Plank *et al.* 2004; Yki Jarvinen *et al.* 2007). However, people still need to be able to apply the information to their personal situations and have the opportunity to practice relevant behaviours. Group education provides a form of peer support and often helps people feel less alone in the problems they face and feelings about diabetes, which can have positive health benefits. Internet-based education programmes are also effective for younger and older people especially when they are interactive and emphasise behavioural and motivational strategies (Bond *et al.* 2007).

Health professionals are often also patient advocates; in fact patient advocacy is listed as in *Role and Scope of Practice for the Credentialed Diabetes Educator in Australia* (Australian Diabetes Educators Association (ADEA) 2007). Specific advocacy actions for diabetes educators and nurses include helping people obtain relevant health care, advocating for services, and interceding with other health professionals on the individual's behalf. Health advocacy is a complex process and nurses are often hindered in their advocacy by issues such as a sense of powerlessness, lack of support from colleagues, lack of time, and insufficient knowledge and skills (Negarandeh *et al.* 2006).

Health literacy

Forty one percent of Australians have inadequate health literacy skills and 59% struggle to understand their health and health choices (Australian Bureau of Statistics 2012). Similar statistics apply in many other countries. Significantly, health literacy encompasses more than the ability to read and write. Considering health literacy and numeracy is

Practice points

(1) Listening is an essential element of education and care and heals (Dunning 2013b, 62–76).
(2) Diabetes education is not about getting the individual to do what the health professional wants.
(3) Even if the health professional is not trying to control the individual's life, it often feels that way to the person concerned. Most people's instinct is to resist. Core beliefs and values are held more strongly when people feel they have lost control over aspects of their life (Thomas 2001; Speight 2013) and affect readiness and ability to make relevant behaviour changes.
(4) Emotions need to be acknowledged not solved. Health professionals' instinct is to try to solve the problem. The art of teaching is to help the individual find the solution themselves.

essential to the success of person-focused interventions (Coulter & Ellins 2007). Health literacy and numeracy are complex concepts. Nutbeam (2000) defined three levels of health literacy from a 'risk factor' perspective, where most previous definitions were based on a biomedical perspective of health and ill health. Individuals may not fall neatly into Nutbeam's levels:

(1) Functional health literacy that includes basic reading and writing skills needed to function in daily life.
(2) Communicative/interactive health literacy that includes more advanced literacy and cognitive skills that combine with social skill and enable people to participate in a range of activities and apply information in changing circumstances.
(3) Critical health literacy that encompasses even more advanced cognitive and social skills an individual uses to have control over their lives.

More recent definitions of health literacy encompass an asset-based perspective and encompass health system literacy and the individual's ability to understand and interact with the social determinants of health and navigate the health system (de Leeuw 2012), which might also be a requirement of health professionals.

People with low health literacy have poorer health outcomes, less self-care knowledge and self-care skills lower medicine adherence rates, more admissions to hospital and are less likely to engage in healthy eating and exercise (de Walt *et al.* 2004). In addition, cross-sectional studies indicate poor numeracy skills are common in people with diabetes and might be associated with inadequate glycaemic control as well as low self-efficacy and inadequate knowledge (Cavanaugh *et al.* 2008) and increase the risk of hypoglycaemia (Sarkar *et al.* 2008).

Likewise Kerr & Varshneya (2012) undertook a confidential online survey of health professionals who provide diabetes education to people with diabetes in the UK, Australia and Germany (n = 328). Health professionals believed people with diabetes have trouble with spelling and grammar; find it difficult to understand graphs and tables as well as fractions, decimals and percentages. The health professionals estimated 3–4 people in 10 had difficulty following instructions and felt people struggled to understand the behavioural aspects of diabetes care such as diet and activity advice and managing insulin doses and dose adjustments. Interestingly health professionals scored themselves highly on their ability to effectively meet people with diabetes needs. Thus, it is essential to understand health literacy and numeracy when designing care plans with people with diabetes and when making decisions about their behaviours including risk-taking behaviours.

People with limited health literacy often feel ashamed and try to hide the fact from other people. For example, Parikh *et al.* (1996) found two thirds of patients had never disclosed their low health literacy to their spouses, more than half had never told their children, and one in five had never disclosed to anybody. Clues to low health literacy include the individual's response to written information, for example, 'I forgot my glasses, I will read it when I get home', responses to questions about health care behaviours, for example, inability to name medicines, actual behaviours, for example, missing appointments or not adhering to medicine regimens. However, these are clues to explore the issue: they are not diagnostic (Davis *et al.* 1993; Weiss 2007).

Methods of assessing health literacy include:

- Newest Vital Sign (NVS) (Johnson &Weiss *et al.* 2008) is used to screen for limited health literacy by answering questions about a nutrition label for ice cream.
- Rapid Estimate of Adult Literacy in Medicine (REALM) (Davis *et al.* 1993) is a word recognition test and is one of the oldest and most widely used health literacy assessment instruments. Variations on the original REAL include a version for adolescents (REALM-Teen), a shorter version than the original 66 questions (REALM-7). Other versions are under development, for example, for dentistry.
- Test of Functional Health Literacy in Adults (TOHLA) is more complex and is often used for research purposes (Parker *et al.* 1998). It takes ~20 minutes to complete but a shorter version is available that can be completed in 12 minutes. It assesses numeracy as well as literacy.
- National Assessment of Adult Literacy (NAAL) can be used as a population screening tool and identifies four levels of health literacy from basic to proficient (Kutner *et al.* 2007).
- The eHealth Literacy Scale (eHEALS) is a measure of knowledge, comfort and skill at using information technology to obtain health information from electronic sources and has been validated with adolescents (Norman & Skinner 2006).
- Nutrition Literacy Scale, which is specific to nutrition.
- Health Literacy Skills Instrument (McCormack *et al.* 2010), which measures people's ability to obtain and use information and adopts a skills based approach.

It may be possible to incorporate health literacy assessments into routine clinical practice but it can be time consuming and patients may not be willing to undergo such testing. If time and resources permit, a health literacy point prevalence survey may provide a guide to the prevalence of the problem in a given target population. It may be more useful to ensure written health information is at grade 8 or 9 level by undertaking various readability and usability tests on the information commonly provided such as:

- The Simple Measure of Gobbledegook (SMOG).
- CLOZE.
- DISCERN designed to evaluate the quality of written patient health information (Coulter *et al.* 1998).
- Fry Readability Graph, which is commonly used and can be found on the Iowa Department of Health Fry's readability Graph page.
- Gunning FOG, which can also be obtained from the Iowa Department of Health.
- Material for Informed Choice-Evaluation (MICE) designed to assess the readability of scientific information for patients (Charnock 1998).
- PMOSE/KIRSCH, which focuses on material that use lists, charts and graphs

- Flesch Reading Ease, which is used in the Microsoft word grammar checker. However scores can be 2–3 grades lower than results obtained using valid assessment tools. For example a score of 7 would most likely be 10 on the SMOG.
- Suitability Assessment of Materials (SAM) developed by Doak and Doak (Doak *et al.*1996) and assesses readability, usability and suitability of materials.

It is very likely that a great deal of information is not at an appropriate literacy level to promote informed health decision-making and may not suit all learning styles. Godolphin *et al.* (2001) found 50% of the pamphlets on display in doctor's consulting rooms was well below the required level on the DISCERN scale. Generally, people want health information and if their information needs are met in a form appropriate to their needs they are more likely to actively participate in their care (Larson *et al.* 1996; Coulter *et al.* 1998; McKenna *et al.* 2003) yet doctors often underestimate people's desire for information and are less likely to provide information for older people (McKenna *et al.* 2003).

Other design issues are also important such as colour contrast, font size, font type (sans serif fonts, e.g., Arial and all capital letters are harder to read than serif fonts, e.g., Times New Roman and sentence case), the amount of 'white space', and the graphics used. Interestingly, a recent study found people taking antiepileptic medicines (n = 60 000) were more likely to miss doses if they were given generic medicine that was a different colour from their usual medicines (Kesselheim *et al.* 2013).

Survival skills

While the preceding information largely addresses the need to consider the mental and social aspects of learning and teaching, there are some tasks that need to be mastered for safe, effective self-care. Survival skills are taught at diagnosis and throughout life as the need arises. The family should be involved whenever necessary if possible. Survival skills education refers to providing minimal information to enable the person to manage their medicines, eat an appropriate diet, monitor blood glucose and ketones, prevent and/or manage hypoglycaemia, safely dispose of used equipment and obtain relevant supplies. Written information can support verbal teaching and is more effective if the health professional gives the information to the individual and points out important information relevant to the individual. However, the individual's specific concerns/questions must be addressed. The person should be able to:

- demonstrate correct insulin care and administration techniques (if appropriate);
- know the effect of medications, exercise and food on their blood glucose levels;
- know the names of their insulin/oral glucose lowering medicines (GLM) (if relevant);
- demonstrate correct blood glucose monitoring techniques (and blood and ketone testing in Type 1 diabetes) and appropriately documenting the results;
- know the significance of ketones (Type 1);
- recognise the signs and symptoms, causes and appropriate treatment of hypoglycaemia if on insulin or GLMs;
- know that regular meals containing the appropriate amount of carbohydrate are important;
- have an emergency contact telephone number if help is required;
- demonstrate safe disposal of sharps;
- enrol in the NDSS (in Australia).

Thus, acquiring even the basic diabetes information (survival information) is a significant burden. Significantly, many health professionals do not understand these issues (Livingstone & Dunning 2010; Dunning *et al.* 2010). Dunning *et al.* (2013c) used the ADKNOWL (Bradley 2003) to determine health professionals' diabetes knowledge in two Australian regional aged care facilities. The response rate was disappointingly low: conversations in follow up interviews with nurses revealed 'the questions were too hard for general nurses.' This is a major concern considering the ADKNOWL was designed to be used with people with diabetes (and health professionals) and one would expect nurses caring for people with diabetes to have *at least* an equivalent level of knowledge about diabetes and its care, especially when caring for some of the most vulnerable people in society—older people living in aged care homes. It is not surprising many people with diabetes worry health professionals '*will bugger it* [diabetes care] *up*' when they are in hospital (Savage *et al.* 2012).

A sample diabetes education record that could be used to document 'survival information' and plan for further teaching follows.

Sample diabetes education record chart

DIABETES EDUCATION RECORD

Date of referral ....
Referred by Dr/RN ....
Language spoken ....
Literacy level ....
Other communication issues (e.g. hearing problems, wears
  spectacles)..
Method used to address issues ....
Perceived level of skill and understanding attained ....
Follow-up requirements ....

Information supplied

1. What is diabetes? ....
2. How it is controlled:
   • diet ....
   • tablets/insulin ....
   • activity/exercise ....
3. Ketone testing ....
4. Home blood glucose monitoring ....
5. Diet and nutrition ....
6. Insulin and GLMs:
   • care of ....
   • insulin administration ....
   • when to take OHA/insulin ....
   • sharps disposal ....
7. Hypos ....   8. Sick days ....
9. Foot care ....   10. Sport & exercise ....
11. Dentist ....   12. Travel & Driving ....

Other information ....
Family support: good/fair/inadequate (if the latter why e.g. spouse is old and has multiple
  comorbidities)
Carer health status (especially older partners) ....
Follow-up care needed from practice, home care or community nurses or the GP ....
  ....
  ....

Discharge checklist

1. Education material supplied – itemise ....

2. List of medicines that includes self-prescribed and complementary medicines ....
....

3. Record book .or other means of documenting blood glucose levels e.g. meter.................
....

4. Blood testing equipment ....

5. Ketone testing ....   6. Specific diet advice ....

6. Medic alert ....

7. Starter pack: syringes/needles/lancets ....

8. Medicines ....

9. Discharged to: diabetic clinic/GP/specialist ....

10. Referred for further education ....

11. Any Alerts that need to be recorded e.g. low literacy

Enrolment in Diabetes Association ....

Plan for next session ....

Signature ....   Date ....

Ongoing education

Education can be continued on an individual basis or in group programmes. Education is a lifelong process, thus both methods are usually employed. Survival information should be reviewed and further information given. The person should gradually be able to perform the following depending on their individual care plan:

- Demonstrate appropriate insulin adjustment considering the effects of factors such as food, activity, medicines and illness on blood glucose as relevant.
- Manage illnesses at home, especially continue insulin/diabetes tablets, continue to drink fluids and test for ketones, especially Type 1.
- Recognise the signs and symptoms of hypoglycaemia and treat appropriately.
- Cope in special situations, such as eating out, during travel and playing sports.
- Understand that appropriate complication screening such as foot care will help prevent long-term complications and hospital admissions.
- Know that normoglycaemia and regular examination of the eyes, feet, blood pressure, cardiovascular system and kidney function can prevent or delay the development of long-term diabetic complications.
- Understand that certain jobs and activities are unsuitable/risky for people with diabetes on insulin, for example, scuba diving, driving heavy vehicles.
- Wear some form of medical alert system identifying them as having diabetes.
- Understand they should not neglect general health care such as mammograms, prostate checks, breast self-examination, regular dental checks, and preventative vaccinations.
- In order to recognise 'abnormal', for example, hypoglycaemia or signs of a complication, the individual needs to recognise what 'normal' is *for them*. This involves learning to listen to their bodies, interpret body cues, self-diagnose and make a decision about what to do. They may or may not seek assistance to interpret the body cues. They usually test their theories (legitimisation).

Practice points

(1) Education methods that incorporate behavioural strategies, experiential learning, co-negotiated goal setting, and use reinforcement are more likely to be effective.
(2) Patient satisfaction is a key element of adherence.
(3) Helping the person reflect on events and consider future strategies make education more personal.
(4) The therapeutic relationship between the patient and health professional is important to effective education and care.

Empowerment

There is no doubt that diabetes education is essential, but knowledge alone does not predict health behaviour. Beliefs, attitudes and satisfaction are some of the intervening variables between knowledge, behaviour, and disease status. These are not constants and they need to be assessed on a regular basis, for example, deciding what is happening at the time, what could/will change and how will the change affect the individual and their significant others.

Empowerment models of diabetes education are based on shared governance considering the whole person and their life situation and personal environment. These issues are not a new concept. Hippocrates is credited with saying, 'In order to cure the human body it is necessary to have knowledge of the whole.' Likewise, the psychiatrist in T.S. Elliot's play *The Cocktail Party* states that he needed to know a great deal more about the patient than the patient himself could always tell him.

Empowerment models recognise that people with diabetes must, and mostly want to be responsible for their own care. Empowerment is based on three characteristics:

(1) The person with diabetes makes choices affecting their healthcare.
(2) The individual is in control of their care.
(3) The consequences of the choices affect the person with diabetes.

Empowerment then, is a collaborative approach to care where management is designed to help the individual make informed choices and maximise their knowledge, skills, and self-awareness. It requires the individual to make deliberate conscious choices on a daily basis. In reality, most people are not disempowered; they make decisions and act on them every day including deciding to attend or not attend a consultation (Speight 2013).

Empowerment education requires health professionals to accept the legitimacy of an individual's goals even if they result in suboptimal control (Anderson *et al.* 1996; Skinner 2013, 49–61) and the individual to accept responsibility for the consequences of their decisions. Not everybody is capable of taking control. Some people require specific instructions, for example, an individual who has an external locus of control. In addition, stress and anxiety at specific times can impair an individual's ability to take control.

An empowerment model of diabetes education seeks to determine what the person with diabetes wants, and to reach agreement between what should be done and what the individual wants or is capable of achieving in order to balance the burden of treatment and quality of life (see Chapter 15). Diabetes is only one aspect of people's lives and affects them on many levels:

- observable, for example, signs and symptoms of hyper/hypoglycaemia;
- not directly observable, for example, personhood, self-concept, body image;
- insights into their disease;
- relationships.

Special issues

The individual's questions should be addressed as they arise and planned into teaching programmes as appropriate to the individual. Questions may relate to:

- pregnancy and diabetes;
- sexuality and diabetes;
- exercise;
- diet;
- weight control;
- how to manage their medicines;
- a range of other issues such as diabetes information the person hears or reads in media reports.

Clinical observation

It is not absolutely necessary for people with diabetes to have a detailed knowledge about the causes and pathophysiology of diabetes to undertake appropriate self-care and achieve good control.

The nurses' role in diabetes education

Patient teaching is a recognised independent nursing function and education is a vital part of the diabetic treatment plan. Therefore, teaching patients in acute, aged care and extended care facilities is within the scope of professional nursing practice. Some key points should be kept in mind when educating people with diabetes:

(1) the aim of diabetes education is autonomy and empowerment;
(2) consider the psychological and social aspects when discussing diabetes;
(3) encourage questions and dialogue;
(4) ask open questions and use active listening;
(5) teach specific skills and allow the patient time to practice new skills (e.g. insulin administration);
(6) allow time for patients to discuss difficulties and concerns about diabetes;
(7) relate new information to the patient's experience;
(8) make sure the information provided is consistent with the information provided by the diabetes team;
(9) refer to a diabetes educator when necessary, especially if you do not know the answer.

Practice point

Although there are many disadvantages to bedside teaching, e.g. noise, distractions, illness, other priorities and concerns, and lack of privacy, it can enable teaching to occur at a 'teachable moment' and effectively reinforce information. The information must be consistent with hospital policies/procedures and the nurse must have the appropriate knowledge in order to teach effectively. Nurses make a substantial contribution to the health and well being of the patient by allowing them to participate in decision-making about their care in hospital and to make appropriate decisions at home.

Teaching in the ward effectively reinforces the information supplied by the diabetes nurse specialist/diabetes educator, doctor, podiatrist and dietitian. However, ward teaching *must* be consistent with that of the diabetes team and procedures such as insulin technique and blood glucose monitoring performed correctly according to the agreed protocols. Patients are quick to perceive inconsistencies and may become confused or loose faith in the staff if they perceive inconsistencies.

Learning is facilitated when the need/readiness to learn is perceived and immediately applied in a given situation: that is, 'teaching at a teachable moment'. Teachable moments often occur when the ward staff is performing routine nursing care, such as blood glucose tests, or giving injections.

Teaching is non-verbal as well as verbal. In fact >60% of communication is non-verbal. People learn by observation, therefore the nurse is a role model and care should be taken to perform procedures correctly and to refer questions to another person if they do not know the answer. In this way, formal and informal ongoing education in the ward is possible and desirable. The nurse's own knowledge about diabetes will influence their willingness and ability to participate in patient teaching. Theories of teaching and learning were not traditionally part of the nurse training. This is changing as empowerment in chronic disease management is recognised and accepted along with a focus on preventative healthcare.

Many factors can influence teaching and learning. Some of these are shown in Table 16.3. It is the responsibility of the teacher to ensure that the environment is not distracting. Noise in a busy ward can make conversation difficult and hinder learning. The patient should be as comfortable as possible and free from pain and other distractions.

The following basic principles need to be considered when planning a teaching session, whether it is for an individual or a group:

- the aim of the session;
- the patient's needs/goals and learning style;
- objectives should be realistic and achievable;
- the environment must be conducive to learning;
- ascertain and build on the patient's existing knowledge;
- relate teaching to patient's own experience;
- demonstrate the skills to be acquired;
- provide opportunities for the patient to practice the skill (return demonstration);
- evaluate the skill and knowledge;
- provide positive reinforcement;
- review information before commencing the next teaching session.

It is usual to begin with the simple concepts and proceed to more complex ones.

Table 16.3 Some common patient and health professional factors that influence teaching and learning.

Factor	Patient	Health professional
Health beliefs	√	√
Social support	√	
Well-being/illness	√	√
Environment	√	√
Knowledge	√	√
Skills	√	√
Time	√	√
Perceived responsibility	√	√
Work priority		√
Perception of teaching role		√
Learning style	√	√

The Instruction Sheets at the end of the chapter are examples of information material used in teaching, which is often available in several languages. In some cases the medical terms may need to be replaced with the patient's words. Blood glucose monitoring is discussed in Chapter 3. Specific patient instruction will depend on the testing system being used.

Insulin administration

Insulin can be administered using a range of insulin delivery systems including syringes, insulin pens, and insulin pumps. Syringes are not used as often as the other devices in some countries, because other devices offer greater flexibility and portability, reduce dosing errors and are discreet, thus avoiding some of the stigma attached to using syringes. The person should be shown a range of options and helped to choose one that suits them. The short fine needles in use today mean injections are relatively painless – less painful than blood glucose testing.

Insulin should be given subcutaneously (see how to give an injection). IM injections, through incorrect technique, cause erratic blood glucose levels because the insulin is absorbed faster than via the subcutaneous route (Vaag *et al*. 1990). Reusing needles and syringes causes local trauma, microscopic damage to the needle tip and increases the likelihood that the needle will bend and/or break off in the injection site; it should therefore be discouraged. Needles left on insulin pens form a conduit to the outside allowing air to enter the vial and dose inaccuracies (Ginsberg *et al*. 1994).

These factors may not be an issue in developed countries where needles are supplied under the NDSS scheme, but they still occur in other countries where access is difficult or costly.

Guidelines for teaching people about insulin delivery systems

Patient learning requirements

The patient should be familiar with the structure and function of the particular insulin device chosen. They must be able to:

- assemble the device in the correct sequence;
- load the insulin correctly if necessary;
- ensure insulin is expelled from the needle after loading the insulin;
- know when to replace the insulin cartridge/device;
- know how to inject the insulin according to the particular device chosen;
- know how to store and transport the device;
- know the appropriate method of cleaning and maintaining the device;
- recognise signs that the device may be malfunctioning and know what action to take to remedy the situation.

It is important to discuss with and advise the individual about safe disposal of used equipment, especially sharps disposal at home. Guidelines for sharps disposal in the home can be found in Chapter 17.

Documenting diabetes education

Documentation was discussed in Chapter 2. Documentation is a legal requirement as well as a method of communication. Documenting diabetes education can be very time-consuming, thus using templates or teaching records that list standard education and make provision for individual differences to be recorded can save time.

Examples of patient instruction sheets appear on the following pages.

Example instruction sheets

These Instruction Sheets are designed for use with a practical demonstration of the procedure/s. They should not be handed out without adequate discussion. *They are examples only.*

The following two information sheets about drawing up insulin in syringes are included because syringes are still used in other countries and in many hospital settings, although most people with diabetes do not use syringes to self-inject in Australia. Likewise, short/rapid acting and Isophane insulins are still used in some places although premixed insulins are more common in others (Chapter 5).

Example Instruction Sheet 3: How to draw up insulin from one bottle

Your insulin is called ....
It can be useful to indicate the particular insulin colour code especially if the person is not literate.

(1) Remove insulin bottle from fridge. Check expiry date – do not use if exceeded.
    Cloudy insulin must be mixed before drawing up.
(2) Gently invert insulin bottle or roll between hands until well mixed (do not shake). Insulin should be 'milky'; there should be no lumps.
    Clear insulin should be clear and colourless.
(3) Clean bottle top with spirit.
(4) Draw back plunger to .... units of air.
(5) Inject air into insulin bottle, invert bottle and draw back .... units of insulin, ensuring that all air bubbles are removed from the syringe.
(6) Administer insulin.

Example Instruction Sheet 4: How to draw up insulin from two bottles (usually a short/rapid acting and an intermediate acting insulin)

Your insulins are called .... (clear)
.... (cloudy)

(1) Remove insulin bottles from fridge. Check expiry date and do not use if exceeded.
(2) Gently invert or roll bottle of 'cloudy' insulin between hands, until 'milky' (do not shake).
(3) Clean bottle tops with spirit.
(4) Draw back plunger to .... units of air.
(5) Inject air into cloudy insulin and remove needle from the bottle.
(6) Draw back plunger to .... units of air.
(7) Inject air into clear insulin.
(8) Invert bottle and draw back .... units of clear insulin, ensuring that all air bubbles are removed from syringe.
(9) Put needle into cloudy bottle and withdraw .... units of cloudy insulin to the exact required dose of the syringe.
(10) If more cloudy insulin is accidentally drawn up, discard contents of the syringe and start again.
(11) Total clear and cloudy insulin equals .... units.

Example Instruction Sheet 5: How to give an insulin injection using syringes or insulin pens

(1) Insulin can be injected into the abdomen, thighs, buttock or upper arm. The abdomen is the preferred site.
(2) Inject into a different spot each time.
(3) Pinch up a fold of skin between two fingers.
(4) Quickly push the needle into the skin at right angles.
(5) Gently push the plunger all the way to inject your insulin.
(6) Leave the needle while you count to five to reduce the flow of some insulin out the needle track.
(7) Pull the syringe/device out quickly and apply pressure to the injection site.

Insulin should be stored away from heat and light. The bottle/cartridge in use can be kept at room temperature.
Stores should be kept in the refrigerator.
The same injection technique applies to insulin pens.

Example Instruction Sheet 6a: Managing your diabetes when you are ill: patients with Type 1 diabetes

Illness (such as colds and flu) cause the body to make hormones which help the body fight the illness. These hormones usually also cause the blood glucose to go high. High blood glucose levels can lead to unpleasant symptoms like thirst, tiredness and passing a lot of urine.
  By taking some simple precautions the minor illness can usually be treated at home.

What to do

(1) Tell a family member or friend you are unwell.
(2) Continue to take your insulin. You may need to increase the dose during illness to control the blood glucose and prevent ketones from developing.
(3) Test your blood glucose every 2–4 hours. Write down the test results.
(4) Test your blood for ketones. If moderate to heavy ketones are detected consult your doctor.
(5) Continue to drink fluids or eat if possible (see recommended food list).
(6) Read the labels on any medication you take to treat the illness because it may contain sugar, sugar substitutes or other ingredients that cause the blood glucose to go high.
(7) Rest.
(8) Keep the telephone number of your doctor, diabetes clinic or diabetes nurse specialist/ diabetes educator beside the telephone.

When to call the doctor

(1) If you have diarrhoea and/or vomiting.
(2) If ketones develop.
(3) If the blood glucose continues to rise.
(4) If you develop signs of dehydration (loss of skin tone, sunken eyes, dry mouth).
(5) If the illness does not get better in 2–3 days.
(6) If you feel you need advice.

What to tell the doctor when you call

(1) How long you have been sick.
(2) What the blood glucose level is.
(3) How long the blood glucose has been high.
(4) The level of ketones in the blood.
(5) How frequently you are passing urine and how much.
(6) If you are thirsty, tired or have a temperature.
(7) What medications you have taken to treat the illness.
(8) If you have vomiting or diarrhoea, how frequently and how much.

Food for days when you are sick

It is important to continue to eat and drink. Small frequent meals may be easier to digest.

Suggested foods

- sweetened jelly (not low cal)
- ice cream (1/2 cup)
- custard with sugar (1/2 cup)
- honey (3 teaspoons)
- sugar (1 tablespoon)
- sweetened ice block (one small or 90 mL)
- egg flip – sweetened (similar to eggnog but less creamy 8 oz)
- milk (10 oz)
- Coke, lemonade or other sweetened soft drink (3/4 cup – not low cal)
- unsweetened tinned fruit (3/4 cup)
- orange juice (3/4 cup)
- apple juice (1/2 cup)
- pineapple juice (1/2 cup)
- orange (one medium)
- banana (one small)
- unflavoured yoghurt (100 g or 1/2 carton)
- flavoured (sweetened) yoghurt (200 g or one carton)
- broth or soup

Continuing care

(1) If the doctor prescribes antibiotics to treat the illness it is important to complete the full course.
(2) Continue to test for ketones until they show clear for 24 hours.
(3) Continue to test your blood glucose 2–4 hourly and record the results until you recover and then go back to your usual routine.
(4) Go back to your usual food plan when you recover.
(5) If your insulin has been increased during the illness decrease it again when you recover to avoid hypoglycaemia.
(6) Develop a sick day management plan.
(7) Consider writing down a medical history for quick reference in times of illness or in an emergency.
List:
- all the medications you are taking
- past illnesses
- blood group
- date of last tetanus and flu injection
- illnesses that run in the family.

This can be worn in an identification tag or be kept with your diabetes record book.

Example Instruction Sheet 6b: Managing your diabetes when you are ill: patients with Type 2 diabetes

Illnesses (such as colds and flu) cause the body to make hormones which help the body fight the illness. These hormones usually also cause the blood glucose to go high. High blood glucose levels can lead to unpleasant symptoms like thirst, tiredness and passing a lot of urine.
  By taking some simple precautions the minor illness can usually be treated at home.

What to do

(1) Tell a family member or friend you are unwell.
(2) Continue to take your diabetes tablets. This is very important, because the blood glucose usually goes high. In severe illnesses or during an operation insulin injections may be needed until you recover.
(3) Test your blood glucose every 2–4 hours. Write down the test results.
(4) Continue to drink fluids or eat if possible (see recommended food list).
(5) Read the labels on any medication you take to treat the illness because it may contain sugar, sugar substitutes or other ingredients which cause the blood glucose to go high.
(6) Rest.
(7) Keep the phone number of your doctor, diabetes clinic or diabetes nurse specialist/ diabetes educator beside the telephone.

When to call the doctor

(1) If you have diarrhoea and/or vomiting.
(2) If the blood glucose continues to rise.
(3) If you develop signs of dehydration (loss of skin tone, sunken eyes, dry mouth).
(4) If the illness does not get better in 2–3 days.
(5) If you feel you need advice.

What to tell the doctor when you call

(1) How long you have been sick.
(2) What the blood glucose level is.

(3) How long the blood glucose has been high.
(4) How frequently you are passing urine and how much.
(5) If you are thirsty, tired or have a temperature.
(6) What medications you have taken to treat the illness.
(7) If you have vomiting or diarrhoea, how frequently and how much.

Food for days when you are sick

It is important to continue to eat and drink. Small frequent meals may be easier to digest.

Suggested foods

- sweetened jelly (not low cal)
- ice cream (1/2 cup)
- custard with sugar (1/2 cup)
- honey (3 teaspoons)
- sugar (1 tablespoon)
- sweetened ice block (one small or 90 mL)
- egg flip – sweetened (8 oz)
- milk (10 oz)
- Coke, lemonade or other sweetened soft drink (3/4 cup – not low cal)
- unsweetened tinned fruit (3/4 cup)
- orange juice (3/4 cup)
- apple juice (1/2 cup)
- pineapple juice (1/2 cup)
- orange (one medium)
- banana (one small)
- unflavoured yoghurt (100 g or 1/2 carton)
- flavoured (sweetened) yoghurt (200 g or one carton)
- broth or soup

Continuing care

(1) If the doctor prescribes antibiotics to treat the illness it is important to complete the full course.
(2) Continue to test your blood glucose 2–4 hourly and record the results until you recover and then go back to your usual routine.
(3) Go back to your usual food plan when you recover.
(4) Develop a sick day management plan.
(5) Consider writing down a medical history for quick reference in times of illness or in an emergency.
    List:
    - all the medications you are taking
    - past illnesses
    - blood group
    - date of last tetanus and flu injection
    - illnesses which run in the family.

This can be worn in an identification tag or be kept with your diabetes record book.

Evaluating diabetes education

It is important to evaluate diabetes education delivered to individuals and in education programmes. Likewise, it is important to use appropriate evaluation processes and outcome measures and to value audit, evaluation and translational research and ensure some ethical oversight is in place. The evaluation method used depends on the aim/s of the evaluation, which might not be the same as the aims of the programme.

Clinicians are more likely to evaluate the individual's progress, which typically involves measuring:

- Knowledge change (but knowledge does not necessarily translate into action).
- Biochemical parameters such as HbA_{1c} and lipids: bearing in mind these factors are influenced by a host of inter-related confounding variables and may not be a primary outcome of diabetes education.
- Psychosocial variables (see Chapter 15).
- Satisfaction, recognising high patient satisfaction scores could be an artifact and many satisfaction questionnaires may not ask an appropriate range of questions.
- Other outcomes according to the initial nursing assessment.

Programme evaluation is only briefly described here. It is an essential element of diabetes education programmes and should be considered when the programme is *being developed, not planned after the programme has been delivered*. The evaluation method depends on the purpose of the evaluation (aim/s), which will influence the measurement tools and procedures used in the evaluation. In some cases permission is needed to use copyright tools and some copyright holders charge a fee to use their tools. It is professional courtesy to acknowledge the authors.

Some reasons programme evaluations are undertaken include:

- Cost-benefit/effectiveness to ensure continued funding for the programme
- Determine programme outcomes, bearing in mind it is difficult to interpret the outcomes if the structure and process variables are not considered. Outcomes might be short term or long term.
- Health professional performance should be a component of most evaluation programmes and is usually part of the process variables. Most current patient satisfaction surveys are not adequate to evaluate health professional performance
- Needs analysis to determine the characteristics of the target population so the programme can be appropriately planned to suit their need.
- A combination of these broad aims.
- Determine the public health impact of the programme in the short and/or long term.

Glasgow & Osteen (1992) suggested many diabetes education programme evaluations have a narrow focus on HbA_{1c} and knowledge acquisition and do not assess other important variables and do not report important information in research reports and publications readers need to interpret the findings. Although there has been some improvement in diabetes education evaluation research since 1992, many publications still contain methodological flaws and adopt a narrow focus that does not take account of the many factors and confounders likely to affect the outcome. Glasgow & Osteen recommended assessing outcomes in all relevant aspects of the programme and collecting standardised, objective and specific measures in each stage of the evaluation and in each of the following categories:

- The social and environment context because these issues impact on people's capabilities e.g.:
  - social support and available community resources;
  - living arrangements;
  - health insurance;
  - organisation of the diabetes clinic or service;
  - time, cost, location and access to the programme.
- Participant characteristics, which is important to determine whether participants in the programme are representative of the sampling or whole population:
  - description of the target population (sampling population including the approximate size of the population;

- ○ individual's demographic characteristics;
- ○ medical history such as diabetes complications and other comorbdities;
- ○ cognitive functioning;
- ○ physical functioning especially older people and people with disabilities;
- ○ measures might include knowledge, attitudes and beliefs, self-efficacy, spirituality, problem-solving ability, health literacy and numeracy, well being and quality of life and metabolic data such as HbA_{1c}, lipids, weight, smoking and might be measured before and after the programme or at set intervals of time e.g. before, 3–4 months after the programme and again 12–18 months or in the longer term over years.
- Processes:
  - ○ was the programme delivered as planned?
  - ○ if changes were needed, why were the needed and how did the change affect participants?
  - ○ what did participants think about the programme: content, delivery methods, health professional performance and the materials used in the programme and may include the parameters listed under participant characteristics?
- Outcomes of the programme, usually also measured before and after the programme:
  - ○ participation and attrition rates;
  - ○ representativeness of the final sample;
  - ○ changes in diabetes self-care behaviours such as blood glucose monitoring, medicine management, accessing resources, admission to hospital, attending scheduled appointments, morbidity and mortality.

Most importantly, people with diabetes should be involved in designing education programmes, evaluation processes and quality metrics that are valuable to them (Jones 2013) or the care to be person-centred. Most people want their health professionals to be knowledgeable and competent and to know the care they receive is evidence based, but they value effective communication, empathy, trust, and the health professional being present in the moment.

References

Alston, C., Paget, L., Halvorson, G. *et al.* (2012) *Communicating with Patients on Health Care Evidence*. Washington State Institute of Medicine of the National Academies, Washington DC.

Anderson, R., Funnell, M. & Arnold, M. (1996) Using the empowerment approach to help patients change behaviour, in *Practical Psychology for Clinicians* (eds B. Anderson & R. Rubin). American Diabetes Association, Alexandria, VA, pp. 163–172.

Anderson, B. & Funnell, M. (2005) *The Art of Empowerment*, 2nd edn. American Diabetes Association, Virginia, USA.

Anderson, R., Funnell, M., Burkhart, N., Gillard, M. & Nwankwo, R. (2002a) 101 *Tips for Behaviour Change in Diabetes Education*. American Diabetes Association, Virginia, USA.

Anderson, R., Funnell, M., Burkhart, N., Gillard, M. & Nwankwo, R. (2002b) 101 *Tips for Diabetes Self-Management Education*. American Diabetes Association, Virginia, USA.

Arora, N., Mchorney, C. & Rao, S. (2000) Medical decision-making: Who really wants to participate? *Medical Care*, **38** (3), 335–341.

Assal, J-P. & Assal, T. (2013) Role and use of creative arts in diabetes care, in *Diabetes Education: Art, Science and Evidence*. (ed. T. Dunning) Wiley Blackwell, Chichester pp 98–115.

Australian Bureau of Statistics (ABS) (2012) Data quoted during the Centre for Culture, Ethnicity and Health forum *Curing the Cultural Barrier: Health Literacy Forum*, Fitzroy Town Hall Melbourne 28th February 2012.

Australian Diabetes Educators Association (ADEA) (2007) *The Credentialled Diabetes Educator in Australia: Role and Scope of Practice*. ADEA, Canberra.

Ajzen, I. & Fishbein, M. (1980) *Understanding Attitudes and Predicting Social Behaviour*. Prentice Hall, Englewood Cliffs NJ.

Bandura, A. (1986). *Social Foundations of Thought and Action*. Prentice Hall, Englewood Cliffs NJ.

Becker, M. & Maiman, L. (1975). Sociobehavioral determinants of compliance with health and medical care recommendations. *Medical Care*, **13** (1),10–24.

Bert G. (2011) *Treating with words: Narrative medicine*. ZOE Foundation http://www.foundazionezoe.it/code/13426/11279 (accessed August 2012).

Bertakis, K. (1977) The communication of information from physician to patient: a method for increasing patient and physician satisfaction. *Journal of Family Practice*, 5, 217–222.

Bond, G., Burr, R., Wolf, F. & McCurry, S. & Teri, L. (2007) The effects of a web-based intervention on physical outcomes associated with diabetes among adults age 60 and older: A randomised trial. *Diabetes Technology Therapy*, **9** (1), 52–59.

Bosch-Capblanch, X., Abba, K., Prictor, M. & Garner, P. (2007) Contracts between patients and health care practitioners for improving adherence to treatment, prevention and health promotion activities. *Cochrane Database of Systematic Reviews*, Art. No. CD004808. DOI: 10.1002/1451858.CD004808.pub3.

Bradley C. (2003). *The audit of diabetes knowledge (ADKnowl) user guidelines*, 4th draft. Health Psychology Research, Royal Holloway University of London, Egham, Surrey, UK. Downloaded 26th November, 2009. http://www.healthpsychologyresearch.com/Admin/uploaded/Guidelines/adknowl%20user%20guidelines%20rev24.9.03.pdf.

Cavanaugh K, Huizinga M, Wallston K. (2008) Association of numeracy and diabetes control. *Annals of Internal Medicine* **148**, 737–746.

Cochrane Library (2004) *Internet Use Has Negative Effect on Health*. Cochrane Library issue 4, London. evidence-informed-musings.blogspot.com/.../national-free-access-to-cochrane.html (accessed August 2012).

Charnock, D. (1998) *The DISCERN Handbook. Quality Criteria for Consumer Health Information on Treatment Choices*. Radcliffe Medical Press, Oxford.

Coulter, A., Entwhistle, V. & Gilbert, D. (1998) *Informing Patients. Assessment of the Quality of Patient Information Materials*. King's College, London.

Coulter, A. & Ellins, J. (2007) Effectiveness of strategies for informing, educating and involving patients. *British Medical Journal*, **335** (7609), 24–27.

Cousins, N. (2005) *Anatomy of an Illness as Perceived by the Patient*. WW Norton, New York.

Cox, D. & Gonder-Frederick, L. (1992) Major developments in behavioural diabetes research. *Journal of Consulting Clinical Psychologists*, **60**, 628–638.

Cox, D., Gonder-Frederick, L., Ritterband, L. *et al.* (2006) Blood glucose awareness training: What is it, where is it, and where is it going? *Diabetes Spectrum*, **19**, 43–49.

Davis, T., Long, S. & Jackson, R. (1993) Rapid estimate of adult literacy in medicine: A shortened screening instrument. *Family Medicine*, **25**, 391–395.

Doak, C., Doak, L. & Root, J. (1996) *Teaching Patients with Low Literacy Skills*. JB Lippincott, Philadelphia, PA.

Donan, P., MacDonald, T. & Morris, A. (2002) Adherence to prescribed oral hypoglycaemic medication in a population of patients with Type 2 diabetes: A retrospective cohort study. *Diabetic Medicine*, **19**, 279–284.

Dunning, T. (2007) Complementary therapies and diabetes: Perfect partners or dangerous liaisons? Integrative Medicine Perspectives. Australasian Integrative Medicine Association (AIMA) Annual Conference, Peppers Fairmont Resort, Blue Mountains, Sydney.

Dunning, T. (2010) Chronic disease self-management: What do we measure? *Nursing and Healthcare of Chronic Illness* **2**, 251–253.

Dunning, T. (2013a) Teaching and learning: The art and science of making connections, in *Diabetes Education: Art, Science and Evidence* (ed. Dunning, T.), Wiley Blackwell, Chichester pp. 28–46.

Dunning, T. (2013b) The teacher: Moving from good to exceptional, in *Diabetes Education: Art, Science and Evidence* (ed. T. Dunning) Wiley Blackwell, Chichester pp 62–76.

Dunning, P., Wellard, S., Rasmussen, B. *et al.* (2013) Managing diabetes medicines in regional residential aged care facilities: balancing competing challenges. Abstract number ICN 13ENA–2630 presented at the International Council of Nurses Conference 18–23rd May, Melbourne Australia.

Edelman, D. (2012) *The Funnel is Dead. The New Consumer Decision Journey*. http://www.linkedin.com/today/post/article/2012018110732=1816165 (accessed October 2012).

Fisher, E., Brownson, C., O'Toole, M. *et al.* (2005) Ecological approaches to self-management: The care for diabetes. *American Journal of Public Health*, **95** (9), 1523–1535.

Gale, J. (2007) *Health Psychology Meets Coaching Psychology in the Practice Of Health Coaching*. http://www.psychology.org.au/publications/inpsych/health_coaching/ (accessed December 2007).

Ginsberg, B., Parkes, J. & Sparacina, C. (1994) The kinetics of insulin administration by insulin pens. *Hormone Metabolism Research*, **26**, 584–587.

Glasgow, R. & Osteen, V. (1992) Evaluating diabetes education. *Diabetes Care*, **13** (10), 1423–1432.

Godolphin, W., Towle, A. & McKendry, R. (2001) Evaluation of the quality of patient information to support informed shared decision-making. *Health Expectations*, **4**, 325–242.

Fisher, L., Mullan, J. & Arean, P. (2010) Diabetes distress but not clinical depression or depression symptoms is associated with glycaemic control in both cross-sectional and longitudinal analysis *Diabetes Care*, **33**, 23–28.

Funnell, M. & Anderson, R. (2000) The problem with compliance in diabetes. *Journal of the American Medical Association*, **284**, 1709.

Heisler, M., Vijan, S., Anderson, R. *et al.* (2003) When do patients and their physicians agree on diabetes treatment goals and strategies, and what difference does it make? *Journal of General Internal Medicine*, **18**, 909–914.

International Alliance of Patients' Organisations (IAPO) (2005) *Declaration on Patient-Centred Care.* IAPO www.patientsorganisations.org/pchreview (accessed December 2007).

Institute of Medicine (IOM) (2012) Communicating with patients on health care evidence. IOM http://www.iom.edu/evidence (accessed October 2012).

Johnson, K. & Weiss, B. (2008). How long does it take to assess literacy skills in clinical practice? *Journal of the American Board of Family Medicine*, **21**, 211—214.

Jones K. (2013) Patients need to be involved in quality metrics. *Primary care Progress blog* (accessed January 2013).

Jutterstrom, L., Isaksson, U., Sandstrom, H. & Hornsten, A. (2012) Turning points in self-management of Type 2 diabetes. *European Diabetes Nursing*, **9** (2), 46–50.

Kemp, E., Floyd, M., Mc-Cord-Duncan, E. & Lang, F. (2008) Patients prefer the method of 'tell back-collaborative inquiry' to asking for understanding of medical information. *Journal American Board Family Medicine*, **21** (1), 24–30.

Kerr D, Varshneya R. (2012) How education impacts on diabetes patient care. *Practical Diabetes Supplement* S1–S7.

Kesselheim, A., Misono A, Shrank W, *et al.*(2012) Variations in pill appearance of antiepileptic medicines. *Archives of Internal Medicine*, DOI 10 1001/2013.jamaainternmed.997 (accessed January 2013).

Kolb, D. (1984) cited in Arndt, M. & Underwood, B. (eds) (1990) Learning style theory and patient education. *Journal of Continuing Education in Nursing*, **21** (1), 28–31.

Knight, K. & Donan, T. (2006) The diabetes educator: Trying hard, but must concentrate more on behaviour. *Diabetic Medicine*, **23**, 485–501.

Kutner M, Greenberg E, Jin Y, et L. (2007). Literacy in everyday life: Results from the 2003 National Assessment of Adult Literacy. http://nces.ed.gov/pubsearch/pubsinfo.asp?pubid=2007480. (Accessed December 2012).

Larson, C., Nelson, E., Gustafson, D. & Batalden, P. (1996) The relationship between meeting patients' information needs and their satisfaction with hospital care and general health status outcomes. *International Journal Quality Health Care*, **8**, 447–456.

de Leeuw E. (2012) The political ecosystem of health literacies. *Health Promotion International* **27** (1), 1–4.

Lewin, S., Sea, Z., Entwhistle, V., Zwarenstein, M. & Dick, J. (2001) Interventions for providers to promote a patient-centred approach in clinical consultations. *Cochrane Database of Systematic Reviews*, (4), CD003267.

Linder, N., Menzies, D., Kelly, J., Taylor, S. & Shearer, M. (2003) Coaching for behaviour change in chronic disease: a review of the literature and the implications for coaching as a self-management intervention. *Australian Journal of Primary Health*, **9**, 177–185.

Livingston, R. & Dunning, T. (2010) Practice nurses' role and knowledge about diabetes management within rural and remote Australian general practices. *European Diabetes Nursing* **7**, 55–61.

MacKeracher, D. (1996). Making sense of adult learning. Toronto, Culture Concepts. books.google.com/.../Making_Sense_of_Adult_Learning_2nd_ed.html?id.

Mayo Clinic (2009) *Diabetes Medication Choice Decision Aids Cards.* http://www.mayoclinic.org. news2009-rst/5454.html (accessed December 2012).

McKenna, K., Tooth, L., King, D., *et al.* (2003) Older patients request more information: A survey for use of written patient education materials in general practice. *Australian Journal on Aging*, **22** (1), 15–19.

McCormack, L., Bann, C., Squiers, L., *et al.* (2010) Measuring health literacy: A pilot study of a news skills-based instrument. *Journal of Health Communication* **15**, 51–71.

Morris, A., Boyle, D., McMahon, A. *et al.* (1997) Adherence to insulin treatment, glycaemic control, and ketoacidosis in insulin-dependent diabetes mellitus. *Lancet*, **350**, 1505–1510.

National Public Health Institute of Helsinki (2007) *The Goal Lifestyle Implementation Trial*. Helsinki, Finland.

Negarandeh, R., Oskouie, F., Ahmandi, F., Nikraves, M. & Rahmfallberg, I. (2006) Patient advocacy: Barriers and facilitators. *BMC Nursing*, 5, 3. DOI: 10.1186/1472–6955-5–3.

Norman, C. & Skinner, H. (2006) The eHEALS: Health Literacy Scale. *International Medicine Internet Research*, 8, e27.

Nutbeam, D. (2000) Health literacy as a public health goal: A challenge for contemporary health education and communication strategies into the 21st century. *Health Promotion International* **15**, 259–267.

O'Connor, A. (2003) Decision aids for people facing health treatment or screening decisions. *Cochrane Database of Systematic Reviews No* **2** (2003) CD001431.

O'Connor, A., Wennberg, J., Legare, F., *et al.* (2007) Toward the 'tipping point': Decision aids and informed patient choice. *Health Affairs* **26** (3), 716–725.

Parikh, N., Parker, R., Nuss, J., Baker, D. & Williams, M. (1996) Shame and health literacy: The unspoken connection. *Patient Education and Counselling*, **17**, 33–39.

Parker R (1998) Health literacy: a challenge for American patients and their health care providers. *Health Promotion International*, **15** (4), 277–283.

Plank, J., Kohler, G., Rakovac, I., *et al.* (2004) Long term evaluation of a structured outpatient education programme for intensified insulin therapy in patients with Type 1 diabetes: A 12-year follow up. *Diabetologia*, **47**, 1370–1375.

Parkin, T. & Skinner, T. (2003) Discrepancies between patient and professionals' recall and perception of an outpatient consultation. *Diabetic Medicine*, **20**, 909–914.

Phelps, K. & Hassad, C. (2011) *General Practice: The Integrative Approach*. Elsevier, Sydney.

Prochaska, J. & DiClemente, C. (1983). Stages and processes of self-change of smoking: Toward an integrative model of change. *Journal of Consulting and Clinical Psychology*, **51** (3), 390–395.

Rasmussen, B., O'Connell, D. & Dunning, T. (2007) Young women with Type 1 diabetes management of turning points and transitions. *Qualitative Health Research* **17** (3), 300–310.

Redman, B. (2001) *The Practice of Patient Education*. Mosby, Toronto.

Rushford, N., Murphy, B., Worcester, M. *et al.* (2007) Recall of information received in hospital by female cardiac patients. *European Journal of Cardiovascular Prevention & Rehabilitation*, **14** (3), 463–469.

SAM Suitability Assessment of Materials for evaluation of health-related information for adults www.beginningsguides.com/upload/SAM-for-Beginnings.pdf (accessed November 2012).

Sarkar, U. & Schillinger, D. (2008) Does lower diabetes–related literacy lead to increased risk for hypoglycaemic events? *Annals of Internal Medicine*, **149**, 594.

Savage, S., Dunning, T., Duggan, N. & Martin, P. (2012) The experiences and care preferences of people with diabetes at the end of life. *Journal of Hospice and Palliative Nursing*, **14**, 293–302.

Schulman-Green, D., Jaser, S. & Martin, F. (2012) Processes of self-management in chronic illness. *Journal Nursing Scholarship*, **44**, 136–144.

Schwarz, P., Felton, A.M., Cobble, M., Bonilla Islas, A. & Wens, J. (2012) Differences in patient and clinician perspectives in T2DM: The MOTIVATE global survey. Poster 966 presented at the European Association for the Study of Diabetes (EASD) Annual Conference, 2012, Berlin.

Wilkins, S. (2012a) What's behind the patient satisfaction, doc communication disconnect. Hospital Impact. http://www.hospitalimpact.org/index.php/2012/10/17/p4147#more4147 (accessed December 2012).

Skinner T (2013) Making choices, setting goals. Chapter 4 in *Diabetes Education: Art, Science and Evidence*. (ed. T. Dunning) Wiley Blackwell, Chichester pp. 49–61.

Skinner, T., Barnard, K., Craddock, S. & Parkin, T. (2007) Patient and health professional accuracy of recalled treatment decisions in out-patient consultations. *Diabetic Medicine*, **24**, 557–550.

Speight J. (2013) Managing diabetes and preventing complications: What makes the difference? *Medical Journal of Australia*, **198** (1),16–17.

Speight, J., Conn, J., Dunning, T. & Skinner, T. (2012) Diabetes Australia position statement: A new language for diabetes improving communication with and about people with diabetes. *Diabetes Research and Clinical Practice*, **97**, 425–531.

Tankova, T., Dakovska, G. & Koev, D. (2001) Education of diabetic patients – A one year experience. *Patient Education and Counselling*, **45**, 139–145.

Thomas, N. (2001) The importance of culture throughout life and beyond. Holistic nursing practice. *The Science of Health and Healing*, **15** (2), 40–46.

Toobert, D., Hampson, S. & Glasgow, R. (2000) The summary of diabetes self-care activities measure: Results from 7 studies and a revised scale. *Diabetes Care*, **23**, 943–950.

Tope, R. (1998) The impact of interprofessional education in the south west region – A critical analysis. The literature review www.doh.gov.uk/swrp/tope.htm

Vaag, A., Handberg, M., Lauritzen, J., Pedersen, K. & Beck-Neilsen, H. (1990) Variation in absorption of NPH insulin due to intramuscular injection. *Diabetes Care*, **13** (1), 74–76.

Vale, M., Jelinek, M., Best, J., *et al*. (2003) Coaching patients on achieving cardiovascular health (COACH): A multicenter randomized trial in patients with coronary heart disease. *Archives of Internal Medicine*, **163**, 2775–2783.

Wagner, E., Davis, C., Schaefer, J., Von Korff, M. & Austin, B. (2002) A survey of leading chronic disease management programs: Are they consistent with the literature? *Journal of Nursing Care Quality*, **16** (2), 67–80.

Wagner, E., Austin, B. & von Korff, M. (1996) Organizing Care for Patients with Chronic Illness. *The Milbank Quarterly*, **74** (4), 511–44.

Wilkins, S. (2012b) Patient engagement is the holy grail of health care http://www.kevinmd.com/blog/2012/patient-engagement.holy-grail-health-care.html (accessed January 2012).

Woodcock, A. & Kinmonth, A. (2001) Patient concerns in their first year with type 2 diabetes:patient and practice nurse views. *Patient Education and Counseling*, **42**, 257–270.

de Walt, D., Berkman, N., Sheridan, S., Lohr, K. & Pignone, M. (2004) Literacy and health outcomes: A systematic review of the literature. *Journal of General Internal Medicine* **19**, 1228–1239.

Weiss, B. (2007) Assessing health literacy in clinical practice. *Medscape*, http://www.medscape.com/viewprogram/802_pnt (accessed November 2007).

World Health Organization (WHO) (2003) *Adherence to long term therapies: Evidence for action.* WHO, Geneva.

Yki-Jarvinen, H., Juurinen, L., Alvarsson, M. *et al.* (2007) Initiate insulin by aggressive titration and educate (INITIATE). *Diabetes Care*, **30**, 1364–1369.

Young, D., Furler, J., Vale, M., *et al.* (2007) Patient Engagement and Coaching for Health: the PEACH study – A cluster randomised controlled trial using the telephone to coach people with Type 2 diabetes to engage with their GPs to improve diabetes care. *BMC Family Practice*, **8** (20), 8–13.

Further reading

Broom, D. & Whittaker, A. (2003) Controlling diabetes: moral language in the management of Type 2 diabetes. *Social Science and Medicine*, **58**, 2371–2382.

DAFNE Study Group (2002) Training in flexible, intensive insulin management to enable dietary freedom in people with Type 1 diabetes: Dosage Adjustment for Normal Eating (DAFNE) randomised controlled trial. *British Medical Journal*, **325**, 746–751.

Dunning, T. (2013) *Diabetes Education: Art, Science and Evidence.* Wiley Blackwell, Chichester.

Felder, R.M. & Silverman, L.K. (1988) Learning and teaching styles in engineering education. *Engineering Education*, **78** (7), 674–681. (The article that originally defined the Felder–Silverman model and identified teaching practices that should meet the needs of students with the full spectrum of styles. The paper is preceded by a 2002 preface that states and explains changes in the model that have been made since 1988).

Makoul, G. (2001) Essential elements of communication in medical encounters: The Kalamazoo consensus statement. *Academic Medicine*, **76**, 390–393.

Page, P., Verstraete, D., Robb, J. & Etzwiler, D. (1981) Patient recall of self-care recommendations in diabetes. *Diabetes Care*, **4**, 96–98.

Parker, R., Baker, D., Williams, M. & Nuss, J. (1999) The test of functional health literacy in adults (TOFHLA): A new instrument for measuring patients' literacy skills. *Journal of General Internal Medicine*, **10**, 537–545.

Partnership for Clear Health Communication (2006) *What is Health Literacy?* http://www.p4chc.org/health-literacy.aspx (accessed October 2007).

Chapter 17
Nursing Care in the Emergency, Intensive Care, Outpatient Departments, Community and Home-Based Care and Discharge Planning

---

Key points

- Common diabetes-related emergencies include DKA and HHS (Chapter 7) serious hypoglycaemia (Chapter 6), cardiovascular emergencies and foot problems (Chapter 8). Non-diabetes-related emergencies are the same as for people who do not have diabetes but the effects of metabolic derangements need to be considered and managed in emergency settings.
- Practice nurses (nurse who work in general practice settings) play an increasingly important role in community diabetes care and there is a global focus on prevention and early detection of diabetes and its complications.
- Well-established collaboration and referral procedures among health services and health service providers are essential to ensure smooth transitions among and between service settings.

COMMUNITY, PRACTICE AND HOME CARE NURSES ARE IN AN IDEAL POSITION TO DELIVER PREVENTATIVE HEALTH CARE EDUCATION

Rationale

Diabetes accounts for a great many presentations to outpatient clinics and emergency departments and discharges every year. In addition, people present to community centres and general practitioners with potential emergency situations, for example, silent myocardial infarction, see Chapter 8. People are also being managed in general practice settings and practice nurses are playing increasingly important roles in diabetes ambulatory care, and early detection and prevention programs. Practice nurses provide

Care of People with Diabetes: A Manual of Nursing Practice, Fourth Edition. Trisha Dunning.
© 2014 John Wiley & Sons, Ltd. Published 2014 by John Wiley & Sons, Ltd.

important care planning, education, monitoring, and assessments that complement the care the GP and specialist diabetes services provide. Practice nurses often act as the link between the specialist and primary care services and with diabetes educators.

This chapter outlines important issues but other chapters in the book should be cross-referenced for specific information about the conditions mentioned in this chapter for example Chapters 6 and 7, which discuss hyperglycaemic states and hypoglycaemia and chapter 1, which discusses diagnosis and overall management. It is important that diabetes is identified as soon as the individual presents for treatment and their metabolic status is assessed to limit the morbidity and mortality associated with diabetic emergencies. Diabetes might be diagnosed during the emergency, and early referral to the multidisciplinary team is desirable. It is important to be aware that conditions such as myocardial infarction and urinary tract infections can be present with few of the classical signs and symptoms.

The emergency department

Medical emergencies are a major source of morbidity and mortality for people with diabetes. The particular presenting problem may be unrelated to diabetes; however, the existence of diabetes usually affects metabolic control and complicates the management of the presenting problem such as trauma and other medical or surgical emergencies. Extra vigilance is needed to reverse or limit the metabolic abnormalities arising as a consequence of altered glucose metabolism due to stress, illness, or trauma (Chapters 1, 7 and 9). Diabetes-related abnormalities frequently presenting to the emergency department are:

- myocardial infarction;
- cerebrovascular accident;
- severe hypoglycaemia;
- infected/gangrenous feet, cellulitis;
- hyperglycaemia;
- ketoacidosis;
- hyperosmolar coma.

Rapid effective therapy and effective nursing care increase the chance of a good recovery.

Practice points

- In serious emergency situations clear rapid or short-acting insulin administered in an IV infusion is recommended to manage ketoacidosis, hyperosmolar states, cerebrovascular events, myocardial infarction and severe sepsis.
- The target blood glucose range is 5–10 mmol/L to reduce morbidity and mortality. IV glucose might be required to prevent hypoglycaemia e.g. during fasting.
- Blood glucose and ketone testing are necessary to monitor the response to treatment and assist treatment decisions (American Diabetes Association 2011; Australian Diabetes Society (ADS) 2012a,2012b).

Nursing responsibilities

(1) Carry out assessment and observations appropriate to the presenting complaint.
(2) Note medic alert/identification tags.

   (3) Enquire whether the patient has diabetes.
   (4) Record blood glucose.
   (5) Record blood ketones.
   (6) Ascertain time and dose of last diabetes medication.
   (7) Ascertain time and amounts of last meal, especially the amount of carbohydrate consumed.
   (8) Assess usual day-to-day diabetic control and the period of deteriorating control.
   (9) Record any other medication, those prescribed by a doctor and anything taken to treat the present complaint including complementary therapies.
 (10) Seek evidence of any underlying infection.
 (11) Assess pain, severity, site, cause, and relieve appropriately.
 (12) Consider the psychological aspects of the illness. Give a full explanation to the patient and family about the findings of the examination, treatment, and likely outcomes.
 (13) Avoid long delays in assessing the patient if possible, and be aware of the possibility of a hypoglycaemic episode in people on glucose lowering medication who are not eating or who have vomiting and diarrhoea.
 (14) Have appropriate carbohydrate available to treat promptly if hypoglycaemia does occur.
 (15) Assess diabetic knowledge and refer for further education if necessary.
 (16) Ensure that the patient knows when to take their next diabetes medication if discharged from the emergency department, especially if the medication regimen or the dose/s have been adjusted, and that the patient understands the new dose.
 (17) Arrange appropriate follow-up care.

Clinical observations

   (1) Blood glucose can be elevated by infection, pain, and anxiety.
   (2) TPR and BP can also be affected by emotional stress.
   (3) Reassure, rest the patient, repeat the TPR and BP. Older people with cognitive impairment might be hypoglycaemic, hyperglycaemic or have delirium and all three conditions need to be considered.
   (4) Cognitively impaired older people are at risk of injury and falls so extra vigilance is needed.

Practice points

   (1) Hypoglycaemia may be masked by coma from other causes, some medications, and autonomic neuropathy.
   (2) Prolonged hypoglycaemia can result in hypothermia especially in cold weather.
   (3) UTI and myocardial infarction can be present with few, if any, of the usual presenting signs due to autonomic neuropathy.
   (4) Repeated visits to the emergency department especially for hypoglycaemia or ketoacidosis can indicate an underlying psychosocial problem (see Chapters 7 and 15).

Intensive Care (ICU)

People with diabetes area admitted to ICU for a range of reasons, many diabetes-related. The seriousness of the presenting problem influences the priority order and type of care provided. However, hyperglycaemia has adverse effects on outcomes in people with and without diabetes. Chapter 7 discusses the importance of normalising blood glucose and preventing ketosis in acute illness and other emergencies and the value of IV insulin infusions to achieving these aims. The ADA (2011) stated critically ill people with diabetes require an IV insulin infusion using a protocol that has demonstrated efficacy and safety to avoid severe hypoglycaemia. Avoiding hypoglycaemia is important because it also has adverse effects on outcomes.

For example, the Normoglycaemia in Intensive Care Evaluation and Survival Using Glucose Algorithm Regulation trial (NICE-SUGAR) (2009) reported higher mortality and hypoglycaemia rates in ICU patients randomised to intensive glycaemic control than in the conventional care group. However, the conventional care group required insulin 60% of the time to achieve target blood glucose, < 10 mmol/L, which supports the contention that carefully managed insulin therapy is necessary.

Thus, the glycaemic range for critically ill people with diabetes is still controversial, although most experts agree the upper range should be < 10 mmol/L (ADA 2011; ADS 2012). In some cases the target range should be 6.1–7.8 mmol/L provided hypoglycaemia and glucose variability can be avoided (ADA 2011). Most current guidelines recommend individualising the blood glucose targets to suit the individual, enhance safety and maintain comfort.

Glycaemic variability, the amplitude from high (peak) to low (trough) in blood glucose has emerged as an important determinant of hyperglycaemia on outcomes (Schmeltz 2011) and there is a near linear relationship between mortality in mixed medical, cardiac and surgical ICUs and mean blood glucose (Krinsley 2003). In addition, even people with good glycaemic control (mean glucose 7 – 9 mmol/L) and large glucose variability have a 5-fold in mortality compared to people with less glycaemic variability (Krinsley 2003; Egi *et al.* 2009).

An important determinant of care is the terminal end of life stage, which is outlined in Chapter 18.

The outpatient department

People with diabetes may present to the outpatient department for routine appointments or for minor surgical or radiological procedures. They are usually basically well and mobile, although some may require a wheel chair, interpreter and/or guide dog assistance. Water should be provided for guide dogs especially in hot weather.

Nursing responsibilities

(1) Avoid long delays in seeing the doctor if possible.
(2) Be aware of the possibility of hypoglycaemia and know how to recognise and treat it effectively. Know where glucagon and other hypoglycaemic treatments are kept and be sure to restock after use. Have available at least one of the following:
   • dry biscuits
   • sandwiches
   • tea/coffee, sugar
   • glucose gel

- orange juice
- glucose.

(3) Have blood glucose monitoring equipment available.
(4) Test blood of people with Type 1 diabetes for ketones if blood glucose is elevated.
(5) Ensure test results are available in the medical record.
(6) Ensure appropriate examination equipment is available, including:
  - tendon hammer
  - sterile pins
  - Semmens – Weinstein filaments
  - ophthalmoscope
  - tuning fork
  - biothesiometer
  - stethoscope
  - eye chart
  - midriatic drops if still used.
(7) Ensure patient knows the location of toilets, other clinics, pharmacy.

Nurses and other health professionals should ensure that they are up-to-date with emergency procedures such as cardiopulmonary resuscitation especially when they are working in community settings.

COMMUNITY, PRACTICE NURSING, AND HOME-BASED CARE

Introduction

Community care home-based care enables technical and professional care to be provided to acutely and chronically ill patients at home. The provision of specific services will be influenced by the home environment, the person's condition and capabilities, and available home support services. A nursing care plan should be prepared to complement the medical management plan. Supporting people to enable them to remain at home is an important consideration when planning diabetes management with the individual and his or her family. Practice nurses and community and home-care nurses play an important role in this respect.

These nurses also play and important role in supporting carers and identifying carer distress. A recent Australian study showed carers have lowest well being of any large societal group (Australian Unity 2008). Significantly, well being decreases as the number of hours spent providing care increases and women carers have lower levels of well being than male carers. The Australian Unity survey showed unpaid, largely family, carers provide ~ $30.5 billion worth of care per year. Many carers have high levels of worry about their financial situations and their personal health that often results in depression. They often make significant lifestyle, family and work sacrifices in order to provide care. Many do not receive care for their own health issues, which include depression, chronic pain, injuries attributable to caring and many are overweight, which increases their risk of obesity-related diseases.

Diabetes-related care in the home includes:

- preparing insulin doses for people with diabetes to self-administer at the appropriate time;

- administering insulin;
- performing blood glucose and ketone tests;
- assessing the general condition of the patient;
- supporting the continuing education of the patient and of family/carers;
- attending to wound dressings;
- attending to personal hygiene;
- assisting with medication management and noting medicine self-care deficits;
- detecting deteriorating metabolic control, and functional and cognitive decline;
- helping older people remain independent for as long as possible.

Making clinical decisions about the patient in the home situation without advice and support can be stressful and difficult. In addition, the home situation must be carefully assessed to ascertain how to obtain access to the home, and the correct address and telephone number. The safety of the nurse is an important consideration and issues such as the surrounding environment and household members should be assessed before-hand, if possible. The service base should have some idea of the route the nurse is likely to take. Other information (e.g. presence of dogs) should also be noted. This chapter outlines the important diabetes-related information needed to gauge whether medical assessment is necessary.

How to obtain advice

It is important for home care and domiciliary nursing bodies to establish open communication links with the referring agency or practitioner. The referring agency should be the first point of contact for advice.

General points

(1) Ensure diabetes teaching is consistent with that of the diabetes educator.
(2) Before recommending equipment, for example, blood glucose meters and insulin delivery systems, ensure the person will be able to use the product, can afford it and can obtain further supplies. This is particularly important if the person is visiting from another country or is travelling overseas where some brands of equipment may not be available. Assess:
  - vision
  - manual dexterity
  - comprehension.
  There may be costs associated with purchasing diabetes equipment and medications in some countries. It is important that the person understands the costs and any government initiatives to reduce/eliminate those costs.
(3) Ensure the person is enrolled in the National Diabetes Services Scheme so that they can obtain needles, syringes, lancets and test strips at the subsidised price (relevant only in Australia).

Diabetes-related problems commonly encountered in the home

(1) finding an elevated blood glucose level;
(2) hypoglycaemia;
(3) the patient has not taken their insulin/diabetes tablets;
(4) the patient does not follow the diabetes management plan;
(5) managing wounds such as surgical wounds, trauma, and foot ulcers;

(6) disposing of sharps (needles and lancets) in the home situation;

(7) obtaining help/advice about specific patient problems.

Nursing actions

(1) Assess general clinical state (see Chapters 2 and 3).

(2) If the patient appears unwell, record:
  - temperature
  - pulse
  - respiration and presence of respiratory distress
  - blood pressure
  - colour
  - any other symptoms, behaviours or changes from usual.

(3) Assess presence, location, duration and severity of any pain and whether it is increasing or resolving.

(4) Note nausea, diarrhoea, and/or vomiting.

(5) Note presence of any symptoms of urinary tract infection but be aware there are often few, if any symptoms:
  - frequency
  - burning
  - scalding
  - itching.

(6) Assess hydration status.

(7) Note time and dose of last diabetic medication.

(8) Note time and amount of last meal.

(9) Measure blood glucose level and ketones if relevant.

Interpreting the blood glucose level

To assess the diabetic status one must first ascertain whether the patient is in danger because of the blood glucose level. Ascertain:

- The present blood glucose and ketone levels.
- The usual blood glucose range.
- Why the blood glucose is outside the usual range. Whether the patient has suffered any illness, committed a dietary indiscretion, commenced on a new medication, missed a medication dose, or is using a complementary or self-prescribed medication.
- Whether it is likely to go up or down.

When ascertaining the blood glucose level check whether:

- the test was performed correctly;
- there was enough blood on the strip; if using a meter that the meter was calibrated and used correctly;
- the strips have exceeded the expiry date (see Chapter 4, Monitoring 1: Blood Glucose);
- the patient has commenced any new medication that could alter the blood glucose level (see Chapter 3).

The patient may require attention if the blood glucose level is:

- low – hypoglycaemia < 3 mmol/L;
- high – hyperglycaemia > 15 mmol/L for a significant number of tests.

Hypoglycaemia

For more detailed information see Chapter 8.

(1) Treat according to the severity and time of occurrence of hypoglycaemia.
(2) Avoid over-treatment.
(3) Give rapidly absorbed high GI glucose, if symptomatic, for example,:
   - glucose gel
   - orange juice
   - tea/coffee with sugar
   - jelly beans.
(4) Give more slowly absorbed low GI glucose, if the hypoglycaemia is asymptomatic and there is some time before the next meal is due.
(5) Suggest they have their meal if it is due in half an hour.
(6) Ensure patient has recovered before leaving the home. Check the blood glucose. Wash the person's hands before testing the blood glucose if they have been handling glucose to treat the hypoglycaemia.
(7) Record incident.

If severe follow the procedure for managing unconscious hypoglycaemia (Chapter 8). IM glucagon can be administered if it is available. If not, manage the airway and seek medical or ambulance assistance.

Practice point

The next dose of medication is not usually withheld following a mild hypoglycaemic event.

Discuss recognition and treatment of hypoglycaemia with patient and family. Ensure that the person and/or their family and carers know how to manage hypoglycaemia, that there is appropriate food/fluids to manage hypoglycaemia and they know who to call in an emergency.

Hyperglycaemia

For more detailed information, see Chapter 7. Ascertain:

- how long the blood glucose level has been elevated;
- whether the patient is unwell;
- whether there are any symptoms of hyperglycaemia, for example, polyuria, polydipsia, thirst or lethargy;
- whether there are ketones present in the urine.

If moderate/heavy ketones are detected seek medical advice (this usually only occurs in Type 1 people).
   Check for any obvious source of infection:

- urinary tract
- foot ulcer wound
- cold or flu.

> ### Practice point
>
> Infection can be present without any of the usual overt signs and symptoms.

Counsel the patient about managing at home when unwell. (Patient information guidelines are shown in Chapter 5.) The important points are that the patient should:

- continue to take insulin or glucose lowering medicines;
- maintain fluid and carbohydrate intake;
- test and record blood glucose regularly, for example, 2- to 4-hourly.

In addition:

(1) if the patient has type 1 diabetes they should test their blood or urine for ketones every 4 hours;
(2) maintain contact with the patient and liaise with the diabetes team;
(3) advise them to seek medical advice if vomiting and/or diarrhoea occur, if the blood glucose continues to increase, if ketones develop or their conscious state changes.

The person with chest pain

(1) reassure the patient and family;
(2) instruct the patient to stop current activity and to sit or lie down. loosen tight clothing;
(3) instruct patient to take anginine if prescribed by doctor;
(4) assess the severity of the discomfort and the frequency of attacks;
(5) people with long-standing diabetes may have 'silent myocardial infarcts;' complaints of vague chest discomfort should be investigated, the classic pain radiating into the jaw, arm, and chest may be absent;
(6) seek medical advice and call an ambulance service;
(7) record BP;
(8) discuss decreasing risk factors for cardiac disease (see Chapter 8).

The person who has not taken their prebreakfast insulin or diabetes tablets and it is '11 a.m.' or later

More than 80% of people miss medication doses (Morris *et al.* 2000; Gilbert *et al.* 2002). If medication is missed frequently, self-care capability, cognitive functioning and mental status (e.g. depression), beliefs about medications should be assessed. Often medications are missed or taken incorrectly because the person is given inaccurate, hurried or conflicting information or the information is presented in a format the person cannot read or does not understand (Davis *et al.* 2012).

Stopping medications without consulting a doctor and inappropriately altering doses is common (Kriev *et al.* 1999). Older people in particular make more mistakes including incorrect doses when drawing insulin up in a syringe (de Brew *et al.* 1998). Home-based nursing services play a vital role in assisting elderly people to manage their medicines safely.

Medications that have long duration of action are less of a problem if a dose is missed than medications with short duration of action. Missing several consecutive doses of medicines with a narrow therapeutic index may lead to a loss of efficacy, for example, the effect of aspirin on platelet stickiness might be diminished. Time will be required to re-establish therapeutic blood concentrations if consecutive doses of medicines with a long half-life are missed.

(1) check blood glucose level;
(2) ascertain why the medication was omitted; did the person omit other medicines due to prebreakfast?
(3) ascertain whether this is a regular occurrence;
(4) ascertain whether they have eaten breakfast, and what they ate.

In general, medication may need to be modified and the dose reduced. The amount will depend on the dose and types of insulin and the blood glucose level:

(1) If it is not appropriate to administer medicines, seek advice from the referring agency or the person's general practitioner.
(2) Document any medication adjustment.
(3) Have the order signed by the appropriate doctor within the specified time period, for example, 24 hours.
(4) Plan strategies with the individual that set out what to do if a dose is missed in future and set up cues to minimise the number of missed doses, for example, a reminder on the refrigerator door. Medical information leaflets are provided with medications when they are dispensed as part of the Quality Use of Medicines Program in Australia, but this may not be the case in other parts of the world, including the UK. These information leaflets often contain advice about what to do if a dose of the medicine is missed.

Readings <6.0 mmol/L may indicate good control and the usual dose should be taken. If non-diabetic medications have been missed the person should take their normal dose at the usual time.

If it is before 11 AM counsel the patient to check their blood glucose; if it is 6 mmol/L or above the patient should:

• take usual medication dose and eat breakfast;
• eat lunch within 3 to 4 hours then tea 3 to 4 hours after that;
• have medication and breakfast at normal time the next day.

Follow-up visit

Ascertain whether:

• the patient followed advice;
• the management strategy was effective;
• hypo/hyperglycaemia occurred as a result of missed medication and modified dose
• further dietary counselling is necessary.

Managing diabetic foot ulcers at home

Diabetic foot ulcers are a common complication of diabetes and occur as a result of peripheral neuropathy and vascular changes (see Chapter 8).

On first visit
(1) Ascertain the extent to which the individual can be involved in their care, for example, cleanliness, knowledge of foot care.

(2) Check treatment plan and medication prescriptions.
(3) Assess ulcer to obtain a baseline for future comparison:
  - dimensions: width and depth;
  - type and quantity of discharge;
  - colour of surrounding tissue;
  - presence of oedema.
(4) Counsel patient to:
  (a) rest with foot elevated as much as possible.
  (b) protect foot:
    - bed cradle (stiff cardboard or polystyrene box);
    - appropriate footwear;
    - regular inspection.
  (c) complete full course of antibiotics.
(5) Monitor blood glucose tests.

Subsequent visits
(1) Perform the dressing according to the prescription. The dressing may be:
  - dry
  - occlusive
  - or the wound may be cleaned and left open.
(2) Assess progress of the wound using objective documentation such as measuring the depth and width and amount and type of exudate.
(3) If the wound deteriorates:
  - note odour and amount and type of discharge;
  - take a swab for culture and sensitivity;
  - record TPR;
  - record blood glucose level;
  - refer for assessment.

Practice points

If bandages are used ensure they are correctly applied and do not constrict the blood supply. People with neuropathy may not be able to tell if the bandage is too tight.

(1) Bandage from the foot upwards, even if the ulcer is on the leg.
(2) Do not put bandages or tape in a circular fashion around the toes.
(3) Never prick the toes to obtain a blood glucose test.
(4) Small foot wounds can hide deep infection including bone involvement.
(5) Swabs need to be taken from deep in the wound, not from the surface of the wound because mixed anaerobic and aerobic organisims are often present. Superficial swabs may not detect anaerobic organisms and delay appropriate treatment.

The person who does not follow their management plan ('non-adherence'; see Chapters 15 and 16)

'Non-compliant' is a derogatory and negative term. There may well be good reasons why people do not follow prescribed treatment, including:

- inappropriate, insufficient and/or unclear advice from health professionals;
- a complicated regimen that the patient does not understand;

- treatment goals are those of the management team and not the patient;
- inability to comply (patient may not have a refrigerator to put their insulin in, may suffer from low vision, or loss of fine motor skills);
- cultural and language differences;
- economic factors – cost of supplies;
- non-acceptance of diabetes and the constraints it imposes on lifestyle;
- other concerns may outweigh those about diabetes;
- during usual life transitions where other priorities take precedence;
- 'burnout';
- learned helplessness.

Counselling, education and appropriate modification of health professional expectations may help. Behavioural changes may take years; patient, supportive health professionals and family can assist the patient to eventually make some changes (Chapters 5 and 15).

Disposing of sharps in the home situation

In the community the person with diabetes is responsible for the safe disposal of used needles and lancets. Thousands of diabetes needles are discarded every week, outside hospitals. All health professionals have a responsibility to promote the safe disposal of used sharps. The safe disposal of used needles, syringes and lancets should be an integral part of teaching injection technique and blood glucose monitoring.

Practice point

Ensure the patient understands what you mean by a 'sharp'.

Guidelines for handling and disposing of sharps at home

(1) Take care with sharps at all times.
(2) Store needles and lancets out of reach of children.
(3) Use a 'standards approved' container if possible (check with the local council about how to obtain one).
(4) Only recap your own syringe and lancet.
(5) Recapping of syringes and lancets is a good idea if an approved container is not available, for example, at a restaurant.
(6) If testing blood glucose for family/friends always use a new lancet.
(7) Check arrangements for disposal of full containers with:
    - your local diabetes association;
    - your local council.
(8) If an approved container is not available it is advisable to:
    - recap needles and lancets;
    - place immediately into a puncture-proof, unbreakable container, clearly labelled 'used sharps;'
    - keep the container out of the reach of children;
    - keep the lid tightly closed (New South Wales Department of Health 2004).

In the UK people are advised to use a safe-clip device to remove needles and to dispose of lancets in an opaque container.

Storing insulin

Insulin should be stored in the refrigerator if possible; *it should not be frozen*. The vial in use can be stored at room temperature if it is protected from heat and light and should be used within one month of opening. Any unused insulin stored at room temperature should be discarded after one month.

> ### Practice point
> - If there is any change in appearance or consistency of the insulin, or if the expiry date is exceeded, discard the insulin.
> - If the patient has required a period in hospital, unused previously drawn up doses of insulin should be discarded. A new batch should be drawn up when the patient is discharged.

Practice nurses

Practice nurses (PN) are nurses who provide nursing services in general practice. They have a broad and collaborative role with general practitioners (GP), diabetes educators and other health professionals. In Australia their role in diabetes education and management is expanding because of legislative changes and the focus on early detection and prevention and managing Type 2 diabetes in the community. PNs can enhance the range of services available to people with diabetes through changes to the Medicare Benefits schedule that provides funding for nurses to provide services such as wound care and managing chronic illness such as diabetes under GP management plans and team care arrangements, which can improve patient outcomes, deliver cost effective care (Raftery *et al.* 2005), increase the practice income (Australian Divisions of General Practice, undated) and is acceptable to patients (Cheek *et al.* 2002).

GP management plans are developed in collaboration with the individual with a chronic disease and encompass:

- Ensuring the individual does not already have a care plan and that they are eligible under the Medicare benefits schedule
- Discussing the process, benefits and costs with the individual and if relevant their carer.
- Undertaking a thorough assessment to identify current and predict future care needs.
- Developing a plan that is agreed with the patient and that identifies relevant management targets to be met and the self-care the patient needs to undertake in order to meet agreed management targets and the actions the GP needs to undertake.
- Documenting the management in the relevant places and communicate the plan to other relevant health professionals.
- Documenting a date to review the outcomes.

The individual may be eligible for a team care arrangement if they have complex care needs or are at significant risk of complications. In Australia, Medicare items such as team care arrangements provide for interventions from a multidisciplinary team. The arrangements must involve the GP and at least two other health or community care providers. The process is essentially similar to the care plan process. The patient must have a GP management plan and a team care arrangement in place, or a current enhanced primary care plan, or the GP must make a contribution to a care plan developed for an older person in a residential aged care facility to be eligible to access Medicare for allied health and dental services.

Both PNs and GPs have unparalleled access to a large proportion of the population and are in an ideal position to provide structured and opportunistic health promotion and illness prevention messages (Sim 2006). These include general and diabetes-specific primary prevention programmes as well as secondary prevention programmes such as complication screening and early initiation of medicines such as insulin in Type 2 diabetes, antihypertensive and lipid lowering agents when they are indicated.

Discharge Planning

> ### Key points
>
> - Commence early (on admission).
> - Arrange follow-up care.
> - Give relevant contact telephone numbers so people can seek advice after discharge if necessary.
> - Ensure self-care knowledge is adequate.
> - Ensure insulin and monitoring equipment are available.
> - Ensure patient understands how and when to take medication.
> - Communicate with appropriate health professionals/carers.

There is a wealth of information about discharge planning available in the general literature and readers are referred to that literature. Transitions among service settings are high risk times for all patients and particularly people with diabetes and diabetes-related discharge planning should be part of the overall discharge plan and should begin on admission (American Medical Association (ADA) 2011). People discharged how are particularly at risk of adverse events and readmission if they do not have an appropriate discharge plan that is communicated to relevant health professionals and other service providers; in particular to the individual verbally and in writing in a culturally relevant way and in a language suitable to their health literacy and cognitive ability.

That is, discharging planning must be proactive and include the individual and relevant other in the planning process. It is important to incorporate discharge planning into the initial assessment and patient care plan, and to consider social and home needs, for example, risk of falls in older people. The plan should look beyond the current episode of care in order to prevent readmission and relevant health professionals, family and carers. Strategies include:

During the admission

(1) Informing allied health professionals of admission on day one or two of admission (diabetes nurse specialist/diabetes educator, dietitian, podiatrist, social worker).
(2) Ensuring self-care status has been assessed so that the patient is capable of caring for their own diabetes and will be safe at home.
(3) Referring for home assessment early if indicated.
(4) Reconciling medicines on admission, before discharge and after discharge. People with diabetes and relevant others should be educated about safe medicine use fro

newly prescribed medicines. Medication changes such as new medicine commenced, medicines ceased and dose or dose interval adjustments should be included in discharge documentation. Information about managing glucocorticoid medicines especially when prescribed for a short time, for example reducing the dose prescribed for anexacerbation of COPD, and managing GLMs to prevent hypoglycaemia (Chapters 6 and 10). Ensuring the person knows how to manage sick days (Chapter 7).

On day of discharge

(1) Ensure patient has necessary medications and supplies, insulin delivery device, blood glucose testing equipment, fingerprick device and diabetic record book (if relevant) and understands their use, and where to obtain future supplies.
(2) Ensure relevant follow-up appointments have been made, and a discharge letter has been written to the GP and other relevant health professionals. Electronic care systems make such communication easier and should reduce adverse events and misinformation.
(3) If further diagnostic investigations are to be performed on an outpatient basis ensure the patient has written instructions and understands what to do about medications and fasting and knows where to go for any investigations required.
(4) Ensure the patient has a contact telephone numbers for assistance if necessary.
(5) Ensure the patient knows about the services offered by the relevant diabetes association (e.g. Diabetes Australia, Diabetes UK), and other relevant services, for example, meals-on-wheels, low vision clinic, rehabilitation services, community nurse for support especially when new to insulin and liaison with the diabetes nurse specialist/diabetes educator, counselling, and council services, for example, sharps disposal.

Transfer to another service, hospital or nursing home

In addition to the usual information provided relating to nursing and medical management the nursing letter accompanying the patient should contain information about:

- diet;
- progress of diabetes education:
  - skills assessment for performing blood glucose testing and insulin administration;
  - medication regimen;
  - details of medical condition and nursing care.

Ensure transport has been arranged and that the family is aware of the discharge. Some nursing homes and special accommodation facilities may not have cared for people with diabetes in the past, or have done so on an infrequent basis. Diabetes education for the staff of the facility in this situation is desirable.

References

American Diabetes Association (2013) Standards of medical care in diabetes. *Diabetes Care*, **36**, Supp 1, S11–S66.

Australian Diabetes Society (ADS) (2012a) *Guidelines for routine glucose control in hospital*. ADS, Canberra.

Australian Diabetes Society (ADS) (2012b) *Peri-operative Diabetes Management Guidelines*. ADS, Canberra.

Australian Divisions of General Practice (undated). *Nursing in General Practice Business Case Models*. www.adgp.com.au/site/index.cfm?display=4002 (accessed August 2012)

Australian Unity (2008) Carers wellbeing lowest on record. *Australian Unity Journal*, **August**, 10–11.

de Brew, K., Barba, B. & Tesh, S. (1998) Assessing medication knowledge and practices of older adults. *Home Healthcare Nurse*, **16** (10), 688–691.

Cheek, J., Price, K., Dawson, A., *et al.* (2002) *Consumer Perceptions of Nursing and Nurses in General Practice*. University of South Australia. www.joannabriggslibrary.org/index.php/jbisrir/article/download/.../1076 (accessed December 2012)

Davis T, Federman A, Bass P, et al. (2012) Improving patient understanding of prescription drug label instructions. *Journal General Internal Medicine*, **24** (1), 57–52.

Egi M, Bellomo R, Stachowski E. (2006) Variability of blood glucose concentrations and their short term mortality in critically ill patients. *Anaesthesiology*, **195**, 244–252.

Gilbert, A., Roughead, L. & Sanson, L. (2002) I've missed a dose, what should I do? *Australian Prescriber*, **25** (1), 16–18.

Kriev, B., Parker, R., Grayson, D. & Byrd, G. (1999) Effect of diabetes education on glucose control. *Journal of the Louisiana State Medical Society*, **151** (2), 86–92.

Krinsley, J. (2003) Association between hyperglycaemia and increased hospital mortality in a heterogenous population of critically ill patients. *Mayo Clinical Practice* **78**, 1471–1478.

Morris, A., Brennan, G., Macdonald, T. & Donnan, P. (2000) Population-based adherence to prescribed medication in Type 2 diabetes: A cause for concern. *Diabetes*, **40**, A76.

New South Wales Department of Health (2004) Community sharps management guidelines for local councils. New South Wales department of Health www0.health.nsw.gov.au/pubs/2004/pdf/**sharps**.pdf (accessed December 2012).

NICE-SUGAR (Study Investigators) (2009) Intensive versus Conventional Glucose Control in Critically Ill Patients. *New England Journal of Medicine*, **360**,1283–1297.

Raftery, J., Yao, G., Murchie, P., Campbell, N. & Ritchie, L. (2005) Cost effectiveness of nurse led secondary prevention clinics for coronary heart disease in primary care: Follow up of a randomized controlled trial. *British Medical Journal*, **330**, 707–710.

Schmeltz, L. (2011) Management of inpatient hyperglycaemia. *Laboratory Medicine* **42** (7), 427–434.

Sim, M. (2006) Prevention: Building on routine clinical practice. *Australian Family Physician*, **35** (1/2), 12–15.

St Vincent's Hospital (2001) *Drawing Up Insulin Doses for Patients Who Are Unable to Draw Up Their Own Doses*. Department of Endocrinology and Diabetes Policy Manual, Melbourne.

Further reading

United Kingdom Royal College of Nursing Guidelines (1999a) *Guidelines on Premixing and Preloading of Insulin for Patients to Give at a Later Date*. London UK www.rcn.org.**uk**/

United Kingdom Royal College of Nursing Guidelines (1999b) *Guidelines on Preparing and Preloading of Insulin for Patients to Give at a Later Date*. London UK www.rcn.org.**uk**/

Chapter 18
Managing Diabetes at the End of Life

Each person experiences and interprets dying differently.
(Statement by a person with diabetes during an interview about end of life care)

Key points

- A palliative care approach involves implementing aspects of palliative care at appropriate times throughout the life journey with diabetes.
- Palliative care focuses on avoiding burdensome monitoring, managing unpleasant symptoms and addressing spirituality and quality of life to help individuals achieve a 'good death' and supporting carers.
- It is essential that the individual and their family are involved in care decisions so that care can be person-centred and individualised.
- Palliative care is a key aspect of the chronic disease trajectory. Proactive planning for palliative and end of life situations could be incorporated into annual diabetes complication screening processes and other key points in the individual's life journey.
- Hyper- and hypoglycaemia contribute to the distressing symptoms associated with end of life care but their presence and significance is often under-recognised, under-rated and therefore, under-treated.
- Blood glucose monitoring can help identify hypo- and hyperglycaemia and enable appropriate treatment and symptom management.
- The blood glucose range and medicine regimen should be individualised and adjusted as needed, sometimes frequently.
- Psychological and spiritual care is central to dignified end of life care.
- Care and support must also be available to carers who often derive positive benefits from providing care but also experience stress from witnessing a loved one suffer and who may not be well themselves.

Care of People with Diabetes: A Manual of Nursing Practice, Fourth Edition. Trisha Dunning.
© 2014 John Wiley & Sons, Ltd. Published 2014 by John Wiley & Sons, Ltd.

Introduction

Although life expectancy has increased in the past 20 years, diabetes is associated with significant morbidity and mortality and is among the top ten leading causes of death globally, particularly due to cardiovascular disease (McEwen *et al.* 2006; IDF 2012). Palliative care, especially at the end of life, focuses on maintaining comfort and quality of life, minimising unpleasant symptoms, providing effective, timely pain management, and providing spiritual and psychological support to the individual and their family/ carers.

In order to achieve these goals the effect of diabetes on the dying process needs to be considered as well as the effect of other disease processes on glycaemic control. Palliative care now encompasses chronic diseases and experts have described a palliative care approach as well as palliative care (Canadian Hospice Palliative Care Association, undated). A palliative care approach uses aspects of palliative care when appropriate throughout the illness trajectory for example, when a diabetes complication develops or worsens such as renal disease progressing to end stage renal disease requiring dialysis or during periods of unstable blood glucose.

A palliative approach concerns;

- Sensitive and effective communication about the person's disease process, disease course, possible outcomes and prognosis in the early stages of the disease process.
- Setting management goals and advanced care planning (ACP) at an appropriate time.
- Providing psychological support to the individual and their family/carers.
- Managing pain and other symptoms.
- In the later stages and during period of instability the palliative approach focuses on reviewing management and life goals, providing relevant information, adjusting the management and self-care regimens and making relevant referrals where indicated, which might include to the palliative care team. (Canadian Hospice Palliative Care Association, undated).

Palliative care is defined as:

> *An approach that improves the quality of life of patients and their families facing the problems associated with life-threatening illness, through prevention and relief of suffering by means of early identification and impeccable assessment and treatment of pain and other problems, physical, psychosocial and spiritual.*
>
> World Health Organization (WHO) 2005.

Palliative care acknowledges that dying is a normal process where there is no need to hasten or postpone death. Palliative care focuses on managing symptoms to improve comfort and supporting the individual and their family/carers to live active, fulfilling lives for as long as possible (Canadian Hospice Palliative Care Association, undated). Implementing palliative care signifies a transition from a curative approach to managing comfort and quality of life to achieve a dignified death.

It is imperative that end of life care is individualised and agreed in consultation with the person with diabetes and their family/carers, when relevant. As indicated, dying is a normal part of the life trajectory. Encouraging people with diabetes to proactively plan for palliative and end of life care could/should be part of routine diabetes care and complication screening processes (Dunning 2012). In fact, implementing a palliative approach early could improve people with diabetes' quality of life and disease management (Sudore *et al.* 2012).

Palliative care and diabetes

Diabetes is prevalent in most countries and is associated with increased morbidity and mortality and some forms of cancer. Likewise, people with diabetes with long term complications of diabetes such as end stage renal disease and cardiovascular disease may require palliative care or a palliative approach (Emanuel *et al.* 2004; Burge 2012). There is limited research evidence to guide diabetes palliative and end of life care due to the vulnerable nature of people at the end of life and the ethical issues involved in undertaking research in the area (Dunning *et al.* 2012). Thus, existing guidelines such as Dunning *et al.* (2010) and Diabetes UK (2012) are largely based on consensus opinion.

Such diabetes-specific guidelines can be used with other palliative care guidelines such as the *National Guideline for a Palliative Approach in Residential Aged Care* (Commonwealth Department Health and Aging 2006), *Ethical Framework for Integrating Palliative Care principles into the Management of Advanced terminal and Chronic Conditions* National Health and Medical Research Council (2011), End of Life Care Strategy (Diabetes UK 2012) and the Scotland End of Life Care Strategy (2008) (Emanuel *et al.* 2004).

Dunning *et al.* (2010) developed a guiding philosophy as the conceptual framework for their guidelines. The philosophy was derived from the available literature, publicly available narratives written by dying people or relatives, and, significantly, interviews with people with diabetes at the end of life and their families (Savage *et al.* 2012), and the quality use of medicines framework (QUM) (National Prescribing Service 2009) because pharmacovigilance is imperative; especially in palliative and end of life situations (Chapter 5). Figure 18.1 depicts a QUM framework for managing medicine at the end of life.

Key issues in palliative and end of life care

Deciding optimal diabetes-related end of life care is challenging because of the multifactorial, inter-related issues that need to be considered. Table 18.1 outlines some of these issues concerning diabetes. Diabetes may be the underlying cause of symptoms or contribute to or exacerbate symptoms (Quinn *et al* 2006; Dunning 2012). Monitoring blood glucose to detect hyper-and hypoglycaemia can help identify the cause of symptoms, yet many health professionals regard blood glucose monitoring at the end of life and using glucose-lowering medicines (GLM), especially insulin, as intrusive and inappropriate curative management (Quinn *et al.* 2006). However, people with diabetes regard these care aspects as a vital part of appropriate end of life care (Savage *et al.* 2012). Blood glucose monitoring and using GLMs is consistent with the WHO definition of palliative care and the focus on 'early identification and impeccable assessment.'

Many people want to die at home and be cared for by their family: 88% of 1000 people (Palliative Care Australia 2012) but changed family roles mean that is not always possible. Families often prefer hospital/hospice care because 'it preserves personal boundaries of social intimacy' because health professionals deliver care in hospital/hospice settings (Bloomer 2012). Likewise, not all dying people require specialised palliative care services, although they could benefit from a palliative approach to ensure symptoms and pain are managed and ACP are documented (Sudore *et al.* 2012; Pesut *et al* 2012).

Diabetes experts could proactively prepare for and implement a palliative approach or palliative care and ACP planning in regular diabetes assessment, management and

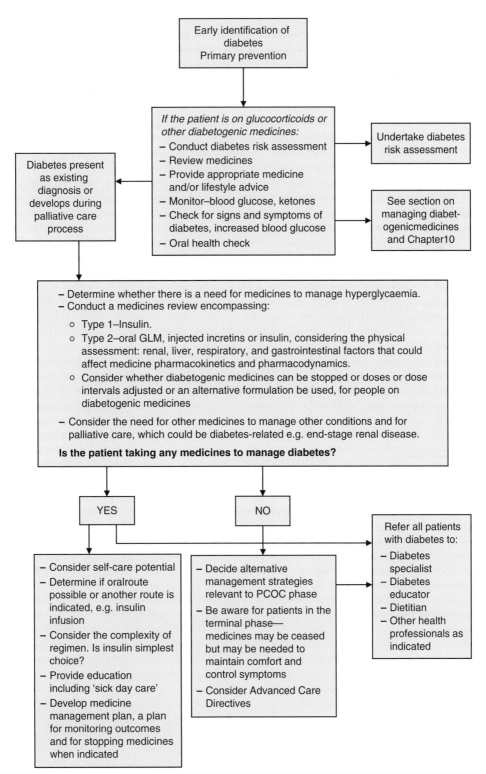

Figure 18.1 Quality Use of Medicines (QUM) Framework for managing diabetes at the end of life. (Dunning T, Savage S, Duggan N, Martin P. [2010] with kind permission.)

Table 18.1 The relationship between common symptoms encountered in people receiving palliative care, the possible impact on diabetes and/or be diabetes-related. (Dunning T, Savage S, Duggan N, Martin P. [2010] with kind permission)

Common palliative care symptoms	Impact on diabetes management	May be diabetes-related
Pain (acute/ chronic)	Increased: – somnolence or confusion/cognitive impairment due to pain/analgesia – risk of hyperventilation – hyperglycaemia Reduced: – intake – mobility – sleep – self-care ability – quality of life	– Peripheral vascular disease – Amyotrophy – Peripheral neuropathy – Myocardial Infarction (MI) – Tissue glycosylation (e.g. carpel tunnel syndrome) – Ketoacidosis (abdominal pain)
Depression/ anxiety	Increased: – fatigue – lethargy, change in performance status – risk of DKA, HHS – social isolation Reduced: – self-care ability, disinterest increased risk of hyperglycaemia – confidence – inadequate nutrition increased risk of hypoglycaemia – communication capacity and self-care	– Associated with diabetes especially hyperglycaemia – Renal disease – Corticosteroid medicines – Hypoglycaemia symptoms can be mistaken for anxiety
Oral Pathology (oral and maxillofacial pathology) Mucositis, ulcers, dry mouth	Increased: – pain – dry mouth – inadequate nutrition, inappropriate weight loss, cachexia, hypoglycaemia if on GLM/insulin Reduced: – intake – self-care deficits – mood	– Diabetic ketoacidosis (DKA), HHS may lead to dry mouth, thirst and clinical dehydration – Risk of dental caries and oral pathology – Risk of hypoglycaemia if on GLM or insulin
Nausea/vomiting	Increased: – confusion – lethargy – disinterest – pain/discomfort – inadequate nutrition → weight loss, cachexia, hyperglycaemia – hypoglycaemia if on GLM/insulin – dehydration and electrolyte imbalance – risk of ketoacidosis Reduced: – intake – energy, depleted energy stores	– May be due to gastric autonomic neuropathy – Renal disease – Hyperglycaemia – DKA, HHS – Medicines: – Metformin – Byetta
Delirium	Increased: – cognitive impairment Reduced: – ability to communicate and detect signs/symptoms of hypo/hyperglycaemia – self-care ability	– May be due to many factors including hyper and hypoglycaemia, dehydration and medicines

(Continued)

Table 18.1   Continued.

Common palliative care symptoms	Impact on diabetes management	May be diabetes-related
Sepsis		– May be silent in diabetes (urinary tract infection (UTI), MI) – May precipitate DKA, HHS
Acute dyspnoea	Increased: – hypoxia contributing to confusion Reduced: – self-management capacity	Increased: – confusion – energy requirements – pain – difficulty interpreting elevated white cell count, which could be caused by hyperglycaemia, sepsis, or other factors – bone marrow failure Reduced: – intake increased DKA, HHS risk – quality of life – wound healing
Diabetes Emergencies	Examples: – Hypoglycaemia – Hyperglycaemia – MI, which is often atypical and/or silent	– Hypoglycaemia – DKA, HHS, Lactic acidosis, which contribute to delirium, especially in older people
Oncology Emergencies	Examples: – Spinal cord compression (corticosteroids) and acute immobility – Superior vena clava (SVC) obstruction (acute dyspnoea and delirium) – high dose of corticosteroids – Febrile neutropenia – Major bronchial obstruction (dyspnoea and use of corticosteroids)	– Hypoglycaemia – DKA, HONK, Lactic acidosis

HHS: hyperosmolar hyperglycaemic states. GLM: glucose-lowering medicines.

monitoring processes, but this does not appear to happen at present and the majority of people with diabetes do not have a documented ACP or other relevant documents. Likewise, addressing symptom burden and palliative care is not included in most current diabetes management guidelines.

Palliative Care Australia (PCA) (2012) undertook a survey during Palliative Care Week (n = 100), which showed 90% of participants did not have an ACP, 78% did not know what an ACP was and 90% of those who did know, had not developed an ACP. In addition, 50% worried that doctors might ignore their wishes. Seventy five percent had discussed end of life issues with their families but 45% felt their families did not really understand their wishes.

Similarly, Dunning *et al.* (2010) found only one of the 14 people with diabetes in the last stages of life they interviewed when they developed guidelines for managing diabetes at the end of life, had documented an ACP. However, the person had not included diabetes management in her ACP, which she later amended to include how she wanted her diabetes managed. A second participant developed an ACP that included how she wanted her diabetes managed after participating in the interview.

Helping people with diabetes develop an ACP is an important aspect of holistic diabetes care because:

'*In the absence of a formal visible record of resident's wishes* [older people in care homes] *places an onerous burden on health care professionals to preserve life, when that may not be the preference of the person or their families* (Allen & Barnett 2010).

People with diabetes often carry a high symptom burden including acute and chronic pain, fatigue, constipation, nausea, lethargy, insomnia, anxiety and depression (Sudore *et al.* 2012). The symptom burden was more prevalent in people with short survival expectancy in Sudore *et al.*'s study, but was evident in all stages of the diabetes life trajectory (n = 13 71 aged 30–74 mean age 60). Interestingly, Sudore *et al.* did not report other uncomfortable symptoms associated with hyperglycaemia such as thirst, dry mouth and hypoglycaemic symptoms, which distress people with diabetes (Savage *et al.* 2012) and contribute to the symptom burden and underlie many of the symptoms Sudore *et al.* described.

The symptom burden is often overlooked in the imperative to achieve glycaemic and other targets. As mentioned, managing symptoms is paramount in end of life care but should be considered throughout the chronic disease trajectory, not only at the end of life (Morrison & Meter 2004). Recognising and managing hypo- and hyperglycaemia-related symptoms in a timely manner is important to people with diabetes (Savage *et al.* 2012) and can reduce the symptom burden.

Dying people expect health professionals to respect 'their ways of being' and understand time is precious at the end of life. They find waiting for appointments and test results distressing and want some indication of 'how much time they have left' in order to put their affairs in order (Pesut *et al.* 2012). People also want health professionals to deliver care without being intrusive and work with and support their supportive family/carers. In addition, people want some general 'signposts' (cues) to help them recognise when they are entering the deteriorating stage to enable them to make realistic decisions about dying (Pesut *et al.* 2012). Loss of privacy during the dying process, especially in hospitals/hospices, but also at home, is a concern for some people.

Family and carers worry about their lack of knowledge and skills to undertake diabetes self-care when their loved ones require help, and worry about unnecessarily hastening death or causing discomfort and pain (Dunning *et al.* 2010). Likewise, carer participants in Pesut *et al*'s (2012) study indicated health professionals often overestimate their knowledge and that they 'do not know what questions to ask [health professionals].' Thus, educating family/carers and helping them ask pertinent questions is part of supportive, personalised care at the end of life.

The end of life process

The end of life process follows a common continuum from stable through unstable, deteriorating and terminal stages and usually lasts ~6–12 months (Palliative Care Outcomes Collaborative (PCOC) (2008); see Table 18.2. However, the stages are not linear, especially in diabetes where episodes of stable/unstable metabolic control occur over years before the individual enters the PCOC end of life stages. Thus, there may be a long progression to terminal care.

It can be difficult to determine an individual's disease trajectory and prognosis and when to begin discussing advance care planning and palliative and end of life care with people with diabetes. However, opportunities for proactive care planning occur during regular consultations and annual complication assessment programs (the annual cycle of care) (RACGP/DA 2011/12), which are part of standard diabetes care. In addition to ACP, making or updating wills, designating power of attorney and making funeral arrangements might be relevant.

Table 18.2 Palliative Care Outcome Collaborative (PCOC) (2008) stages of the dying process and some of the issues health professionals could consider in each stage applied to diabetes.

PCOC stage	Characteristics of the PCOC stage	Brief overview of essential care considerations in addition to managing diabetes
Stable	Includes everybody not in the other four stages. Metabolic status is managed according to an individualised care plan and individualised targets. Symptom burden is managed. Medicines management is reviewed to reduce the medicine burden. The stable period may last for months or years and may become unstable e.g. during an intercurrent illness such as the flu, or the development/worsening of a complication and then revert to stable.	Undertake a proactive risk assessment for hypo-and hyperglycaemia and their consequences as well as other key risk screening such as cardiovascular risk and malnutrition risk, which can contribute to the symptom burden and affect health status. Determine whether the person has an ACP and other relevant documentation such as a will, enduring power of attorney, proxy decision-making arrangements. Consider future symptom and medicine burden and plan to implement an early palliative approach with the individual and their family/carers. Ensure the person knows how to manage intercurrent illnesses and knows how and when to seek advice early. Include family/carers in education sessions.
Unstable	A new, sometimes unexpected, problem or a rapid increase in the severity of existing problem/s such as progression of renal disease or a cardiovascular event occurs and causes metabolic instability. Symptom burden usually increases during the acute episode. Family/carers may need to provide assistance with diabetes self-care and medicine management and other activities of daily living when the person is at home and should be supported to do so in hospitals and hospices.	Adjust management plan to manage the metabolic derangement and associated symptom burden and underlying cause. Decide whether the condition can be stabilised or will proceed to the deteriorating stage. If the condition stabilises, review the management plan and future plans for a palliative approach/care and ACP. Determine family/carers' capacity to care for/support the individual and whether they need education and support themselves.
Deteriorating	The person's condition rapidly or gradually worsens and they often develop new problems and increased symptom burden. Medicines may be a cause of or contribute to the symptom burden e.g. when another medicine is prescribed to manage a medicine side effect, thus pharmacovigilance is essential and deprescribing might be required (Chapter 5).	Decide whether emergency management is needed or whether the Liverpool Care Pathway (Ellershaw 2003) should be activated. Proactively consult with palliative care experts. If warranted, implement the person's ACP. Address the family/carer's needs. Decide when to withdraw treatment.
Terminal	Death is likely in days.	Palliative care should be continued to manage symptoms and promote quality of life and a dignified death. Follow the person's wishes in their ACP. If there is no ACP family/carers should be consulted. Arrange for religious care if relevant and ensure religious conventions regarding treatment of the body after death are adhered to (Healthcare Chaplaincy 2009; The Joint Commission 2010). Support the family/carers and explain what is happening carefully.
Bereaved	The family/carers usually grieve when their loved one dies.	Implement bereavement support or other counselling as needed.

ACP = advanced care plan.

However, people's perspectives change over time, and in different situations; therefore, health professionals need to help the individual make the best possible decision in the moment, and understand that an ACP made several years before may not reflect the individual's wishes at a different time (Geri Pal 2010). Thus, it is important to regularly clarify whether people's values and wishes have changed.

Key management considerations for managing diabetes at the end of life

Diabetes management should be integrated into the overall palliative care plan and should be a collaborative process among relevant diabetes and palliative care clinicians and other clinicians where relevant, and make provision for:

- Providing individualised personalised care that includes preparing an ACP, identifying cultural, religious and spiritual beliefs and customs that influence how palliative care, death and care of the body and family/carers after death should be managed.
- Making provision for communication with the individual and their family/carers and among health professionals throughout the palliative care journey.
- Identifying and managing pre-existing diabetes and diabetes complications that affect management decisions such as medicines choices when renal and liver disease are present and can contribute to pain and discomfort. In addition, corticosteroid-induced hyperglycaemia is common in palliative care situations, in people with pre-existing diabetes and those with diabetes risk factors (Giovannucci *et al.* 2010; Gannon & Dando 2010).
- Identifying individuals at risk of corticosteroid-induced diabetes when people are admitted to palliative care and/or when steroid medicines are prescribed, detecting diabetes early, and managing diabetes that develops following corticosteroid use.
- Identifying risk of and developing strategies to reduce episodes of and manage hypoglycaemia, which can be individually or collectively related to GLMs, low hepatic glucose reserves, particularly if the individual is malnourished or has hepatic metastases, renal impairment or malabsorption due to gastrointestinal disturbance, to anorexia and cachexia syndrome.
- Choosing a safe, effective medicines and medicine regimen to achieve optimal glycaemic targets for the individual and the PCOC stage. Renal and hepatic function is often altered and gastrointestinal disturbance and impaired glucose absorption is common, which, along with the prognosis, and the individual's care decisions, influences medicine choices. Many oral GLM might be contraindicated and insulin might be a safer, simpler option but only consensus evidence is available (Dunning *et al.* 2010, Diabetes UK 2012, Australian Diabetes Society (ADS) 2012).
- Providing adequate nutrition and hydration.
- Avoiding diabetes-related emergencies such as ketoacidosis, hyperosmolar states, lactic acidosis, and severe hypoglycaemia (Chapters 6 and 7).
- Deciding when to withdraw treatment and activating the Liverpool Care Pathway when the individual is dying (Ellershaw 2003).
- Supporting spiritual growth. Spirituality is difficult to define and is a broader concept than religion, although it might encompass religion, and refers to the transformational process of finding meaning and purpose in life and an inner sense of coherence and resilience (Parsian & Dunning 2009; Koren & Papamiditriou 2013). Spirituality enables people to positively cope with life stressors. Significantly, people can find meaning and purpose in life when they are dying. However, people's spirituality and their connectedness to others can be affected by grief and loss (Puchalski 2011).

Spirituality also affects family/carers' ability to cope. The factors that give meaning and purpose to people's lives influences their end of life care decisions. Spirituality should be encompassed in the medical history and regularly evaluated including when there is a change in clinical status. Spiritual distress and depression can overlap and manifest as demoralisation, or people can be depressed and have no hope or become depressed and feel isolated from God (Puchalski 2011). However, people can have spiritual distress without being depressed.

> ### Practice points
>
> Diabetes is a chronic disease of long duration and often has periods of stability and instability. Thus, the general palliative care interpretation of the PCOC stable and unstable phases might need to be reconsidered or specifically defined for diabetes and other similar chronic disease care.

Glycaemic targets

Cardiovascular and renal disease are leading causes of death in people with diabetes; thus, maintaining blood glucose and blood pressure within the normal ranges is important to prevent cardiovascular disease and other diabetes complications in the stable phase and improves outcomes in many unstable phases through an individual's journey with diabetes and are discussed in other chapters in the book

Preventing long term diabetes complications is not a priority of palliative care; however, managing existing complications to manage pain and promote comfort and quality of life and prevent unnecessary admission to hospital, is essential.

Opinions differ about the optimal glycaemic target range and blood glucose monitoring frequency in end of life care. Targets must be individualised, but generally, aiming for a range between 6–11 mmol/L (Dunning *et al.* 2010) and avoiding levels < 6 mmol/L and >15 mmol/L (Diabetes UK 2012) appear reasonable, noting these are consensus targets and there is very little evidence to support them. Likewise, there is no evidence of an optimal HbA_{1c} target, which should be individualised: aiming for ≤ 8% might be reasonable.

Blood glucose monitoring

Opinions vary about the value of monitoring blood glucose at the end of life: it is important to detect hypo- and hyperglycaemia (because of their effect on comfort and symptom burden), which can be difficult without monitoring blood glucose. Many people with diabetes and their families want their usual blood glucose monitoring regimen continued because it helps them maintain stability at a frightening, uncertain time of life and enables unstable glucose levels to be detected (Dunning *et al.* 2010; Savage *et al.* 2012). In addition, some people with diabetes and/or their families regard reduced or no blood glucose monitoring as staff 'giving up', and feel abandoned.

Some staff are concerned that blood glucose monitoring represents a painful, unnecessary intervention (Quinn *et al.* 2006), which is interesting considering the very invasive and painful treatments that are often provided during end of life care.

Monitoring frequency should be decided with the individual and according to their end of life stage, medicine regimen and hypo- and hyperglycaemia risk profile. It may not be necessary in the terminal stage.

Hyperglycaemia

Hyperglycaemia causes distressing osmotic symptoms, exacerbates pain, contributes to malnutrition delirium and confusion, reduces mood, problem-solving and coping ability and quality of life. The symptoms are often attributed to other causes and not appropriately treated. Alternatively, hyperglycaemia can be present without significant symptoms and progress to a diabetes emergency such as ketoacidosis or hyperosmolar states that require urgent care.

Type 2 diabetes is a progressive disease due to loss of beta cell function and declining insulin production and >50 % eventually need insulin (Chapter 1).

The need may be greater in palliative care situations where medicines and other factors are prohyperglycaemic. Thus, preventing hyperglycaemia can enhance comfort and meet a key palliative care goal. Having an appropriate plan for managing intercurrent illness (sick days) and episodes of hyperglycaemia is as important as an appropriate medicine regimen.

Families/carers may need education about how to recognise and manage hyperglycaemia and what blood glucose levels and symptoms should trigger them to seek health professional advice. Sick day management is discussed in Chapter 7.

Hypoglycaemia

The risk of hypoglycaemia is increased in palliative situations due to anorexia, malnourishment, liver disease, low glycogen stores and cachexia syndrome in advanced cancer. Thus, hypoglycaemia risk needs to be considered when deciding medicine management strategies and glycaemic targets.Factors that increase hypoglycaemia risk are:

- GLMs especially sulphonylureas and insulin;
- medicines that interact with GLMs (Chapter 5);
- malnourishment, cachexia, which occurs in 40–90% of the cancer palliative care population, anorexia, which affects endogenous glucose stores;
- anorexia: some medicines affect appetite and food enjoyment;
- renal and/or liver disease;
- weight loss;
- hypoglycaemia unawareness;
- cognitive impairment and delirium, which could be from chronic hypoglycaemia, hyperglycaemia, medicines or dementia;
- unmanaged pain, which affects appetite. adequate pain management is essential and is generally well documented in palliative care plans;
- fasting for procedures or surgical interventions;
- health professionals attributing hypo- hyperglycaemic coma to other causes such as the dying process;
- health professional beliefs about an 'appropriate diabetic diet.'

Hypoglycaemia symptoms and management are described in Chapter 6 but symptoms can be atypical, which makes some degree of regular blood glucose monitoring important, especially in high risk patients. It is also an important diagnostic tool.

It is difficult to treat hypoglycaemia when people are anorexic or have nausea or vomiting (McCoubrie *et al.* 2004; Dunning *et al.* 2010), thus GLMs are often stopped in people who have hypoglycaemic episodes, which may not be the best management choice because of the resultant hyperglycaemia and its adverse effects. A comprehensive medicine review and managing other underlying hypoglycaemia risk factors is advisable. Educating the individual and family/carers (and sometimes health professionals) might also be required; especially if the person's usual hypoglycaemia symptoms change.

The choice of GLM/s, dose and dose frequency needs to be carefully considered and the blood glucose should not fall below 6 mmol/L because of the hypoglycaemia risk (Diabetes UK 2012). In addition, dietetic advice can help health professionals and family/carers plan a diet suitable to the individual and provide supplements if necessary to reduce the effects of malnutrition and minimise weight loss.

Medicine management

Pharmacovigilance and adopting a quality use of medicines approach is essential to achieving optimal glycaemic control with minimal risk, see figure 19.1 and Chapter 5. Pharmacovigilance encompasses proactively monitoring medicines and deprescribing where necessary/possible (Rowett *et al.* 2012). Pharmacovigilance encompasses QUM, which concerns deciding whether a medicine is needed and selecting medicine options wisely, if a medicine is indicated (National Prescribing Service (NPS) 2009). In addition, medicine choices depend on the prognosis, health status, oral intake, risk profile and co-existing diseases as well as the type of diabetes.

> ### *Practice points*
>
> Insulin is:
> - Not a cure for diabetes or any other condition.
> - Is essential treatment for people with Type 1 diabetes and LADA.
> - Is required by most people with Type 2 diabetes due to progressive beta cell loss.
> - Is an effective way of managing blood glucose levels including at the end of life and may be simpler and safer to use than other GLMs and reduce the medicine burden.

Type 1 diabetes

People with Type 1 diabetes who are in the stable phase should continue their usual insulin regimens but doses should be adjusted if renal disease is present and if weight loss occurs depending on the eating pattern to avoid hypo- and hyperglycaemia. In the terminal phase medicines are usually ceased. Generally, basal bolus regimens are used unless contraindicated. A daily dose of a long acting insulin analogue and/or small doses of rapid acting insulin when the individual eats might be appropriate in the unstable and deteriorating stages and when nausea, vomiting and anorexia are present.

However, management in the unstable stage will depend on the likely outcome: recovery and return to the stable phase, or deteriorate. In the former case an IV insulin infusion might be warranted to manage acute illnesses and during surgical procedures Chapters 7 and 9.

Many people use insulin pumps, which enable the insulin regimen to be flexible in changing situations such as palliative care. People who use insulin pumps are very competent at managing their pumps in the stable phase but may need help during the other PCOC stages. Basal rates can be set to mange predictable circumstances and to prevent ketosis and bolus doses can be administered with food or as correctional doses. Health professionals must have the technical expertise and competence to manage insulin pumps and the advice of expert diabetes health professionals should be sought early.

Blood ketone tests should be performed if the blood glucose is >15 mmol/L, especially if the individual has nausea, vomiting and signs of dehydration, which could indicate remediable ketoacidosis.

Type 2 diabetes

The individual's GLM regimen can usually be continued in the stable phase but doses may need to be reduced or insulin initiated to simplify the medicine regimen and/or reduce the risk of hypoglycaemia, when the person is at high risk of hypoglycaemia and in the unstable and deteriorating PCOC phases. The choice of GLM or GLM combinations depends on the individual's health status and blood glucose pattern.

However, gastrointestinal problems and malabsorption syndromes may mean oral GLMs are not absorbed appropriately and will be ineffective.

Metformin

Metformin is the most commonly used oral GLM especially in overweight people. Renal function needs to be monitored and metformin doses adjusted or the medicine ceased if renal function declines (creatinine >150 mmol/L or eGFR <30 ml/min/1.73 metres squared). Metformin may also be contraindicated it the person has risk factors for lactic acidosis (Chapter 7), distressing gastrointestinal symptoms such as nausea and flatulence and significant weight loss.

Sulphonylureas

Sulphonylureas may be contraindicated if renal and/or liver disease is present if the person is malnourished and when there is a high risk of hypoglycaemia.

Thiazolididiones

Thiazolididiones are not indicated if liver and/or congestive heart failure is present. They cause oedema, which can cause uncomfortable symptoms. Pioglitazone is contraindicated in people at risk of bladder cancer and people who already have bladder cancer.

Incretins

GLP-1 and DPP-4 analogues may be appropriate depending on prescribing indications in the relevant country. GLP-1 and sulphonylurea combination increases the risk of hypoglycaemia. GLP-1 often cause nausea and weight loss and may be contraindicated. Both GLP-1 and DPP-4 have been associated with pancreatitis. Thus, they may not be the best choice in people with pancreatic disease and should be stopped if they cause abdominal pain.

Insulin

As indicated, the majority of people with Type 2 diabetes eventually require insulin and may already be on insulin when they commence palliative care. Insulin doses are easier to adjust than oral GLMs. Initiating insulin can reduce the tablet burden and simplify the medicine regimen.

Sodium-glucose cotransporter-2 inhibitors (SGLT-2)

There is not enough clinical experience with the SGLT-2 medicines to recommend their use in palliative care situations at present and they are not approved for use in many countries. They are associated with urinary tract and genital infections and polyuria.

Other medicines

Most people with diabetes will also be using antihypertensive and lipid lowering medicines and many will be using anticoagulant medicines and the benefits and risks of continuing these medicines need to be considered (Chapters 5 and 8). The gastrointestinal effects of aspirin can be more prominent when the individual is anorexic or using corticosteroids. If these medicines are continued, a proton pump inhibitor or other gastroprotective medicine might be indicated.

Complementary and alternative therapies (CAM)

CAM is discussed in Chapter 19. Many people at the end of life use CAM to relieve pain, improve quality of life and manage the spiritual aspects of dying to achieve a good death (free from pain) (Running *et al.* 2008). CAM can also reduce restlessness, agitation and mental stress. Commonly used CAM include:

- massage, with and without essential oils;
- music therapy including thanatology;
- guided imagery;
- essential oils in vapourisers, baths or massage;
- acupuncture;
- pet therapy: those who know the book, *Making Rounds with Oscar*, by David Dosa (Dosa 2010) will understand the power of pets at the end of life;
- meditation;
- art therapy;
- reflexology (Horowitz 2009).

However, CAM use can interact with conventional medicines and needs to be integrated into the care plan and monitored as part of the care plan.

Nutrition and hydration

People requiring palliative care often have anorexia, cachexia and dysphagia and at some point will be unable to consume oral food and fluids, which can distress family and carers. Nutrition to sustain energy reserves and provide essential nutrition and fluids needs to be considered on an individual basis and tailored to the end of life stage. Actively dying people do not experience hunger, largely due to the effects of starvation and consequent ketone production; although they may experience thirst. However, thirst is not alleviated by artificial hydration. Comfort care should be provided to manage dry mouth (mouth care) (Kedziera 2001).

The risks and benefits of artificial nutrition need to be carefully considered when it is indicated, including the risk of accelerating death.

Diabetogenetic medicines

Several medicines can cause or exacerbate hyperglycaemia especially antipsychotic medicines, thiazide diuretics and corticosteroids (Chapters 5 and 10). Corticosteroids are an essential part of the management of many disease processes such as haematological malignancies, inflammatory diseases, COPD, allergies and shock, and are commonly used in palliative care to manage symptoms, often dexamethasone or prednisolone.

However, long term use and high doses of corticosteroids cause hyperglycaemia in people with diagnosed diabetes and predispose people at risk of diabetes to corticosteroid-induced diabetes: incidence of new onset diabetes 2–12% (Oyer *et al.* 2006; Donihi *et al.* 2006) and appears to be proportional to the dose, dose form and dose regimen and duration of treatment (Dunning 1996; Diabetes UK 2012). Ocular formulations, inhalers and topical corticosteroid preparations do not cause diabetes (Donihi *et al.* 2006). Hyperglycaemia usually occurs when doses of Prednisolone or equivalent medicines exceeds 7.5 mg/day. In contrast, short courses may not cause hyperglycaemia or only have a short-term effect on the blood glucose.

Screening people for diabetes risk factors on admission to palliative care and monitoring blood glucose when people commence corticosteroids will identify corticosteroid-induced hyperglycaemia early and enable treatment to initiate to reduce the impact on comfort, cognitive function and other symptoms.

Several mechanisms have been proposed for the diabetogenic effects of corticosteroids; these include:

- Enhancing hepatic gluconeogenesis by upregulating key regulatory hormones that contribute to hyperglycaemia such as glucose-6-phoshatase and phosphoenolpyruvate carboxylase (PEPCK).
- Suppressing insulin release from the beta cells.
- Inducing peripheral insulin resistance by inhibiting production of glucose transporters in adipose and skeletal muscle cells. Insulin resistance and impaired glucose tolerance can occur within 48 hours of commencing corticosteroids.
- Corticosteroids appear to cause both fasting and postprandial hyperglycaemia (Du 2008). However, a morning daily dose tends to cause hyperglycaemia in the late afternoon or early evening.

> ### Practice point
>
> People should be informed they could develop diabetes when they are prescribed oral corticosteroid medicines, especially when they are risk of developing diabetes.

In addition to causing hyperglycaemia, corticosteroids can mask the signs and symptoms of infections, which are often atypical in people with diabetes. The skin can become thin and fragile and prone to tears, especially in older people, which causes considerable discomfort and distress. Corticosteroids also have variable effects on bone formation and reduce calcium absorption from the intestine, which predisposes susceptible individuals to osteoporotic fractures and pain. Mental changes can also occur ranging from mild psychosis to significant psychiatric pathology. Mild psychological effects may be difficult to distinguish from delirium and other cognitive deficits.

Managing corticosteroid-induced diabetes in palliative care patients

Balancing the benefits of corticosteroid medicines with their effects on glucose homeostasis is multifactorial and challenging and is affected by individual susceptibility, meal schedules, whether dosing is intermittent or continuous and the diabetogenic effects of the individual medicines. The aim is to maintain stable blood glucose, limit glucose variability, prevent ketoacidosis and hyperosmolar states, minimise the risk of hypoglycaemia, and limit the care burden on the individual and their family/carers.

Management consists of monitoring blood glucose especially in the afternoon, but more frequently if insulin is prescribed, using the lowest effective corticosteroid dose and the least diabetogenic corticosteroid formulation for the shortest possible time, and proactively treating hyperglycaemia. An acceptable blood glucose range is fasting ~ 6 mmol/L and postprandial < 11 mmol/L (Du 2008). People managed using diet may require medicines to manage fasting and/or postprandial hyperglycaemia and its symptoms.

The choice of GLM depends on the person's health status, corticosteroid regimen and relevant medicine precautions and contraindications. For example (Du 2008; Dunning *et al.* 2010; ADS 2012; Diabetes UK 2012):

Morning corticosteroid:

Morning sulphonylurea such as Glipizide OR

Prebreakfast or BD Isophane insulin.

BD or TDS corticosteroid:

BD sulphonylurea such as Glipizide OR

Daily long-acting insulin analogue.

Bolus doses of rapid acting insulin may be required with some or all meals depending on the blood glucose and the individual's food intake.

GLM doses may need to be reduced if the corticosteroid dose is reduced or ceased. As indicated, blood glucose monitoring is essential to manage GLMs and prevent hypoglycaemia and the associated adverse events including MI and falls. In addition, large doses of corticosteroid for more than two weeks can induce adrenal insufficiency, which dramatically reduces insulin requirements. The signs of adrenal insufficiency are similar to other palliative care symptoms: increased fatigue, weight loss, nausea and diarrhoea (Fowler 2009).

Antipsychotic medicines

Depression and anxiety are common in people with diabetes and may occasionally be treated with antipsychotic medicines. Antipsychotic medicines are sometimes used to manage pain associated with peripheral neuropathy, which is a common complication of diabetes, and to manage refractory nausea and delirium (Llorente & Urrutia2006).

Antipsychotic medicines induce hyperglycaemia. Blood glucose monitoring may be required and oral GLMs or insulin might be required depending on the emerging blood glucose pattern.

Corticosteroid like antipsychotic medicines should be used for the shortest possible period of time, at the lowest effective dose and using the least diabetogenic medication in the class where possible. People with diabetes and their carers should be informed about the likely effects of corticosteroids and possible effects of antipsychotic medicines on their blood glucose levels and given advice about blood glucose testing and managing hyperglycaemia. Likewise, it is advisable for clinicians to document their advice in the individual's medical record and other relevant documentation.

Supporting family/carers

It is important to inform carers about the person with diabetes' care plan and health status and involve them in decisions where appropriate. Some family/carers may require diabetes education if they need to take on the person's usual diabetes self-care tasks such as blood glucose monitoring and administering insulin (Savage *et al.* 2012). There are positive beneficial effects of care giving, although the stress of witnessing a loved one suffer can be significant (The Joint Commission 2010).

The severity of the individual's distress is the strongest predictor of end of life family/carer strain (Fromme *et al.* 2005). Men are less likely to report caregiver strain than women and use fewer words to describe their strain and distress. Caregiver Strain Index (Hartford Institute for Geriatric Nursing) might be useful to monitor family/carer strain. Dunning *et al.* in collaboration with Diabetes Australia and Palliative Care Australia (2012) published brochures for people with diabetes and family/carers to inform them about diabetes and end of life issues (the brochures can be accessed from www.palliativecare.org.au or www.caresearch.com.au).

Health professionals can support family/cares by offering them the opportunity to discuss their concerns and enabling them to express their grief. Enabling family/carers to participate in end of life care such as helping with feeds, providing CAM and being present, and scheduling rounds to coincide with family/carer visits if possible.

Withdrawing treatment

Withdrawing treatment is an essential aspect of palliative care and peoples' wishes can be documented in ACPs, which help health professionals make decisions about withdrawing treatment. The deteriorating and terminal phases are often key decision points for initiating the Liverpool Care Pathway and withdrawing treatment. Savage *et al.* (2012) found most people with diabetes do not want unnecessary treatment continued in the terminal phase but they want to be comfortable and die with dignity.

Knowing the prognosis can aid decisions about when to withdraw treatment, but it is difficult to predict prognosis although The Gold Standard Prognostic Indicator (Royal College of General Practitioners 2008) and the PCOC stages (PCOC 2008) are helpful. Factors that indicate limited prognosis include:

- Multiple comorbidities.
- More than 10% weight loss in a short period of time.
- Failure to thrive and/or general decline.
- Serum albumin < 25 g/L.
- Reduced performance e.g. Karnofsky score < 50% and requiring significant help to undertake usual activities of daily living and diabetes self-care tasks.
- Will to live, which is a strong predictor of survival in older people regardless of their age, gender and comorbidities (Karppinen *et al.* 2012).
- Social factors such as satisfaction, support from family, friends and health professionals might have an important effect on will to live. Will to live could be explored as part of the spiritual history.

GLMs should be stopped when they cause frequent, severe hypoglycaemia associated with other risks such as falls, especially in the deteriorating and terminal phases when the risks outweigh the benefits. However, the discomfort and risks associated with hyperglycaemia need to be considered in light of the prognosis.

There are ethical issues associated with stopping any treatment, even in end of life settings (Ford-Dunn *et al.* 2006) and the wishes of the patient and their family and ACP, if they are available, must be considered. Family/carers may be concerned about euthanasia and worry that withdrawing food and fluids will cause pain and discomfort. Thus, timely, careful, clear communication is essential.

Diabetes education

Education and support, including bereavement support is essential for individuals with diabetes, their families and often health professional carers. Sensitive discussion about the need to adjust medicines and other changes to established self-management routines is essential. In addition, diabetes specialists are in an ideal position to identify regular opportunities when to begin discussing palliative care and other end of life issues.

References

Allen S. & Barnett A. (2011) Exploring advanced care planning in rural aged care. *Australian Nursing Journal*, **17** (9), 41.

Australian Diabetes Society (ADS) (2012) *Guideline for Routine Glucose Control in Hospital*. ADS, Canberra.

Australian Government Department of Health and Ageing (2006). *Guidelines for a Palliative Approach to Residential Aged Care. Enhanced Version.* www.nhmrc.gov.au/_files_nhmrc/publications/attachments/ac14.pdf *(accessed December 2012)*.

Bloomer, M. (2012) Care in final days. *Nursing Review*, **August**, 20.

Burge, F. (2012) How to move to a palliative approach to care for people with multimorbidity *British Medical Journal* 345 doi: http://dx.doi.org/10.1136/bmj.e6324 (Published 21 September 2012).

Canadian Hospice Palliative Care Association (CHPCA) (undated) The Palliative Care Approach. CHPCA, www.hpintegration.ca (accessed January 2013).

Diabetes UK (2012) End of Life Care Strategy: A strategy document commissioned by Diabetes UK Clinical care recommendations, www.diabetes.nhs.uk/document.php?o=3730 (accessed December 2012).

Donihi, A., Raval, D., Saul, M. *et al.* (2006) Prevalence and predictors of corticosteroid-related hyperglycemia in hospitalized patients. *Endocrine Practice*, **12** (4), 358–362.

Dosa D. (2010) *Making Rounds With Oscar*. Hyperion Books, New York City.

Du, L. (2008) Management of steroid-induced diabetes in patients with COPD. *Medscape Diabetes and Endocrinology* http://www.medscape.com/viewarticle/458619 (accessed October 2012).

Dunning, T. (1996) Corticosteroid medications and diabetes mellitus. *Practical Diabetes International*, **13** (6), 186–188.

Dunning, T. (2012) Managing diabetes at the end of life. *Diabetes Management Journal*, **39**, 6–8.

Dunning, T., Savage, S., Duggan, N. & Martin, P. (2010) *Guidelines for Managing Diabetes at the End of Life*. Centre for Nursing and Allied Health Research, Geelong Australia.

Dunning, T., Savage, S., Duggan, N. & Martin, P. (2012) Diabetes and end of life: Ethical and methodological issues in gathering evidence. *Scandinavian Journal Caring Sciences*, DOI: 10.111/j.1471.612.2012.01016.x.

Ellershaw, J. (2003) Introduction, in *Care of the Dying. A Pathway to Excellence*, (eds J. Ellershaw & S. Wilkinson). Oxford University Press, Oxford.

Emanuel, L., Alexander, C., Arnold, R. *et al.* (2004) Integrating palliative care into disease management guidelines. *Journal of Palliative Medicine*, **7** (6), 774–783.

Ford-Dunn, S., & Quin, J. (2004). Management of diabetes in the terminal phase of life. *Practical Diabetes International*, **21** (5), 175–176.

Ford-Dunn, S., Smith, A., & Quin, J. (2006) Management of diabetes during the last days of life: Attitudes of consultant diabetologists and consultant palliative care physicians in the UK. *Palliative Medicine*, **20**, 197–203.

Fowler M. (2009) Pitfalls in diabetes outpatient management. *Clinical Diabetes Journals*, http://clinical diabetesjournals.org (accessed May 2012).

Fromme, E., Drach, L., Tollle, S. *et al.* (2005) Men as caregivers at the end of life. *Journal of Palliative Medicine*, **8** (6), 1167–1175.

Gannon, C. & Dando, N. (2010) Dose-sensitive steroid-induced hyperglycaemia. *Palliative Medicine*, **24** (7), 737–739.

GeriPal (2010) Advanced Care Planning: Accounting for Changing Perspectives. http://www.thecamreport.com2010/09/advanced-care-planning-accounting-for-changing-perspectives (accessed August 2012).

Giovannucci, E., Harlan, D., Archer, M. *et al.* (2010) Diabetes and Cancer. *Diabetes Care*, **7**, 1674–1685.

Hartford Institute for Geriatric Nursing Geriatric Assessment tools www.hartfordign.org/publications/trythis/issue14 (accessed April 2012).

HealthCare Chaplaincy (2009) *A Dictionary of Patients' Spiritual and Cultural Values for Health Care Professionals*. New York, HealthCare Chaplaincy, http://www.healthcarechaplaincy.org/userimages/doc/Cultural%20Dictionary.pdf (accessed December 2012).

Horowitz, S. (2009) Complementary therapies for end of life. *Alternative and Complementary Therapies*, **15** (5), 226–230.

International Diabetes Federation (IDF) (2012) *The Diabetes Atlas*. IDF Brussels,

Karppinen, H., Laakonen, M.L., Strandberg, T., Tilvis, R. & Pitkala, K. (2012) Will-to-live and survival in a 10-year follow-up among older people. *Age and Aging*, **41** (6), 789–794.

Kedziera P. (2001) Hydration, thirst and nutrition, in *Textbook of Palliative Nursing* (eds Ferrell, B. & Coyle, N.) Oxford University Press, New York.

Koren, M. & Papamiditriou, C. (2013) Spirituality of staff nurses: Application of modeling and role modeling theory. *Holistic Nursing Practice*, **27** (1), 37–44.

Llorente, M. & Urrutia, V. (2006) Diabetes, psychiatric disorders, and metabolic effects of antipsychotic medications. *Clinical Diabetes*, **24**, 18–24.

McCoubrie, R., Jeffrey, D., Paton C, Dawes L. (2004) Managing diabetes mellitus in patients with advanced cancer: A case note audit and guidelines. *European Journal Cancer Care*, **14** (3), 244–248.

McEwen, N., Kim, C., Hann, M. & Ghosh, D. (2006) Diabetes reporting as a cause of death: Results from the translating research into action for diabetes (TRIAD) study. *Diabetes Care*, **29**, 247–251.

Morrison, R. & Meter, D. (2004) Clinical practice palliative care. *New England Journal of Medicine*, **350** (25), 2582–2590.

National Health and Medical Research Council (1999) *A Guide to the Development, Implementation and Evaluation of Clinical Practice Guidelines*. National Health and Medical Research Council, Canberra.

National Prescribing Service Ltd and Palliative Care Australia (2009) *Achieving quality use of medicines in the community for palliative and end of life care: A consultation report*. National Prescribing Service, Sydney.

National Prescribing Service (NPS) (2009) National Strategy for the Quality Use of Medicines (QUM) www.health.gov.au/internet/main/publishing.nsf/content/.../natstrateng.pdf (accessed October 2012).

Oyer, D., Shah, A. & Bettenhausen, S. (2006) How to manage steroid diabetes in the patient with cancer *Journal Supportive Oncology*, **4**, 479–483.

Palliative Care Australia (PCA) (2012) *National Palliative Care Week Survey*. PCA, Canberra.

Palliative Care Outcomes Collaboration (PCOC) (2008): *PCOC Assessment Tool Definitions: Phase V 1.2.* Centre for **Palliative Care** : **Palliative Care Outcomes Collaboration** *centreforpallcare.org/... palliative_care.../palliative_care_outcomes_collaboration/* (accessed january 2013).

Parsian, N. & Dunning, T. (2009) Spirituality and coping in young adults with diabetes: A cross-sectional survey. *European Diabetes Nursing*, **6**, 100–1004.

Pesut, B., McLeod, B., Hole, R. & Dalhuisen, M. (2012) Rural nursing and quality end-of-life care: Palliative care, palliative approach or somewhere in between *Advances in Nursing Science*, **35** (4), 288–304.

Puchalski, C. (2011) *Spirituality is an Important Component of Patient Care*. WebMD Professional http://www.medscape.com/viewarticle/738237 (accessed August 2012).

Quinn, K., Hudson, P., & Dunning, T. (2006) Diabetes management in patients receiving palliative care. *Journal of Pain and Symptom Management*, **32** (3), 275–286.

Royal Australian College of General Practitioners (RACGP), Diabetes Australia (DA) (2011/12) *Diabetes Management in General Practice*. RACGP/DA, Canberra.

Royal College of General Practitioners (2008) Prognostic Indicator Guidance (version 5), in: National Gold Standards Framework Centre England. Available from: http://www.goldstandardsframework. nhs.uk (accessed December 2012).

Rowett, D., Currow, D., Fazekas, B., *et al.* (2012) *Prescribing at the end of life, pharmacovigilance and palliative care*. National Medicine Symposium, Sydney 2012.

Running, A., Grant, J. & Andrews, W. (2008) A survey of hospice use of complementary therapy. *Journal of Hospice Palliative Nursing*, **16** (4), 394–312.

Savage S, Dunning T, Duggan N, Martin P. (2012) The experiences and care preferences of people with diabetes at the end of life. *Journal of Hospice and Palliative Nursing*, **14** (4), 293–302.

Scotland End of Life Care Strategy (2008) www.scotland.gov.uk/Resource/0040/00400709.pdf (accessed November 2012).

Sudore, R., Karter, A., Huang, E. *et al.* (2012) Symptom Burden of Adults with Type 2 Diabetes Across the Disease Course: Diabetes and Aging Study. *Journal of General Internal Medicine*, **27** (12), 1674–1681.

The Joint Commission (2010) *Advancing Effective Communication, Cultural Competence, and Patient- and Family-Centered Care: A Roadmap for Hospitals*. The Joint Commission, Oakbrook Terrace, IL.

World Health Organization (WHO) (2005) World Health Organisation Definition of Palliative Care www.who.int/cancer/palliative/definition/ (accessed March 2013).

Chapter 19
Complementary and Alternative Therapies

Key points

Modern diabetes management philosophy is consistent with complementary therapy (CAM) philosophy, specifically, prevention, the central role of the individual in their care and empowerment.

- The acronym CAM encompasses a wide range of therapies as well as herbal medicines.
- People with diabetes are high CAM users and are entitled to unbiased, evidence-based information about the benefits and risks CAM.
- CAM can work synergistically with conventional care to improve diabetes balance and quality of life provided the benefits and risks are considered in the context of the individual's health and social situation.
- Many herbal medicines have hypoglycaemic effects, and people use glucose lowering herbal medicines; but do not assume every person with diabetes using CAM is doing so to control their blood glucose.
- Herb/medicine and herb/herb interactions and other adverse events can occur.
- Health professionals should ask about and document CAM use during routine diabetes assessments especially when medicines are initiated, when doses are adjusted and prior to surgical and investigative procedures.

Rationale

Complementary therapy (CAM) use is increasing, as is the interest in integrative medicine (IM). If used appropriately within a quality use of medicines (QUM) framework some CAM can help people with diabetes heal and become proactive and empowered participants in their diabetes management. CAM use is associated with both benefits and risks. An essential aspect of any management strategy is making informed decisions

Care of People with Diabetes: A Manual of Nursing Practice, Fourth Edition. Trisha Dunning.
© 2014 John Wiley & Sons, Ltd. Published 2014 by John Wiley & Sons, Ltd.

with the individual about their personal level of risk and tailoring treatment to meet their needs.

CAM has both risks and benefits for people with diabetes including when undergoing surgery and having investigations. Not all CAM people use medicines and not all CAM carry the same level of risk or confer equal benefits. Adopting an holistic QUM approach, including using non-medicine options first when appropriate, can optimise the benefits and reduce the risks. A key aspect of QUM is asking about and documenting CAM use. People with diabetes who use CAM need written advice about how to manage their CAM including during the surgical/investigative period. People with diabetes who have renal disease and those on anticoagulants and other medicines with a narrow therapeutic index and those designated high risk medicines are at particular risk if they use some CAM medicines (Dunning 2007).

Introduction

CAM use is increasing, possibly as part of the evolution of a new health paradigm as people try to solve modern health problems such as chronic lifestyle diseases and depression. When people consider their therapeutic options they are likely to make choices that are congruent with their life philosophy, knowledge, experience, societal norms, and culture. Depending on these factors they may or may not choose to be actively involved in their care. Understanding these associations is important to understanding an individual's self-care, adherence, and empowerment potential. For example, there is a high correlation among health beliefs, spirituality and CAM use (Hildreth & Elman 2007). In addition, there is good evidence that CAM users adopt health-promoting self-care strategies, undertake preventative health care (Kelner & Welman 1997; Garrow & Egede2006) and believe responsibility for their health ultimately rests with them.

CAM is used by >50% of the general population in most countries and the rate of use is increasing, particularly by people with chronic diseases, especially women educated to high school level or higher, those with poor health who often have a chronic disease, are employed, and are interested in self-care (Lloyd *et al.* 1993; MacLennan *et al.* 1996; Eisenberg 1998; Egede *et al.* 2002; MacLennan *et al.* 2002). However, there is some evidence that the profile of Cam users is changing and many younger people use CAM (Manya *et al.* 2012).

The true prevalence of CAM use by people with diabetes is largely unknown. Old studies in the general population (Leese *et al.* 1997; Ryan *et al.* 1999) found approximately 17% of people with diabetes in diabetic outpatient settings used a range of CAM, particularly herbs, massage, and vitamin and mineral supplements such as zinc. People using CAM were satisfied with their chosen therapy even if it 'did not work'. Satisfaction with treatment improves well being (see Chapters 15 and 16). These researchers appeared to assume people used CAM to 'control their diabetes', however, the individuals concerned may have had different reasons for using CAM from those assumed by researchers and health professionals. Controlling blood glucose may not have been their primary aim. The author's experience in a diabetes service suggests that, in many cases, people use CAM to maintain health (prevention) as well as to manage conditions such as arthritis, stress, and the unpleasant symptoms of intercurrent illness and diabetes complications, for example, nausea, pain, anxiety, and depression.

More recently, Egede *et al.* (2002) found people with diabetes were more likely to use CAM than non-diabetics, as were people with other chronic conditions, in a national study in the USA. In particular, people with diabetes over 65 years were the most likely group to use CAM. The most commonly used CAM was nutritional advice, spiritual healing, herbal medicine, massage, and meditation (see Table 19.1). The high usage rates

Table 19.1   Commonly used complementary therapies.

Acupuncture	Meditation
Aromatherapy using essential oils for therapeutic purposes	Music
	Naturopathy
Ayurveda	Nutritional therapies including vitamin and mineral and antioxidant supplements
Chinese Medicine	Pet therapy
Chiropractic	Reflexology
Counselling (a range of techniques)	Reiki
Herbal medicine (from several traditions – Indian, Chinese, North American, Australian Aboriginal, Japanese)	Therapeutic Touch
Homoeopathy	Ayurveda and Chinese Medicine (uses several techniques such as herbs, cupping, moxibustion, essential oils diet and exercise)

[a]Now referred to as Chinese medicine in some countries. Many therapies are combined, for example, aromatherapy and massage. Likewise, traditional medical systems use a range of strategies in combination (CAM within CAM) and different diagnostic techniques instead of or in addition to conventional diagnostic processes, for example, tongue and pulse diagnosis. Often they are also combined with conventional care, formally and informally, in self-prescribed regimens.

in people with diabetes are hardly surprising and accord with the established demographics of CAM users. Recently, Dunning *et al.* (unpublished findings) conducted a point prevalence survey of CAM use in a large regional hospital and residential aged care facility (400 acute care beds and 410 aged care beds). Fifty five percent and 38% respectively reported using CAM and significantly, although the majority stated they informed their doctors and nurses, CAM use was not document in the medical records audited as part of the study.

Many health professionals, especially nurses and general practitioners (GPs) are incorporating CAM into their practice to enrich and extend their practice and provide holistic integrated care (Phelps & Hassad 2011;Kotsirilos et al. 2011). Many nurses and GPs who use CAM in their practices do not have formal CAM qualifications and do not effectively document or monitor the outcomes of CAM usage. In addition, they often use CAM in their own healthcare. Dunning (unpublished findings) found that 50% of a sample of 37 diabetes nurse specialists/diabetes educators indicated they used CAM in their practice, but none had a CAM qualification.

There are a great many CAMs ranging from well-accepted therapies with an acceptable research basis to 'fringe' therapies with little or no scientific evidence to support their use. The public interprets the term 'CAM' differently from health professionals and CAM and conventional practitioners and researchers use different definitions, which makes it difficult to compare studies. Several definitions and categories exist. The Cochrane collaboration defined CAM as:

All health systems, modalities and practices and their accompanying theories and beliefs, other than those intrinsic to the politically dominant health system of a particular society or culture in a given historical period. They include all such practices and ideas self-defined by their users as preventing or treating illness or promoting health and well being. *The boundaries within and between* complementary therapies are not always sharp or fixed.

(Cochrane Collaboration 2000).

Likewise, several terms are used to refer to CAM including complementary and alternative medicine (CAM), traditional medicine and non-scientific therapies. These terms are generally understood to mean therapies that are not part of conventional medicine. As the Cochrane definition indicates, the status of CAM is not fixed and some CAM become part of conventional medicine as the evidence base for the safety and efficacy accumulates, for example, acupuncture for some conditions.

CAM philosophy

The various CAM have a common underlying philosophy. Current diabetes person-centred empowerment strategies that focus on effective professional–patient partnerships, good communication, and preventative healthcare are consistent with this philosophy. CAM philosophy embodies the notion that:

- Each individual is unique, thus there is no one 'right' way to manage their health problems.
- Balance is important.
- The body has the capacity to heal itself. Healing is not synonymous with treating, managing or curing. The word is derived from the Anglo Saxon 'haelen', to make whole. Likewise, health is derived from the Anglo Saxon 'haelth' from 'hal', which also means to make whole. To achieve healing, all parts and polarities need to be integrated – mind, body, and spirit within the individual's social environment and context.
- Healing occurs by intent. Healing intent is an important component of the therapeutic relationship (Dunning 2013a, 28–48).
- A positive attitude is important to health and well being. Increasing importance is placed on positive psychology, including incorporating it into school curricula. Positivity encompasses resilience, the capacity to overcome adversity and find meaning and purpose in life (transcendence). Thus, resilience is an essential aspect of healing, particularly in chronic diseases (Lloyd *et al.* 1993; Dunning 2013b, 117–132).
- The client–therapist relationship is a key aspect of the healing process and has a significant effect on outcomes.
- The therapist's role is to support the individual's innate healing potential.
- The mind, body, and spirit cannot be separated – what affects one affects the others (mind–body medicine). The mind-body-spirit model is embodied in eastern medical philosophy and 'encompasses fundamental and universal elements of well-being' (Chan *et al.* 2006).
- Illness represents an opportunity for positive change (transcendence) (Bridges 1991).

The following core Hippocratic tenets underpin CAM philosophy, particularly naturopathy, but they apply to all health care:

1. *Vis medicatrix naturae* – the healing power of nature.
2. *Primum non nocere* – first do no harm.
3. *Tolle causam* – treat the cause.
4. Treat the whole person.
5. *Docere* – the doctor is a teacher.
6. Prevention is the best cure.

> **Practice point**
>
> Healing does not mean curing. It refers to a process of bringing the physical, mental, emotional, spiritual, and relationship aspects of an individual's self together to achieve an integrated balance where each part is of equal importance and value (Dossey *et al.* 1998). Disruption to any aspect affects the others, and consequently affects outcomes.

Understanding CAM philosophy is important to understanding why people use CAM. People seek answers to their health problems that match their existing beliefs and explanatory models. People's health choices are part of their larger life orientation and are not made in isolation from their beliefs and attitudes. They frequently mix and match CAM with CAM and CAM with conventional therapies to suit their needs. Adverse events can arise when due consideration is not given to the potential effects of such combinations, for example, potentially damaging medicine/herb interactions. Alternatively, CAM can enhance the effects of conventional medicines, enable lower doses of medicines to be used, reduce unwanted side effects and improve healing rates (Braun 2001).

Integrating complementary and conventional care

Quality use of medicines (QUM) is a useful framework for safely integrating health options including the broad categories of CAM and conventional care (see Chapter 5). QUM is congruent with CAM philosophy. QUM can be a helpful decision-making framework to achieve optimal heath care including medicines if medicines are indicated. QUM encompasses, prevention, lifestyle strategies, and risk management. IT is an holistic, integrated framework that recognises not everybody requires medicines to maintain health.

Integrative medicine (IM) is becoming increasingly popular among health professionals, although it was originally consumer-driven. CAM and integrative medicine (IM) are not synonymous terms. IM focuses on providing best practice conventional medicine and includes prevention, and emotional wellbeing, thus it might encompass CAM. Likewise, QUM is not concerned with either/or choices but with providing holistic care by helping the individual make informed choices about the best way to maintain optional health. IM is defined as:

> The blending of conventional medicine and complementary medicines and/or therapies with the aim of using the most appropriate of either or both modalities to care for the patient as a whole.

> (Australasian Integrative Medicine Association)

IM is concerned with wellness and is a flexible approach to responding to the individual and societal factors impacting on health care. The specific therapies used in IM depend on the individual, objective evidence for benefit and risk, consideration of alternative choices (QUM), cost/benefit, practitioner experience and knowledge, and/or the need to refer to other practitioners (Phelps *et al.* 2011; Kotsirilos *et al.* 2011).

Significantly, almost 80% of the global population depends on herbal medicines and traditional medical systems (WHO 2002) although the medicines and systems may be different among countries and cultures. Migration and refugee displacement through war and natural disasters mean the types of CAM available outside the country of origin is increasing. Individuals import some products into their new countries and these products may not be subject to stringent regulatory processes such as good manufacturing practices and other relevant regulations that control many of the system-related risks.

Many health institutions are concerned with regulatory and supply issues as well as benefits and risks and safe CAM use. The degree and processes for regulating CAM therapies, products and practitioners varies from country-to-country and from therapy-to-therapy. Frequently there are no formal regulatory processes in place but some CAM professional associations have stringent training and ongoing professional development requirements as part of self-regulation. Some such associations require competence in first aid, for example, the International Aromatherapy and Aromatic Medicine Association.

The safe, effective combination of conventional and CAM care involves considering the following issues:

- The safety of the client, allowing for their personal choices.
- Facilitating people to make informed choices based on understanding the risks and benefits involved when using CAM, especially combining CAM and conventional care. When the patient is not competent to consent, guardianship issues may arise.
- The knowledge and competence of health professionals to give advice about CAM and how to refer to a suitably qualified practitioner if indicated. CAM needs to be appropriate to the individual's physical, mental, and spiritual status and selected after considering all the options and after a thorough assessment considering potential interactions with conventional therapies. The continued suitability of CAM, like all management strategies, should be reviewed regularly because diabetes is a progressive disease and continued use may be unnecessary or dangerous, e.g. in people with renal and liver disease (see Chapters 8 and 10). Conventional medicine doses should be monitored and may need to be changed.
- Guidelines should be followed where they exist, and consent to use CAM is required in some settings. Policies and guidelines need to include processes for communication between CAM and conventional practitioners and for collaboration and referral mechanisms to prevent fragmented care (Dunning 2001). Where possible, guidelines should be evidence-based to support best practice. They should not be prescriptive and inflexible.
- Processes for monitoring outcomes and accurately documenting the effects of the therapy should be in place and objective data relevant to the aims of the therapy, should be collected.
- Ensuring that safe quality products are used is important. Dose variations, contamination and/or adulteration with potentially toxic substances such as heavy metals and animal parts, and unsubstantiated claims made about the product can lead to serious adverse events including irreversible kidney failure (Ko 1998; Bjelakovic & Nikolova 2007). The *Sydney Morning Herald* reported some Chinese medicines confiscated by customs officials contained 'potentially poisonous plants, unlabelled ingredients and bits of endangered animals' concerning pant species included *Aristolochia* species, which have been linked to cancer (Phillips 2012).
- Safety data information should be available where possible and could be included with research papers or medication reference books/electronic databases in a portfolio in areas where CAM is used.
- It is important that an accurate diagnosis is made and a thorough health history and assessment are undertaken prior to using any therapy. These considerations are often

overlooked, especially when the person with diabetes self-diagnoses and self-treats. Such practices can mask or mimic important symptoms and result in delays in instituting appropriate management and, consequently deteriorating metabolic control.

These considerations apply equally to selecting and using conventional therapies.

Practice points

1. There is an increasing body of scientific evidence as well as a large body of traditional evidence for many CAM. However, evidence about the *combination* of CAM and conventional medicines is not well documented.
2. Many, but not all, CAM have a strong evidence base of traditional use but this is not the same as 'scientific evidence'. In addition, modern technology has changed the traditional method of manufacturing, administering, and monitoring some CAM therapies. Therefore, the traditional evidence base needs to be considered in the light of any such changes.
3. There are methodological flaws in a great deal of CAM research. The same is true of a great deal of conventional research.

Can complementary therapies benefit people with diabetes?

Managing diabetes effectively is about achieving balance. To achieve balance a range of therapies used holistically, is usually needed. For example Type 2 diabetes is a progressive, multifactorial disease, thus a single strategy is unlikely to address the underlying metabolic abnormalities or the consequent effects on mental health and well being. From a general perspective, and based on the premise people need to be mentally well to achieve physical outcomes including care targets, CAM can assist people with diabetes to:

- Incorporate diabetes into the framework of their lives, which encompasses two key aspects of spirituality: transformation and connectedness.
- Accept and manage their diabetes to achieve balance in their lives by reducing stress and depression, which can help them achieve management targets (balance) and reduce hepatic glucose output and insulin resistance. That is address spirituality, resilience and coping.
- Develop strategies to recognise the factors that cause stress and methods to manage or prevent stress from occurring.
- Take part in decision-making, increase their self-esteem, self-efficacy and sense of being in control by improving their quality of life and enabling personal growth and transformation.
- Increase insulin production and reduce insulin resistance, either by the direct effects of the therapy, or by managing stress, or by enhancing the effects of conventional medications.
- Manage the unpleasant symptoms of diabetic complications such as pain and nausea.
- Prevent some associated problems, for example, foot care to maintain skin integrity and prevent problems such as cracks that increase the potential for infection and its consequences.
- Learn and retain information.

Some specific benefits for people with diabetes have also been reported. They include:

1. A reduction in blood glucose levels in children being given regular massage by their parents. The parents who reported reduced anxiety levels in themselves (Field *et al.* 1997). Massage has also been shown to reduce pain intensity, unpleasantness, and anxiety in postoperative patients in the short term, especially in the first four days (Mitchinson *et al.* 2007). Likewise, yoga and meditation reduce features of the metabolic syndrome such as waist circumference, systolic blood pressure, fasting blood glucose and triglycerides, as well as improve mental health (Agrawal 2007).

2. Many herbs have been shown to lower blood glucose by various mechanisms, HbA_{1c} and lipids, for example, American ginseng (*Panex quinquefolius*) (Vuksan *et al.* 2000); Gymnema/gurmar (*Gymnema sylvestre*) (Baskaran *et al.* 1990), fenugreek (*Trigonella foenum-graecum*) (Sharma *et al.* 1990, 1996), chromium picolinate (Finney & Gonzalez-Campoy 1997). These herbs and supplements have primarily been used in Type 2 diabetes, but fenugreek has also been shown to lower blood glucose in Type 1 diabetes (Sharma *et al.* 1990). Chromium possibly has a role in reducing insulin resistance. It is excreted in urine at a faster rate in people with diabetes than non-diabetics, thus a relative chromium deficiency could contribute to insulin resistance (Udani *et al.* 2006). The evidence for a glucose lowering effect of chromium is confusing and may depend on the formulation used and the dosage. People who use chromium report improved blood glucose levels but the required dose may be higher than that usually used ($400\,\mu g$): at least $5000\,\mu g$ chromium picolinate is probably required (Udani *et al.* 2006). Martin *et al.* (2006) compared chromium picolinate $1000\,\mu g$ plus either glipizide or placebo for 24 weeks and reported lower fasting and post prandial glucose, HbA_{1c} less weight gain and less body fat measured using DEXA in the intervention groups. Herbal medicines are also used in diabetes-related conditions such as heart failure *Crataegus species* (hawthorn) (Pittler *et al.* (2007); gastrointestinal reflux (peppermint) (Chaudhary 2007) and CQ-10.

3. Manage weight. Some CAM weight loss medicines and dietary strategies are beneficial, others are associated with significant risks and they should not be self-prescribed or used indiscriminately. Both the FDA in the US and the AMA in Australia have warned the public about the safety of many weight loss preparations. Weight loss requires and integrated approach that encompasses diet and exercise (see Chapter 4). The Diet-Pill-Study group (http://www.diet-pill-study.com/product-reviews.htm) regularly monitors conventional and complementary 'diet pills' and evaluates them according to set criteria for safety and efficacy and also evaluates the company marketing the product. Three products recently met the criteria: (*Hoodia gordonii* plus, Dietrine, and herbal Phentermine. In particular, products containing ephedra may lead to adverse events (Bent *et al.* 2003). Einerhand (2006) found conjugated linoleic acid (CLA) led to weight loss from the abdomen in men and women and women also lost weight from the thighs. Insulin sensitivity was not affected. The clinical significance of this finding is not clear. CAM therapies frequently used to enhance weight loss include herbal medicines, yoga, meditation, acupuncture, massage and Eastern martial arts (Sharpe *et al.* 2007). There is good pooled data to support small weight loss associated with Chromium picolinate but it is not a replacement for diet and exercise.

4. Remain active. The benefits if Tai Chi in improving strength, balance, and mood in older people is well documented (Chou *et al.* 2004). Muscle wasting and reduced strength in the lower limbs is associated with advancing age and can lead to

inactivity and contribute to falls. Tai Chi can be combined with a healthy diet, resistance training, correcting malnutrition, and controlling blood glucose and lipids. Recent research suggests creatine supplementation may enhance the effects of resistance training but the clinical relevance has yet to be determined (O'sathuna 2007).

5. Acupuncture can improve the pain of diabetic peripheral neuropathy (Abuaisha *et al*. 1998). Acupuncture has also been shown to be equivalent to monotherapy at reducing mild to moderate hypertension if it is performed by expert practitioners (Flachskampf 2007). Glucosamine and chondroitin are widely used to manage arthritic and joint pain. There is little evidence that oral dosing contributes significantly to hyperglycaemia.

6. A range of biofeedback, relaxation and counselling therapies can reduce stress by attenuating the effects of increased autonomic activity and catecholamine production. Improved mood and reduced blood glucose levels have been reported with biofeedback (McGrady *et al*. 1991). Exercise also plays a key role. There is good evidence that St John's Wort (*Hypericum perforatum*) effectively improves mild-to-moderate depression and is better tolerated than conventional antidepressants. Recent research suggests it is as effective as paroxetine in moderate to severe depression (Szegede *et al*. 2005). However, St John's Wort interacts with many conventional medicines, thus a medication review should be performed before commencing the medicine and its use should be monitored.

7. Antioxidant therapies receive significant press coverage. There is accumulating evidence that oxidation plays a role in the development of many diseases including vascular disease due to the development of oxidative stress and reactive oxygen species (ROS) (see Chapter 8). For example, O'Brien & Timmins (1999) and Verdejo *et al*. (1999) suggested antioxidants may delay the progression of retinopathy by increasing blood flow to eyes and kidneys (vitamin E) and/or replenishing vitamin E (vitamin C) and/or improving nerve function (the B group vitamins). Other researchers suggest free radicals might be markers of disease rather than the cause, and that eliminating them may interfere with normal defense mechanisms (Bjelakovic *et al*. 2007). Antioxidants are also associated with adverse events and medicine interactions especially in the high doses often used. However, consensus has not been reached about the benefits of using antioxidants, the dose needed or when in the course of diabetes they should be used.

8. Prevent illness. For example cranberry preparations, which prevents bacteria sticking to the bladder wall can reduce UTIs over a 12-month period particularly in women who suffer recurrent UTIs (Jepson & Craig 2008). Cranberry juice may also effectively control *Helicobacter pylori* (Zhang *et al*. 2005).

9. In 2000 the media reported that baths could help reduce blood glucose levels. The claims have not been substantiated and there could be risks such as postural hypotension, falls, and burns to neuropathic feet if the water is too hot. Faster uptake of injected insulin or reduced stress levels could be methods whereby blood glucose is reduced.

10. Aromatherapy can be used to enhance well being and relaxation and to reduce stress, which benefits metabolic control. It can also be used for physical conditions such as alleviating pain, reducing blood pressure, improving sleep, and foot care. Aromatherapy may also alleviate stress during procedures such as CAT scans, and post-cardiac surgery (Stevenson 1994; Buckle 1997). Managing stress improves the individual's quality of life and psychological wellbeing. Aromatherapy is beneficial for fragrancing the environment to increase work performance, reduce absenteeism and reduce keyboard errors. In this respect the benefit is for the health professionals and organisations rather than an individual but it can

have a role in diabetes education sessions. Aromatherapy is often combined with music and massage. There is a strong link between touch, aroma and wellbeing. In aged care settings aromatherapy is used to reduce pain, improve sleep, maintain skin integrity and manage behavioural problems (Thomson 2001). Significantly, difficulty identifying odours may be an early sign of Alzheimer's disease and precedes signs of cognitive dysfunction (Wilson 2007). Wilson showed that every 1 point decrease in the odour identification score represents an 18% risk of mild cognitive impairment progressing to Alzheimer's disease.

Clinical observation

The powerful effect of odour on physical and mental well being is often overlooked. On a practical level, several media reports in 2001 concerning dogs being able to recognise when their owners with diabetes were hypoglycaemic and alert them early enough to enable the person to manage the episode themselves, or to alert another person. Guide dogs for visually impaired people are standard therapy and help visually impaired people lead independent lives, likewise, dogs have alerted individuals or their families to epileptic seizures and horse riding for the disabled is well established in many countries.

Spirituality

Spirituality is a neglected aspect of conventional health care and is often confused with religion. The two are quite different although spirituality may encompass religion and prayer and religion may be used as spiritual tools. Information already presented in this chapter demonstrates that spirituality is central to optimal self-care. There are many definitions of spirituality. Most encompass the following core aspects:

- positive empowering aspect of being human;
- quest for meaning and purpose in life;
- transcendence;
- holistic perspective;
- connectedness;
- resilience and confidence to turn crises into opportunities for personal growth;
- synergy – all components work together and small changes in one component can positively or negatively affect all other components.

These are essential to effective diabetes management. Parsian & Dunning (2008a, 2008b) validated a tool for assessing spirituality and coping in young people with diabetes and demonstrated a significant association among spirituality, coping, and lower HbA_{1c}. Females were more spiritual than males and there was no significant association between religion and spirituality. Several other researchers around the world are currently using the tool.

CAM and surgery

CAM usage is high among surgical patients, >51%; especially women aged 40–60 years, and is often used on the advice of friends (Tsen *et al.* 2000; Norred *et al.* 2000) (see Chapter 9). There are some well-documented benefits of using CAM to improve the health outcomes of people undergoing surgery. For example, foot massage using essential oils reduced stress and anxiety post CAGS (Stevenson 1994) and MRI-associated claustrophobia and stress. Massage reduced postoperative pain intensity, pain unpleasantness, and anxiety during the first four post operative days (Mitchinson 2007). Acupuncture and peppermint or ginger tea reduces nausea, and a range of strategies can relieve pain and improve sleep. Prophylactic CQ_{10} prior to cardiac surgery improves postoperative cardiac outcomes (Rosenfeldt *et al*. 2005).

However, the risks also need to be considered in the context of the individual, the type of procedure and the overall management plan. Significant risks include bleeding, hypo or hypertension, sedation, cardiac dysrhythmias, renal damage, and electrolyte disturbances (Norred *et al*. 2000). Many conventional medicines need to be adjusted or ceased prior to surgery. There is less information about managing CAM medicines in surgical settings but there is a growing body of evidence to suggest that many CAM medicines may also need to be stopped or adjusted before surgery. Thus, it is important for conventional practitioners to ask about CAM use, although most do not (Braun *et al*. 2006).

The following general information is relevant to people already using CAM medicines and those considering using them before or after surgery. People are advised to consult a qualified CAM practitioner for specific advice. Self-prescribing is not recommended because many CAM medicines require supervised use especially in the context of the complex metabolic and neuroendocrine response to surgery.

Before surgery

People need written information about how to manage CAM medicines in the operative period. Conventional health professionals can provide such information if they are qualified to do so. They should refer the person to a qualified CAM practitioner if they do not have the relevant information. People also require written instructions about how to manage their conventional medicines as well as any special preparation needed for the surgery or investigation.

Great care is needed if the surgery is major or high risk such as heart, orthopaedic, or neurosurgery, if the person has renal or liver disease, or is very young or elderly. Most people's conventional medication list is unlikely to include CAM medicines or supplements, although it should: thus, health professionals should discuss CAM use with people during a structured medicines preoperative health assessment.

Some CAM medicines such as evening primrose oil, bilberry, cranberry, fish oils, ginger, Gingko, liquorice, guarana, willow bark, meadowsweet, and ginseng need to be stopped at least one week before surgery. St John's Wort and supplements such as vitamin E should be stopped two weeks before surgery, primarily because of the risk of bleeding. Some, such as *Hypericum perforatum (*St John's Wort), may need to be stopped gradually (like conventional antidepressants). However, where CAM medicines are the main form of treatment, alternative management may be required to prevent the condition deteriorating and affecting the surgical outcome, for example, glucose lowering herbal medicines.

Some commonly used CAM medicines might/do interact with some anaesthetic agents and prolong their sedative effects, others increase the risk of bleeding, some affect blood pressure and the heart rate, others cause changes in the major electrolytes, potassium, calcium and sodium, levels in the blood. Grapefruit juice interferes with the action of some antibiotics such as cyclosporine, which may be needed pre or postoperatively. Not everybody experiences such problems and it is sometimes difficult to predict who will or will not have problems. General safety issues also need to be considered.

Some hospitals have policies about using CAM although they may not address surgery, investigations or diabetes specifically. People who wish to continue using CAM in hospital should clarify the hospital's policies and procedures with the relevant hospital before they are admitted. Most hospital do not prescribe or supply CAM in Australia.

In addition to managing medicines, achieving the best possible health status before surgery improves recovery afterwards. The preoperative assessment is an ideal time to revise the importance of eating a healthy balanced diet and exercise within the individual's capability to control blood glucose and lipids as well as to support the immune system and enhance wound healing. Most people should continue their usual physical activity unless it is contraindicated to maintain strength and flexibility. Stress management strategies such as meditation, guided imagery, essential oil massage or inhalations, and music can help reduce anxiety and fear about the surgery. Ginger capsules or tablets taken one hour before surgery reduces postoperative nausea (Gupta & Sharma 2001).

The preoperative assessment is also an ideal time to discuss postoperative recovery including pain and sleep management. CAM may be a useful alternative to some conventional medicines provided a quality use of medicines framework is adopted.

After surgery

A range of CAM strategies can be used to manage post operative pain and most are less likely to cause constipation and drowsiness than pethidine and morphine-based medicines. Alternatively, if these medicines are the best method of managing pain, high-fibre CAM medicines such as *Aloe vera* juice, probiotics, and psyllium can reduce constipation once oral feeding is allowed. Probiotics also increase bowel health and support natural bowel flora. Peppermint or ginger tea reduces mild-to-moderate nausea. Lymphatic drainage massage is very effective after some surgery to reduce swelling and relieve pain. Valerian, hops and lavender in a vapourised essential oil blend or massage might promote restful sleep without the side effects of some conventional sedatives.

Some CAM products promote wound healing, for example, *Aloe vera*, Medihoney, and calendula and could be used depending on the wound. Arnica ointment reduces bruising but should not be used on open wounds. Comfrey poultices are very effective at reducing local oedema and local pain but should not be used on open wounds or taken internally.

After surgery, the person needs information about whether and when it is safe to start using CAM again. New conventional medicines might be prescribed or dose and or dose intervals of medicines taken preoperatively might change, for example, anticoagulants, which could influence the choice of CAM medicines or the dose. Likewise, some non-medicine CAM might need to be used with care such as needle acupuncture and deep tissue massage because they can cause bruising and/or bleeding.

Adverse events

Adverse events encompass safety, which is a complex multifactorial issue (see Table 19.2). Using QUM strategies significantly reduces the risk of adverse events. These may be general or diabetes specific. Diabetes-specific adverse events associated with CAM reported in the literature include:

- Stopping insulin in a person with Type 1 diabetes leading to ketoacidosis (Gill *et al.* 1994).
- Trauma and burns to neuropathic feet and legs from cupping and moxibustion (Ewins *et al.* 1993).
- Allergies, drug/herb interactions and hospital admissions, largely from adulterated traditional Chinese medicine (Biegel & Schoenfeld 1998; Ko 1998).

Table 19.2   Medicine-related safety and quality use of CAM and conventional medicines that need to be considerd as inter-related factors that impact on outcomes.

Issue	Considerations for practitioners
Health system at global, national and local levels	Degree of product regulation including manufacture and marketing Affordability and accessibility of medicines Support for research Evidence-based guidelines to support use Adverse event monitoring systems Pre- and post-market surveillance systems including adverse event reporting systems Medicine scheduling systems Marketing processes Methods of communicating important medicine-related information to the public
Practitioner	Education and competence including ongoing professional development Regulation and self-regulatory processes, which includes scope of practice Licences to practice Professional liability insurance Communication, documentation, and referral processes Attitudes towards and beliefs about medicines and CAM
Herbal medicines	Research and development Pre- and post-market testing surveillance Manufacturing practices including herb identification, handling, storing, and infection control procedures, and whether the herb is prepared according to the traditional method Adulteration and contamination Labels Adverse event monitoring including interactions Inappropriate dose and/or dose interval Prescribing to at risk groups Contraindicated
Person with diabetes	Age Physical and mental health status Knowledge Not disclosing herbal medicine use Self-diagnosis and self-treatment, which can delay treating serious problems Storage and handling of medicines Inappropriate use of medicines and CAM Monitoring defined outcomes False hope of cure or control Polypharmacy Cost

- Hypoglycaemia following prolonged massage and using herbal therapies.
- Bleeding from herb/anticoagulant interactions, (see Table 19.3).
- Kidney and liver damage, see Chapter 8. (National Library of **Medicine** Kidney Diseases: MedlinePlus).
- Heavy metal poisoning (Keen *et al.* 1994).

A number of initiatives have been taken to limit some of these problems, for example, in 1991 the World Health Organisation developed guidelines for the safe use, manufacturing and labelling of plant medicines, the Chinese Government introduced strategies for identifying the content of Chinese herbal medicines and global strategies are in place to

Table 19.3 Commonly used herbs and supplements, their potential interactions, reported adverse events and some management strategies to use should an adverse event occur. (Data from Braun 2010).

Herb	Potential interactions	Reported adverse events	Management strategies
Echinacea	Hepatoxic medicines, for example, anabolic steroids, amiodarone, methotrexate, ketaconazole Immunosuppressants, for example, corticosteroids, cyclosporin	Allergic reactions especially in atopic people Impairs the action of immunosuppressive drugs Can cause immunosuppression if taken long-term In acute surgery impairs wound healing	Do not use continuously for >8 weeks at a time
Fenugreek	Anticoagulants Oral hypoglycaemic agents	Bleeding Hypoglycaemia	Do not use concurrently Monitor Adjust dose of OHA or the herb
Feverfew	NSAIDS, warfarin, offset the herb's effect for migraine and might alter bleeding time	Changed bleeding time	
Garlic	Aspirin Warfarin Cholesterol lowering agents	Risk of bleeding especially when taken with anticoagulants Increased GIT activity Decreased effectiveness of antacids Inhibits platelet aggregation Additive effects	Discontinue 7 days before surgery Do not use concomitantly with antacids
Ginger	Antacids Warfarin	Decreased effectiveness of antacids	Do not use at the same time
Gingko biloba	Aspirin Warfarin SSRI MAO inhibitors	Bleeding risk if used with anticoagulants	Stop 36 hours before surgery Do not use concurrently
Ginseng Note: there are several species in common use	Corticosteroids Oral contraceptives Warfarin Digoxin Oral hypoglycaemic agents MAO inhibitors and tricyclic antidepressants	Increased risk of bleeding with anticoagulants Suppresses immune system – infections risk Hypoglycaemia Headache Additive effects	Stop 7 days before surgery Do not use concomitantly
Glucosamine		GIT complaints Allergy if allergic to seafoods Nausea, vomiting abdominal pain Sleepiness Hyperglycaemia	Avoid with seafoods
Guar and bulking agents	Antibiotics Alpha-glucosidase inhibitors	Decreased food absorption – hypoglycaemia risk	Do not administer at the same time

(Continued)

Table 19.3 Continued.

Herb	Potential interactions	Reported adverse events	Management strategies
Hawthorn	Antihypertensive agents Digoxin Alcohol, Antipsychotics	Hypotension Dizziness Falls	
Kelp (contains iodine)	Thyroid hormones Antithyroid hormones	Altered thyroid function	
Liquorices	Corticosteroids Antihypertensive agents Oral contraceptives Digoxin	Fluid retention Electrolyte imbalance Block oestrogen in contraception Digoxin toxicity	
Slippery elm		Decrease GIT absorption Hypoglycaemia	
St John's Wort	MAO inhibitors SSRI Decreases effect of HIV medications Warfarin Anticonvulsants Activates liver enzyme, hastening drug metabolism and reducing their effectiveness	Alters metabolism of some medicines, for example, cyclosporin, warfarin, steroids Interacts with psychotrophic drugs and can increase their effect Skin allergies	Stop 5 days before operation Do not use concomitantly
Valerian, hops	Anaesthetic agents Barbiturates Hypnotics Antidepressive medicines	Enhance/potentiate the effects of sedatives With long-term use the amount of anaesthetic needed is increased	Withdrawal – symptoms resemble valium addiction Taper dose preoperatively
Vitamin supplements C & E, B group; often as antioxidants	Vitamin toxicity Niacin	Decreases the beneficial effects of statins on HDL levels	
Zinc	Increased HbA_{1c} in Type 1Type 1 diabetes		

Many of these interactions are theoretical, others are well documented. When considering the likelihood of an interaction, the total individual situation and medication regimen must be considered. In addition, although 'medicine interactions' is usually used to denote negative interactions, the term itself is objective and non-judgmental. Many interactions may actually be beneficial and it is just as important to document these.

protect endangered animal and plant species as well as to improve the quality of CAM research. Another initiative, the Convention on International Trade in Endangered Species of Wild Fauna and Flora (CITES) was established in Washington DC in 1975 in response to growing concerns that over-exploitation of wildlife through the international trade could contribute to the rapid decimation of many plant and animal species in the world.

Herb/medicine interactions

There are four main potential mechanisms for herb/medicine interactions. Herbs can:

1. Induce production of liver enzymes, especially the cytochrome P450 system, which reduces medicine bioavailability.
2. Induce intestinal D-glycoprotein, which inhibits medicine absorption and metabolism.
3. Stimulate neurotransmitter production especially serotonin enhancing the effects of some medicines, i.e. they both do the same thing. Others decrease the effects of serotonin-inhibiting medicines (Braun 2001).
4. Compete with medicines for binding sites on serum protein increasing the amount of free medicine available. People with low serum albumin are especially at risk, for example, the older people and those with malnutrition.

Herb/medicine interactions are a two-way street – alone neither the medicine nor the herb might be a problem, but when used together, the *combination* can be potentially dangerous. However, ingredients in the CAM or conventional medicine beside the active ingredient/s might also be responsible for the adverse effects, for example, incipients, preservatives, and contaminants. It should also be noted that liver failure (20–30%) and kidney damage (30%) are recognised serious side effects of readily available conventional medicines, but the benefits are considered to outweigh the risks.

People most at risk of herb/medicine interactions are those who:

- are taking medicines with a narrow therapeutic index such as lithium, phenytoin, barbiturates, warfarin and digoxin and high risk medicines such as insulin;
- are at risk of, or have, renal and/or liver damage and therefore, have altered ability to metabolise and excrete medicine;
- have atopic conditions such as allergies, asthma or dermatitis;
- are older;
- are children;
- are taking >5 medicines (polypharmacy);
- use alcohol or drugs of addiction;
- lack knowledge or consult CAM and/or conventional practitioners who lack knowledge about appropriate therapies to use, consult health professionals who do not ask them about CAM use
- self-diagnose, delay seeking medical advice, do not tell conventional or CAM practitioners about the therapies/medicines they are using;
- import products or use products when travelling that are not subject to regulations governing good manufacturing practices; the danger of contamination of products from some countries is significant.

People with diabetes are at increased risk because they usually have more than one risk factor present and risk factors could be additive.

How can complementary therapies be used safely?

Giving people appropriate advice so they can make informed decisions is an important aspect of nursing care (see Table 19.4). The following information could help nurses assist people with diabetes to use CAM safely and choose therapies appropriate for the problem they want to treat. Patients need to know there could be risks if they do not follow conventional evidence-based diabetes management practices. They should not be made to feel guilty or lacking in judgment if they choose to use CAM. People can be advised to:

- Develop an holistic health plan and decide what they hope to achieve by using CAM and use a therapy that is best suited to achieve these goals, for example, to reduce stress: use massage, counselling or time-line therapy.
- Find out as much about the therapy as they can before using it. Seek information from unbiased sources and be wary of information they find in chat rooms on the Internet and advertising material.
- Consult a reputable practitioner, for example, a member of the relevant professional association, and buy products from reputable sources that are approved and have relevant safety data available.
- Store and maintain products appropriately and consider safety issues if children and confused elderly people are part of the household. This also applies to storage of products in healthcare settings.
- Ensure the condition for which they want to use CAM is correctly diagnosed before they treat it, otherwise appropriate treatment could be delayed and the condition deteriorate.
- Be aware that there are risks if they do not follow conventional evidence-based diabetes management recommendations.

Table 19.4   Advice health professionals can provide to people with diabetes to help them use CAM safely.

- Consider what you want to achieve by using CAM.
- Decide on your general life and health goals and your diabetes goals.
- Select a therapy that is likely to achieve these goals.
- Learn all there is about it/then so you can use the therapy from an informed perspective.
- Consult reputable practitioners for example a member of a professional association that has training standards and requires practitioners to keep up-to-date.
- Buy products from reputable sources that comply with good manufacturing and regulatory processes and are stored appropriately before purchase. Be wary of importing other medicines or buying on the Internet.
- Read labels carefully and look for Aust L or Aust R on the label.
- Have a correct diagnosis before using any therapy. Inform conventional and complementary practitioners about all the therapies you are using and understand there may be risks associated with not following evidence based conventional care.
- Monitor the effects against the health goals you set.
- Keep a list of all the CAM medicines and therapies you use, update it regularly and make sure your CAM and conventional health professionals have a copy.
- Realise that some CAM may take longer to show an effect than conventional medicines.
- Do not stop conventional medicines without consulting your doctor or diabetes educator. CAM medicines may need to be adjusted or stopped temporarily before surgery, illness, investigations, and changes in conventional medicines. You should seek advice in these circumstances.
- Seek advice quickly if any of the following occur: hypo or hyperglycaemia, mental changes, abdominal pain, skin rashes, nausea, vomiting, diarrhoea, falls.

- Be aware that they should not stop or change recommended conventional treatments without the advice of their doctor.
- Inform all practitioners, conventional and complementary, about the therapies they are using so the health plan can be coordinated.
- Some CAM should not be used continuously for long periods.
- Take extra care if they are old, very young, pregnant, breastfeeding, have kidney or liver damage or are using a lot of other treatments, because these people are at increased risk of adverse events.
- Seek advice about how to manage the therapy if they need surgery or an investigative procedure especially if radio contrast media are required (see Chapters 3 and 8), or starting any new conventional treatment.
- Seek advice quickly if any of the following occur:
  - hypo/hyperglycaemia
  - mental changes
  - abdominal pain
  - skin rashes
  - nausea, vomiting, diarrhoea.
- Monitor the effects on their diabetes, for example, blood glucose, lipids and HbA_{1c} as well as their response with respect to the reason they chose the therapy, for example, to manage pain.

Nursing responsibilities

Nurses have a responsibility to respect people's choices and not to be judgmental about the choices they make. They also have responsibilities to their employer, other patients, visitors and staff. Nurses can use CAM as part of holistic nursing care but they have a duty of care to practice at the level of their education and competence and use safe therapies. The following general advice applies. Specific information about individual CAM should be sought before using CAM or giving advice about it.

- Reflect on own attitudes towards and beliefs about CAM.
- Be sensitive to the philosophical and cultural views of people with diabetes and be aware that they may perceive risks and benefits differently from health professionals.
- Follow guidelines for using CAM where they exist, for example, those of the NMC in the UK. In Australia the state nurse registering authorities, the Australian Nursing Federation and Royal College of Nursing, Australia, all have produced guidelines for nurses using CAM (McCabe 2001).
- Ensure CAM practitioners are appropriately qualified and competent if you decide to use, recommend or offer advice about CAM to a person with diabetes.
- Look for evidence of safety and efficiency but do not be too quick to accept or reject 'evidence'.
- Communicate the risks and benefits to people with diabetes and their families/carers. If the person chooses not to follow advice, documentation should outline the information that was given.
- Develop a portfolio of evidence for reference in clinical areas where CAM is used.
- Use herbs and essential oils within the philosophy of QUM and prescribe, administer, document and monitor within that philosophy. Nursing assessment should ask about CAM. People are not always willing to disclose such information and skilful questioning is required. Questions should be asked in a framework of acceptance. The patient has a responsibility to disclose. Nurses can make it easier for them to do so.
- Value the nurse–patient relationship as an essential aspect of the healing process.

Table 19.5 Scale for assessing the likelihood of a CAM-conventional interaction and information that should be included in the report. One point is allocated to each of the following criteria.

Interpreting the score:

0–3: Insufficient information to be able to assessed/attribute the event to CAM use.

4–7: Interaction is possible but other explanations for the event need to be excluded.

8–10: Interaction is likely.

(1) The health history is well documented.
(2) The person has:
    a. renal disease
    b. liver disease
    c. atopic conditions
    d. significant alcohol or illegal drug use
    e. is very young or elderly.
(3) The AE[a] was associated with using a CAM medicine or therapy.
(4) The medication regimen is documented and includes conventional medicines, CAM medicines, and over-the-counter medicines and doses and dose frequency.
(5) Alternative explanations for the event are excluded.
(6) The AE is adequately described, for example, time of onset of symptoms in relation to taking the medicine, what actually happened, what else was occurring at the time the event occurred.
(7) The time between taking the medicine and the onset of the event is reasonable considering the medicine usual action profile.
(8) The reaction resolves when the CAM medicine is stopped.
(9) The sequence of events is consistent with an AE.
(10) The event recurs when the medicine is used again.

[a]AE: adverse event. The event should be noted in the individual's health history and an adverse event report forwarded through the relevant process in the country of origin. In Australia reports go to the Adverse Drug Reactions Advisory Committee (ADRAC) on the 'blue' reporting form (www.tga.gov.au/addr/bluecard.pdf). In the US, suspected interactions can be reported via the MedWatch program (www.fda.gov/medwatch/how.htm). In the UK reports can be submitted on the yellow card to the MHRA and the Commission Human Medicine (CHM) (www.yellowcard.gov.au). The information is based on Fugh-Berman & Ernst (2001) and the websites cited above.

- Consider the effect of CAM on other staff, visitors and patients, for example, vapourising essential oils, playing music.
- Know how to contact the Poisons Advisory Service in the area.
- Have mechanisms in place to clean and maintain any equipment needed, for example, aromatherapy vapourisers. Processes should be in place to deal with any CAM products the patient brings with them.
- Document appropriately, in the same manner as conventional treatment, the type, dose and duration of the therapy, condition it is used for, advice given, expected outcome, actual outcome and report any adverse events.
- Reliably report suspected or actual CAM adverse events (see Table 19.5).

Identifying quality health information on the Internet

Many people gain information about CAM from the media. Generally, the media and pharmaceutical bodies are careful to only make medium to general level claims consistent with regulations. They often rely on information published in quality peer-reviewed conventional journals often as meta-analysis or systematic reviews or presented at conferences and frequently use 'experts' to promote their message. These experts should declare any conflict of interest, which is increasingly required in publications but is not common in other media. However, the media also specialises in telling stories and sensationalising information, therefore, you may need to verify the source of the information and be wary of sites that quote 'experts' to gain credibility. In addition, the media often reports 'exciting breakthroughs' but the product may not actually be available for many years.

When accessing Internet information carefully scrutinise the site – the quality and reliability varies a great deal. Non-sponsored sites are likely to be more objective. Questions to ask include:

- What is the name of the individual or organisation that produced the site? Information produced by reputable organisations is likely to be more reliable than that produced by individuals.
- What are their credentials?
- Are their links to other sources I can use to verify the information?
- Is the information presented in an objective way and does it discuss a range of options and their benefits and risks?
- Is the discussion comprehensive or does it only discuss one or two options all available from one manufacturer; i.e. is the information actually advertising/marketing?
- Is the site clearly selling products? As a general rule of thumb, if the site is selling or promoting a product and has a number of glowing testimonials from 'happy, satisfied customers', be wary, and check the information in another source.
- Is there evidence the information has been verified in any way e.g. there is a list of peer-reviewed references or links to other reputable sites.
- Is any conflict of interest declared?

Various guidelines have also been developed to evaluate Internet health information but some may not be applicable to CAM (Cooke & Gray 2002). The following are examples that might be useful when assessing the reliability of Internet information:

- Biome Evaluation Guidelines;
- Sandvik Score;
- European Commission Guidelines;
- Discern instrument, which was developed for use by the general public;
- eHealth Code of Ethics.

The following processes are commonly used to grade evidence into a hierarchy according to the quality of the science:

- JADAD score (formulated for CAM);
- National Health and Medical Research Council levels of evidence;
- Cochrane Data base process;
- Joanna Briggs Center for Evidence Based Nursing.

Other factors to consider are advertising codes.

Self-reflection

1. How will you respond to a person with diabetes who asks you about taking a Chinese herbal medicine to control their blood glucose?
2. What will you do when a person with diabetes and end stage renal failure elects to use herbal medicine?
3. How would you advise a person with diabetes who asks you can she use aromatherapy to help her sleep?

Clinical observation

A young Aboriginal man from Central Australia was studying research methods at a University. At the same time he was being educated about traditional tribal practices. He fractured his tibia and fibula playing football. It was a simple fracture but he became depressed and the bones were not mending as well as expected.

The young man's mother took him to consult with the Tribal Elders. On his return the doctor said to the mother, 'That won's cure him you know'. The mother replied, 'No, but it will put him in a frame of mind to accept your medicine. That will work now'.

References

Abuaisha, B., Boulton, A. & Costanz, J. (1998) Acupuncture for the treatment of chronic painful diabetic peripheral neuropathy: a long-term study. *Diabetes Research and Clinical Practice*, **39** (2), 115–121.

Agrawal, R. (2007) Yoga improves sense of well-being, reverses changes in metabolic syndrome. *Diabetes Research and Clinical Practice*, **78**, e9–e10.

Australian Integrative Medicine Association. 0000 www.aima.net.au

Baskaran, K., Kizar, A., Radha, K. & Shanmugasundaram, E. (1990) Antidiabetic effect of leaf extract from *Gymnema sylvestre* in non insulin-dependant diabetes mellitus patients. *Journal of Ethnopharmacology*, **30** (3), 295–300.

Bent, S., Tiedt, T., Odden, M. & Shipak, M. (2003) The relative safety of ephedra compared with other products. *Annals of Internal Medicine* **138** (6), 468 – 467.

Biegel, Y. & Schoenfeld, N. (1998) A leading question. *New England Journal of Medicine*, **339**, 827–830.

Bjelakovic, G. & Nikolova, D. (2007) Mortality in randomized controlled trials of antioxidant supplements for primary and secondary prevention: systematic review and meta-analysis. *Journal of the American Medical Association*, **297**, 842–857.

Braun, L. (2001) Herb – drug interactions: A danger or an advantage? *Diversity*, **2** (6), 31–34.

Braun, L. (2006) Use of complementary medicines by surgical patients. Undetected and unsupervised, in *Proceedings of the Fourth Australasian Conference on Safety and Quality in Health Care*, Melbourne.

Braun, L. & Cohen, M, (2010) *Herbs and Natural Supplements: An Evidence-based Guide*. Churchill Livingstone, Chatswood, Sydney.

Bridges, W. (1991) *Transitions: Making Sense of Life's Changes*. Addison Wesley, Reading MA, USA.

Buckle, J. (1997) *Clinical Aromatherapy in Nursing*. Arnold, London.

Chan, C., Ng, S., Rainbow, T. & Chow, A. (2006) Making sense of spirituality. *Journal of Clinical Nursing*, **15**, 822–834.

Chaudhary, S. (2007) Peppermint oil may relieve digestive symptoms, headaches. *American Family Physician*, **75**, 1027–1030.

Chou, K., Lee, P. & Yu, E. (2004) Tai Chi on depressive symptoms amongst Chinese older patients with depressive disorders: A randomized clinical trial. *International Journal of Geriatric Psychiatry*, **19** (11), 1105–1107.

Cochrane Collaboration (2000) *Complementary Medicine Field* www.cochrane.org/.../topic-list-cochrane-complementary-medicine-field-related-reviews-cochraneorg (accessed November 2012).

0000 *Convention on International Trade in Endangered Species of Wild Fauna and Flora* (CITES) www.cites.org/eng/disc/species.php (accessed November 2012).

Cooke, A. & Gray, L. (2002) Evaluating the quality of internet based information about alternative therapies: Development of the BIOME guidelines. *Journal of Public Health Medicine*, **24**, 261–267.

Department of Health and Aging (2002) *National Strategy for the Quality Use of Medicines*. anberra http://www.health.gov.au/haf/nmp/advisory/pharm.htm

Diet-Pill-Study http://www.diet-pill-study.com/product-reviews.htm (accessed December 2007).

Dossey, B., Keegan, L., Guzzetta, C. & Kolkmeier, L. (1998) *Holistic Nursing: A Handbook for Practice*. Gaithersburg, Maryland US,Aspen Publications,

Dunning, T. (2001) Developing clinical practice guidelines, in *Complementary Therapies in Nursing and Midwifery* (ed. P. McCabe). Melbourne VIC Ausmed Publications, pp. 37–48.

Dunning T. (2007) Quality use of medicines: Does the concept apply to complementary medicines? *The Australian Diabetes Educator*, **5**, 20–49.

Dunning T. (2013a) Teaching and learning: the art and science of making connections Chapter 3 in *Diabetes Education Art Science and Evidence* (ed. T. Dunning). Wiley-Blackwell, Chichester, pp 28–48.

Dunning T. (2013b) Turning points and transition crises and opportunities, Chapter 8 in *Diabetes Education Art Science and Evidence* (ed. T. Dunning). Wiley-Blackwell, Chichester, pp 117–132.

Dunning, T., Chan, S.P., Hew, F.L. *et al.* (2001) A cautionary tale on the use of complementary therapies. *Diabetes in Primary Care*, **3** (2), 58–63.

Egede, L., Xiaobou, Y., Zheng, D. & Silverstein, M. (2002) The prevalence and pattern of complementary and alternative medicine use in individuals with diabetes. *Diabetes Care*, **25**, 324–329.

Einerhand, S. (2006) CLA weight loss debate continues. *WebMD Health News* 2006. www.webmd.com/.../news/20060522/cla-weight-loss-debate-continues (accessed December 2012).

Eisenberg, D. (1998) Advising patients who seek alternative medical therapies. *American Journal of Health Medicine*, **127** (1), 61–69.

Ewins, D., Bakker, K., Youn, M. & Boulton, A. (1993) Alternative medicine: Potential dangers for the diabetic foot. *Diabetic Medicine*, **10**, 980–982.

Fetrow, C. & Avila, J. (1999) *Professional's Handbook of Complementary and Alternative Medicines*. Springhouse Corporation, Pennsylvania.

Field, T., Hernandez-Reif, M., LaGreca, A. *et al.* (1997) Massage lowers blood glucose levels in children with diabetes. *Diabetes Spectrum*, **10**, 237–239.

Finney, L. & Gonzalez-Campoy, J. (1997) Dietary chromium and diabetes: Is there a relationship? *Clinical Diabetes*, Jan/Feb, 6–8.

Flachskampf, F. (2007) Blood pressure changes with acupuncture comparable to those with ACE inhibitor monotherapy. *Circulation*, online June 4, weblogdofraga.blogspot.com/2007/.../blood-pressure-changes-with-acupuncture.html (accessed December 2012).

Fugh-Berman, A. & Ernst, E. (2001) Herb–drug interactions: Review and assessment of report reliability. *British Journal of Clinical Pharmacology*, **52**, 587–595.

Garrow, D. & Egede, L. (2006) Association between complementary and alternative medicine use, preventative care practices, and use of conventional medical services among adults with diabetes. *Diabetes Care*, **29**, 15–19.

Gill, G., Redmond, S., Garratt, F. & Paisley, R. (1994) Diabetes and alternative medicine: Cause for concern. *Diabetic Medicine*, **11**, 210–213.

Gupta, Y. & Sharma, M. (2001) Reversal of pyrogallol-induced gastric emptying in rats by ginger (*Zingiber officinalis*). *Experimental Clinical Pharmacology*, **23** (9), 501–503.

Hildreth, K. & Elman, C. (2007) Alternative worldviews and the utilization of conventional and complementary medicine. *Sociological Inquiry*, **77** (1), 76–103.

Jepson, R. & Craig, J. (2008) Cranberries for preventing urinary tract infections. *Cochrane Database of Systematic Reviews*, Issue 1, Art. No. CD001321. DOI: 10: 1002/14651858. CD001321. pub4.

Keen, R., Deacon, A., Delves, H., Morton, J. & Frost, P. (1994) Indian herbal remedies for diabetes as a cause of lead poisoning. *Postgraduate Medicine Journal*, **70**, 113–114.

Kelner, M. & Wellman, B. (1997) Health care and consumer choices: Medical and alternative therapies. *Social Science and Medicine*, **45**, 203–212.

Ko, R. (1998) Adulterants in Asian patent medicines. *New England Journal of Medicine*, **339**, 847.

Kotsirilos, V., Vitetta, L. & Sali, A. (2011) *An Evidence-based Guide to Integrative and Complementary Medicine*. Churchill Livingstone, Chatswood NSW, Australia.

Leese, G., Gill, G. & Houghton, G. (1997) Prevalence of complementary medicine usage within a diabetic clinic. *Practical Diabetes International*, **14** (7), 207–208.

Lloyd, P., Lupton, D., Wiesner, D. & Hasleton, S. (1993) Choosing on alternative therapy: An exploratory study of sociodemographic characteristics and motives of patients resident in Sydney. *Australian Journal of Public Health*, **17** (2), 135–144.

MacLennan, A., Wilson, D. & Taylor, A. (1996) Prevalence and cost of alternative medicine in Australia. *The Lancet*, **347**, 569–573.

MacLennan, A., Wilson, D. & Taylor, A. (2002) The escalating cost and prevalence of alternative medicine. *Preventative Medicine*, **35** (2), 166–173.

Manya, K., Champion, B. & Dunning, T. (2012) The use of complementary and alternative medicines among people living with diabetes in Western Sydney. *BMC Complementary Medicines*, **12**, 1–5.

Martin, J., Wang, Z., Zhang, X. *et al.* (2006) Chromium picolinate supplementation attenuates body weight gain and increases insulin sensitivity in subjects with Type 2 diabetes. *Diabetes Care*, **29** (8), 1826–1832.

McCabe, P. (ed.) (2001) *Complementary Therapies in Nursing and Midwifery*. Ausmed Publications, Melbourne.

McGrady, A., Bailey, B. & Good, M. (1991) Controlled study of biofeedback assisted relaxation in Type 1 diabetes. *Diabetes Care*, **14** (5), 360–365.

Mitchinson A, Kim H, Rosenberg J, *et al.* (2007) Acute postoperative pain management using massage as an adjuvant therapy: a randomized trial. *Archives Surgery*, **142** (12), 1158–1167.

National Library of Medicine Kidney Diseases: MedlinePlus. www.nlm.nih.gov/medlineplus/kidneydiseases.html (accessed January 2013).

Norred, C., Zamudio, S. & Palmer, S. (2000).Use of complementary and alternative medicines by surgical patients. *American Association of Nurse Anesthetists Journal*, **68** (1), 13–18.

O'srien, R. & Timmins, K. (1999) Trends. *Endocrinology and Metabolism*, 5, 329–334.

O'sathuna, D. (2007) Creatinine and resistance training for older adults. *Alternative Medicine Alert*, **10** (11), 121–124.

Parsian, N. & Dunning, T. (2008a) Validation tool to assess spirituality and coping in young adults with diabetes. *Proceedings of the 3rd International Congress of Complementary Medicine Research*, (ICMR). ICMR, Sydney, Australia.

Parsian, N. & Dunning, T. (2008b) Spirituality and coping in young adults with diabetes. *Proceedings of the 7th International Diabetes Federation Western Pacific Region Congress*, (IDFWPR). IDFWPR, Wellington, New Zealand.

Phelps, K. &, Hassad, C. (2011) *General Practice: The Integrative Approach*. Churchill Livingstone, Chatswood NSW, Australia.

Phillips N. (2012) Bits of black bear found in Chinese medicines. *Sydney Morning Herald* 13th April p24.

Pittler, M., Guo, R. & Ernst, E. (2008) Hawthorn extract for treating chronic heart failure. *Cochrane Database of Systematic Reviews*, Issue 1, Art. No. CD005312. DOI: 10.1002/14651858.CD005312

Ryan, E., Pick, M. & Marceau, C. (1999) Use of alternative therapies in diabetes mellitus. *Proceedings of the American Diabetes Association Conference (ADA)*, ADA, San Diego, CA, USA.

Rosenfeldt, F., Marasco, S., Lyon, W. *et al.* (2005) Coenzyme Q10 therapy before cardiac surgery improves mitochondrial function and in vitro contractility of myocardial tissue. *Journal of Thoracic Cardiovascular Surgery*, **129**, 25–32.

Sharma, R., Raghuram, T. & Rao, N. (1990) Effect of fenugreek seeds on blood glucose and serum lipids in Type 1 diabetes. *European Journal of Clinical Nutrition*, **44**, 301–306.

Sharma, R., Sarkar, A. & Hazra, D. (1996) Use of fenugreek seeds powder in the management of non insulin-dependent diabetes mellitus. *Nutritional Research*, **16**, 1331–1339.

Sharpe, P., Blanck, H., Williams, J., Ainsworth, B. & Conway, J. (2007) Use of complementary and alternative medicine for weight control in the United States. *The Journal of Complementary and Alternative Medicine*, **13** (2), 217–222.

Szegede, A., Kohnen, R. & Dienel, A. (2005) Acute treatment of moderate to severe depression with hypericum extract WS 5570 (St John's Wort): Randomized controlled double blind non-inferiority trial versus paroxetine. *British Medical Journal*, **330** (7490), 503.

Thomson, S. (2001) Complementary therapies in aged care, in *Complementary Therapies in Nursing and Midwifery* (ed. P. McCabe). Ausmed Publications, Melbourne, pp. 257–275.

Tsen, L., Segal, S., Pothier, M. *et al.* (2000). Alternative medicine use in presurgical patients. *Anesthesiology*, **93**, 148–151.

Udani, J., Kavoussi, B. & Hardy, M. (2006) Chromium for Type 2 diabetes mellitus and weight loss. *Alternative Medicine Alert*, **9** (7), 78–82.

Verdejo, C., Marco, P., Renau-Piqueras, J. & Pinazo-Duran, M. (1999) Lipid peroxidation in proliferative vitreoretinopathies. *EYE*, **13** (Part 2), 183–188.

Vuksan, V., Stavro, M. & Seivenpiper, J. *et al.* (2000) Similar postprandial glycaemic reductions with escalation of dose and administration time of American ginseng in Type 2 diabetes. *Diabetes Care*, **23**, 1221–1226.

Wilson, R. (2007) Difficulty identifying odours may herald mild cognitive impairment. *Archives of General Psychiatry*, **64**, 802–808.

World Health Organization (WHO) (2002) *Traditional Medicine Strategy 2002–2005*. WHO, Geneva.

Zhang, L., Ma, J. & Pan, K. (2005) Efficacy of Cranberry juice on *Helicobacter pylori* infection: A double-blind randomized placebo-controlled trial. *Helicobacter*, **10**, 139–145.

Index

Note: Page numbers in *italics* refer to Figures; those in **bold** to Tables.

Care of People with Diabetes: A Manual of Nursing Practice, Fourth Edition. Trisha Dunning.
© 2014 John Wiley & Sons, Ltd. Published 2014 by John Wiley & Sons, Ltd.